RCL 23

GOVERNORS STATE UNIVERSITY LIBRARY

W9-BFU-682

3 1611 00225 7597

This important new reference book on human cancer provides a global perspective on the epidemiology of cancer and its environmental causes. By summarising geographical, environmental and ethnic factors on a cancer-by-cancer basis, the volume collates a wealth of useful information which, taken together, provides valuable insights into the causes of cancer and the scope for its control and elimination. Sufficient information is included to enable the scientist, interested in environmental carcinogenesis, to understand those causes for which there is some degree of agreement regarding their role in human carcinogenesis, and to recognise that, for many neoplasms, no single critical cause has been identified. The growing roles of molecular, biochemical and genetics approaches in epidemiology is emphasized. The contents include: (1) general epidemiological methods (2) a review of known or suspected causes (3) a detailed review of specific cancers (4) a brief review of legal and ethical implications.

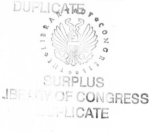

DUPLICATE

SURPLUS
LIBRARY OF CONGRESS
DUPLICATE

GOVERNORS STATE UNIVERSITY
LIBRARY

DEMCO

Cambridge Monographs on Cancer Research

LIBRARY OF CONGRESS

JAN 1 0 2006 E

COPY
COPYRIGHT OFFICE

Human cancer: epidemiology and environmental
causes

Cambridge Monographs on Cancer Research

Scientific Editors
M. M. Coombs, Imperial Cancer Research Fund Laboratories, London
J. Ashby, Imperial Chemical Industries, Macclesfield, Cheshire
R. M. Hicks, United Biscuits (UK) Ltd, Maidenhead, Berkshire

Executive Editor
H. Baxter, formerly at the Laboratory of the Government Chemist, London

Books in this Series
Martin R. Osborne and Neil T. Crosby
Benzopyrenes

Maurice M. Coombs and Tarlochan S. Bhatt
Cyclopenta[a]phenanthrenes

M. S. Newman, B. Tierney and S. Veeraraghavan
The chemistry and biology of benz(a)anthracenes

Jürgen Jacob *Sulfur analogues of polycyclic aromatic hydrocarbons (thiaarenes)*

Forthcoming Volumes
Ronald G. Harvey *Polycyclic aromatic hydrocarbons: chemistry and carcinogenicity*

W. Lijinsky *The chemistry and biology of N-nitroso compounds*

W. F. Karcher *Dibenzanthracenes and environment carcinogenesis*

Human cancer: epidemiology and environmental causes

JOHN HIGGINSON

Clinical Professor, Department of Community and Family Medicine
Georgetown University Medical Center
Washington, DC USA
Former Director of the International Agency for Research on Cancer
Lyon, France

CALUM S. MUIR

Director of Cancer Registration in Scotland, Information and Statistics Division
Common Services Agency for the Scottish Health Service
Former Deputy Director of the International Agency for Research on Cancer
Lyon, France

NUBIA MUÑOZ

Chief, Unit of Field and Intervention Studies
International Agency for Research on Cancer
Lyon, France

GOVERNORS STATE UNIVERSITY
UNIVERSITY PARK
IL 60466

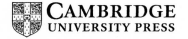
CAMBRIDGE
UNIVERSITY PRESS

RC
261.48
.H54
1992

CAMBRIDGE UNIVERSITY PRESS
Cambridge, New York, Melbourne, Madrid, Cape Town, Singapore, São Paulo

Cambridge University Press
The Edinburgh Building, Cambridge CB2 2RU, UK

Published in the United States of America by Cambridge University Press, New York

www.cambridge.org
Information on this title: www.cambridge.org/9780521412889

© Cambridge University Press 1992

This publication is in copyright. Subject to statutory exception
and to the provisions of relevant collective licensing agreements,
no reproduction of any part may take place without
the written permission of Cambridge University Press.

First published 1992
This digitally printed first paperback version 2005

A catalogue record for this publication is available from the British Library

Library of Congress Cataloguing in Publication data
Higginson, John, 1922–
Human cancer: epidemiology and environmental causes/John
Higginson, Calum S. Muir, Nubia Muñoz.
    p.   cm.–(Cambridge monographs on cancer research)
Includes bibliographical references.
ISBN 0-521-41288-9 (hardback)
1. Cancer–Etiology. 2. Cancer–Epidemiology. 3. Cancer–
Environmental aspects.   I. Muir, C. S.   II. Muñoz, N.   III. Title.
IV. Series.
[DNLM: 1. Environmental Exposure. 2. Neoplasms–epidemiology.
QZ 202 H637h]
RC261.48.H54 1992
614.5′999–dc20
DNLM/DLC
for Library of Congress   91-23259   CIP

ISBN-13 978-0-521-41288-9 hardback
ISBN-10 0-521-41288-9 hardback

ISBN-13 978-0-521-02196-8 paperback
ISBN-10 0-521-02196-0 paperback

Dedication
Dr Harold L. Stewart

Every research worker meets, at some time during his career, an individual whose knowledge, character, and way of looking at problems have a lasting influence. For the three editors of this book, that individual was Dr Harold L. Stewart, known to his friends as 'Red'. He was, for several decades, Chief of the Laboratory of Pathology of the National Cancer Institute of the United States (NCI) and, for many years, Chairman of the UICC Committee on Geographical Pathology. He remains active as Chairman of the Animal Tumor Registry of the NCI. His iconoclasm, enquiring spirit, intellectual prowess and constant encouragement to those working in that borderland between pathology and epidemiology, denoted as geographical pathology, marked him as a leader in the field. He never lost sight of its *raison d'être*, so aptly summarized by Sir Richard Doll as '... to increase knowledge of the incidence of specific diseases in population groups living in different environments and having different habits, customs and working conditions in the hope that the knowledge may provide clues to the causation of disease'.

Contents

Contributors

HELMUT BARTSCH
International Agency for Research on Cancer

ELIZABETH CARDIS
International Agency for Research on Cancer

MICHAEL SHERIDAN
Georgetown University Medical Center

LORENZO SIMONATO
Tumour Registry of Veneto, University of Padova, Italy

Preface

This monograph attempts to summarize the epidemiology of human cancer, including not only its geographical distribution in various environments and ethnic groups, but also known or suspected causes. The aim is to make available a compact source of data and a summary consensus of current views on etiology and thus provide a background, not only for evaluating cancer control and preventive policies, but also for developing strategies for research into the causes of specific tumors. The authors wish to emphasize that epidemiology remains the only discipline which can provide definitive data as to the existence, extent and nature of cancer risks in humans and the impact of preventive and intervention strategies. The term *environmental carcinogenesis*, as used here, reflects the Hippocratic view that the environment covers all exogenous factors that impinge on human health, whether they be physical, biological, cultural or chemical. The techniques used by epidemiologists to identify and measure the determinants of human neoplastic disease are described briefly.

No attempt is made to explore in depth the sophisticated biomathematical techniques now used in the analysis of epidemiological data. Their correct application is not simple and requires collaboration between the epidemiologist and biostatistician. The mere statement that an observation is statistically significant has little meaning unless the many variables that may complicate a study have been taken into account. These issues have been extensively reviewed by Breslow and Day (1980, 1987).

Human cancers usually have a long induction period, some possibly beginning in childhood, and levels of exposure to carcinogenic factors tend to be very low compared to those in animal experimentation. This means that years must elapse before epidemiological methods can show a causal link, if at all. Conclusions on the level of risk associated with exposure to a carcinogen or carcinogenic risk factor as a basis of cancer control in humans also requires considerable scientific judgment and recourse to experimental and epidemiological data which may often be incomplete.

However, this short monograph cannot cover the detailed epidemiology of human cancer or discuss all the possible etiological hypotheses that have been put forward for individual tumors. Rather, the intention is to provide sufficient information to enable the general scientist, interested in environmental carcinogenesis, to understand those causes for which there is some degree of agreement regarding their role for humans, and to recognize that for many neoplasms no single critical cause has been identified. When an association is described as causal in this monograph, it implies that the epidemiological and biological criteria deemed necessary to justify the conclusion have been taken into consideration as well as statistical significance.

The problem facing the authors has been limiting the discussion so that the reader can appreciate the broad etiological picture without being confused by unverified epidemiological or experimental hypotheses. Thus, certain arbitrary decisions have been made and the monograph may appear in part overly didactic or simplistic, reflecting biases. Failure to discuss many potential mechanisms and etiological hypotheses does not mean that they should be regarded as unimportant or irrelevant, but rather they are believed to be insufficiently developed to justify a detailed discussion in a book of limited size.

No attempt is made to review or discuss the early literature in depth, as the general epidemiological literature is adequately covered in the admirable monograph of Schottenfeld and Fraumeni (1982), and the descriptive data in Volume V of *Cancer Incidence in Five Continents* (Muir *et al.*, 1987). The bibliography is generally limited to recent key references and reviews providing further information on etiology. The authors hope, however, sufficient information has been provided to enable the reader to go to more detailed sources if so desired.

Experimental laboratory studies have added much information on potential cancer causes and the mechanisms whereby different factors may influence carcinogenesis in humans. A brief introduction (Chapter 3) on the application of laboratory techniques to epidemiological studies is included. This approach often described as 'molecular' epidemiology, is of increasing importance in human studies (Harris *et al.*, 1987).

Lastly, it is not possible to adequately summarize the detailed information in the IARC monograph series on the *Evaluation of Carcinogenic Risks of Chemicals to Humans*, which are an essential component of the library of any environmental or occupational epidemiologist. However, a useful summary of the earlier volumes is contained in Supplement 7 (IARC, 1987). The IARC has also produced a recent monograph covering control strategies (Tomatis *et al.*, 1990).

References

Breslow, N.E. & Day, N.E. (1980). *Statistical Methods in Cancer Research. Volume I. The Analysis of Case-Control Studies*. IARC Scientific Publications No 32. Lyon: International Agency for Research on Cancer.

Breslow, N.E. & Day, N.E. (1987). *Statistical Methods in Cancer Research. Volume II. The Design and Analysis of Cohort Studies*. IARC Scientific Publications No. 82. Lyon: International Agency for Research on Cancer.

Harris, C.C., Weston, A., Willey, J.C., Trivers, G.E. & Mann, D.L. (1987). Biochemical and molecular epidemiology of human cancer: indicators of carcinogen exposure, DNA damage, and genetic predisposition. *Environ. Health Perspect.*, **75**, 109–19.

IARC (1987). *IARC Monographs on the Evaluation of Carcinogenic Risks to Humans*, Overall evaluations of carcinogenicity: an updating of IARC monographs volumes 1 to 42, Supplement 7. Lyon: International Agency for Research on Cancer.

Muir, C., Waterhouse, J., Mack, T., Powell, J. & Whelan, S. (eds) (1987). *Cancer Incidence in Five Continents*, volume V. IARC Scientific Publication No. 88. Lyon: International Agency for Research on Cancer.

Schottenfeld, D. & Fraumeni, J.F., Jr (eds) (1982). *Cancer Epidemiology and Prevention*. Philadelphia: W.B. Saunders.

Tomatis, L., Aitio, A., Day, N.E., Heseltine, E., Kaldor, J., Miller, A.B., Parkin, D.M. & Riboli, E. (eds) (1990). *Cancer: Causes, Occurrence and Control*. IARC Scientific Publications 100. Lyon: International Agency for Research on Cancer.

Acknowledgements

The authors wish to express their gratitude to Drs. Helmut Bartsch and Elizabeth Cardis of the International Agency for Research on Cancer (IARC), Michael Sheridan of the Georgetown University Medical Center and Lorenzo Simonato of the University of Padova, for writing specific sections relating to their experience. Dr. Sheridan also assisted in editing. Our thanks are due, as well, to Dr. H. Vainio of the International Agency for Research on Cancer for his review of Chapter 8.

We specifically wish to thank Captain Leonard Young USN (Ret.) for his careful and competent compilation and editing of the bibliography.

The authors wish to state that the views expressed in this monograph are not necessarily those of the International Agency for Research on Cancer.

The authors also wish to thank the Georgetown University Medical Center and those organizations which supported the Program of Advanced Studies.

Historical introduction

Background

Although cancer was known to the ancient Egyptians and the symptoms of what can be assumed to be malignant disease were described in Chinese and Arabic medical writings, nothing was known of its causes or geographical distribution. Cancer was first mentioned as a cause of death in 1629 in the annual Bills of Mortality produced in London. Scattered reports also came from Paris and from some other European countries. The fact that few individuals survived into their 50s probably explains its apparent rareness. The majority of reports on cancer were essentially clinical observations and concepts of etiology were rudimentary.

While Hippocrates had emphasized the role of environmental factors in human disease causation, little real data was available about such exogenous factors. With developments in microbiology in the late nineteenth century, the situation changed as the major communicable diseases began to be identified and controlled. However, for non-communicable chronic diseases, including cancer, knowledge remained inadequate although theories, often far-fetched, abounded. In 1775, Percival Pott demonstrated the relationship between scrotal cancer in chimney sweeps and soot, raising the possibility of prevention. Recognized as a milestone today, Pott's work had relatively little impact during the following century. Clemmesen (1965) provides an excellent introductory review to this early period.

This monograph is not the place to discuss the historical development of the many theories of carcinogenesis that were considered possible until the 60s. Later, the concept of somatic mutation induced either directly or indirectly, was first introduced by Bauer (1928) and became widely accepted. This concept led to intensive research on mutagens as putative carcinogens in the early seventies and emphasis later on their regulation as a major approach to cancer control. However, today it is widely agreed that, while genome damage is critical in many neoplasms, carcinogenesis is highly complex and many different mechanisms may be involved, which interact both with host and with exogenous/environmental modulating factors.

Nineteenth century

The first significant attempts to determine the geographical distribution of cancer and its causes appeared in the nineteenth century. The Society for Investigating the Nature and Cure of Cancer published the findings of a questionnaire about the disease in the Edinburgh Medical and Surgical Journal (1806) commenting, 'with regard to cancer, it is not only necessary to observe the effects of climate and local situation but to extend our views to different employments, as those in various metals and manufactures; in mines and collieries; in the army and navy; in those who lead sedentary or active lives; in the married or single; in the different sexes, and many other circumstances. Should it be proved that women are more subject to cancer than men, then we may enquire whether married women are more liable to have the uterus or breast affected; those who have suckled or those who did not; and the same observations may be made of the single.' This statement could scarcely be improved upon today.

In 1844, Rigoni Stern, in Verona, Italy, compared the incidence of cancer of the breast and uterus among married and unmarried females and showed the relationship of marital status to these cancers. Clemmesen (1965) regarded this report as the first to give results of lasting value regarding the etiology of these tumors and to underscore the concept of lifestyle factors.

August Hirsch (1864) pointed out in his textbook of geographic pathology that, although cancer seemed frequent in autopsy series, there was insufficient data to permit assessment of its true incidence. Better statistical studies began to appear in many European countries in the last decades of the nineteenth century.

The first International Statistical Congress was held in Brussels in 1853. It requested William Farr of London and Marc d'Espine of Geneva to prepare '*une nomenclature uniforme des causes de décès applicable à tous les pays*'. The resulting classification formed the basis of the current International Classification of Diseases published by the World Health Organization, of which the most recent appeared in 1976 (WHO, 1977).

The emergence of histopathology as a rigorous discipline favored the more accurate and consistent diagnosis of malignant disease. With the growth of experimental carcinogenesis and recognition of occupational cancer, views on the etiology and biology of cancer and the possibility of its prevention began to change. Nevertheless, for many years most cancers were generally considered to be the inevitable result of ageing and heredity, even by physicians.

Twentieth century

Although Pierre Louis introduced statistics into medicine in 1833 (Beclard, 1875), the use of rigorous statistical techniques to investigate chronic diseases is barely 50 years old. Early in the century, a major review of descriptive cancer mortality statistics of great historical interest was made by Hoffman (1915), an actuary for the Prudential Insurance Company. While a number of work-place associated cancers were identified and control measures begun, the potential of epidemiological case-control studies in culturally related cancers remained largely undeveloped. Outside the work-place, early studies had little impact on cancer prevention policies. Despite the pioneering epidemiological studies by Lane-Claypon (1926) on reproductive behavior and breast cancer, by Orr (1933) on betel chewing and oral cavity neoplasms, and by Muller (1940) on cigarettes and lung cancer, lifestyle remained largely ignored by oncologists. Experimental studies in chemical and viral carcinogenesis, however, expanded enormously in the early twentieth century and provided more sophisticated scientific approaches for the investigation of cancer causation in animals.

The modern era of cancer epidemiology began after World War II with the application of advanced statistical and experimental methods to the study of cancer and its pathogenesis. The general scientific opinion on the nature of human cancer and its causes at mid-century was well summarized in an exhaustive review by Willis (1948). His discussion of etiology was largely confined to occupational cancers, with mention of aromatic amines, asbestos and dusts, ionizing radiation, and UV light. Willis agreed with Wilhelm Hueper that a new artificial environment was in the making in the modern world, 'an arresting reminder of the complexity of the chemical carcinogenic hazards of modern life'. Both Willis and Hueper approached cancer causation essentially from the experimental viewpoint. Both dismissed the role of cigarettes in lung cancer, Willis stating that proof of a causal association would be impossible. Such attitudes were then widespread in the scientific community and explained much of the delay in accepting the causal association between cigarette smoking and lung cancer in the fifties. However, Willis could not offer any convincing hypothesis for most cancers of the human gastrointestinal tract, breast and prostate.

The Oxford Meeting, 1950

The first major international effort in the post-World War II era to study systematically cancer causes in humans using a combined experimental and epidemiological approach arose out of a symposium organized in Oxford in 1950 by the Council for the Coordination of International Congresses of Medical Sciences (CIOMS) and the World Health Organization (WHO) (Clemmesen, 1950). The membership included many of the major research workers of that period from a wide range of disciplines. The objective was to examine the distribution of human cancer in various communities and geographic areas and to correlate laboratory and field findings in order to provide clues as to causation. The group accepted the Hippocratic view that not only chemicals, but any cultural, biological, nutritional, physical or other factor which impinged on humans should be considered.

At the meeting a preliminary report on the role of cigarette smoking in lung cancer was presented by Doll, but the hypothesis was not accepted without caveats. Clemmesen pointed out that there was no increase in lung cancer incidence among Danes, who were notoriously heavy smokers. The impact of changing smoking habits and the long latency period for lung cancer were still inadequately appreciated and a primary role for ambient air pollution had strong advocates.

The concept of multistage carcinogenesis and modulation was clearly accepted, if not specifically defined. There was considerable discussion on diet and Kennaway pointed out that its composition could modify carcinogenesis. In retrospect, the major concepts of carcinogenesis in humans, as understood today, were implicit in the transactions of this symposium.

In conclusion, the symposium recommended multidisciplinary systematic studies of the role of race, nutrition and environment on carcinogenesis, and stated that special efforts should be made to examine the interaction of such factors in all future epidemiological studies on humans. The concept of what is now known as molecular epidemiology was clearly foreseen. The Oxford group recommended that the WHO investigate cancer and emphasized that there was a need to organize some international coordinating body. This recommendation was eventually realized by the creation of the International Agency for Research on Cancer (IARC) by the World Health Assembly in 1965 (IARC, 1968).

At that time the major voluntary body coordinating international cancer research was the International Union Against Cancer (UICC), founded in 1924, through which cancer workers collaborated by symposia, publication and limited research. As a result of the Oxford Symposium, a Committee of Geographical Pathology was established in 1954 by the UICC, with Dr Harold Stewart as Chairman, to systematically explore and develop multidisciplinary investigations on the epidemiology and causes of cancer. A program of workshops was established over the next decade. These covered primary cancer of the liver, Burkitt's lymphoma, Kaposi's hemangiosarcoma, gastrointestinal, skin and bladder cancer, cancer of the genital system and nasopharyngeal among others (Clemmesen, 1965). In 1966, the Committee published the first volume of *Cancer Incidence in Five Continents*, summarizing the latest cancer morbidity data from 26 registries around the world. After Volume II, this series was continued under the IARC and the International Association of Cancer Registries (IACR) and remains the essential reference source for the study of the global distribution of human cancer (Muir *et al.*, 1987).

The impact of new scientific developments on etiological concepts and prevention strategies

Beginning in the 1960s, new developments in carcinogenesis began to modify scientific attitudes toward cancer prevention.

The emphasis of the Oxford meeting was on chemical carcinogens, the earlier work on oncogenic viruses by Peyton Rous and others having been largely neglected. In the early 1950s, however, the identification of vertical transmission of leukemia viruses in mice had a major impact on concepts of cancer causation and the direction of research. Despite the lack of supportive evidence, the view became widespread that many cancers in humans were due to viruses so that research on such agents, including anti-cancer vaccines, led to playing down the role of chemicals, and, more importantly, tobacco.

Despite the strength of the epidemiological evidence of Wynder and Graham (1950) in the United States and that of Doll and Hill (1950) in the United Kingdom, the role of tobacco smoking in human lung cancer was discounted by many scientists as being merely statistical and not experimental. Despite an earlier report by the Royal College of Physicians in the United Kingdom, it was not until the publication of the Surgeon General's report (1964) that the role of tobacco in cancer began to be accepted seriously by scientists in the United States. Epidemiology (including geographical pathology) slowly became accepted as a potent tool in studying such chronic diseases as human cancer and the role of causal factors. Gradually, experimental interest in chemical carcinogenesis revived and this discipline, in association with modern epidemiology, became predominant in environmental research on causation and prevention in the late 1960s and early 1970s. In retrospect, it is difficult to appreciate the enormous boost given to cancer epidemiology and prevention by the identification of the role of cigarette smoking in lung cancer.

Chemical carcinogenesis and environmental issues

Even prior to 1939, control measures had been established to prevent excessive exposures of the general population to certain animal carcinogens, e.g. butter-yellow. Since World War II, the joint FAO/WHO committee had kept food additives under constant review. In the 1950s, comparative geographical pathology between African, European and North American populations suggested that there was an exogenous component in about 70–80% of cancers (Higginson & Oettlé, 1960) and these estimates were gradually accepted as valid over the next two decades. This observation implied that cancer was not predominantly hereditary or familial but, at least in theory, could be prevented by environmental control. With the post-war growth in petrochemicals, the possible damaging role of man-made chemical pollution in the ambient environment gave rise to increased public concern, focused by Rachel Carson (1962). Her book drew attention to possible damage to the environment and health by the growing use of herbicides and pesticides, some of which were carcinogenic in animals. Unfortunately, the term 'environment' came to be interpreted by many as synonymous with man-made chemicals and the fact that it also covered diet and cultural habits (lifestyle) – as emphasized by early workers – was ignored.

Environmental concerns were further strengthened in the mid-1960s by the increasing recognition of asbestos as an ubiquitous carcinogen. Asbestosis had been diagnosed in the asbestos manufacturing industry since the 1930s but although asbestosis was suspected as a factor in lung cancer, this was not confirmed epidemiologically until the mid-fifties (Doll, 1955). In 1960, a disturbing report by Wagner et al. (1960) from South Africa showed that very low levels of exposure could cause mesothelioma. These findings were extended by Selikoff et al. (1964) who demonstrated increased lung cancer and mesothelioma in insulation workers. By 1966 it was widely recognized that what had been considered a limited occupational hazard could extend both to downstream industries and to a large segment of the general population. In December 1964, the UICC set up a committee on asbestos and cancer to study this problem

(Bogovski *et al.*, 1973). Later it was found that exposure to asbestos and smoking cigarettes were synergistic.

By the late 1960s, two major directions were appearing in the study of environmental carcinogenesis. The first was the potential impact of low level chemical exposures on cancer patterns. The second was the recognition that the many factors comprising 'lifestyle', notably tobacco, were probably responsible for the greater fraction of the cancer burden. The mechanisms underlying these cancers received increasing attention and, thus, environmental carcinogenesis came of age as a recognized discipline.

International Agency for Research on Cancer (IARC)

The growing global concern on the issues of environmental cancer, notably chemicals, and the resultant political and economic implications emphasized the need for international cooperation specifically directed to the study of human populations. In 1965, the International Agency for Research on Cancer (IARC) was established, under the direction of Dr John Higginson, as a result of the initiative of a number of French intellectuals only one of whom was a scientist. The agency began immediately to develop a multidisciplinary program in environmental carcinogenesis with an experimental, epidemiological and educational content. The scientific program was designed to cover all aspects of the causation of human cancer, including lifestyle, diet and basic biology, and to build systematically on the base provided by the UICC during the 1950s and the 1960s (IARC, 1968).

The epidemiological programs were aimed to assess the reasons for unusual differences in cancer incidence between communities and approximately 70 field projects were established around the world, including Africa and Asia. Special emphasis was given to lifestyle cancers such as breast and large intestine; viruses in primary liver cancer, Burkitt's lymphoma and nasopharyngeal cancer; and diet in esophageal and gastric cancer.

An early program which came to have a major impact in environmental carcinogenesis was the publication of a series of monographs summarizing the available experimental and epidemiological data on chemicals potentially carcinogenic to humans. Originally intended as a research tool for scientists, the monographs by providing objective and accurate evaluation of chemicals to which human exposure was likely, came to be widely used by governments and public health officials as an important element in drafting legislation.

Conclusions

Writing in retrospect in 1980, Maclure and MacMahon (1980) concluded that by 1950 there was solid evidence for cancer induction in humans by soot, arsenic, coal-tar, X-rays, tobacco, mineral oil, radium, naphthylamine, nickel compounds and UV light; and suggestive evidence for benzidine, auramine, 4-aminobiphenyl, asbestos, alcohol, benzene, radon daughters and thorotrast. Of the latter eight, most were confirmed as human carcinogens by the early 1970s, and, in many countries, significant control steps were taken.

The fact that control of the tobacco habit has never reached its full potential must be regarded as reflecting political realities and human frailties in relation to a pleasurable cultural habit, not scientific inadequacy of proof of causation. The existing insufficiency of knowledge on the causes of many human cancers, especially lifestyle related tumors, does not justify the accusation that efforts in the past were inadequate. Rather, it reflects the complexities of the carcinogenic process which have continued to prove more difficult to unravel and control than anticipated. The concept of metabolic or biochemical epidemiology had been developed earlier in the post-World War II period, although for years progress was limited by the lack of sophisticated techniques (Higginson, 1973). The present concentration on metabolic or molecular epidemiology has arisen out of the progress made in molecular biology, which has provided new techniques which can be applied to the study of carcinogenesis in humans, including the identification of biomarkers, adducts, oncogenes, metabolites and DNA mutations.

It is hoped that the users of this monograph will take note of a large volume of early work which, although not reviewed here, forms the foundation of present and future epidemiological research and preventive strategies.

References

Bauer, K.H. (1928). *Mutationstheorie der Geschwulst-Entstehung*. Berlin: Verlag Von Julius Springer.

Beclard, M.J. (1875). The Eloge de M. Louis. Mem. Acad. Med., **31**, I-XX.

Bogovski, P., Gilson, J.C., Timbrell, V. & Wagner, J.C., eds. (1973). *Biological Effects of Asbestos*, IARC Scientific Publications No. 8. Lyon: International Agency for Research on Cancer.

Carson, R.L. (1962). *Silent Spring*. Boston: Houghton Mifflin.

Clemmesen, J. ed. (1950). *Symposium on Geographical Pathology and Demography of Cancer*, session held at Regent's Park College, Oxford, England, July 29 to August 5, 1950. Copenhagen: Council for the Coordination of International Congresses of Medical Science.

Clemmesen, J. (1965). *Statistical Studies in the Aetiology of Malignant Neoplasms*, vol. 1. Copenhagen: Danish Cancer Registry.

Doll, R. (1955). Mortality from lung cancer in asbestos workers. *Brit. J. Ind. Med.*, **12**, 81–6.

Doll, R. & Hill, A.B. (1950). Smoking and carcinoma of the lung: Preliminary report. *Br. Med. J.*, **ii**, 739–48.

Higginson, J. (1973). Metabolic aspects of host–environmental relationships: An overview. In *Host Environment Interactions in the Etiology of Cancer in Man*, Proceedings of a meeting held at Primosten, Yugoslavia, 27 August - 2 September 1972, ed. R. Doll & I. Vodopija, pp. 201–12. Lyon: International Agency for Research on Cancer.

Higginson, J. & Oettlé, A.G. (1960). Cancer incidence in the Bantu and 'Cape Colored' races of South Africa: Report of cancer survey in Transvaal (1953–55). *J. Natl. Cancer Inst.*, **24**, 589–671.

Hirsch, A. (1860–1864). *Handbuch der pathologischen und historischen Pathologie*. Erlangen, Germany: F.Enke.

Hoffman, F.L. (1915). *The Mortality from Cancer Throughout the World*. Newark, NJ: Prudential Press.

IARC (1968). *Annual Report*. Lyon: International Agency for Research on Cancer.

Lane-Claypon, E.J. (1926). *A Further Report on Cancer of the Breast, with Special Reference to its Associated Antecedent Conditions*, Ministry of Health report No. 32. London: Ministry of Health.

Maclure, K.M. and MacMahon, B. (1980). An epidemiologic perspective of environmental carcinogenesis. *Epidemol. Reviews*, **2**, 19–48.

Muir, C., Waterhouse, J., Mack, T., Powell, J. & Whelan, S., eds. (1987). *Cancer Incidence in Five Continents*, volume V, IARC Scientific Publication No. 88. Lyon: International Agency for Research on Cancer.

Muller, F.H. (1940). Tabaksmisbrauch und Lungenlkarzinom. *Z.f. Krebsforsch*, **49**, 57–85.

Orr, J.M. (1933). Oral cancer in betel nut chewers in Travancore. *Lancet*, **ii**, 575.

Selikoff, I.J., Churg, J. & Hammond, E.C. (1964). Asbestos exposure and neoplasia. *JAMA*, **188**, 22–6.

Society for Investigating the Nature and Cure of Cancer (1806). *Edinburgh Med. Surg. J.* **2**, 382–9.

Surgeon General (1964). *Smoking and Health. Report of the Advisory Committee to the Surgeon General of the Public Health Service*. Washington: US Dept. of Health, Education and Welfare.

Wagner, J.C., Sleggs, C.A. & Marchand, P. (1960). Diffuse pleural mesothelioma and asbestos exposure in the north western Cape Province. *Brit. J. Ind. Med.*, **17**, 260–71.

WHO (1977). *Manual of the International Statistical Classification of Diseases, Injuries and Causes of Death*, vol. I (Tabular list) and vol. II (Index), 1975 revision. Geneva: World Health Organization.

Willis, R.A. (1948). *Pathology of Tumours*. London: Butterworth & Co. Ltd.

Wynder, E.L. & Graham, E.A. (1950). Tobacco smoking as a possible etiological factor in bronchiogenic carcinoma. A study of six hundred and eighty four proved cases. JAMA, **143**, 329–36.

Part I

Epidemiological methods

1

Introduction to cancer epidemiology

1.1   Introduction

The recording of mortality and morbidity from communicable diseases has a long history. However, although Pierre Louis described the importance of cancer statistics in the 1830s, the need to measure accurately chronic diseases in humans, such as cancer, was not recognized until the twentieth century.

1.2   Definition of epidemiology

Epidemiology, a science based on population measurements, can be described as the study of the distribution and determinants of diseases in human populations and the application of the results to their prevention or control. Unlike the experimentalist who controls risk factors and then observes their effects, the epidemiologist, in general, measures effects and then tries to determine the risk factors. In the traditional observational study, the investigator has no direct control over the assignment of risk factors and must rely on somewhat less efficient methods of design and analysis to uncover associations between the factors and disease end-points. However, epidemiological methods can also be used to assess the impact of active interventions, introducing the concept of experimentation. The major types of epidemiological studies are:

(a) *Descriptive*: These studies examine differences in the distribution of disease occurrence with respect to population, place and time. These investigations include correlational analysis, case series and case reports. In general, such studies cannot address specific causal hypotheses, but may generate them.

(b) *Analytic*: These studies compare risk factors and disease status and can be used to test specific and causal hypotheses. There are two types of analytic studies:

(i) ***Observational*** or non-experimental studies, including case-control and cohort, in which the investigator examines the relation between disease and exposure without active intervention;

(ii) ***Interventional*** or experimental studies, such as clinical trials, in which the investigator actively intervenes and then observes the intervention's effects on the disease process.

Although these two approaches are complementary components of the same discipline, the methods used differ. While consistency of results among all approaches provides the strongest evidence as to causation, e.g. tobacco and lung cancer, data often may be obtainable only through one approach.

In descriptive studies (Chapter 2), information on both risk factors and disease outcomes for each individual is not available. Although an etiologic hypothesis for a disease of previously unknown cause may emerge from examination of descriptive data, such as the latitude gradients seen in the distribution of non-melanoma skin cancer (Chapter 37) and the link between pleural mesothelioma and asbestos exposure (Chapter 35), such studies are valuable chiefly in evaluating the relative impact of different diseases on a community. In *analytical* studies (Chapter 3), information on risk factors and disease outcome for each *individual* is available and consequently these studies can explore one or more causal hypotheses.

1.3   Biostatistical considerations

No attempt is made to discuss the complex biostatistical methods relevant to epidemiology which have been mentioned in this monograph. Reference should be made to specific texts for more detailed discussion and bibliography (Breslow & Day, 1980, 1987).

1.4   References

Breslow, N.E. & Day, N.E. (1980). *Statistical Methods in Cancer Research. Volume 1. The Analysis of Case-Control Studies*. IARC Scientific Publications No 32. Lyon: International Agency for Research on Cancer.

Breslow, N.E. & Day, N.E. (1987). *Statistical Methods in Cancer Research. Volume II. The Design and Analysis of Cohort Studies*. IARC Scientific Publications No. 82. Lyon: International Agency for Research on Cancer.

2

Descriptive epidemiology: the measurement of human cancer

2.1 Introduction

It is customary to assess the distribution of disease, including cancer, by age, sex, place and time. The most informative estimate of the frequency and distribution of cancer in a population comes from the cancer registry, an organization which measures incidence by recording all newly diagnosed cases of cancer occurring in a defined population. If incidence data are not available, then mortality, the number of persons in a defined population certified as dying from cancer, is used as a surrogate index of the cancer burden. The relation between incidence and mortality varies by cancer site and is influenced by the effectiveness and success of therapy and level of medical services. Many of the issues in measuring human cancer have been summarized by Muir *et al.* (1987) in CI5V (a commonly used abbreviation for Volume V of the monograph series *Cancer Incidence in Five Continents*).

The *International Classification of Diseases* (*ICD*) of the World Health Organization, now in its ninth revision, is universally used to present cancer occurrence data. The classification is largely organized on an anatomical basis since location influences cancer treatment, histological type and other factors. Indeed, the causal agent often determines the organ involved. A few cancers are primarily classified on histological or cytological criteria rather than anatomical location, e.g. choriocarcinoma, malignant melanoma of skin, malignant lymphomas and leukemia. A triaxial specialized adaption, the ICD-O (International Classification of Diseases – Oncology), provides code numbers for topographical location of the tumor, histological type, and behavior (malignant, benign, in situ, uncertain, etc). This flexible system, which is available in many languages, is readily converted into the parent ICD.

2.2   Incidence and mortality

Incidence and mortality data are presented in the form of rates per 100,000 population per annum (and represent the most useful form of cancer data for research and public health purposes). Thus, the incidence of lung cancer in males in Scotland in 1978–82 was 132.3 per 100,000 per annum (16,503 diagnosed in a population of 2,494,860 males) (Kemp *et al.*, 1985). This rate is denoted the *crude* rate as it takes no account of the age structure of the population nor of the age at which the cancers occurred. As cancer rates increase with age, *age-specific* rates are calculated by five-year age intervals to assess the latter relationship.

2.3   Incidence according to age group

The World Health Organization has recommended the use of three age classifications:

(a) under 1 year, 1 year to 4 years, 5–9, 10–14 and similar five year groups to 84 years, and 85 years and over;

(b) under 1 year, 1 to 4 years, 5–14, 15–24 and similar 10 years age group to 74, and 75 years and over;

(c) under 1 year, 1 to 14 years, 15–44 years, 45–64, and 65 years and over.

Whenever possible, data should be presented by the first classification. Should the number of cases be rather small, the use of the second grouping is permissible. Where the age of an appreciable proportion of the population is not known with any precision, the third classification is to be preferred.

2.4   Age standardized rates

Crude rates do not reflect the ages at which cancers are occurring. Thus, crude rates may be highly misleading for comparison between countries if the age structures vary widely. Since few people survived over 50 years of age in Africa, it was erroneously assumed for many years that cancer was rare in that continent. Computation of an *age-adjusted rate* corrects for age structure of populations so that the experience of populations of differing age-structure can be validly compared. In essence, age-adjustment applies the age-specific rates for each age-group for a given cancer in a country or region to the comparable age group in a selected *standard population*. This assumes the latter had experienced the same age-specific rates as the country or region in question. The number of cancers are then summed from all-age groups, and the resultant figure is expressed as the *age-adjusted* rate per 100,000 standardized for the specific population selected. The most commonly used standard population, the world standard population, was derived by Segi (1960), based on the age structure of 46 countries around 1950, and later modified by Doll *et al.* (1966).

Age-adjustment is technically easy (Muir *et al.*, 1987) (Table 2.1). The resulting rate is, like the crude rate, synoptic and a full appreciation of all the interactions with age requires study of the individual age-specific rates for each age group. Since diagnosis tends to be most accurate in those less than 65 years of age, a *truncated standard* rate may be computed for the age group 35–64.

Another increasingly used measure is the *cumulative rate* which estimates the probability of developing or dying from cancer over a defined age-span, normally 0–64 or 0–74 years. For example, in 1978–1982 the cumulative rate for lung cancer in Norwegian males aged 0–74 was 4.1%, or one in 25. This corresponds to the cumulative risk used in most animal studies.

Accuracy issues: Population at risk

Rates depend not only on an accurate numerator, i.e. all newly diagnosed cases of cancer registered or persons certified as dying from cancer, but also on an accurate estimation of the population at risk. For the calculation of rates, a census population is probably the most reliable. Although most vital statistics administrations issue mid-year or end-of-year estimates taking into account births and deaths, such estimates for districts within a country may be distorted by migration in and out of a particular district. This migration is unlikely to be uniform for all age-groups. For example, those moving to urban centers to seek work are likely to be younger than those moving to clement regions on retirement. To obtain as accurate a picture as possible, the number of cancers recorded over a five year period is frequently related to the population at risk derived from a census taken towards the middle of the third year. Muir *et al.* (1987) provide a further discussion on census accuracy. Rates based on a million person – years of observation are likely to be statistically robust, even for rare sites.

Survival from cancer

Mortality is an acceptable surrogate for incidence for a few sites of cancer such as the pancreas and very poor for others, such as non-melanoma skin cancer. To give the reader a notion of current survival patterns, the data for corrected five-year survival for the major sites of cancer treated in the canton of Geneva between 1978–1982 are presented

Table 2.1. *Computation of age-standardized incidence rates: stomach cancer all males in Scotland in 1978–1982.*

Age in Years	Number of cancers in 5 years (*n*)	Number of males in Scotland[a] (*P*)	Age-specific incidence per 100,000 per year[b] (*I*)	Number of persons in standard (world) population (*W*)	Expected cases in standard population[c] (*E*)
0–4	—	90,190	—	12,000	—
5–9	—	98,794	—	10,000	—
10–14	—	125,477	—	9,000	—
15–19	—	132,134	—	9,000	—
20–24	1	114,408	0.2	8,000	0.02
25–29	2	95,751	0.4	8,000	0.03
30–34	3	96,967	0.6	6,000	0.04
35–39	12	82,984	2.9	6,000	0.17
40–44	29	78,890	7.4	6,000	0.44
45–49	75	78,572	19.1	6,000	1.15
50–54	133	78,776	33.8	5,000	1.69
55–59	211	77,420	54.5	4,000	2.18
60–64	250	65,155	76.7	4,000	3.07
65–69	406	58,310	139.3	3,000	4.18
70–74	413	44,701	184.8	2,000	3.70
75–79	289	26,744	216.1-	1,000	2.16
80–84	181	11,768	307.6	500	1.54
85+	72	5,297	271.9	500	1.36
	2077	1,362,338	30.5[d]	100,000	21.73[e]

[a] Average population 1978–1982

[b] Incidence $= I = n \times \dfrac{100,000}{P \times 5}$

[c] $E = \dfrac{I \times W}{100,000}$

[d] Crude rate $= 30.5$ per 10^5 per year

[e] Standardized rate $= 21.73$ per 10^5 per year

(Fig. 2.1.). With a relatively small population, most cancer patients in the Canton of Geneva are treated at one center and the standards of medical care are very high. These figures could thus be considered as representing excellent results. The poor survival for lung and stomach cancer are particularly striking. These figures, which relate to a total population and to all persons with cancer, whether treated or not, must be distinguished from those resulting from controlled clinical trials in which carefully selected patients are allocated to two or more treatment regimes.

Fig. 2.1 Rates for corrected five-year survivals for the principal cancer sites, by sex (1978–1982), Geneva.

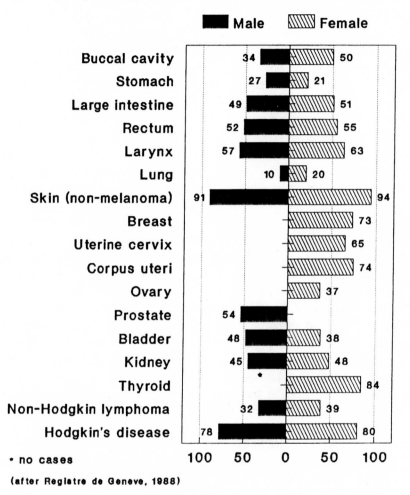

2.5 **Local and national registration**

Today, the cancer registry especially directed to measuring cancer morbidity, is regarded as an essential tool for cancer research and control (Parkin *et al.*, 1985). Incidence registration may be: national, e.g. the Nordic countries (Clemmesen, 1977; Hakulinen *et al.*, 1986); local, e.g. Alameda County, California; or regional, e.g. the West Midlands, (UK). The SEER Program (US Dept of Health and Human Services, 1986; Young *et al.*, 1981) covers a number of different regions of the USA representing about 11% of the total population. Registration of specific segments of a community may prove valuable, such as the registry which the DuPont company maintains of its staff and retirees in the USA, or the church registry of seventh Day Adventists or ethnic minorities (US Dept of Health, Education and Welfare, 1975). Registries expend considerable efforts to ensure complete coverage; however, there are few that can be certain that all cancer cases are in fact included in their records. The diverse problems of registration are fully discussed by MacLennan *et al.* (1978) and Jensen *et al.* (1991). However, those wishing to use data from a cancer registry should discuss possible sources of error and bias with the registry staff. Despite many efforts at international standardization of methods of data collection, there may be inter-registry differences.

Cancer registry data fall into two major groups: *core* items and *optional* information. The former include the anatomical location and histological type of the tumor, if known, also the most valid basis of diagnosis, e.g. biopsy, autopsy, surgical operation, biochemical tests, radiology or other methods of diagnostic imaging, or clinical diagnosis. Optional data frequently include information on stage and therapy. Good identification data for the cancer patient are essential and should permit the unequivocal identification of the same individual on different records systems. For example, in hospitals a new registration form is usually completed at each contact, so that it is essential to know if a form relates to a new or an already registered patient. When assessing survival, lists of diagnosed patients need to be accurately matched with lists of deaths. The Victorian Cancer Registry (Australia) provides an example (Giles, 1987) of an attractive informative presentation of cancer registry data.

Kurihara *et al.* (1984) have published a general summary of cancer mortality statistics following up on the earlier Segi studies.

2.6   Cancer incidence in five continents (CI5C)

Cancer registries normally publish an annual report, presenting incidence by sex, site and five year age-group. The most useful international compilations are contained in the *Cancer Incidence in Five Continents* monographs, the fifth volume (CI5V) of which was published in 1987 by the International Agency for Research on Cancer (IARC) and the International Association of Cancer Registries (IACR) (Muir *et al.*, 1987). This provides data presented in a standard manner for 187 populations in 36 countries during the years 1978–1982. Supporting data include indices of reliability with comments on interpretation; age-specific incidence rates, by five-year age-group; standardized rates for world and truncated populations; cumulative rates for the age periods 0–64 and 0–74. Rates are also given for four digit divisions of selected ICD rubrics, e.g. parts of the colon. These monographs are essential to anyone evaluating regional and national differences. Appendix I, Table 1, provides incidence rates for major sites from a representative sample of 35 registries from CI5V. For each individual site discussed in this book, a histogram is presented giving the incidence rates from registers representative of the four major continents. Due to unstable conditions in recent years, however, African rates are drawn from the fourth Edition (CI5IV) (Waterhouse *et al.*, 1982).

Volumes I and II were edited by Doll *et al.* (1966, 1970) and Volume III by Waterhouse *et al.* (1976). The different monographs do not necessarily cover the same registries.

Accepting that no registry is perfect, and that it would be unwise to give much significance to minor differences, incidence data for cancer are more likely to approximate the truth than for other major disease.

2.7 Other types of measurement
Relative frequency

Where cancer patients cannot be linked to a defined population, useful information may be derived by expressing the frequency of individual sites as a proportion of all cancers, the so-called *relative frequency* (Parkin *et al.*, 1985). Such relative frequencies can be based on series of biopsies, autopsies or hospital admissions as for example the early studies of Steiner (1954).

In a relative frequency series an increase of one cancer automatically decreases the relative frequency of another cancer without changing the latter's absolute rate in the population. A high relative frequency does not necessarily mean a high incidence, but may be due to a relative absence of other cancers.

Distortion is also due to population age-structure. For example, a young population will have proportionately more sarcomas, an older population more prostate cancer. A method for the age correction of relative frequency series has been devised (Tuyns, 1968). However, this method corrects only for the influence of age and the procedure should not be used for a small number of cases.

Despite limitations, when relative frequency data show a consistently high proportion for a given site, and there are no obvious sources of bias, the cancer in question is likely to be truly common. The converse is less likely to be true.

Biopsy series

In most countries, over three-quarters of patients with recognized cancer are biopsied. Biopsy series, while having more precise diagnosis,

Table 2.2. *Relative frequency of selected cancer sites in population-based vs. hospital registry, expressed as a percentage of all tumors observed.*

| | Bombay Cancer Registry 1968–1972 | | Tata Memorial Hospital 1970–1972 | |
	M	F	M	F
Tongue	9.2	2.4	15.1	2.2
Mouth	5.7	4.6	10.3	6.6
Pharynx	10.8	2.7	23.6	4.5
Oesophagus	9.6	7.8	11.3	8.1
Stomach	5.7	3.8	1.7	1.0
Colon–rectum	5.7	4.0	2.9	1.7
Larynx	9.4	2.0	1.8	0.8
Lung	8.9	2.1	5.7	0.9
Breast	0.1	17.2	0.1	17.9
Cervix uteri	—	21.7	—	35.5
Prostate	2.6	—	0.7	—
Bladder	1.6	0.8	1.1	0.3
Lymphoma	3.3	1.8	4.3	1.9
Leukaemia	3.8	3.0	1.6	0.9

(After Parkin *et al.*, 1986.)

are usually weighted by the more accessible neoplasms and inevitably reflect the interests of local surgeons. Unless all histological material in an area is pooled, considerable distortion can be caused by hospital admission policies, facilities, the existence of special departments, etc. This is readily demonstrated by comparing data from the Tata Memorial Hospital in Bombay, which draws cancer patients from all over India, notably those with head and neck tumors, with data covering the total Bombay population (Table 2.2).

Autopsies

Autopsy series can be valuable but also are somewhat biased. Not only are hospital admissions selected but not all deaths are autopsied. In many countries, autopsy is rarely practised. Curable cancers, e.g. skin and cervix, are poorly represented. Males are more likely to be autopsied than females and the rate of autopsies tends to decline after the age of 40.

It may be possible to pool biopsy and autopsy material from the same population to provide a more balanced picture. In Africa, a high frequency of liver cancer was previously shown on autopsy, but cancer of the cervix was rare; whereas biopsies showed the opposite pattern. In contrast, both autopsy and biopsy studies demonstrated a high frequency of esophagus and liver cancers which are highly fatal. Evaluation of *all* the data, however, led to conclusions that were very similar to those produced by later incidence studies.

2.8   Minimum incidence rate

If the population of a region or a city is known approximately, and genuine residents can be identified in biopsy, autopsy and other material, it may be possible to calculate a *minimum incidence* rate, i.e. the true rate cannot be less. This may be useful in certain developing countries. Yaker (1980) has used this technique for Algiers, Constantine and Oran.

2.9   Comparison of incidence, mortality and relative frequency

Incidence and mortality data are complementary. Incidence is not influenced by survival but is frequently not available for entire populations. Mortality data generally cover an entire country and have been collected since the beginning of this century for much of the developed world. However, cancer mortality statistics are, as pointed out by Smithers, 'a summary of what thousands of doctors of varying skill have, under very different conditions and opportunities for accurate diagnosis, seen fit to write as their opinion of the cause of death' (Boyle *et al.*, 1989). The accuracy of death certificates has been a subject of study. It has been shown that cancers are not only missed, but also over-diagnosed, but that these errors tend to cancel out (Heasman & Lipworth, 1966; Puffer & Wynn-Griffith, 1967; James *et al.*, 1955). The coding of death certificates, for both the eighth and ninth revisions of ICD also varies between countries, coders interpreting the underlying cause of death for the same certificate differently (Percy & Muir, 1989). Even when the diagnosis of cancer has been made during life and cancer mentioned as a cause of death, the death certificate statement tends to be less precise, e.g. leukemia rather than myeloid leukemia.

2.10   Time trends and cohort analysis

Variations in time trends

The fact that cancer incidence and mortality change over time is of the greatest significance. A change in burden of cancer as represented by the absolute number of cases in a community resulting from demographic factors, such as the increasing age of the population, must be distinguished from a change in incidence as reflected in the standardized rates. Changes may be artefactual. An 'epidemic' of cancer in the United States, described in the mid-1970s, was eventually shown to be due to the late arrival of an accumulation of several months of death certificates at the National Center for Health Statistics. Following the diagnosis of

Note: In Fig 2.2 to 2.5, the overall average annual rate of increase, or decrease, is given at the lower left of each diagram for males, and that for females on the right, in the box appearing above the time-scale which runs from 1960 to 1980. The age-adjusted incidence rates are given on the vertical axes. The upper curve is usually that for males; the lower that for females. A comment for each site is given above the figure.

Fig. 2.2 Esophagus (ICD 150). The rise in the black (B) population of Detroit in both sexes contrasts with the virtual stability observed in whites (W). In the other populations the rate is either stable or falls.

ESOPHAGUS

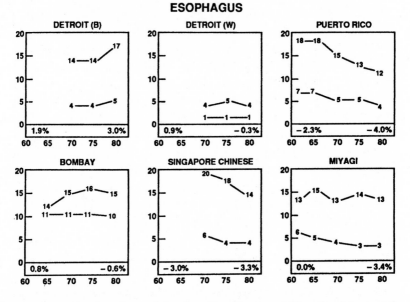

breast cancer in the wives of the then President and Vice-President of the United States, a sudden increase in the incidence of mammary cancer was reported that year which in later years reverted to normal levels. None the less, a steady rise in incidence, for example, as for lung cancer, may imply that intensity of exposure to a carcinogen may have increased, that more people are exposed, or that a new factor has entered the environment. A fall in risk suggests reduced exposure to a carcinogenic agent, even if its nature is unknown, as for cancer in the stomach. A fall in mortality in the presence of stable incidence suggests improved survival.

Time trends can be presented in many ways. The conventional and most usual approach is to graph the age-standardized incidence or mortality rate for a given site, sex, and registry, country or region, for a series of years. This approach takes care of the changing age-structure of a population and, if rolling three years averages are used, most random year-to-year fluctuation. Such cross-sectional time-trends derived from incidence data in the *Cancer Incidence in Five Continents* Monographs

Fig. 2.3 Lung (ICD 162). While rates are rising sharply in many countries in both sexes, eg. Detroit and Singapore Chinese, in Birmingham (UK) there has been a substantial decline in males. However, in females, the rates continue to rise.

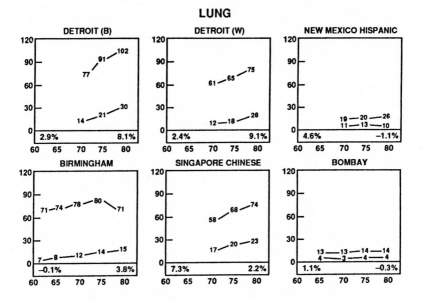

(Doll *et al.*, 1966, 1970; Waterhouse *et al.*, 1976, 1982; Muir *et al.*, 1987) are presented in Figs. 2.2 to 2.5 for several common sites from selected registries.

This cross-sectional approach using a synoptic figure, namely the age-standardized incidence or mortality rate, answers the question 'is the overall risk increasing or decreasing?' from year to year, but none the less conceals a great deal of information. As those developing or dying from cancer in a given year were born at different times, their exposures are by definition likely to have been different. For this reason it is often useful to look at the age-specific rates by calendar period. In other words, what was the risk, for example, in, 50 to 54 year olds, in 1940, 1945, 1950 and so on. This approach is most useful in that changes in risk, in either direction, are often observed first in the younger age-groups. Thus, at a time when the crude mortality rates from gastric cancer for all ages combined in Japan was rising, it was already falling in the younger group aged 40–44 years (Muir *et al.*, 1980). Other epidemiological techniques are necessary to ascertain whether the decline is due to lower exposures to carcinogens in the younger age-groups or, less likely, to the success of screening programs. Age-specific rates for mortality from cancer of the prostate in the United States blacks show that for generations born

Fig. 2.4 Melanoma of skin (ICD 172). Melanoma of skin shows the highest rates of increase of any form of cancer. Rates, although too small to plot in the black population of Detroit and in Puerto Rico, are however increasing.

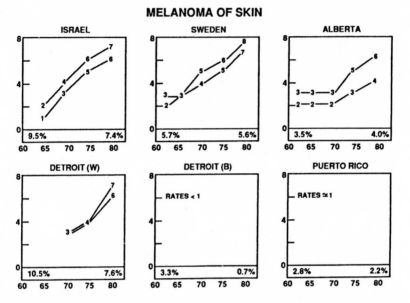

Fig. 2.5 Breast (ICD 174). In all populations considered, the incidence of breast cancer is rising, the rate of increase being greatest in Hawaiian Japanese. The level of breast cancer in Hawaii in 1960, was not reached until 1980 in Miyagi Prefecture (Japan). This suggests that the relevant risk occurred 20 years later in Japan.

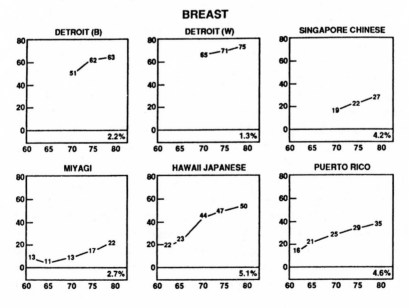

Fig. 2.6 Age-specific mortality rates for cancer of the prostate in the United States (blacks) by year of birth (1846–1925).

PROSTATE CANCER

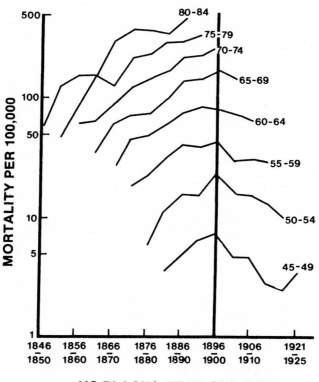

US BLACKS: YEAR OF BIRTH

between 1850 and 1900 the risk continued to rise as successive cohorts attained a given age (Fig. 2.6). After 1900 the risk began to fall. If these trends continue, one can envisage a gradual fall in the age-standardized mortality rates for all ages combined in the US black population, the population with the world's highest published incidence rates of prostatic cancer.

This type of information can be presented graphically in a somewhat different way, namely, the age-specific incidence rates for each birth cohort. This portrayal enables one to examine the cancer experience of a group of people born at one point of time as they grow older and compare this with those born earlier or later. Possibly the clearest examples of a strong year-of-birth effect are for malignant melanoma and lung cancer (Fig. 2.7). The increase of mortality from malignant melanoma in

Fig. 2.7 Lung cancer incidence in successive birth cohorts in Detroit (females), 1969–1982.

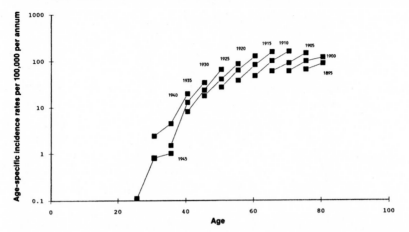

successive birth cohorts, irrespective of the current level for all ages combined, in all countries with a fair-skinned population, suggests a major cause has been operating with increasing intensity all over the world on those born 1880 and later (Muir & Nectoux, 1982) (Chapter 37).

Birth cohort analysis

Any age-specific incidence or mortality curve in a birth cohort diagram of the type shown in Figure 2.7 has three components. One, which is assumed to be parallel for all populations, is the increase with advancing age (which may be equated to the end result of the cumulative exposure to the risk factors); the second is the effect of the year of birth which frequently governs the level of exposure; the third the time of diagnosis or death which may influence the likelihood of the disease being diagnosed. There has been a great deal of interest in trying to determine the relative contributions from each of these components (Schifflers *et al.*, 1985). Unfortunately, due to problems of identification no statistical technique to solve this problem has yet gained universal acceptance.

2.11   Cancer maps

A cancer map can bring out features of cancer distribution not readily discernible in a table (Boyle *et al.*, 1989). The earliest cancer atlas presented information for females in England and Wales in 1875. More recently, maps have been made for Scotland (Kemp *et al.*, 1985), France (Rezvani *et al.*, 1985), the United States (Mason *et al.*, 1975; Pickle *et al.*, 1987) the European Economic Community (Boyle *et al.*, 1991) and the Nordic countries (NCU, 1988).

There are problems, however, in the interpretation of cartographic patterns, including distortions due to large areas with small populations, arbitrary administrative boundaries and regional variations in registration efficiency.

A common practice is to map statistically significant differences from the national standard mortality ratio (SMR). Statistical significance is, however, heavily influenced by population numbers. Thus, contiguous areas with similar age-adjusted incidence rates may have different levels of significance. It is thus preferable to map the age-adjusted rate to bring out the pattern of risk and provide information on statistical significance in supporting tables. None the less, despite these limitations, the cancer atlas is a valuable point of departure readily appreciated by non-specialists as illustrated by the maps for cancer of the esophagus (Chapter 25).

Urban–rural differences

Some cancer registries provide data for the urban and rural portions of their registration area; thus in England and Wales the urban mortality rate was 241, that for rural areas being 207. In females, however, not only are overall rates lower, but the urban/rural differential is not so marked, 193 and 183 respectively. Comparable differences are seen in the urban and rural portions of the Saarland and the Federal Republic of Germany. Urban–rural differences have been held to reflect the influence of atmospheric and other forms of pollution. It is difficult to conceive how atmospheric pollution in Cracow could plausibly give rise to a higher rate for breast cancer (29.6) than in rural Nowy Sacz (18.4) in the same region of Poland. A further complication arises from differing definitions of urban and rural (Chapter 7). Other factors such as smoking, reproductive habits, selective migration, etc, must be considered.

2.12   Clusters

Unusual distributions of rare cancers in a small area are of great etiological interest. Such clusters may occur within a restricted geo-graphical area, a school, near a suspected source of industrial pollution or toxic waste dump, or nuclear installations and frequently over a fairly short time span. The problem is well illustrated by the reports of leukemic clusters near Sellafield in England which were attributed to radiation from nuclear installations. While clusters had occurred, there is no convincing evidence yet that they are due to radiation (Chapter 16). Rothman (1990) is of the opinion that too much   attention has been given to the demonstration of clustering and not enough to the clustering of causes. Of some 60 reported occupational clusters investigated, only 16 showed that

Table 2.3. *Change in mortality on migration from Japan to the USA.*

Group	Stomach (M)	Colon (M)	Lung (M)	Breast (F)
Japan	100	100	100	100
Japan-born Americans	72	374	306	166
US Whites	17	489	316	591

Note: The mortality rate in Japan is considered to be 100 and the other rates are given as percentages of this reference rate.
(After Haenszel and Kurihara, 1968.)

Table 2.4. *Change in mortality rate[a] on migration from Poland to the United States*

Group	Stomach (M)	Colon (M)	Lung (M)	Breast (F)
Poland (1959–1961)	38	3	17	6
Polish-born Americans (1950)	34	14	36	19
US native whites (1950)	10	13	31	22
	–			

[a] Age-standardized to the world population standard
(After Muir & Staszewski, 1986.)

there was a real excess of cases and for none of these was the etiology uncovered (Schulte *et al.*, 1987). Clusters may yield information on cause if the clusters are recent or extremely rare (see also Neutra, 1990).

2.13   Migrants

The significance of changes in cancer risk after migration was first recognized by Kennaway (1944), who stated 'The very high incidence of primary cancer of the liver found among Negroes in Africa, does not appear in Negroes in the United States of America and is therefore not of purely racial character. Hence, the prevalence of this form of cancer in Africans may be due to some extrinsic factor, which could be identified.' The classic papers of Haenszel (1961) and Haenszel and Kurihara (1968) led to the value of migrant studies becoming more widely appreciated. Cancer mortality patterns in migrants to the US from such diverse countries as Japan (Table 2.3) and Poland (Table 2.4) have indicated that events early in life determine the risk of stomach cancer, whereas risk for cancer of the colon seem to depend on factors acting in adulthood. A rapid increase in risk would suggest that promoters were acting on cells which had already been initiated. A rise following a long induction period would suggest exposure to initiators which did not exist in the country of origin. The risk of developing the superficial spreading variant of malignant melanoma in migrants to Australia was largely determined by their age at migration: for persons who migrated below the age of 10, the risk was the same as that for the Australian born. After the age of 25, the risk was that of the country of origin. For some cancers, such as the breast, changes in migration are somewhat more complicated. In Polish-born migrants to the USA, the mortality from breast cancer increased within their lifetime to the high level of native American women. In Japanese migrants, mortality remained low for breast cancer and the high incidence characteristic of US-born white American females was probably first reached by the third generation of American–Japanese, a finding consistent with slow changes in dietary patterns influencing, in turn, hormonal patterns. For an account of more recent migrant studies, see Muir and Staszweski (1986).

Migrant studies have certain inherent problems. Migrants are seldom a random sample of the population of the country of origin. Among many other differences, they are usually landless farmers, skilled workers or professionals, refugees, members of an ethnic or religious minority, etc. They often originate from a specific location. When variation in cancer risk within a country is large, as in China, knowledge of the place of origin of the international migrants is crucial, as illustrated by the variations for several common cancers in various southern Chinese dialect groups in Singapore (Table 2.5). Steiner (1954) speaking of migrants, has said 'factors such as climate, altitude, temperature ... may differ at once.... On the other hand, certain environmental factors, some of which may be cultural, change more slowly after migration. The choice of food and culinary practice, occupational exposures, sanitary habits, economic levels, and other factors may gradually change over a period of years ...'. If much of breast, large bowel and prostate cancer is in some way linked to diet, the advent, in high-risk countries, of migrant groups at low risk for these cancers should be quickly followed by appropriate studies. Yet investigations on migrants have been very few in number.

2.14 Correlation or ecological studies

Patterns of cancer distribution between, and within, countries are frequently correlated with such environmental factors as alcohol consumption, tobacco use and dietary fat. Such correlations, commonly called ecological studies, may suggest hypotheses for further testing. However, they have many pitfalls, notably the correlation of cancer

Table 2.5. *Relative risks (RR) for selected cancers for Chinese dialect groups, adjusted for age, with Hokkien (1968–1982) rate as baseline.*

Site	Baseline (Hokkien) M	F	Teochew M	F	Cantonese M	F	Hainanese M	F	Hakka M	F	Others M	F
Nasopharynx	16.6	6.3	1.01	1.03	1.84	1.80	1.05	1.02	0.89	0.87	0.86	0.70
Esophagus	23.4	6.6	1.23	1.10	0.20	0.27	0.27	0.18	0.30	0.46	0.61	0.80
Stomach	53.2	21.3	0.91	0.81	0.38	0.59	0.54	0.53	0.43	0.69	1.32	1.44
Colon	13.2	13.0	1.16	0.90	1.25	1.14	1.00	0.48	0.96	0.88	0.77	1.01
Rectum	13.0	8.6	0.94	0.99	0.88	1.04	1.19	0.75	0.69	0.82	1.01	1.06
Liver	36.7	8.2	0.79	0.97	0.83	0.99	0.82	0.50	0.72	0.68	1.01	0.85
Larynx	10.1		0.86		0.95		0.57		1.13		0.42	
Lung	77.1	17.7	0.91	0.84	0.76	1.59	0.49	0.60	0.59	0.78	0.97	1.29
Skin (ex. melanoma)	10.9	7.5	0.78	0.68	0.56	0.81	0.29	0.50	0.37	0.77	0.58	0.41
Prostate	3.9		1.15		1.62		1.11		1.40		1.57	
Bladder	6.9		1.39		0.92		0.62		0.63		0.64	
Breast		24.1		0.77		1.25		0.62		0.66		0.79
Cervix uteri		21.4		0.78		0.77		0.55		0.91		1.01
Ovary		7.2		0.83		1.12		0.73		0.65		0.96
Thyroid		3.9		1.19		1.21		0.86		0.63		0.98
All sites	311.9	181.2	0.95	0.86	0.77	1.03	0.65	0.62	0.62	0.77	0.99	1.05

(After Lee *et al.*, 1988.)

patterns and suspected parameters at the same time, ignoring the latent period, and rather poor quality of environmental and lifestyle data in the past. None the less, several interesting hypotheses have emerged from findings, such as the correlation between large bowel cancer and the proportion of calorie intake consumed as fat. However, there is no guarantee that those getting the colon cancer were those who ate larger quantities of fat. The pertinence of such studies can be improved by correlating the cancer level with environmental variables measured from a probability sample of the population at risk, as in the Denmark–Finland large bowel cancer study (Jensen *et al.*, 1982) (Chapter 28).

The correlation techniques mentioned above use no more than the age and sex of cancer patients and total population environmental or consumption data for several geographical locations. If other items of information are available for the individual or the population at risk, further studies become possible.

2.15   Proportional mortality rates

In many countries, the occupation at the time of death is recorded on the death certificate, which makes it possible to calculate a Proportionate Mortality Ratio (PMR) showing for example, whether lung cancer is more or less a common cause of death among farmers than

Table 2.6. *General advantages and disadvantages of descriptive epidemiology.*

Characteristics or Study Type	Advantages	Disadvantages
Mapping of incidence or mortality rates by small areas.	May point to existence of suspected 'hot spots', i.e. neighborhood plants, toxic waste dumps, ethnic groups, etc.	Seldom convincing due to potential confounding variables. If areas are very small, significant random clusters may occur by chance; if areas are large, effects of localized exposure may be diluted out. Individuals cannot be identified and appropriate records are often not available.
Correlation between disease levels and various environmental factors or attributes such as occupation.	Frequently based on data already available. May be useful to generate and check on hypotheses, e.g. aflatoxin/liver cancer association. May show that an association is unlikely.	Correlations observed may be due to other confounding variables, such as smoking; or socio-economic variations. Individual variations may be diluted out.
Case reports.	May indicate cause if exposure and/or resulting disease are unique and rare, e.g. angiosarcoma, acute tubular necrosis.	Situation rare.

teachers or metal workers. Such PMRs can be age-adjusted to take into account the possible differences in the age-structure of those in a particular occupational group, but they are still subject to arithmetic bias. A low or high proportion may be due to an unusual incidence of another cancer in an occupational group. If there is some measure of the distribution of these occupations for the population-at-risk, as from a census, then it becomes possible to calculate observed and expected numbers and compute a standardized mortality rate (SMR), again taking age into account. Probably the best known of such analyses is *Occupational Cancer Mortality* published by the Office of Population Censuses and Survey in England and Wales (Chapter 8).

Those following a given occupation are normally assignable to a socio-economic group. When SMRs are compared within socio-economic groups, many of the differences between occupations disappear. Occupations falling into the same socio-economic group, no matter how diverse, often have an SMR in the same range. Further, comparison of the cancer and general mortality of wives with that of their husbands following a certain occupation often shows a remarkable correlation, suggesting that factors other than the exposures to potential hazards at work are likely to be responsible. Cancers due to at-work exposures do, of course, exist (Chapter 8).

2.16   Conclusion

Descriptive epidemiology studies are an essential tool in the study of human cancer. The advantages and disadvantages are listed in Table 2.6. They provide valuable information on the distribution of the disease in human populations living under a variety of national and cultural environments giving rise to causal hypotheses. A hypothesis inconsistent with the observed distribution of cancer is either incorrect or incomplete (Muir, 1973).

2.17   References

Boyle, P., Muir, C.S. & Grundmann, E. (eds.) (1991). Cancer Mapping, *Recent Results in Cancer Research*, vol. 114. Heidelberg: Springer.

Clemmesen, J. (1977). *Statistical Studies in Malignant Neoplasms II: Basic Tables.* Denmark: Aarhuus Stiftsbogtrykkerie.

Doll, R., Payne, P. & Waterhouse, J. (eds.) (1966). *Cancer Incidence in Five Continents,* A technical report, UICC. Berlin: Springer Verlag.

Doll, R., Muir, C. & Waterhouse, J. (eds.) (1970). *Cancer Incidence in Five Continents,* volume II. Geneva: UICC.

Giles, G.G. (1987). 1983 *Statistical Report, Victorian Cancer Registry.* Melbourne: Anticancer Council of Victoria.

Hakulinen, T., Andersen, A.A., Malker, B., Pukkala, E., Schou, G. & Tulinius, A. (1986). Trends in Cancer Incidence in the Nordic Countries: A Collaborative Study of the Five Nordic Cancer Registeries. *Acta Pathologica, Microbiologica et Immunologica Scandinavica,* Section A, Supplement No. 288, 94.

Haenszel, W. (1961). Cancer among the foreign-born in the United States. *J. Natl. Cancer Inst.,* **26**, 37.

Haenszel, W. & Kurihara, M. (1968). Studies of Japanese migrants: Mortality from cancer and other diseases among Japanese in the United States. *J. Natl. Cancer Inst.,* **40**, 43–68.

Heasman, M.A. & Lipworth, L. (1966). *Accuracy of Certification of Cause of Death (Studies on Medical and Population Subjects,* No. 20). London: Her Majesty's Stationery Office.

James, G., Patton, R.E. & Healin, A.S. (1955). Accuracy of Cancer Death Statement on Death Certificates. *US Pub. Health Res.* (Washington). **70**, 39–51.

Jensen, O.M., McLennan, R. & Wahrendorf, J. (1982). Diet, bowel function, fecal characteristic and large bowel cancer in Denmark and Finland. *Nutr. Cancer,* **4**, 5–19.

Jensen, O., Parkin, D.M., McLennan, R., Muir, C.S. & Skee, R. (1991). *Cancer Registration: Principles and Methods.* IARC Scientific Publications No. 95. Lyon: International Agency for Research on Cancer.

Kemp, I., Boyle, P., Simons, M. & Muir C.S. (eds.) (1985). *Atlas of Cancer in Scotland 1975–1980. Incidence and Epidemiological Perspectives*. IARC Scientific Publications No. 72. Lyon: International Agency for Research on Cancer.

Kennaway, E.L. (1944). Cancer of the liver in the negroes in Africa and America. *Cancer Res.*, **4**, 571–7.

Kurihara, M., Aoki, K. & Tominaga, S. (1984). *Cancer Mortality Statistics in the World*. Japan: University of Nagoya Press.

Lee, H.P., Day, N.E. & Shanmugaratnam, K. (1988). *Trends in Cancer Incidence in Singapore*. IARC Scientific Publications No. 91. Lyon: International Agency for Research on Cancer.

MacLennan, R., Muir, C.S., Steinitz, R. & Winkler, A. (eds.) (1978). *Cancer Registration and Its Techniques*. IARC Scientific Publications No. 21. Lyon: International Agency for Research on Cancer.

Mason, T.J., McKay, F.W., Hoover, R. & Fraumeni, J.F. (1975). *Atlas of Cancer Mortality for U.S. Counties*. 1950–1969. HEW Publication, pp. 751–80. Washington: U.S. Government Printing Office.

Muir, C.S. (1973). Geographical differences in cancer patterns. In *Host Environmental Interactions in the Etiology of Cancer in Man*, IARC Scientific Publications No. 7, ed. R. Doll & I. Vodopija, pp. 1–13. Lyon: International Agency for Research on Cancer.

Muir, C.S., Choi, N.W. & Schifflers, E. (1980). Time trends in cancer mortality in some countries: Their possible causes and significance. In *Proceedings of the Skandia International Symposium*, pp. 269–309. Stockholm.

Muir, C.S. & Nectoux, J. (1982). Time trends in malignant melanoma of the skin. In *Trends in Cancer Incidence*, ed. K. Magnus, UICC and Norwegian Cancer Society, pp. 365–85. New York: Hemisphere.

Muir, C.S. & Staszweski, J. (1986). Geographical Epidemiology and Migrant Studies. *In Biochemical and Molecular Epidemiology*, ed. C.C. Harris, pp. 135–48. New York: Arliss.

Muir, C.S., Waterhouse, J., Mack, T., Powell, J. & Whelan, S. (eds.) (1987). *Cancer Incidence in Five Continents*, volume V, IARC Scientific Publications No. 88. Lyon: International Agency for Research on Cancer.

NCU (1988). *Atlas of Cancer Incidence in the Nordic countries*. ed. O.M. Jensen, B. Carstensen, E. Glattre, B. Malker, E. Pukkala & H. Tulinius. Helsinki: Nordic Cancer Union.

Neutra, R.R. (1990). Reviews and commentary. Counterpoint from a cluster buster. *Am. J. Epidemiol.*, **132**, 1–8.

Parkin, D.M. (ed.) (1986). *Cancer Occurrence in Developing Countries*. IARC Scientific Publications No. 75. Lyon: International Agency for Research on Cancer.

Parkin, D.M., Wagner, G. & Muir, C.S. (eds.) (1985). *The Role of the Registry in Cancer Control*. IARC Scientific Publications No. 66. Lyon: International Agency for Research on Cancer.

Percy, C. & Muir, C.S. (1989). The international comparability of cancer mortality data. Results of an international death certificate study. *Am. J. Epidemiol.*, **129**, 934–46.

Pickle, L.W., Mason, T.J., Howard, N., Hoover, R. & Fraumeni, J.F. (1987). *Atlas of US Cancer Mortality among Whites*: 1950–1980. NIH Publication 87–2900). Washington: U.S. Government Printing Office.

Puffer, R.R. & Wynne-Griffith, G.G. (1967). *Patterns of Urban Mortality: Report of the Inter-American Investigation of Mortality*. Pan-American Health Organization Scientific Publication No. 151. Washington: Pan-American Health Organization.

Registre Genevois des Tumeurs (1988). *Cancer à Génève. Geneve*.

Rezvani, A., Doyon, F., Flament R. & de Ryeke Y. (1985). *Atlas de la Mortalité par Cancer en France*. Paris: Edition, INSERM.

Rothman, K.J. (1990). A sobering start for the cluster busters conference. Keynote presentation. *Am. J. Epidemiol.*, **132**, S6-S13.

Schifflers, E., Smans, M. & Muir, C.S. (1985). Birth cohort analysis using irregular cross-sectional data: a technical note. *Stat. Med.*, **4**, 63–75.

Schulte, P.A., Ehrenberg, R.L. & Singal, M. (1987). Investigation of occupational cancer clusters: Theory and practice. *Am. J. Pub Health*, **77**, 52–6.

Segi, M. (1960). *Cancer Mortality for Selected Sites in 24 Countries* (1950–1957). Sendai, Japan: Department of Public Health, Tohoku University School of Medicine.

Steiner, P.E. (1954). *Cancer: Race and Geography*. Baltimore: Williams and Wilkins.

Tuyns, A.J. (1968), Studies on relative cancer frequencies (ratio studies): a method for computing an age standardized cancer ratio. *Int. J. Cancer*, **67**, 625–32.

US Dept. of Health and Human Services (1986). *Cancer Among Blacks and Other Minorities: Statistical Profiles*. NIH Publication No. 86–2785. Bethesda, MD: National Institutes of Health (NCI).

US Dept. of Health, Education and Welfare (1975). *Third National Cancer Survey: Incidence Data*. National Cancer Institute Monograph 41. DHEW Publication No. (NIH) 75–787. Bethesda, MD: National Institutes of Health (NCI).

Waterhouse, J., Muir, C., Correa, P. & Powell, J. (eds.) (1976). *Cancer Incidence in Five Continents*, volume III, IARC Scientific Publications No. 15. Lyon: International Agency for Research on Cancer.

Waterhouse, J., Muir, C.S., Shanmugaratnam, K. & Powell, J. (eds.) (1982). *Cancer Incidence in Five Continents*, volume IV, IARC Scientific Publications No. 42. Lyon: International Agency for Research on Cancer.

Yaker (1980). *Profil de la Morbidité Cancereuse en Algerie* (1966, 75). Societé Nationale d'Edition et de Diffusion.

Young, J.L., Percy, C.L., Asire, A.J. (eds.) (1981). *Surveillance, Epidemiology and End Results: Incidence and Mortality Data*, 1973–77. National Cancer Institute Monogr. 57, DHEW Publication No. (NIH) 81–2330, Bethesda, MD. National Institute of Health NCI.

3

Analytical epidemiology: techniques to determine causal relationships

MICHAEL J. SHERIDAN
Georgetown University Medical Center

In an analytic study, information on exposure to risk factors and on disease outcome are known for each individual in the investigation. Two analytical strategies are available to the epidemiologist for exploring causal cancer relationships. First, is the experimental or interventional approach, in which the investigator can determine the randomized entrance of an individual into the exposed (treatment) and nonexposed (control) groups. This type of study can most accurately address the question of causation.

The second type of study is the non-experimental or observational approach, in which the investigator has no active control over risk factors, but must assess such factors and disease outcome in the natural setting of the study. Study groups to be compared are based either on the presence or absence of disease (case-control) or of risk factors (cohort). On their own, these studies are generally less persuasive in addressing causation than experimental studies. Nevertheless, non-experimental studies do permit examination both of multiple etiological causes for a single disease (case-control) and of multiple diseases for a single cause (cohort).

A considerable literature exists on the techniques of analytical epidemiology which can only be outlined here. Reference should be made to the standard texts for further information (Breslow & Day, 1980, 1987; Lilienfeld & Lilienfeld, 1980; Schlesselman, 1982; Kelsey *et al.*, 1986; Meinert, 1986; Rothman, 1986; Weiss, 1986; Hennekens & Burning, 1987; Checkoway *et al.*, 1989; Kahn & Sempos, 1989). Associated laboratory studies are described in Chapter 5.

3.1   Experimental or interventional studies

An experimental study is the most direct and conclusive method for establishing a causal association between a risk factor and a disease.

Controlled experiments in human populations are seldom possible or ethical and so epidemiologic strategies most often rely on observations of non-institutionalized members of a population. However, it may be possible to assess the consequences of a change in exposure resulting from a 'natural experiment' or from a specific clinical intervention believed to offer benefit to the participant. Such 'natural interventions' – such as children given poliomyelitis vaccine accidentally contaminated by SV40 virus – approximate the experimental situation and should be exploited wherever possible.

A tragic example of human intervention is provided by the survivors of the atomic bombs dropped on Hiroshima and Nagasaki at the end of World War II. Here, it was possible to assess the relationship between estimated dose of radiation exposure and the subsequent frequency and latency of leukemia and a wide variety of cancers in the exposed group and their progeny.

Examples of a specific clinical intervention to alter individual risk by influencing the carcinogenic process are provided in studies in China and Africa. Based on evidence that certain vitamin deficiencies may influence esophageal cancer, Muñoz *et al.* (1985) provided vitamin supplements or placebos to randomly selected members of a Chinese population at high risk for esophageal cancer. Since hepatitis-B carriers are believed at high risk for primary liver cancer, the Gambian Hepatitis Intervention Study (GHIS, 1987) vaccinated a large population in Gambia against hepatitis-B virus to ascertain whether the high risk of primary liver cancer is eventually reduced in vaccinated but not in non-vaccinated individuals.

The use of intervention studies utilizing some form of chemoprevention probably will become more frequent as knowledge of carcinogenic mechanisms grows. For example, certain oral contraceptives have been shown to reduce ovarian cancer risk through suppression of ovulation. In view of the protective impact of early pregnancy on breast cancer, the development of a hormonal regime to mimic such a state in young women has been suggested as a potential chemopreventive technique. Theoretically, such interventions can be designed to affect either the early or later stages of carcinogenesis and this was the rationale for a proposed study on low fat diets to reduce the frequency of metastases after mastectomy for breast cancer. To date, however, clear reductions in specific cancers through interventions have been observed only for smoking cessation and in certain occupations where efforts to control exposures have been instituted.

Despite their methodologic superiority, intervention studies pose ethical, economic and logistical limitations which result from the

Table 3.1. *Major advantages and disadvantages of case-control studies.*

Advantages	Disadvantages
Latent period has elapsed and risk factors have produced their disease effects.	Requires a causal hypothesis and usually can focus only on one type of cancer at a time.
Suitable for the study of rare diseases in relation to a hypothesis or for the examination of a large number of potential risk factors.	Past exposures difficult to identify, validate, measure, e.g. dust levels, diet, hormonal patterns.
Very efficient and cost effective, especially for studying common exposures which produce a large proportion of a specific cancers.	For certain exposures (occupational, chemical) attributable risk may be very small and effect difficult to detect.
'Rapid' answer: normally two to three years.	Selection of appropriate control group may be difficult. Selection and recall bias may be present, seriously reducing the validity of the study.
Needs a relatively small number of subjects.	No direct estimate of the risk of developing a disease among exposed and non-exposed is possible. An estimate of relative risk can be obtained indirectly.

investigator's assignment of subjects to experimental (treatment) and control groups. Interventions known to be harmful should not be allocated nor should those known to be beneficial withheld. It may be difficult also to persuade a large group to give up a therapeutic regimen perceived to be beneficial or if it has gained widespread medical acceptance. Finally, subjects enrolled in a trial must be treated and evaluated individually, which frequently requires repeated visits to a clinic or hospital for examination. The result is a trial which can cost thousands of dollars per subject and be prohibitively expensive. Such considerations can seriously reduce the feasibility of conducting a trial even if scientifically justifiable.

3.2 Non-experimental or observational studies

Most carcinogens were first discovered by an alert clinician who observed an unusual number of cancers in a group. Even a small number of unique cases may present evidence so strong as to establish the existence of a causal association (Hill, 1965). Examples include vaginal adenocarcinomas in the daughters of women receiving diethylstilbestrol during pregnancy (Herbst *et al.*, 1971), adenocarcinoma of the nasal sinuses in the furniture-making industry and mesothelioma due to asbestos. Today, however, observational studies primarily depend on the systematic investigation of large populations designed to test specific hypotheses.

Observational studies remain the most common approach used by epidemiologists to identify causative factors. They permit testing of a wide variety of hypotheses and are less affected by the logistical and ethical limitations of experimental studies. Individually, observational studies cannot specify the mechanisms by which risk factors produce cancer, but they can confer a judgment of causality, if not a claim of proof.

The major disadvantages of observational studies usually include inability to control extraneous factors and less precise quantification of suspected risk factors than in intervention studies. Individuals are daily exposed to a host of potential carcinogenic factors but the epidemiologist may sometimes be able to identify subjects for investigation who vary widely in their exposure to the suspected risk factors of interest.

Two major observational designs are used in analytic epidemiology to assess causal relationships: the case-control study and the cohort study. They differ according to the method of selecting study subjects. Both methods allow estimation of the effect of a factor on the risk of disease and the results of the two approaches for a given hypothesis are usually consistent.

Case-control studies

The advantages and disadvantages of the case-control method are summarized in Table 3.1 and are considered in detail by Breslow and Day (1980) and Schlesselman (1982). Certain general principles are discussed below.

The case-control study, which proceeds from effect-to-cause, is the work-horse of the epidemiologist. This technique begins by selecting individuals with a particular disease (cases) and comparing them to individuals in whom the disease is absent (controls). Cases and controls are then compared on the basis of present or past risk factors considered relevant by the investigator. While study subjects theoretically are derived from a population of individuals who eventually will be the cancer cases or controls, it is not essential, although desirable, that cases or controls be representative of a general population. The principal objective is validity, not generalization, and this requires the ability to measure differences in disease frequency (*relative risk*) between exposed and non-exposed groups.

Subjects can be chosen from a variety of sources, frequently from hospital or disease registries. In a hospital-based study, for example, all patients with the cancer under study admitted to a hospital or network of hospitals, or a random sample of such cancers, are ascertained during a specific time period. Controls can be selected from persons admitted to the same hospitals for conditions other than the cancer under study. However, controls with diseases possibly associated with the suspected risk factors should be avoided. Thus, patients with coronary heart disease would be inappropriate controls for a study of lung cancer since both diseases are tobacco related.

In a population-based study, all newly diagnosed cases, or a random sample thereof, are selected for the study of a specific cancer occurring within a defined geographic area during a specified time. Controls are then selected from a random sample of individuals, free of the cancer of interest, in the same area. Incident (new) cases are to be preferred to prevalent (existing) or decedent cases since they will minimize selection bias.

The size of the control group is also a major consideration. If the number of cases and controls is large and the cost of gathering information relatively equal, then a 1 :1 ratio will be acceptable (Gail *et al.*, 1976). If only a small number of cancers are available, the ratio of cases-to-controls should be increased, bearing in mind that little statistical power will be gained beyond a ratio of 1 :4. To ensure the validity of results, an effort should be made to anticipate the most likely sources of error (bias) at the beginning of the study as well as the sample size required to detect the postulated differences between groups (power).

Case-control studies provide a great deal of information and can assess interaction between common causal factors such as alcohol and tobacco. Such studies can also evaluate the causal significance of a rare risk factor, since it is the prevalence of the risk factor in the cases and not in the controls which is important. A common factor accounting for a high proportion of a cancer at a specific site requires a case control approach (Cole & MacMahon, 1971). If a risk factor is rare, and accounts for a small proportion of a specific cancer, that is, it carries a low population attributable risk as in most occupational exposures, a cohort approach is required.

Limitations to the case-control approach include its high susceptibility to biases which tend to make cases and controls non-comparable. The selection of cases and controls can be biased through improper ascertainment, diagnosis or selection of study subjects. For example, it would be unwise to choose cases from a teaching hospital serving a wide area and controls from a limited geographical area. Errors in estimating past exposures can result from absence of exposure measurements,

Table 3.2. *Major advantages and disadvantages of prospective cohort studies.*

Advantages	Disadvantages
Complete cohort usually easier to assemble than historical cohort.	Follow-up may be difficult and expensive.
Provides a direct estimate of the risk of developing cancer in individuals with a risk factor relative to those without the risk factor.	Losses to follow-up may seriously impair validity of study. If protocol too detailed, logistical problems may become unmanageable.
As protocol is established in advance, the possibility of subjective bias in obtaining the required information, e.g. smoking habits, occupation, 'lifestyle' behaviors, etc. is decreased.	Generally more expensive, more time-consuming and of longer duration than case-control or historical cohort studies.
Economical only if records can be readily and unequivocally linked to outcome.	Storage and analysis of biological materials (e.g. sera, tissues) collected may be costly, even if done only on a case-control basis.
Permits investigation of a wide spectrum of morbidity and mortality, as well as a wide range of cancers.	Inefficient for studying rare diseases.
	If periodic examination required, participation in the study may influence the development of the disease in individuals.
Possible to measure change in risk factors and disease effects during course of study. Biological and biochemical materials (e.g. tissue, sera, etc.) can be collected and stored.	Large populations ($> 20,000$) required to yield reasonable risk estimates of even common cancers.
Nested case-control study may be feasible to assess relationship of risk factors to disease if sufficient cancer cases can be assembled.	Measurement of confounding variables can be difficult or incomplete.

incomplete records, faulty recall, improper interviewing techniques or prevarication.

Cohort studies

In exploring causal association between specific exposures and cancer, an epidemiologist also may proceed from cause-to-effect. Individuals in a defined population with one or more risk factors suspected to be associated with a cancer are selected and followed for a period deemed sufficient for the development of an adequate number of cancers. Cancer rates then can be calculated in subgroups of the population with known differences in exposure. The essential feature is

Table 3.3. *Major advantages and disadvantages of historical cohort studies.*

Advantages	Disadvantages
Latent period has elapsed and risk factors have produced their disease effects.	Numbers of cases with over 20 years exposure may be small, even in a large cohort.
Results may be achieved fairly rapidly – two years.	Risk factors may not be measurable retrospectively and may change in nature and intensity over years.
Can be applied to the study of all chronic disease effects for which appropriate data has been collected in the past.	Rarely possible to assess effects of other variables unless a nested case-control study can be conducted.
Can provide direct estimate of risk.	May be difficult to complete follow-up.
Economical if suitable records are available and can be readily and unequivocally linked with outcome, e.g. cancer registry or death certificates, drug surveillance registration.	Death certificates frequently inaccurate.
Study of many cancer sites and wide spectrum of morbidity and mortality possible.	Appropriate comparison groups not always easy to identify.

that each individual's subsequent cancer experience can be related to prior risk factor information permitting the testing of specific hypotheses. The advantages and disadvantages of cohort studies are summarized in Tables 3.2 and 3.3 and are reviewed by Breslow and Day (1987).

Cohort studies are appropriate when risk factors can be characterized and an adequate number of persons identified and followed to the cancer end-point. Success depends on complete characterization of the cohort and thorough follow-up which should exceed 90%. Such cohort studies are often undertaken in an industrial setting, e.g. brewery workers (Jensen, 1980) or in man-made mineral fiber plants (Saracci, 1986), where exposures are not only likely to be higher, but variations may be easier to measure. For an industrial cohort, follow-up should include those employed for at least six months, as well as those leaving employment or retiring before the end of the period. Generally, only a few cancers related to the suspected carcinogen will appear under 20 years which is usually regarded as the minimum desirable follow-up interval.

(i)   Prospective and historical cohort studies

In a *prospective cohort* study, the cohort is assembled in the present and individual cohort members followed prospectively into the future. A prospective study can convincingly demonstrate differences in risks between groups since incidence rates for the exposed and non-exposed can be calculated. Such a study is very efficient for examining risk factors that are both rare in the general population and which are responsible for only a small fraction of a specific cancer. While the precise information needed may be collected, the approach has the disadvantage that many years may elapse before sufficient cases arise for analysis, and it may be difficult to trace all cohort members.

In a *historical cohort* study, records existing 20 or more years earlier are used to identify a group with certain exposure characteristics, at a previously defined time period, e.g. those employed between 1910–1914. The cancer experience of the group is then followed to a selected date. The advantage of this approach is that the results are potentially available immediately and a prolonged and expensive investigation can be avoided since an adequate period of exposure has already elapsed. However, the quality of historical information, notably for previous exposure and/or personal habits, such as smoking, may be unsatisfactory or missing. Using this approach, Case *et al.* (1954*a*, 1984*b*) showed that an excess of bladder cancer in the chemical industry was largely confined to workers who distilled certain aromatic amines. If a cohort is historical, the listed cohort members can be matched against mortality records or cancer registry data. The focus is still forward in time, and reference to such studies as 'retrospective' is misleading.

On occasion, a historical cohort study may comprise both a retrospective and a prospective element in the same cohort (Jensen, 1980; Engholm *et al.*, 1982). This method has several advantages in that the induction period may have largely elapsed and any findings emerging from the historical cohort portion can be probed in greater detail and with greater confidence during the prospective period, e.g. exposure to man-made mineral fibers.

Results of cohort studies are often presented as standard mortality ratios (SMRs) or standard incidence ratios (SIRs). The number of cases arising in the study group is compared with those expected to occur in the general population of the same age and sex composition during the same period of time. Such ratios have a number of limitations and local populations may provide better data for comparison than national data, if, for example, the work-force comes from a particular ethnic population.

It should be noted that case-control and cohort methods are

complementary. As pointed out by Mantel and Haenszel (1959), 'While the study techniques are different, a case control study examines the risk factor in the cancer cases and appropriate controls arising from a cohort over a limited period of time.' The case-control approach concentrates effort on the informative individuals (cases) and a suitable set of controls, on whom extensive information on confounding variables may be obtainable. The cohort approach provides a well-defined population from which cases can be identified in an unbiased manner.

The case-control method is more efficient for the study of rare cancers than the cohort study which 'wastes' substantial effort in following up the many individuals who remain free of the disease for the period of follow-up. The case-control approach is highly appropriate for studying cancer since cases can be recruited immediately and the problems of long latency avoided. Generally, a case-control study will almost always require less time, less money and fewer subjects than a prospective cohort design. However, a historical cohort study may be superior in cost and time if appropriate valid data have already been collected.

The prospective cohort study design confers some advantages in assessing the causal association between risk factors and disease outcomes. First, recall and selection bias, a major problem in case-control studies, can usually be greatly reduced. Occasionally, some pertinent direct measurement on biological samples may be available, e.g. chemical or metabolic in blood or body fluids. Second, such samples may reflect certain physiological or biochemical parameters prior to the onset of cancer. Third, serial measurements of a risk factor can be obtained, assuring greater accuracy in recording the effects of changing levels of risk and providing an unbiased assessment both of misclassification rates and confounding variables. Fourth, cohort studies provide direct estimates of incidence rates and absolute measures of risk which may be preferable to relative measures of risk for making public health decisions.

Finally, the long-term health effects of a given risk factor can be provided only by a cohort study, as illustrated by the wide range and variations in the time of cancer appearance in the follow-up of atomic bomb survivors in Japan (BEIR, 1980).

(ii) Nested studies

The cohort study design has several limitations, including the necessity to commit substantial resources over many years. Evaluating the significance of moderate excesses in cancer risk is difficult in cohorts for whom accurate exposure records cannot be guaranteed, and for which follow-up is not virtually complete. Finally, it is difficult to estimate a population attributable risk from cohorts assembled from groups with a much higher prevalence of the relevant exposure than the general population.

Increasingly, 'nested' case-control designs are being used which incorporate the case-control approach within a cohort study, to take advantage of the merits of both. In these hybrid designs, the cohort component would usually identify the group, collect information or biological specimens to assess exposure and ascertain the disease experience in the follow-up period; the exposures would then be assessed and measured using the case-control approach. In this way, one ensures strict definition of the study cohort, but the effort and resources devoted to assessing accurate exposure can be concentrated on the most informative sample of individuals, i.e. those with cancer and their controls, i.e. other cohort members.

3.3   Monitoring and surveillance studies

In areas with a national health service, such as Northern Ireland or with specific monitoring systems, such as the Boston Collaborative Drug Surveillance Program, information on the use of prescription medication may be available through a drug registry. It may then be possible to identify chronic effects, such as cancer, using a methodology similar to follow-up studies on chemotherapeutic agents used to treat a first cancer (Kaldor *et al.*, 1987). In contrast, investigating the linkage between cancer of the renal pelvis and analgesic abuse has proved difficult due to the rarity of the disease, the frequency of analgesic usage and uncertainties of dose. In theory, governmental financing of medical care should provide records which facilitate such studies, but the logistic and financial burdens on the investigator often outweigh the advantages.

Only recently have long-term cancer registries been available covering large populations in many countries. The use of such registries in identifying causal associations is still fairly unusual, but will almost certainly become more common in the future as registries provide a very useful and economical method of monitoring and surveying specific populations suspected to be at high risk. Thus, local cancer registries and the Registrar General for England and Wales enter cohort members in the alphabetical list comprising all persons covered by National Health Insurance (virtually the entire population), and of all deaths, informing investigators when a cancer notification (or death) for a cohort member is received. To ensure unequivocal matching, good identifying information is essential. Computerized record linkage programs such as those developed by Statistics Canada (GIRLS) are powerful aids in making such matches. Although theoretically promising, routine record linkage for cancer studies in occupational settings has yet to fulfil expectations because cancer registries have been relatively unsuccessful in obtaining accurate exposure histories. In a series of publications, Malker and Gemne (1987) demonstrated what can be derived from this approach, e.g. in the printing industry.

3.4   References

BEIR (National Research Council, Committee on the Biological Effects of Ionizing Radiation) (1980). *The Effects on Populations of Exposure to Low Levels of Ionizing Radiation.* National Academy of Science. Washington: National Academy Press.

Breslow, N.E. & Day, N.E. (1980). *Statistical Methods in Cancer Research, Volume 1, The Analysis of Case-Control Studies,* IARC Scientific Publication No. 32. Lyon: International Agency for Research on Cancer.

Breslow, N.E. & Day, N.E. (1987). *Statistical Methods in Cancer Research, Volume II, The Design and Analysis of Cohort Studies,* IARC Scientific Publication No. 82. Lyon: International Agency for Research on Cancer.

Case, R.A.M., Hosker M.E., McDonald D.B. & Pearson, J.T. (1954*a*). Tumours of the urinary bladder in workmen engaged in the manufacture and use of certain dyestuff intermediates in the British chemical industry. Part I. The role of aniline, benzidine, alpha-naphthylamine and beta-naphthylamine. *Brit. J. Ind. Med.,* 11, 75–104.

Case, R.A.M., Hosker M.E., McDonald D.B. & Pearson, J.T. (1954*b*). Tumours of the urinary bladder in workmen engaged in the manufacture and use of certain dyestuff intermediates in the British chemical industry. Part II. Further considerations on the role of aniline and of the manufacture of auramine and magenta (fuchsine) as possible causative agents. *Brit. J. Ind. Med.,* 11, 213–16.

Checkoway, H., Pearce, N.E. & Crawford-Brown, D.J. (1989). *Research Methods in Occupational Epidemiology.* Monographs in Epidemiology and Biostatistics, Volume 13. New York: Oxford University Press.

Cole, P. & MacMahon, B. (1971). Attributable risk percent in case-control studies. *Brit. J. Prev. Soc. Med.,* 25, 242–4.

Engholm, G., Englund, A., Hallin, N. & von Schmalensee, G. (1982). Respiratory cancer incidence in Swedish construction workers exposed to man-made mineral fibers (MMMF). In *Proceedings of the Conference on Biological Man-Made Mineral Fibers.* WHO EURO Reports and Studies, No. 81, 20–22 April. Copenhagen: World Health Organization.

Gail, M., Williams, R., Byar, D.P. & Brown, C. (1976). How many controls? *J. Chron. Dis.,* 29, 723–31.

GHIS (Gambia Hepatitis Study Group) (1987). The Gambia Hepatitis Intervention Study. *Cancer Res.,* 47, 5782–7.

Herbst, A.L., Ulfelder, H., & Poskanzer, D.C. (1971). Adenocarcinoma of the vagina. *New Engl. J. Med.,* 284, 878–81.

Hill, A.B. (1965). The environment and disease: association or causation? *Proceedings of the Royal Society of Medicine,* 58, 295–300.

Hennekens, C.H. & Burning J.E. (1987). *Epidemiology in Medicine.* Boston: Little, Brown and Company.

Jensen, O.M. (1980). *Cancer Morbidity and Causes of Death Among Danish Brewery Workers.* Lyon: International Agency for Research on Cancer.

Kahn, H.A. & Sempos, C.T. (1989). *Statistical Methods in Epidemiology.* Monographs in Epidemiology and Biostatistics, Volume 12. New York: Oxford University Press.

Kaldor, J.M., Day, N.E., Band, P., Choi, N.W., Clark, E.A., Coleman, M.P., Hakama, M., Koch, M., Langmark, F., Neal, F.E., Peterson, F., Pompe-Kirn, V., Prior, P., & Storm,

H.H. (1987). Second malignancies following testicular cancer, ovarian cancer and Hodgkin's disease: an international collaborative study among cancer registries of the long-term effects of therapy. *Int. J. Cancer*, **39**, 571–85.

Kelsey, J.L., Thompson, W.D. & Evans, A.S (1986). *Methods in Observational Epidemiology.* Monographs in Epidemiology and Biostatistics, Volume 10. New York: Oxford University Press.

Lilienfeld, A.M. & Lilienfeld, D.E. (1980). *Foundations of Epidemiology*, 2nd edition. New York: Oxford University Press.

Malker, H.S. & Gemne, G. (1987). A register-epidemiology study on cancer among Swedish printing industry workers. *Arch. Environ. Health*, **42**, 73–82.

Mantel, N., & Haenszel, W. (1959). Statistical aspects of the analysis of data from a retrospective study of disease. *J. Natl. Cancer Inst.*, **22**, 719–48.

Meinert, C.L. (1986). *Clinical Trials: Design, Conduct and Analysis.* Monographs in Epidemiology and Biostatistics, Volume 8. New York: Oxford University Press.

Muñoz, N., Wahrendorf, J., Lu Jian Bank, Crespi, M., Thurnham, D.I., Day, N.E., Zheng Hong Ji, Grassi, A., Li Wen Yan, Liu Gui Lin, Lang Yu Wuan, Zhang Cai Yun, Zheng Su Fang, Li Jun Yao, Correa, P., O'Conor, G.T. & Bosch, X. (1985). No effect of riboflavine, retinol and zinc on prevalence of precancerous lesions of oesophagus: a randomized double-blind intervention study in a high-risk population of China. *Lancet*, **ii**, 111–14.

Rothman, K.J. (1986). *Modern Epidemiology.* Boston: Little, Brown and Company.

Saracci, R. (1986). Ten years of epidemiological investigations on man-made mineral fibres and health. *Scand. J. Work Environ. Health*, **12**(Suppl. 1), 5–11.

Schlesselman, J.J. (1982). *Case-Control Studies: Design, Conduct, Analysis.* Monographs in Epidemiology and Biostatistics, Volume 2. New York: Oxford University Press.

Weiss, N. (1986). *Clinical Epidemiology: The Study of the Outcome of Illness.* Monographs in Epidemiology and Biostatistics, Volume 11. New York: Oxford University Press.

4

Limitations of epidemiological methods in cancer studies : study of low-level risks : negative studies

Epidemiological studies of cancer have well-recognized limitations, including: (i) lack of sensitivity; (ii) difficulty in discriminating between several plausible risk factors; (iii) the inadequacy of past exposure data; (iv) inability to evaluate the impact of recent exposures; and (v) uncertainties in interpreting negative studies or inverse relationships. Only the first and last points will be discussed below.

4.1   Low-level exposures and negative studies

Much of the information suggesting a lack of response to suspected carcinogenic exposures at low doses is dependent on the evaluation of negative epidemiological studies. A negative study is one of adequate statistical power in which the relative risk for a suspected factor is not significantly different from unity at the 5% level of statistical significance. The interpretation of apparently negative data is complicated by the impossibility of proving a true negative – no matter how large a study, there remains some chance of missing a carcinogenic effect. These statistical limitations are also inherent even in large scale animal bioassays, where lack of carcinogenic activity is unprovable. Study of low-level potential carcinogenic hazards in the general environment, such as air, water or soil pollution from waste sites or industry, is fraught with many uncertainties (Grisham, 1986). It is not always possible to define the exposed population precisely in order to establish an accurate baseline for the presumed health effect. Bias, confounding and chance can easily produce spurious weak associations and thus the interpretation of negative or weak associations in epidemiological studies requires considerable expertise, as illustrated by controversy on the interpretation of borderline health effects whether investigating low-level radiation

(Cook-Mozaffari *et al.*, 1989 ; Roman *et al.*, 1987), toxic waste deposits (Grisham, 1986), socio-economic variations (Logan, 1982), or dietary components (Zaridze *et al.*, 1985). It is thus essential to decide whether a negative study represents a true non-effect or simply a lack of sensitivity (Day, 1985). As this author has pointed out, 'If one takes 1000 events of interest [i.e. cases of cancer] as representing a large study – in fact, an order of magnitude larger than most industrial cohort studies – and ignoring all considerations other than chance, a negative study [i.e. one with a relative risk estimate of one] will usually be compatible with a 20% increase in risk and almost always be compatible with a 5% increase in risk.'

'For many of the industrial exposures that are suspected of being hazardous, on the basis usually of experimental results, studies of this size are unlikely to be possible, and one will be left, even if the estimated excess risk is zero, with confidence intervals containing risks of appreciable size (20 to 30%). Proposed legislation in some countries aims at reducing exposures to levels at which the excess risk, based on extrapolation procedures using data from animal carcinogenicity experiments, is of the order of 10^{-6}. It is clear that epidemiology will never be able to determine whether such levels have been attained.' The above limitations are equally applicable to inverse relationships.

The same limitations apply also to attempts to demonstrate a threshold. Thus, while observations in Africa and elsewhere suggest a threshold for aflatoxin in liver cancer, there are confounding variables. Observations on radiation and stomach cancer are consistent with both a threshold and a linear quadratic response (Day, 1985). Such uncertainties are inherent for most human and animal data at low-level exposures, although experimental studies suggest that a threshold is biologically plausible for non-genotoxic carcinogens. These issues should be considered by the epidemiologist in evaluating data to be used for the promulgation of exposure standards.

In evaluating negative epidemiological data, little can be added to Doll's (1985) comments at the IARC workshop in 1983, 'Negative human evidence may mean very little, unless it relates to prolonged and heavy exposure. If, however, it does and is consistent in a variety of studies (correlation studies over time, cohort studies of exposed individuals, and case-control studies of affected patients) whereas the laboratory evidence is limited in scope to, for instance, a particular type of tumour in a few species, negative human evidence may justify the conclusion that for practical purposes the agent need not be treated as a human carcinogen. In practice it is, of course, not usual for such perfect negative evidence to

Fig. 4.1 Lung cancer and environmental tobacco smoke exposure in non-smokers: Results of 13 studies.

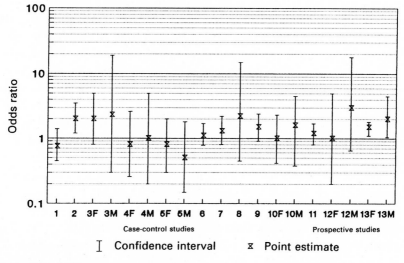

(after NRC, 1986)

be available, but even less conclusive negative human evidence may help determine priorities between different lines of action.'

This author also concludes that the only safe rule is to consider the totality of the evidence available, and emphasises the view of the Royal Society's Study Group in 1983 that some induced events are '...of so low a frequency that the manager or regulator of risk can reasonably regard them as negligible in their overall impact on society even though the consequences to the rare individual may be serious'.

4.2 Meta-analysis

Several systematic approaches, including meta-analysis (Mann, 1990), have been suggested for summarizing, evaluating and comparing epidemiological evidence with respect to human carcinogenicity (NTP, 1985; EPA, 1986; IARC, 1987), especially where numbers are small and equivocal.

Epidemiologists are usually compelled to carry out studies on populations where the total number of individuals observed, and number of cancers or years of observation are more limited than desirable. Thus, consideration has been given to combining data from a number of separate studies to determine whether limited or uncertain conclusions can be further extended or strengthened. As Buffler (1989) has pointed out, pooling of data which are not treated specifically as meta-analyses has been routine in epidemiology. Properly conducted analysis of pooled data to test for consistency of the individual study results can provide summary estimates of risk. In the National Research Council report (1986) on the health consequences of exposure to environmental tobacco smoke, data from ten case-control studies and three prospective studies, conducted in seven countries, were pooled to develop summary estimates of risk which indicated an overall lung cancer risk in non-smokers associated with exposure to environmental tobacco smoke of 1.34, (95% CI : 1.18–1.53) (Fig. 4.1). For the United States, the relative risk was 1.14 (95% CI : 0.92–1.40). None the less the role of passive smoking remains controversial (Chapters 9 and 34).

The present form of meta-analysis comprises a set of statistical techniques and methods for combining evidence from a number of well-controlled quantitative studies to address a specific research question. Buffler (1989) states that 'meta-analysis is to a primary research study what a primary research study is to its study subjects in that the unit of observation for the meta-analysis is a primary research report. Meta-analyses differ from careful literature reviews in that they address more focused questions and the meta-analyst formulates and analyzes at least one numeric summary from each primary study. Methods for specifying the numeric summary include the use of p-values related to null hypotheses, t-statistics, correlation coefficients and effect scores. Suitable weights can be given to the scores for individual studies as determined by the reliability or the sample size of the primary study.'

In summarizing the literature, Louis *et al.* (1985) found only four examples of formal meta-analyses prior to 1985, two of which were concerned with known or suspected environmental carcinogens – lead and vinyl chloride. Although ten studies were available for lead, the authors concluded that the evidence was insufficient to exonerate lead as a human carcinogen, although the results from some studies were consistent with such a conclusion. Recently 100 studies in the petroleum industry were reviewed by quantitative meta-analysis (Wong & Rabbe, 1989).

Unfortunately, meta-analytical approaches are often handicapped by publication bias (Begg & Berlin, 1989). On the one hand, investigators may be reluctant to publish negative studies, even if reproducible, on the grounds that perhaps an increase in study size or its extension over time might uncover an adverse effect. On the other hand, many journals do not accept such studies as being uninformative or due to lack of space.

Meta-analysis probably will be used to a greater degree in the future. By following an agreed protocol and undertaking central analysis, this approach obviates some of the problems of meta-analysis of studies of different designs while enjoying the advantages of adequate numbers and the ability to assess consistency of effect in differing study locations. Statistical and scientific credibility can be increased because of the variety of circumstances considered in the summary analysis, which can also characterize study-to-study variations in underlying effects. The SEARCH program of the IARC (1989) is essentially a well-organized meta-analytical study, on the same cancers, in a number of different locations to provide more detailed understanding of potentially carcinogenic risk factors.

Undoubtedly, more could be learned from available epidemiological studies and meta-analysis is a potentially powerful tool for reviewing of such data. Unfortunately, negative data are probably under-represented in the available literature and may bias the conclusions of a meta-analytical study.

4.3   References

Begg, C.B. & Berlin, J.A. (1989). Publication bias and dissemination of clinical research. *J. Natl. Cancer Inst.*, **81**, 107–15.

Buffler, P. (1989). The evaluation of negative epidemiologic studies : The importance of all available evidence in risk characterization. *Regul. Toxicol. Pharmacol.*, **9**, 34–43.

Cook-Mozaffari, P., Darby, S. & Doll, R. (1989). Cancer near potential sites of nuclear installations. *Lancet*, **i**, 855–6.

Day, N.E. (1985). Statistical Considerations. In *Interpretation of Negative Epidemiological Evidence for Carcinogenicity*, IARC Scientific Publications No. 65, ed. N.J. Wald & R. Doll, pp. 13–27. Lyon : International Agency for Research on Cancer.

Doll, R. (1985). Purpose of symposium. In *Interpretation of Negative Epidemiological Evidence for Carcinogenicity*, IARC Scientific Publication No. 65, ed. N.J. Wald & R. Doll, pp.3–10. Lyon : International Agency for Research on Cancer.

EPA (Environmental Protection Agency) (1986). *Human Health and the Environment : Some Research Needs*, Volume III. Washington : US Department of Health and Human Services.

Grisham, J.W. (1986). *Health Aspects of the Disposal of Waste Chemicals*. Elmsford, NY : Pergamon Press.

IARC (1987). *Overall Evaluations of Carcinogenicity : An Updating of IARC Monographs Volumes 1–42*, IARC Monographs, Supplement No. 7. Lyon : International Agency for Research on Cancer.

IARC (1989). *Biennial Report 88–89*, for the Period 1 July 1987 to 30 June 1989, pp. 68–98. Lyon : International Agency for Research on Cancer.

Logan, W.P.D. (1982). *Cancer Mortality by Occupation and Social Class 1851–1971*. IARC Scientific Publications No. 36. Lyon : International Agency for Cancer Research.

Louis, T.A., Fineberg, H.V. & Mosteller, F. (1985). Findings for public health from meta-analyses. *Annu. Rev. Public Health*, **6**, 1–20.

Mann, C. (1990). Meta-analysis in the breech. *Science*, **249**, 476–80.

NRC (National Research Council) (1986). *Environmental Tobacco Smoke : Measuring Exposures and Assessing Health Effects*. Report from Committee on Passive Smoking. Washington : National Academy Press.

NTP (National Toxicology Program) (1985). *Fourth Annual Report on Carcinogens*, NTP 85–002. Washington : U.S. Department of Health and Human Services.

Roman, E., Beral, V., Carpenter, L., Watson, A., Barton, C., Ryder H. & Aston, D.L. (1987). Childhood leukemia in the West Berkshire and Basingstoke and North Hampshire District Health Authorities in relation to nuclear establishments in the vicinity. *Br. Med. J.*, **294**, 597–602.

Wong, O. & Raabe, G.K. (1989). Critical review of cancer epidemiology in petroleum industry employees, with a quantitative meta-analysis by cancer site. *Am. J. Ind. Med.*, **15**, 283–310.

Zaridze, D.G., Muir, C.S. & McMichael, A.J. (1985). Diet and cancer : value of different types of epidemiological studies. In *Diet and Human Carcinogenesis*, ed. J.V. Joossens, M.J. Hill and J. Geboers, pp. 221–33. New York : Excerpta Medica.

5

Laboratory methods in epidemiology

5.1   Introduction

Carcinogenesis is a multi-factorial, multistep process involving cancer induction by a range of mechanisms which may vary both by agent and neoplasm. While it is considered that some form of DNA damage is essential to the process and that a cascade of other events is involved, the extent and nature of the damage and the specific role of many phenomena seen in carcinogenesis remain to be elucidated. In this context, there is a growing body of laboratory methods that can be utilized to amplify the role of epidemiology in the study of carcinogenic processes. Such approaches are relevant to the following areas:

(a) The diagnosis and determination of the pathogenesis of neoplasms, including preneoplastic end-points.

(b) Methods to measure present and past exposures to suspected carcinogenic agents, both quantitatively and qualitatively, that is, biomarkers of exposure.

(c) Methods to measure exposure to certain nutrients potentially associated with human cancer, i.e. biomarkers that reflect dietary influences with varying degrees of specificity.

(d) Provision of objective end-points for determining individual and tissue susceptibility.

(e) Provision of data on the carcinogenic mechanisms involved, including metabolic pathways.

This chapter discusses certain general concepts and techniques. Other aspects are discussed under individual cancer sites, as well as in Chapters 17 and 18.

5.2   Application of morphological and cytological techniques
Diagnosis of cancer

The validity of descriptive and analytical epidemiological data is greatly influenced by the accuracy of the diagnosis. Accurate diagnosis of tumors reduces misclassification, permits sub-classification and thus improves the possibility of demonstrating causal associations. For many years, the accuracy of cancer diagnosis has rested on cyto-histopathological and hematological techniques. These still form the basic criteria for determining the quality of cancer registration data. Formerly, considerable autopsy material was available, but today in most countries the proportion of diagnoses made at autopsy is small. Diagnosis is increasingly dependent on biopsy supplemented by imaging or other sophisticated clinical laboratory technologies, such as CAT scans.

The most widely used classification today is the *International Classification of Diseases* (WHO, 1977). A specialized adaption for Oncology or ICD-0 was published in 1976 which, in addition to the classification of tumors by site, lists code numbers for the various histological types. The code numbers used are identical to those appearing in SNOMED (College of American Pathologists, 1979); these also appear in the so-called 'Blue Books' of WHO, i.e. the *International Histological Classification of Tumors*, which classify, describe and illustrate the neoplasms arising in a given organ or tissue. Histological subclassification within a given site has been found to be of epidemiological value, e.g. the relationship of cigarette smoking to certain types of the lung carcinoma (Chapter 34). Subclassification of lymphomas has been shown to be important both in terms of etiology and especially clinical course and therapy. Stomach cancer has been classified into intestinal and diffuse types which appear to have different causes and clinical courses (Chapter 26). Despite the many elegant new techniques available, including histo- and cyto- chemistry, monoclonal antibodies, and electron microscopy, these, in many instances, while permitting better and easier diagnosis of tumor origin and cell type, have not yielded significant information on causation except where a specific agent or marker is demonstrable (see below).

Precancerous endpoints and pathogenesis

During the development of human cancer, there is a latent period, usually of many years, during which overt neoplasia cannot be clinically detected. However, histological abnormalities have been recognized in some organs which are associated with an increased risk of developing cancer. In a probabilistic sense such lesions, i.e. dysplasia can be regarded as precancerous at many sites such as the skin and uterine cervix. In certain sites, e.g. mouth and oesophagus, such lesions are preceded by epithelial atrophy and chronic inflammation of the sub-epithelial tissues. While only a small proportion of these lesions progress to cancer, in general, the more advanced the lesions, the higher is the risk of malignant transformation. So far, ultra-structural changes in cells have usually not proven of value in human studies, in contrast to some experimental situations, e.g. peroxisome proliferation as a precursor of rodent hepatoma. This is partly due to logistic problems, lack of specificity and absence of background data. Other cytological lesions considered as precancerous are described further under chromosomal abnormalities.

The study of individuals with precancerous lesions may provide valuable information on pathogenesis as in the following:

(a) In case-control studies, such lesions may increase the possibility of identifying etiological factors due to the shorter interval between exposure and appearance. Thus, individuals with lesions suspected as precancerous for the stomach or the cervix show the same risk factors as those with clinical cancer.

(b) They may identify individuals at high-risk for certain cancers, e.g. cervix and oral cavity, and thus be used in screening programs leading to earlier and more effective treatment.

(c) Their value in the evaluation of primary preventive methods in carcinogenesis is now receiving considerable attention. Thus, factors inducing regression of precancerous lesions may possibly be used as end-points in intervention trials. (Chapter 25).

(d) Such lesions may provide clues to the pathogenic mechanisms. Thus, studies of liver biopsies have demonstrated the progression of viral or alcoholic hepatitis to cirrhosis and occasionally liver cancer.

Morphological and cytological identification of exposure to carcinogenic agents

The techniques used to assess exposure to carcinogenic agents in humans can be considered at various levels (Table 5.1). Such markers range from detection of the agent itself in tissues or body fluids of exposed humans to detection of molecular changes specific to such exposures. Many of these approaches have been recently reviewed (Bartsch *et al.*, 1988*a*).

Table 5.1. *Biomarkers of exposure to carcinogenic agents.*

1. Morphological techniques
    – Specific histological characteristics, e.g. alcoholic hepatitis
    – Presence of defined agents or products (specific exposure):
        physical: asbestos fibers
        chemicals: specific DNA adducts
        biological:
            viruses: specific antigens or DNA fragments
            parasites: worms or ova
2. Sperm abnormalities (non-specific exposures)
3. Chromosomal abnormalities (non-specific exposures)
    – chromosomal aberrations: produced by ionizing radiation and radiomimetic chemicals
    – sister chromatid exchanges: produced by chemicals
    – numerical abnormalities: produced by chemicals
    – micronuclei formation: produced by chemicals
4. Detection of biomarkers in body fluids
    Biomarkers excreted in urine
    – mutagenicity of urine: (non-specific)
    – excretion of *N*-nitrosoproline and other nitroso aminoacids (as an index of endogenous nitrosation)
    – excretion of thioethers: (non-specific) exposure to compounds that conjugate with glutathione
    – 3-methyladenine levels: (non-specific) exposure to methylating agents
    – aflatoxin metabolites and adducts
    Biomarkers in blood
    – hemoglobin adducts (non-specific)
    – albumin adducts (aflatoxin albumin adducts)
    – DNA adducts in white blood cells
5. Detection of biomarkers in target tissue
    – DNA adducts to carcinogens
    – oncogenes

Morphological techniques

These offer several approaches. Thus, certain carcinogenic agents can induce relatively specific morphological changes, e.g. 'alcoholic hepatitis'. Secondly, parasites such as *Clonorchis sinensis, Opisthorchis viverrini,* or schistosomal ova can be identified in the target tissues as can be asbestos bodies or fibers, copper or iron deposits, etc. Ordinary light microscopy can be supplemented by immuno-histochemical techniques, radioactive probes and recently developed techniques of *in situ* hybridization and gene amplification, to identify specific antigens, unusual proteins, DNA fragments or carcinogen DNA adducts. Electron microscopy can separate types of asbestos fibers and the intracellular sites of mineral deposits. The polymerase chain reaction (PCR) can also be used in fixed tissue sections to uncover the presence of viral genomes or DNA modification. These techniques have turned out to be very sensitive and specific.

Sperm abnormalities

Such abnormalities have been used to indicate possible adverse effects on male fertility, especially in occupational exposures, but need further validation. There may be difficulties in obtaining samples and the confounding effect of other exposures, e.g. cigarette smoking, should be considered in interpreting the results.

Chromosomal abnormalities

Damage to chromosomes can take various forms: structural aberrations, sister chromatid exchange (SCE), numerical abnormalities and micronuclei formation. The alteration produced depends on the type of chromosomal damage induced by the genotoxic agent. Chromosomal aberrations result from breakage and rearrangement of whole chromosomes. They are produced by agents that directly break the DNA such as ionizing radiation and radiomimetic chemicals.

Sister Chromatid Exchange (SCE) can result from breakage and rejoining of DNA strands. They are produced by chemicals that form covalent adducts with DNA or interfere with DNA synthesis.

Numerical abnormalities or aneuploidy results from gains or losses of whole chromosomes following exposure to substances that interfere with the apparatus of cell division.

The Micronucleus Test (MN) detects chromosomal fragments not incorporated into the nucleus during cell division following chromosomal breakage. Micronuclei can be identified in peripheral blood lymphocytes and exfoliated epithelial cells, e.g. colon, using special stains for DNA. In theory, MN reflect exposure to clastogens or agents that affect the spindle apparatus.

The above techniques have been used to monitor exposure to occupational carcinogens, chemotherapeutic agents and in subjects exposed to tobacco smoking, alcohol or betel nut chewing. Recently, the MN test has been used as an early and easily identifiable end-point in an intervention study on precancerous lesions of the esophagus (Muñoz *et al.*, 1987).

The major limitation of these end-points is their lack of specificity and the fact that background lesions may not be insignificant. Further, they show considerable intra- and inter-individual variations. Thus their

Fig. 5.1 Steps in Chemical Carcinogenesis and control.

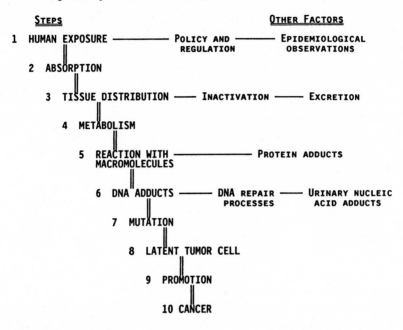

(after Wogan and Tannenbaum, 1987)

significance as specific predictors for later cancer development usually remains to be determined. They are possibly of greatest value in well-defined populations as indicative of exposure to considerable levels of a suspected chemical hazard. Accordingly, there is more interest today in studying specific DNA damage at the molecular level as as means of developing molecular dosimetry to carcinogen exposure.

5.3   Biomarkers

The term biomarker, as used here, refers to either a direct or indirect measure of exposure to a carcinogen or as a predictive marker of increased cancer risk or both.

The great majority of mutagens and chemical carcinogens exert their effects only after metabolic conversion to chemically reactive forms which bind to cellular macromolecules such as nucleic acids (DNA and RNA) and proteins to form adducts. While not all adducts are necessarily related to carcinogenesis, their formation is frequently considered as an indicator of critical damage to DNA which initiates the cascade of events eventually leading to transformation and neoplasia. Figure 5.1 (Wogan & Tannenbaum, 1987) summarizes the carcinogenic process for a hypothetical chemical and many of these steps are identifiable in tissues, even if their exact significance in carcinogenesis is unknown. This simplified model is of help in considering the various steps at which exposures to suspected chemical carcinogens may be measured. However, in only a relatively few situations in humans can a single chemical carcinogen be anticipated as the only causal agent, such as in an occupation where possible high level exposures to a single factor may be of concern. Indeed, a background of multiple DNA adducts can be demonstrated in human and animal tissues, the origin and relevance of which is uncertain.

Detection of biomarkers in target tissues

There are two approaches to the use of DNA adducts in determining the tissue dose: the indirect approach using accessible cells such as blood leukocytes as surrogates for the direct target cells, or the direct approach using the target cells obtained from biopsy or autopsy specimens.

DNA adducts to carcinogens

The detection of DNA adducts in target cells or tissues is considered as the most accurate and direct measure of exposure to carcinogenic agents since this represents an integrated measure of a complex series of events including tissue distribution, metabolism and DNA repair. These methods, however, have serious logistic limitations in application to epidemiological studies due to the inability or difficulty in obtaining cell or tissue specimens from appropriate control population groups, i.e. healthy individuals. Poly- and monoclonal antibodies and physicochemical methods are now available to detect various DNA adducts, e.g. DNA alkylation adducts as index of exposure to *N*-nitroso compounds and other alkylating agents, DNA adducts to aflatoxin, benzo[a]pyrene and other polycyclic aromatic hydrocarbons. The method of ^{32}P-postlabelling, developed by Randérath, has also been used to detect non-specific exposures to environmental genotoxic agents, e.g. in non-smokers or foundry workers, through the detection of DNA adducts in lung, bladder, placenta or leukocytes. Some of the applications of this method in humans are summarized in Tables 5.2 and 5.3 (Wogan, 1988).

Detection of biomarkers in blood (molecular dosimetry)
DNA adducts in white blood cells

The measurement of DNA adducts in peripheral lymphocytes, has been used to assess occupational exposure to benzo[a]pyrene in workers in foundries, aluminum manufacturing plants, coke oven workers

Table 5.2. *Detection of aromatic DNA adducts by ^{32}P-postlabelling^a.*

Source of exposure	DNA analyzed	Principal findings	
Cigarette smoke	Placenta	Smokers (16/17)	Major adduct (designated 1) 1.4 per 10^8 nucleotides (postlabelling) 2.0 per 10^6 nucleotides (ELISA)
		Non-smokers (3/14)	Major adduct
Cigarette smoke	Bronchus, larynx	Smokers (2)	Total adducts: 1 per (1.7–2.9×10^7 nucleotides) (0.10–0.18 fmol/μg DNA) Adduct 1: 8–14 % of total
Betel chewing, tobacco chewing, inverted smoking	Oral mucosa	Exposed (59)	Adducts found in 30–95 % (1 per 10^9 nucleotides to 1 per 10^7 nucleotides)
Cigarette smoke	Oral mucosa	Smokers (11/14)	Total adducts: 0.1–210 amol/μg DNA
		Non-smokers (2.8)	Total adducts: 0.4–1.7 amol/μg DNA
Foundry workers	WBC		Total adducts:
		Exposed (10/10)	0.2–11.6 per 10^8 nucleotides
		Controls (5/10)	0.4 per 10^8 nucleotides
Wood smoke	Placenta, WBC		Total adducts:
		Exposed: Placenta (4) WBC (8)	12 per 10^9 nucleotides ND
		Control: Placenta (5) WBC (8)	12 per 10^9 nucleotides ND

^{a} WBC, white blood cells; ND, not determined
(After Wogan, 1988.)

and cigarette smokers. It has also been used to detect DNA adducts of cisplatinum in leukocytes of ovarian cancer patients treated with chemotherapy, and to detect O^6-methylguanine in the leukocytes of subjects at high risk for esophageal cancer. Poly- or monoclonal antibodies can be used to detect the various DNA adducts.

Table 5.3. *Detection of DNA adducts in target tissues.*

DNA adducts analyzed	Source of DNA	Type of assay	Subjects studied		Principal findings
			Type	No	
BPDE[a]	Lung	ELISA	Cancer/non cancer	5/27	$0.14–0.18$ fmol/g DNA
O^6-methyl-guanine	Oesophagus, stomach	RIA	Cancer/non cancer: China: Europe:	27/37 5/12	$25–160$ fmol/g DNA $25–45$ fmol/g DNA
Unknown	Placenta	ELISA	Smokers	16/17	1 per 2.0 per 10^6 nucleotides
		^{32}P-post-labelling	Smokers	16/17	1 per 1.4 per 10^8 nucleotides
Unknown	Bronchus, larynx	Postlabelling	Smokers	2	1 per $1.7–2.9 \times 10^7$ nucleotides
Unknown	Oral mucosa	^{32}P-post-labelling	Smokers	11/14	$0.1–210$ amol/g DNA
			Non-smokers	2/8	$0.4–1.7$ amol/g DNA
Unknown	Oral mucosa	^{32}P-post-labelling	Betel and tobacco chewers	59	1 per 10^9 nucleotides to 1 per 10^7 nucleotides

[a] BPDE = Benzo[a]pyrene-7,8-diol-9,10-epoxide
(After Wogan, 1988.)

Table 5.4. *Indicators of genotoxic exposure: hemoglobin adducts.*

Compound analyzed	Exposure source	Method of analysis[a]	Principal findings	
N-3-(2-Hydroxy-ethyl)histidine	Ethylene oxide (occupational)	GC–MS	Exposed subjects (5) Control subjects (2)	0.5–13.5 nmol/g Hb 0.5 nmol/g Hb
N-3-(2-Hydroxy-ethyl)histidine	Ethylene oxide (occupational)	GC–MS	Exposed subjects (32) Control subjects (31)	2.08 nmol/g Hb 1.59 nmol/g Hb
N-3-(2-Hydroxy-ethyl)histidine	Ethylene oxide (occupational)	Ion exchange +GC–MS	Exposed subjects (7) Contro subjects (3)	0.68–8.0 nmol/g Hb 0.53–1.6 nmol/g Hb
N-(2-Hydroxy-ethyl)valine	Ethylene oxide (occupational)	Edman degradation +GC–MS	Exposed subjects (7) Control subjects (3)	0.02–7.7 nmol/g Hb 0.03–0.93 nmol/g Hb
N-(2-Hydroxy-ethyl)valine	Cigarette smoke	Edman degradation +GC–MS	Smokers (11) Nonsmokers (14)	389 pmol/g Hb 58 pmol/g Hb
4-Amino-biphenyl	Cigarette	GC–MS (NCI)	Smokers (15) Nonsmokers (26)	154 pg/g Hb 28 pg/g Hb

[a] GC–MS, gas chromatography – mass spectrometry
NCI, negative-ion chemical ionization
(After Wogan, 1988.)

Hemoglobin adducts

The use of hemoglobin alkylative products as an index of exposure to genotoxic agents was introduced by Ehrenberg's group in Sweden in 1978. They have been used to monitor occupational exposure to ethylene oxide and to tobacco smoke. Some of the studies using this biomarker are summarized in Table 5.4.

The fact that a good correlation has been observed between levels of hemoglobin adducts and levels of DNA adducts in other tissues indicates the potential value of using the former as a surrogate measure in epidemiologic studies, especially since relatively large amounts of hemoglobin can be easily obtained from individuals. Further, since the life of a hemoglobin adduct is 120 days, they can advantageously be used as indicators of subacute or chronic exposure.

Albumin adducts

Aflatoxin binds poorly to hemoglobin but does bind to plasma albumin forming an aflatoxin–lysine residue. Since the half-life of human albumin is over 120 days, this adduct may be a satisfactory indicator of DNA adducts formed in the liver. Assays to measure aflatoxin–albumin adducts have been developed but they have not yet been applied to large scale epidemiological studies.

Biomarkers excreted in urine (Table 5.5)

Mutagenicity tests using bacteria such as the Ames test measure non-specific exposure to mutagenic agents. Results of such studies when used to monitor occupational exposures have been inconsistent due to the confounding effects of diet and tobacco smoking and also to technological problems (Rannug *et al.*, 1988). When controlled for diet, mutagenic activity in the urine of smokers of black tobacco was higher than that of blond tobacco smokers and showed a clear dose–response relationship (Malaveille *et al.*, 1989).

N-nitrosoproline(NPRO) and other nitrosoamino acids

The urinary excretion of these compounds has been used as an index of endogenous nitrosation. Formation of endogenous *N*-nitroso-compounds (NOC) was assessed by the formation of NPRO in: (i) subjects living in high- and low-incidence areas for stomach cancer in northern Japan and in Poland, (ii) subjects from high- and low-incidence areas for esophageal cancer in the People's Republic of China, (iii) subjects with different habits of betel quid chewing and tobacco use, (iv)

Table 5.5. *Markers of genotoxic exposure: urinary excretions.*

Compound analyzed	Exposure source	Method of analysis[a]	Principal findings[b]	
Nitrosoamino acids	Unknown	GC-TEA	High-risk area (44)	21.2 μg/day
			Low-risk area (40)	5.6 μg/day
N-Nitrosoproline	Cigarette smoke	GC-TEA	Smokers (13)	5.9 μg/day
			Non-smokers (24)	3.6 μg/day
N-Nitrosoproline	Unexposed	GC-MS	Non-smokers (24)	3.3 μg/day
Aflatoxin B_1, Aflatoxin B_1-7-guanine	Diet	IA-HPLC	Exposed subjects (20)	0.1–10 μg/day aflatoxin B_1 equivalent
Aflatoxin B-7-guanine	Diet	HPLC-SSFS	Low/high-risk areas (983)	12% positive
3-Methyladenine	Unexposed	GC-MS (SIM)	Excretion rate (9)	1.5–16.1 μg/day
Thymine glycol, Thymidine glycol	Unexposed	HPLC	Excretion rate (9)	0.39 nmol/kg/day 0.10 nmol/kg/day

[a] GC, gas chromatography; IA, infra-red analysis; TEA, thermal energy analysis; HPLC, high-performance liquid chromatography; MS, mass spectrometry; SSFS, synchronous scanning fluorescence spectrophotometry
[b] Number of subjects, in parentheses
(After Wogan, 1988.)

European patients with urinary bladder infection, (v) subjects infested with liver fluke in Thailand. In all instances, higher exposure to endogenous NOC was found in high-risk subjects, but individual exposure was greatly affected by dietary modifiers or disease state. Vitamin C efficiently lowered the body burden of intragastrically formed NOC (Bartsch *et al.*, 1988b).

Aflatoxin metabolites and adducts

Aflatoxin metabolites and DNA adducts (guanine adducts) have been measured in urine and breast milk specimens from population groups at varying risk for liver cancer (Groopman, 1988; Wild *et al.*, 1988). The major drawback of these urinary assays is that they only measure recent exposure and that they require sophisticated analytical instrumentation (see albumin adducts above). The major advantage of using adducts is that they are more informative than simple measurement of carcinogens or their metabolites in the environment or body fluids because they assess the amount of carcinogen which has interacted with presumed critical macromolecules (DNA, RNA or proteins) in the target tissues or surrogates.

Thioethers

The level of thioethers in urine has been used extensively to monitor human exposure to compounds that conjugate with glutathione such as ethylene oxide and acrylonitrile. Complementary to the non-specific thioether assay, methods to determine specific thioethers have been developed.

3-methyladenine levels in urine are used as an indicator of exposure to methylating or alkylating agents (Shuker & Farmer, 1988). Thymine glycol, thymidine glycol and 8-hydroxyguanine are used as indicators of oxidative DNA damage. Further development and validation of these methods are necessary before they can be applied in large-scale epidemiological studies.

Table 5.5 summarizes results from studies in which urinary excretion of biomarkers were used as indices of a carcinogenic exposure (Wogan, 1988). In addition, levels of other substances such as steroid hormones suspected to be related to specific cancer sites, can be measured in the urine. In interpreting assays based on the level of urinary excretion of various biomarkers it should be noted that a high level in urine does not necessarily reflect a high target organ dose. Thus, the latter may be very low if most of the compound or its metabolites are excreted.

Limitations to use of biomarkers

The extreme sensitivity of the methods used to identify these molecular markers, however, subjects their evaluation to the biostatistical limitations inherent in studying any low level discriminator. In general, it is necessary that exposures be sufficiently high to permit separation from other confounding exposures, or that the techniques are being used to test a specific hypothesis. It may prove difficult to evaluate a single biomarker, such as a DNA adduct, as predicting cancer in the presence of many other adducts of ambient carcinogens of equal plausibility. While DNA adducts are receiving great attention and, although they measure DNA lesions considered important in carcinogenesis, DNA damage reflects only one aspect in a complex process. Thus, while it is possible to measure DNA adducts in cells of individuals exposed to carcinogenic chemicals and therapeutic agents, it is unlikely that they all will be quantitative predictors of cancer risk. Inconsistencies between adduct formation, transformation and cancer induction have also been reported. Accordingly, their use in epidemiological studies is still limited since many are still under development, and others require checking for reproducibility and validity. Furthermore, the difficulties of applying intervention techniques to healthy populations requires careful consideration (Chapter 21).

Development of highly sensitive techniques to measure exposure to agents such as the gene amplification techniques, including the polymerase chain reaction (PCR) test, are of great value provided they are applied with the greatest care to avoid the common problem of contamination.

5.4   The role of oncogenes

Oncogenes are genes which are capable of inducing malignant transformation of cells. They are derived from normal cellular genes (proto-oncogenes) that regulate cell growth and differentiation which are present in all human and animal cells. Structural or functional alterations of these proto-oncogenes have been of great help in the understanding of mechanisms of carcinogenesis. Experimental studies in animals have shown that certain chemical carcinogens are able to activate proto-oncogenes and that there is considerable chemical specificity in this activation. Activation of specific oncogenes may be one of the initiating events in carcinogenesis. The two basic mechanisms of oncogene activation are deregulation and modification of the gene. Deregulation implies that the gene is altered in its expression, usually over-expressed, and it is caused most commonly by chromosomal translocation and gene amplification. Gene modification can be produced by mutation, deletion or chromosomal translocations. Oncogene activation results from changes

Table 5.6. *Some examples of oncogenes found in some human tumors.*
(*a*)

Oncogene	Human malignancy	Mechanism of activation
abl	Leukemias (CML, ALL)	Translocation
erb B	Gliomas, esophageal cancer	Amplification
c-*myc*	Burkitt's lymphoma	Translocation
L-*myc*	Small cell lung cancer (SCLC)	Amplification
N-*myc*	Neuroblastoma, SCLC	Amplification
p53	Multiple tumors, colon	Mutation
H-*ras*	Bladder cancer	Mutation
K-*ras*	Cancer of the colon and pancreas	Mutation
N-*ras*	Leukemia (ALL)	Mutation
trk	Thyroid carcinoma	
erb B-2/*neu*	Cancers of the breast and ovary	Amplification

(*b*)

Suppressor genes	Human malignancy	Mechanism of suppression
RB	Retinoblastoma	Deletion
Wilms	Wilms' tumor, hepatoblastoma, rhabdomyosarcoma	Deletion
Acoustic neuroma	Acoustic neuroma	Deletion

to a single allele of a gene that will act in a dominant fashion. There is another class of cancer-associated genes which appear to require changes in both alleles. They are called tumor suppressor genes on the basis that they inhibit transformation. In this case, deletion or deactivation of a tumor suppressor gene will be one of the initiating events in carcinogenesis. There are many reviews on the role of oncogenes in human cancer (Bos, 1989), and the subject is continually being updated.

To date, about 50 oncogenes have been identified from a variety of animal and human tumors, and the proto-oncogenes of 28 of these have been mapped to specific regions within human chromosomes (Gordon, 1985). Oncogenes have been detected in practically all major human cancers, although the frequency with which they are found varies with the type of tumor and the sensitivity of the assay used to detect the genes. Examples of oncogenes found in human tumors are given in Table 5.6.

The potential implications of oncogene alterations in our understanding of disease susceptibility, etiology, diagnosis, prognosis and therapy have been recently reviewed by Taylor (1989) (Chapter 18). At present oncogenes are used and exploited mainly as diagnostic and prognostic markers. For example, radiolabelled [^{131}I]-antibodies to protein products of c-*myc* have been used to localize small tumors of various types (Chan *et al.*, 1986). Amplification of HER-2/*neu* in breast cancer patients has been found to be a good predictor of overall survival, even after adjusting for other prognostic factors (Slamon *et al.*, 1987). Oncogenes may also serve as indicators of tumor etiology, since chemical carcinogens produce highly specific oncogene alterations associated with tumor production in laboratory animals. However, since their role in the mechanisms of carcinogenesis is not yet fully clarified, their application and use in epidemiological studies in humans cannot be determined with certainty.

5.5   Biomarkers of dietary intake

As discussed in Chapter 12, the human diet contains a large number of macro- and micro-nutrients which are notoriously difficult to measure retrospectively. Several methods have been developed to assess dietary intake. They are based on the recall of recent or past diet with or without models or photographs of portion size or on records of food consumption. However, these methods have serious limitations. Bio-markers of intake of certain nutrients may help in a better assessment of the role of nutritional factors in human cancer. Some of these bio-markers with potential use in epidemiological studies have been recently reviewed (Riboli *et al.*, 1987) and are summarized in Table 5.7. The most widely used marker of protein intake is 24 hours urinary nitrogen. Since it reflects the protein intake in the preceding 24 hours and shows large individual variations, it is of limited value in prospective epidemiological studies unless periodic measurements are made. Urinary excretion of 3-methylhistidine is used as a marker of protein derived from skeletal muscle. Its application to field studies is also limited because it reflects only a recent exposure and shows considerable individual variation. On the other hand, markers of fat intake such as fatty acids in adipose tissue and cell membranes, reflect relatively long-term intakes and may give reliable results from a single measurement. They have, however, some limitations in epidemiology as they require various invasive procedures to obtain samples. Levels of fatty acids in exfoliated cells from the buccal mucosa have been proposed as an alternative method. Due to the high turnover rate of these cells, however, such levels reflect rather recent exposure. While liposoluble vitamins can be stored in tissues, the hydrosoluble vitamins are excreted rapidly. Such properties determine at least partially their value as markers of long- or short-term exposures.

Table 5.7. *Selected biomarkers of diet.*

Nutrient	Biomarker	Nutrient	Biomarker
Protein	24 h urinary nitrogen 24 h 3-methylhistidine	Vit A	retinol, carotenes in plasma
Fat cells, erythrocyte	Fatty acids in adipose membranes, other cell membranes and in plasma lipids	Vit C	Vit C in plasma, tissue, leukocytes or saliva
		Vit B$_2$	Glutathione reductase activity in erythrocytes, urinary loading test
Fiber	Total fiber or fractions in feces		
		Selenium	Levels in plasma, erythrocytes, hair, nails, 24 h urine

The above biomarkers have been used mainly in nutritional and cardiovascular investigations, and their potential application in cancer epidemiological studies is very recent.

5.6   Conclusion

Over the last two decades, a range of laboratory techniques has been developed which can supplement and strengthen epidemiological investigations on cancer (Harris *et al.*, 1987). This promising field, however, is still developing and it is premature to be definitive relative to its full potential in terms of molecular dosimetry, identification of xenobiotic carcinogens, and critical carcinogenic mechanisms.

5.7   References

Bartsch, H., Hemminki, K. & O'Neill, I.K.(eds.) (1988*a*). *Methods for Detecting DNA Damaging Agents in Humans: Applications in Cancer Epidemiology and Prevention*, IARC Scientific Publications No 89. Lyon: International Agency for Research on Cancer.

Bartsch, H., Ohshima, H. & Pignatelli, B. (1988*b*). Inhibitors of endogenous nitrosation. Mechanisms and implications in human cancer prevention. *Mutat. Res.*, **202**, 307–24.

Bos, J.L. (1989). *ras* Oncogenes in human cancer: A review. *Cancer Res.*, **49**, 4682–9.

Chan, S.Y.T., Evan, G.I., Ritson, A. *et al.* (1986). Localization of lung cancer by a radiolabelled monoclonal antibody against the c-*myc* oncogene product. *Br. J. Cancer*, **54**, 761–9.

College of American Pathologists (1979). *Systematized Nomenclature of Medicine*, 2nd edition, Skokie, IL: College of American Pathologists.

Gordon, H. (1985). Oncogenes. *Mayo Clin. Proc.*, **60**, 697–713.

Groopman, J.D. (1988). Do aflatoxin–DNA adducts measurements in humans provide accurate data for cancer risk assessment? In *Methods for Detecting DNA Damaging Agents in Humans: Applications in Cancer Epidemiology and Prevention*, IARC Scientific Publications No 89, ed. H. Bartsch, K. Hemminki, & I.K. O'Neill, pp. 55–62. Lyon: International Agency for Research on Cancer.

Harris, C.C., Weston, A., Willey, J.C., Trivers, G.E. & Mann, D.L. (1987). Biochemical and molecular epidemiology of human cancer: Indicators of carcinogen exposure, DNA damage, and genetic predisposition. *Environ. Health Perspect.*, **75**, 109–19.

Malaveille, C., Vineis, P., Estève, J., Ohshima, H. *et al.* (1989). Levels of mutagens in the urine of smokers of black and blond tobacco correlate with their risk of bladder cancer. *Carcinogenesis*, **10**, 577–89.

Muñoz, N. Hayashi, M. Lu, J.B., Wahrendorf, J., Crespi, M. & Bosch, F.X. (1987). Effect of riboflavin, retinol and zinc on micronuclei of buccal mucosa and of oesophagus: A randomized double-blind intervention study in China. *J. Natl. Cancer Inst.*, **79**, 687–91.

Rannug, A., Olsson, M., Aringer, L. & Brunius, G. (1988). An improved standardized procedure for urine mutagenicity testing. In *Methods for Detecting DNA Damaging Agents in Humans: Applications in Cancer Epidemiology and Prevention*, ed. H. Bartsch, K. Hemminki, and I.K. O'Neill, IARC Scientific Publications No. 89, pp. 396–400. Lyon: International Agency for Research on Cancer.

Riboli, E., Rönnholm, H. & Saracci, R. (1987). Biological markers of diet. *Cancer Surveys*, **6**, 685–718.

Shuker, D.E.G. & Farmer, P.B. (1988). Urinary excretion of 3-methyladenine in humans as a marker of nucleic acid methylation. In *Methods for Detecting DNA Damaging Agents in Humans: Applications in Cancer Epidemiology and Prevention*, IARC Scientific Publications No 89, ed. H. Bartsch, K. Hemminki, & I.K. O'Neill, pp. 92–6. Lyon: International Agency for Research on Cancer.

Slamon, D.J., Clark, G.M, Wong, S.G. *et al.* (1987). Human breast cancer: correlation of relapse and survival with amplification of the HER-2/*neu* oncogene. *Science*, **235**, 177–82.

Taylor, J.A. (1989). Oncogenes and their applications in epidemiologic studies. *Am. J. Epidemiol.*, **130**, 6–13.

Wild, C.P., Chapot, B., Scherer, E., Den Engelse, L. & Montesano, R. (1988). Application of antibody methods to the detection of aflatoxin in human body fluids. In *Methods for Detecting DNA Damaging Agents in Humans: Applications in Cancer Epidemiology and Prevention*, IARC Scientific Publications No. 89, ed. H. Bartsch, K. Hemminki, & I.K. O'Neill, pp. 67–74. Lyon: International Agency for Research on Cancer.

Wogan, G.N. (1988). Detection of DNA damage in studies on cancer etiology and prevention. In *Methods for Detecting DNA Damaging Agents in Humans: Applications in Cancer Epidemiology and Prevention*, IARC Scientific Publications No 89, ed. H. Bartsch, K. Hemminki, & I.K. O'Neill, pp. 32–51. Lyon: International Agency for Research on Cancer.

Wogan, G.N. & Tannenbaum, S.R. (1987). Biological monitoring of environmental toxic chemicals. In *Toxic Chemicals, Health, and the Environment*, ed. L.B. Lave & A.C. Upton, pp. 142–69. Baltimore: Johns Hopkins University Press.

World Health Organization (WHO) (1977). *Manual of the International Statistical Classification of Diseases, Injuries and Causes of Death*, volume I, Tabular List, volume II, Index. Geneva: World Health Organization.

Part II

Causative factors in human cancer

6

The concept of cause: epidemiological considerations

6.1   Nature of carcinogenesis

Clinical cancer reflects the outcome of a multistage process involving a cascade of biochemical and biophysical events which involve the individual cell and its micro-environment (Weinstein *et al.*, 1984; Cline, 1989; Sharp, 1989; Bohr *et al.*, 1989; Weinberg, 1989). Such events include mutation, gene damage and repair, gene insertion, and gene activation and repression as well as epigenetic events such as membrane and receptor changes, and variations in the metabolic and immunologic status of the host. In general, the molecular nature of many such events is not known with certainty, nor whether they are sequential or irreversible. It is generally assumed that some events are limiting steps and are critical or necessary for cancer induction; others may be epiphenomena. Changes in certain oncogenes may be an essential mechanistic step in some tumors, in others they may have relevance as biomarkers of use in diagnosis and prediction. It is accepted that the whole process can be directly or indirectly triggered by one or more exogenous or endogenous, including genetic, factors. These cover a range of stimuli varying from defined complete carcinogens to multiple as yet poorly identified enhancing factors which modulate carcinogenesis. The statement in the IARC monographs that 'cancer can be induced by a range of different mechanisms which cannot as yet be defined or accurately measured' (IARC, 1982) probably still remains true for the majority of tumors.

The objective of this chapter is to review briefly a number of general conceptual issues which are pertinent to any discussion on the causes of human cancer, and which may have impact not only on the design and interpretation of epidemiological studies, but also on developing strategies for prevention and control. Some aspects are further covered in Chapter

17. Reference should also be made to several recent reviews concerning epidemiology and relevant molecular biological data (Harris, 1986; IARC, 1984*a,b*; Seemayer & Cavenee, 1989). No attempt is made to examine carcinogenic mechanisms in depth.

6.2   Major or avoidable causes

A major contribution of epidemiology in cancer prevention and control is evaluation of suspected triggering factors (causal determinants). It is recognized that cancer is unlikely to result from a single exogenous or endogenous factor, or an isolated molecular mutational event, but rather that it is a reflection of an individual's lifetime exposures and reactions to multiple stimuli, including possible polygenic host factors. None the less, from the practical viewpoint, a single identifiable factor(s), irrespective of its nature, may be so important or critical to transformation that in its absence a significant number of cancers at a specific site would not occur.

Such a factor can be regarded as a critical cause or trigger from an operational or public health viewpoint. Such factors have been referred to as 'major causes' (Higginson & Muir, 1979), or 'avoidable causes' (Doll and Peto, 1981). Thus, work-place studies have shown that some human cancers are preventable by the control of exposures to certain chemicals. A high proportion (80–85%) of all lung cancers would not occur in the absence of smoking, whether other carcinogenic or co-carcinogenic stimuli, e.g. asbestos, are present or not. Identification of a cause in this sense does not imply complete knowledge of all the complex events involved, nor even some of the key molecular mechanisms. Accordingly, the belief that effective primary cancer prevention requires the control of all potentially contributing factors and an understanding of basic mechanisms is not sustainable.

In view of our limited knowledge of the complexities of the carcinogenic process, it is undesirable at present to describe any individual mechanistic event or step in transformation – critical or otherwise as a cause. Only if such an event can unequivocally be recognized as an integral part of a triggering factor, would such a usage be appropriate.

6.3   Classification of carcinogens and carcinogenic risk factors

A generally accepted classification of carcinogens and carcinogenic factors based only on objective mechanistic criteria is not yet feasible, and categorization is basically pragmatic and based on inferences from epidemiological and experimental studies (Harris, 1986; Williams & Weisburger, 1986, 1988).

Theoretically, any chemical which could enhance or increase tumor incidence in man or animals could be described as a chemical carcinogen (Higginson, 1987). Such a wide use would make the term meaningless. The following general classification, used by the authors, may prove helpful in interpreting epidemiological studies. The term *carcinogen* is confined to any reasonably definable agent, which appears causally associated with an increase in cancer risk, in animals or humans, i.e. chemical, virus, or cultural risk factor, such as tobacco. In contrast, the term *carcinogenic risk factor* covers a range of determinants such as age at first pregnancy, absence of dietary fiber or excess macronutrients in diet, etc., which are associated with changes in cancer frequency, but which cannot readily be described at present as discrete carcinogens in a physico-chemical sense (Higginson & Muir, 1979).

Genotoxic carcinogenic agents

A discrete chemical, or chemical mixture which is sufficient per se to induce cancer in humans or animals represents the classical type of such agents. Almost all such chemicals act through mechanisms which cause, either directly or following activation, significant damage to cellular genetic material and are positive in short-term genotoxic tests (Williams & Weisburger, 1988; Ashby *et al.*, 1989; Bartsch & Malaveille, 1989). Such compounds can be described as complete carcinogens, initiators or genotoxic carcinogens. Certain physical or biological factors may also fall into this category, e.g. ionizing radiation, or hepatitis B virus (HBV). The term *carcinogen* can readily be applied to this group without caveat since they are distinct determinants and from a pragmatic viewpoint are easily characterized. Many of the chemicals or chemical mixtures in this class, which are believed relevant to humans, have been reviewed in the IARC monograph series (Chapter 7), and are discussed under the individual cancer sites. It should be noted, however, that many chemicals are regarded as precarcinogens and require bioactivation to a reactive molecule by such enzymes as P-450. The induction of such enzymes is moreover, controlled by a wide range of factors such as barbiturates, steroids, smoking, charcoal broiled steaks, etc. (Shimada *et al.*, 1989), thus illustrating the multifactorial nature of the carcinogenic process even for a single defined carcinogen.

Non-genotoxic agents

Numerous factors, both exogenous and endogenous, have been identified which modulate the action of carcinogenesis through a variety of biological and biochemical mechanisms (IARC, 1984*a*), including agents which effect DNA repair (Bohr *et al.*, 1989). Promoters fall into this group. Since in humans the sequence initiator/promoter cannot rigorously be established, the non-specific term cancer 'enhancer' or 'modulator' is probably preferable. Moreover, no mechanism has been demonstrated as common to all the factors which fall into this group, including promoters. Many promoters, however, may show generic properties such as impairing cell to cell communication (Yamasaki, 1989). It is to be noted that the terms 'promoter' and 'enhancer' are used by molecular biologists with a different connotation.

Pragmatically, factors in this group can be subdivided on an *ad hoc* basis according to whether the evidence suggests that their role in cancer induction is predominantly specific and organotrophic or is a general non-specific effect on the carcinogenic process.

Specific enhancing factors
Experimentally, much information has been collected regarding these agents, some of which may be relatively organ specific. This group includes promoters as well as enhancers or co-carcinogens. Such factors may operate epigenetically through a variety of mechanisms, such as peroxisome proliferation, blocking of receptors, or modification of host status, etc. and resultant DNA damage may be secondary. Some viruses might be included in this group. Hepatitis B virus in liver cancer is an example, for although the virus genome may be incorporated into the liver cells, the possible role of a low grade hepatitis rendering the liver cell susceptible to another exogenous agent cannot be excluded.

In referring to these agents the term *carcinogen* is often justified in an *operational* sense since they are definable, often discrete and their action may be critical or necessary for transformation. Such agents, when they are chemical compounds are often described as non-genotoxic carcinogens and their separation from initiating agents is made largely by use of *in vitro* mutagenic tests, such as that of Ames (Ashby *et al.*, 1989). Many accept such tests as indicative of important qualitative differences which affect dose responses, the possibility of a threshold, etc. It may be difficult in an epidemiological study to separate a strong enhancer or promoter acting on an already 'spontaneously' initiated cell (see below) from a complete carcinogen. The possibility of such mechanisms in human cancer has been largely deduced from animal studies, although human examples exist, e.g. conjugated estrogens and endometrial cancer.

Bartsch and Malaveille (1989) have shown that 80–90% of compounds classified by the IARC as Group(s) 1, 2A or 2B (Chapter 7) show genotoxic effects *in vivo* or *in vitro* systems. The proportion of non-genotoxic agents is relatively constant, irrespective of the IARC grouping. The non-genotoxic agents in Group 1 were steroidal compounds. These authors have also suggested that since several non-genotoxic carcinogens operate through competition for specific cellular receptors, e.g. dioxin (TCDD), the number in the universe which could operate by such mechanisms should be limited on evolutionary grounds.

6.4   Carcinogenic risk factors: lifestyle

If the identification of discrete xenobiotic carcinogens presents difficulties for the epidemiologist, such agents are none the less recognizable as foreign to the human organism. Yet current evidence (pp. 497–9) suggests that perhaps one-quarter to one-half of cancers in occidental males and females, respectively, are influenced by natural food constituents and by chemicals usually regarded as normal cell products or metabolites.

The term *carcinogenic risk factor* covers a range of dietary and reproductive factors the nature of which cannot as yet be expressed in defined biophysical or mechanistic terms. To equate this ill-defined and variegated group with defined operational carcinogens would be overly simplistic and confusing, from both a regulatory and scientific viewpoint. None the less serendipitous clinical or systematic observational studies in patients on drug therapy or experimental data may generate useful hypotheses and guidelines as to their nature and possible biochemical mechanisms involved.

Many of the above factors are commonly encompassed in the term lifestyle. Lifestyle has a wide connotation including, on the one hand, such defined entities as smoking and the use of alcoholic beverages, and, on the other hand, the miscellany of risk factors associated with diet and reproductive habits (Chapters 11 and 12).

For many human cancers, such as those related to diet, the data are often inconsistent with exposure to a single causal agent and multiple direct and indirect interacting factors of diverse nature including modulators, enhancers and inhibitors are probably involved (IARC, 1984b; United States Interagency Staff Group on Carcinogens, 1986; Ames *et al.*, 1987). Due to the complexity of the interactions involved it may be difficult to determine the impact of any single component (Higginson, 1985; 1988). For example, there is a close association between high fat diets and meat intake and obesity all of which may be risk factors for breast cancer.

Factors inhibiting carcinogenesis

In considering non-specific stimuli such as lifestyle, most studies tend to concentrate on factors which enhance tumor induction. Many stimuli, varying from specific chemicals such as progesterone, to non-specific dietary changes such as reduced caloric intake, may inhibit tumor induction. Many chemicals of this type occur in foodstuffs (Chapter 12). Such inhibition can be mediated through a range of mechanisms including activating enzymes, tissue differentiators, radical scavengers, anti-oxidants, etc. Thus, anti-oxidants may induce cancer at one dose level but inhibit at another, e.g. butylated hydroxyanisole (BHA). The absence of such inhibitors in an individual's environment could enhance car-cinogenesis and thus be a contributory cause in cancer induction. Thus, 'lack of dairy products' in patients with stomach cancer or green vegetables in esophageal cancer patients, both which relate to inhibition, could be so defined. Unfortunately, epidemiological studies on inhibiting stimuli are limited, despite their potential importance in dietary modulated carcinogenesis (Chapter 12).

6.5   Known and suspected causes
Classification of cancers according to presumed causes

In addition to their use in identifying discrete carcinogenic agents, descriptive and analytical epidemiological studies may provide evidence on the potential impact on the total cancer burden of environmental risk factors including lifestyle. Further, the possible impact of exogenous as compared to hereditary factors may be evaluated. Thus, the observed differences in sex, age, socio-economic and geographical patterns, including changes in risk or migration over time, can provide evidence from which the existence or absence of risk factors may be inferred. Further, correlation of cancer incidence rates with other variables (e.g. population density, air pollutants, etc.) may support or negate etiological hypotheses. Such ecological associations however, may have more than one interpretation and any theory as to cause should be biologically plausible and be consistent with the observed geographical distribution.

Using such data, human cancers can be categorized by potential cause according to the nature of the epidemiological evidence (Wynder & Gori, 1977; Higginson & Muir, 1979; Doll & Peto, 1981).

Tumors of defined etiology

Tumors with recognizable causes are usually of epithelial cell origin, occur in adults and have been defined with reasonable certainty through case-control or cohort methods. The majority are associated with such personal habits as smoking, excess alcoholic beverage consumption, sunbathing, betel quid chewing, or occupational exposures.

Tumors presumed to have a major environmental component

This group comprises cancers, especially of the gastrointestinal and endocrine dependent systems, for which clearly defined external etiological stimuli have not yet been identified, but for which the most rational interpretation of the available data indicates that exogenous environmental factors are directly or indirectly involved. While the evidence for the role of exogenous factors may be strong, the number and complexity of confounding variables may make the identification of individual factors difficult when evaluating the concept of 'lifestyle' or the role of individual dietary components.

Tumors with major genetic, hereditary or ethnic components

A genetic component may be important in the genesis of certain cancers as leading to increased individual susceptibility to cancer (Knudson, 1986) (Chapter 18). Where susceptibility is polygenic, it may be difficult or impossible to identify susceptible individuals in a population.

Tumors not attributable to exogenous factors (spontaneous)

Both in animals and humans, certain cancers occur, especially in childhood (Chapter 58), for which no plausible etiological hypotheses are as yet available and for which the absence of significant geographic or temporal variations suggests that detection of environmental influences are not important. There is experimental evidence that a background level of transformed or initiated cells may exist in tissues, attributable possibly to background radiation, ambient mutagens, latent oncogenic viruses, etc. Such cells do not undergo visible transformation unless randomly stimulated to clonal expansion by an unidentified enhancing or promoting factor or even a further initiation.

Deductions from epidemiological and animal data

Experimental and epidemiological data may provide both direct and indirect evidence in support of plausible hypotheses as to the nature of the trigger (chemical or viral) and possible mechanisms (Day & Brown, 1980). Examples are the role of hepatitis B virus as a co-factor in human liver cancer (Chapter 29), and the promotive effects of estrogen on endometrial carcinogenesis (Chapter 43). Pharmacokinetic and metabolic pathways, of relevance to humans, have been identified, such as increased enzymal carcinogen activation, peroxisomal proliferation in the liver, etc. There is a growing literature on the role of oncogenes and anti-oncogenes and other molecular markers (Cline, 1989; Sharp, 1989). Such data, in addition to explaining variations in species response, may suggest chemopreventive approaches (Berenblum, 1980). Studies in vinyl chloride metabolism in humans and rats have demonstrated metabolic differences which are consistent with the much lower incidence of angiosarcoma in humans following exposure. The formation of an unusual metabolite, believed necessary for cancer induction in one species but not in another may assist in inter-species extrapolation. Thus a specific alpha-globulin formed in male rat kidney tubules due to aliphatic hydrocarbon exposure is believed to be necessary for renal cancer induction in male rats. The protein is not found, however, in female rats, in which these tumors do not occur, nor in humans, suggesting that the latter would not be susceptible to the suspected carcinogen (Chapter 49). In conclusion, the identification of a 'triggering' factor or co-factors may indicate the possibility of prevention either through elimination or control, e.g. beta-naphthylamine in bladder cancer or through vaccination against hepatitis B virus in African liver cancer even if other important influencing factors are present.

Thus, in evaluating the etiology of a specific cancer and advising on preventive strategies, the epidemiologist should consider the nature of the suspected causes or hypotheses on an ad hoc basis and determine whether the data suggest a single predominant major agent or multiple risk factors. These points have been further discussed (Tomatis, 1990).

6.6   Conclusions

Irrespective of the nature of the original carcinogenic stimulus, all tumors basically have a physico-chemical mechanistic base. Thus, the following sections will tend to emphasize defined or discrete chemicals or cultural habits which have been shown to be operational human carcinogens. In contrast, when considering modulating factors, such as diet, evaluation is more difficult as the role of individual components cannot be defined with certainty.

6.7   References

Ames, B.N., Magaw, R. & Gold, L.S. (1987). Ranking possible carcinogenic hazards. *Science*, **236**, 271–80.

Ashby, J., Tennant, R.W., Zeiger, E. & Stasiewicz, S. (1989). Classification according to chemical structure, mutagenicity to salmonella and level of carcinogenicity of a further 42 chemicals tested for carcinogenicity by the US National Toxicology Program. *Mutat. Res.*, **223**, 73–103.

Bartsch, H. & Malaveille, C. (1989). Prevalence of genotoxic chemicals among animal and human carcinogens evaluated in the IARC Monograph series. *Cell Biol. Toxicol.*, **5**, 115–27.

Berenblum, I. (1980). Cancer prevention as a realizable goal. In *Accomplishments in Cancer Research* 1980, ed. J.G. Fortner & J.E. Rhoads, pp. 101–4. Philadelphia: J. B. Lippincott Co.

Bohr, V.A., Evans, M.K. & Fornace, A.J., Jr. (1989). Biology of disease, DNA repair and its pathogenetic implications. *Lab. Invest.*, **61**, 143–61.

Cline, M.J. (1989). Biology of disease. Molelcular diagnosis of human cancer. *Lab. Invest.*, **61**, 368–80.

Day, N.E. & Brown, C.C. (1980). Multistage models and primary prevention of cancer. *J. Natl. Cancer Inst.*, **64**, 977–89.

Doll, R. & Peto, R. (1981). *The Causes of Cancer: Quantitative Estimates of Avoidable Risks of Cancer in the United States Today.* London: Oxford University Press.

Harris, C.C. (ed.) (1986). *Biochemical and Molecular Epidemiology of Cancer.* New York: Alan R. Liss.

Higginson, J. (1985). Cancer risk factors in human studies. *Natl. Cancer Inst. Monogr.*, **67**, 187–92.

Higginson, J. (1987). Everything is a carcinogen? *Reg. Toxicol. and Pharmacol.*, **7**, 89–95.

Higginson, J. (1988). Changing concepts in cancer prevention: Limitations and implications for future research in environmental carcinogenesis. *Cancer Res.*, **48**, 1381–9.

Higginson, J. & Muir, C.S. (1979). Environmental carcinogenesis: Misconceptions and limitations to cancer control. *J. Natl. Cancer Inst.*, **63**, 1291–8.

IARC (1982). *IARC Monographs on the Evaluation of the Carcinogenic Risk of Chemicals to Humans, Chemicals, Industrial Processes and Industries Associated with Cancer in Humans,* IARC Monographs, volumes 1 to 29, IARC Monographs Supplement 4. Lyon: International Agency for Research on Cancer.

IARC (1984a). *Monitoring Human Exposure to Carcinogenic and Mutagenic Agents,* IARC Scientific Publications No. 59, ed. A. Berlin, M. Draper, K. Hemminki & H. Vainio. Lyon: International Agency for Research on Cancer.

IARC (1984b). *Models, Mechanisms and Etiology of Tumour Promotion,* IARC Scientific Publications No. 56, ed. M. Börzsöny, K. Lapis, N.E. Day, & H. Yamasaki. London: Oxford University Press.

Knudson, A.G., Jr. (1986). Genetics of human cancer. *Ann. Rev. Genet.*, **20**, 231–51.

Seemayer, T.A. & Cavenee, W.K. (1989). Biology of disease, molecular mechanisms of oncogenesis. *Lab. Invest.*, **60**, 585–99.

Sharp, P.A. (ed.) (1989). Gene regulation and oncogenes. AACR special conference in cancer research. (Meeting Report). *Cancer Res.*, **49**, 2188–94.

Shimada, T., Iwasaki, M., Martin, M.V. & Guengerich, F.P. (1989). Human liver microsomal cytochrome P-450 enzymes involved in the bioactivation of procarcinogens detected by *umu* gene response in *Salmonella typhimurium* TA 1535/pSK1002. *Cancer Res.*, **49**, 3218–28.

Tomatis, L. (ed.) (1990). *Cancer: Causes, Occurrence and Control,* IARC Scientific Publications No. 100. Lyon: International Agency for Research on Cancer.

United States Interagency Staff Group on Carcinogens. (1986). Chemical carcinogens: A review of the science and its associated principles. *Environ. Health Perspect.*, **67**, 201–82.

Weinstein, I.B., Caggori-Celli, S., Kurschneuer, P., *et al.* (1984). Multistage carcinogenesis involves multiple genes and multiple mechanisms. In *Cancer Cells. The Transformed Phenotype,* pp. 229–37. Cold Spring Harbor, NY: Cold Spring Harbor Laboratory.

Weinberg, R.A. (1989). Oncogenes, antioncogenes, and the molecular bases of multistep carcinogenesis. *Cancer Res.*, **49**, 3713–21.

Williams, G.M. & Weisburger, J.H. (1986). Chemical carcinogens. In *Casarett and Doull's Toxicology. The Basic Science of Poisons,* 3rd edition, ed. C.D. Klassen, M.O. Amdur & J. Doull. New York: Macmillan.

Williams, G.M. & Weisburger, J.H. (1988). Application of a cellular test battery in the decision point approach to carcinogen identification. *Mutat. Res.*, **205**, 79–90.

Wynder, E.L. & Gori, G.B. (1977). Contribution of the environment to cancer incidence: An epidemiologic exercise. *J. Natl. Cancer Inst.*, **58**, 825–32.

Yamasaki, H. (1989). Short-term assays to detect tumor-promoting activity of environmental chemicals. In *Skin Carcinogenesis: Mechanisms and Human Relevance,* pp. 265–79. New York: Alan R. Liss, Inc.

7

Chemical factors

7.1 Background

The discipline of chemical carcinogenesis originated from Pott's observations on soot and scrotal cancer in chimney sweeps. Later, the identification of other occupational cancers in the nineteenth and early twentieth century followed by the isolation of pure chemical carcinogens established chemical carcinogenesis as an important discipline. In view of the importance of chemicals as environmental carcinogens not only in the work-place but also in the ambient environment, the epidemiologist should be also cognizant with recent laboratory developments and their relevance to cancer prevention and control policies. The object of this chapter is to review certain general issues and principles of epidemiological interest.

The universe of chemicals is believed to constitute 9 to 10 million compounds with over 60,000 in general commercial use. However, less than 4000 comprise over 98% of the total production distributed as in Table 7.1 (Blair & Bowman, 1983). It should be noted that the term *new* chemical in commercial practice does not necessarily denote a new molecule of unknown activity or structure but also encompasses minor structural variations, e.g. new salt, or a new mixture of known chemicals.

While chemicals may influence or cause cancer through many different mechanisms, as pointed out in Chapter 6, a 'chemical carcinogen' can be defined adequately for public health purposes.

Chemical carcinogens of concern to humans can occur in association with the work-place, drug therapy, air and water pollution, and contaminants in food and beverages, such as pesticides and herbicides. While many are man-made, it should be noted that the number of carcinogenic chemicals occurring in the natural world may be large, and human exposure considerable (Ames *et al.*, 1987).

Table 7.1. *Worldwide production, in excess of 1 million lb annually, of chemical and related substances.*

Type of substance	Number of chemicals	Production in millions of lb	Proportion of production
Petroleum, primary derivatives	380	2,258,000	55.4
Inorganics	452	503,000	12.4
Metals, refining residues (ferrous)	20	281,000	6.9
Alakanes	21	272,000	6.7
Organics	1,307	246,000	6.0
Polymer and plastics	893	122,000	3.0
Other	18	95,000	2.3
Coal, primary derivatives	30	90,500	2.2
Natural products and derivatives	254	84,200	2.1
Metals, refining residues (non-ferrous)	52	59,700	1.5
Organics, variable composition	287	27,000	0.7
Metals	24	19,600	0.5
Minerals	29	14,300	0.3
Alloys	13	1,600	0.04
Dyes and pigments	15	133	< 0.01
Living organisms	1	1	< 0.01
Total	3,796	4,074,000	100.00

(After Blair and Bowman, 1983.)

7.2 Monographs of the international agency for research on cancer (IARC)

The most useful and easily accessible source of information on the carcinogenic potential of chemicals is the monograph series entitled *Evaluation of Carcinogenic Risks to Humans* published by the International Agency for Research on Cancer. These monographs were originally intended to facilitate the work of scientists, but are now used in many countries by regulators, public health officials and governments, in developing regulatory and cancer control policies.

These monographs summarize and evaluate published data on the carcinogenic impact of minerals and synthetic chemicals in animals and humans. They cover not only individual chemicals and drugs but also occupational and environmental exposures, and some cultural habits such as tobacco and alcoholic beverages which involve exposure to complex chemical mixtures. A few naturally occurring chemicals are also reviewed (IARC, 1987). Each monograph is prepared by a multidisciplinary international panel of experts. The preamble to each monograph describes the organization of the program, the workings of the expert groups and the criteria used. Compounds are selected for consideration based predominantly on some evidence or suspicion of carcinogenicity in animals or humans and evidence of human exposures. Accordingly, the chemicals reviewed cannot be considered as representative of the chemical universe nor does the order of selection necessarily reflect their importance to humans. Tobacco and alcohol, for example, were reviewed relatively late as they had long been regarded as established human carcinogens.

The evaluation and classification of a chemical is based on the *strength of the evidence* that a compound can cause cancer in humans or animals. With rare exceptions, only data published in the peer reviewed literature are considered.

No attempt is made to determine potency, to classify by mechanism, or to measure the level of risk in humans. The term 'carcinogenic risk' in the IARC monographs series refers to the probability that exposure to an agent will lead to cancer in humans, but it is not expressed in numerical terms. At intervals, the evaluation of earlier monographs are summarized and updated in Supplements. References in the text are usually to IARC monograph Supplement 7 (IARC, 1987) which summarizes and brings up to date information on 628 agents (chemicals, groups of chemicals, industrial processes, occupational exposures and cultural habits). The individual monographs are not referenced but can be identified in Supplement 7. Since 1987 a further five monographs have appeared.

The criteria used by the workshops are summarized in Section 7.3. *No recommendation is given for regulation or legislation on the grounds that such decisions must be made by individual governments and/or appropriate international agencies* (IARC, 1987). The IARC monograph series represents the first step in this context by providing an evaluation of the factual data available in literature.

Classification of epidemiological data: strength of evidence

Epidemiological data are evaluated according to the general criteria described in Chapter 5. Chemicals are categorized by the working party as follows according to the strength of epidemiological evidence:

'Sufficient evidence of carcinogenicity

The Working Group considers that a causal relationship has been established between exposure to the agent and human cancer. That is, a positive relationship has been observed between exposure to the agent and cancer in studies in which chance, bias and confounding could be ruled out with reasonable confidence'.

'Limited evidence of carcinogenicity
A positive association has been observed between exposure to the agent and cancer for which a causal interpretation is considered by the Working Group to be credible, but chance, bias or confounding could not be ruled out with reasonable confidence'.

'Inadequate evidence of carcinogenicity
The available studies are of insufficient quality, consistency or statistical power to permit a conclusion regarding the presence or absence of a causal association'.

Comment   The number of cancers in many occupational studies is usually small so that dose response curves may not be meaningful. Good data on past exposures moreover, are rarely available. These deficiencies limit their use in defining those conditions under which a suspected chemical may or may not represent a significant human cancer risk. Correlation data, whether negative or positive, are seldom accepted by the working party, an exception being aflatoxin. The distinction between *limited* and *inadequate* evidence is relative and open to subjective interpretation, especially for some of the earlier evaluations. The term *inadequate* is sometimes incorrectly interpreted by readers as implying that if more data were available, the conclusion would be positive; the negative alternative is ignored.

'Evidence suggesting lack of carcinogenicity
There are several adequate studies covering the full range of doses to which human beings are known to be exposed, which are mutually consistent in not showing a positive association between exposure to the agent and any studied cancer at any observed level of exposure. A conclusion of "evidence suggesting lack of carcinogenicity" is inevitably limited to the cancer sites, circumstances and doses of exposure and length of observation covered by the available studies. In addition, the possibility of a very small risk at the levels of exposure studied can never be excluded'.

Comment   Unfortunately, seldom can these negative criteria be completely met. Published positive studies, moreover, even if inadequate, may receive more attention since even well-designed and conducted

Table 7.2. *Chemicals or occupations recognized as representing a carcinogenic hazard to humans* (*IARC Group 1*).

A. *Ambient exposures* Arsenic and arsenic compounds Erionite **B. *Cultural habits*** Betel quid with tobacco Tobacco products, smokeless Tobacco smoke Ethanol Maté **C. *Dietary contaminants*** Aflatoxins Arsenic and arsenic compounds **D. *Occupational*** Aluminium production 4-Aminobiphenyl Auramine, manufacture of Benzene Benzidine *N,N-Bis*(2-Chloroethyl)-2-naphthylamine (Chlornaphthazine) *Bis* (chloromethyl) ether and chloromethyl methyl ether (technical grade) Boot and shoe manufacture and repair Chromium compounds, hexavalent Coal gasification Coal-tar pitches Coal-tars Coke production Furniture and cabinet-making Hematite mining, underground with exposure to radon Iron and steel founding Isopropyl alcohol manufacture, strong acid process	Magenta, manufacture of Mineral oils, untreated and mildly treated Mustard gas (Sulphur mustard) 2-Naphthylamine Nickel and nickel compounds Rubber industry Shale oils Soots Vinyl chloride **E. *Therapeutic use*** Analgesic mixtures containing phenacetin Azathioprine 1,4-Butanediol dimethane sulphonate (Myleran 1-(2-Chloroethyl)-3-(4-methylcyclohexyl)-1-nitrosourea (Methyl-CCNU) Cyclophosphamide Diethylstilbestrol Melphalan 8-Methoxypsoralen (Methoaxsalen) plus ultraviolet radiation MOPP (combined therapy with nitrogen mustard, vincristine procarbazine and prednisone) and other combined chemotherapy including alkylating agents Estrogen replacement therapy Estrogen, nonsteroidal Estrogens, steroidal Oral contraceptives, combined oral contraceptives, sequential Treosulphan

(After IARC Monographs.)

studies with no significant findings or an inverse response may not be published (Higginson, 1987). Further, a negative study may still be compatible with a degree of risk (Chapter 4). Negative ecological or other circumstantial data are seldom considered, nor are the effects of multiple exposures within a work-place. Studies to evaluate a specific hypothesis receive greater attention.

Table 7.3. *Chemicals recognized as representing a probable carcinogenic hazard to humans (IARC Group 2A).*

Acrylonitrile	5-Methoxypsoralen
Adriamycin	4,4′-Methylene *bis* (2-chloroaniline)
Androgenic (anabolic) steroids	(MOCA)
Benz[*a*]anthracene	*N*-Methyl-*N*′-nitro *N*-nitrosoguanidine
Benzidine-based dyes	(MNNG)
Beryllium and beryllium compounds	Nitrogen mustard
*Bis*chloroethyl nitrosourea (BCNU)	*N*-Nitrosodiethylamine
Cadmium and cadmium compounds	*N*-Nitrosodimethylamine
1-(2-Chloroethyl)-3-cyclohexyl-1-	Phenacetin
nitrosourea (CCNU)	Polychlorinated biphenyls
Cisplatin	Probacarbazine hydrochloride
Creosotes	Propylene oxide
Dibenz[*a, h*]anthracene	Silica, crystalline
Diethyl sulphate	Styrene oxide
Dimethylcarbamoyl chloride	Tris(1-aziridinyl)phosphine
Dimethyl sulphate	sulphine
Epichlorohydrin	(Thiotepa)
Ethylene dibromide	Tris(2,3-dibromopropyl)
Ethylene oxide	phosphate
N-Ethyl-*N*-nitrosourea	Vinyl bromide
Formaldehyde	

(After IARC, 1987.)

Experimental data

Experimental studies are carefully evaluated and classified according to the strength of the evidence establishing the same principles as for epidemiological data based on number of animals, species, adequacy of the study, etc. (IARC, 1987).

7.3   The overall evaluation

Based on the experimental and human data, an overall summary evaluation is then attempted. This is the most important section of the monographs and that to which regulatory bodies pay greatest attention. The following categories are used:

'Group 1 – The agent is carcinogenic to humans – This category is used only when there is sufficient evidence of carcinogenicity in humans (Table 7.2).

Group 2 – This category includes agents for which, at one extreme, the degree of evidence of carcinogenicity in humans is almost sufficient, as well as agents for which, at the other extreme, there are no human data but for which there is experimental evidence of carcinogenicity. Agents are

Table 7.4. *Chemicals or occupations recognized as representing a possible carcinogenic hazard to humans (IARC Group 2B).*

A-a-C (2-Amino-9*H*-pyrideo[2,3-b]indole)
Acetaldehyde
Acetamide
AF-2[2-(2-Furyl)-3-(5-nitro-2-furyl)] acrylamide
para-Aminoazobenzene
ortho-Aminoazotoluene
2-Amino-5-(5-nitro-2-furyl)1,3,4 thiadiazole
Amitrole
ortho-Anisidine
Aramite

Auramine, technical-grade
Azaserine
Benzo[*b*]fluoranthene
Benzo[*j*]fluoranthene
Benzo[*k*]fluoranthene
Benzyl violet 4*B*
Bitumens, extracts of steam-refined and air-refined
Bleanmycins

Bracken fern
1,3-Butadiene
Butylated hydroxyanisole (BHA)

B-Butyrolactone

Carbon-black extracts
Carbon tetrachloride
Carpentry and joinery
Carrageenan, degraded
Chloramphenicol
Chlordecone (Kepone)
a-Chlorinated toluenes
Chloroform
Chlorophenols
Chlorophenoxy herbicides
4-Chloro-*ortho*-phenylenediamine
para-Chloro-*ortho*-toluidine
Citrus Red No. 2
para-Cresidine
Dicarbazine
Daunomycin
DDT
N,N′-Diacetylbenzidine
2,4-Diaminoanisole
4,4′-Diaminodiphenyl ether
2,4-Diaminotoluene
Dibenz[*a, h*]acridine
7H-Dibenzo[*c, g*]carbazole

Dibenzo[*a, e*]pyrene
Dibenzo[*a, h*]pyrene
Dibenzo[*a, i*]pyrene
Dibenzo[*a, l*]pyrene
1,2-Dibromo-3-chloropropane
para-Dichlorobenzene
3,3′-Dichlorobenzidine
3,3′-Dichloro-4,4′-diaminodiphenyl ether
1,2-Dichloroethane
Dichloromethane
1,3-Dichloropropene (tech. grade)
Diepoxybutane
Di[2-ethylhexy)phthalate
1,2-Diethylhydrazine
Diglycidyl resorcinol ether
Dihydrosafrole
3,3′-Dimethoxybenzidine (*ortho*-Diansidine
para-Dimethylaminoazobenzene
trans-2-[(Dimethylamino)-methylimino]-5-[2-(5-nitro-2-furyl)vinyl]1,3,4-oxadiazole
3,3′Dimethylbenzidine(*ortho*-tolidine)
1,1-Dimethylhydrazine
1,2-Dimethylhydrazine
1,4-Dioxane
Ethyl acrylate
Ethylene thiourea
Ethyl methanesulphonate
2-(2-Formylhydrazino)-4-(5-nitro-2-furyl)thiazole
Glu-P-1 (2-Amino-6-methyldipyrido [*1, 2a : 3′,2′-d*]imidazole)
Glu-P-2 (2-Aminodipyrido[*1,2-a : 3′,2′-d*]imidazole)
Glycidaldehyde
Hexachlorobenzene
Hexachlorocyclohexanes
Hexamethylphosphoramide
Hydrazine
Indeno[*1,2,3-cd*]pyrene
IQ (2-Amino-3-methylimidazo [*4,5-f*]quinoline)
Iron–dextran complex
Lasiocarpine
Lead and lead compounds, inorganic
MeA-a-C (2-Amino-3-methyl-9H-pyrido[*2,3-b*]indole)
Medroxyprogesterone acetate

Table 7.4 (*cont.*)

Merphalan	*N*-Nitrosopiperidine
2-Methylaziridine	*N*-Nitrosopyrrolidine
Methylazoxymethanol and its acetate	*N*-Nitrososarcosine
5-Methylchrysene	Oil Orange SS
4,4′-Methylene *bis*(2-methylaniline)	Panfuran S (containing
4,4′-Methylenedianiline	dihydroxymethylfuratrizine)
Methyl methanesulphonate	Phenazopyridine hydrochloride
2-Methyl-1-nitroanthraquinone	Phenobarbitol
(uncertain purity)	Phenoxybenzamine hydrochloride
N-Methyl-*N*-nitrosourethane	Phenytoin
Methylthiouracil	Polybrominated biphenyls
Metronidazole	Ponceau MX
Mirex	Ponceau 3R
Mitomycin C	Potassium bromate
Monocrotaline	Progestins
5-(Morpholinomethyl)-3-[(5-nitro-	1,3-Propane sultone
furfurylidene)amino]-2-	*β*-Propiolactone
oxazolidinone	Propylthiouracil
Nafenopin	Saccharin
Niridazole	Safrole
5-Nitroacenaphthene	Sodium *ortho*-phenylphenate
Nitrofen (technical grade)	Sterigmatocystin
1-[(5-Nitrofurfurylidene)amino-2-	Streptozotocin
imidazolidinone	Styrene
N-[4-(5-Nitro-2-furyl)-2-	Sulfallate
thiazolyl]acetamide	2,3,7,8-Tetrachlorodibenzo-para-
Nitrogen mustard *N*-oxide	(TCDD)
2-Nitropropane	Tetrachloroethylene
N-Nitrosodi-n-butylamine	Thioacetamide
N-Nitrosodiethanolamine	4,4′-Thiodianiline
N-Nitrosodi-n-propylamine	Thiourea
3-(*N*-	Toluene diisocyanates
Nitrosomethylamino)propionitrile	*ortho*-Toluidine
4-(*N*-Nitrosomethylamino)-1-(3-	Toxa (Polychlorinated camphenes)
pyridyl)-1-butanone (NNK)	Trp-P-1 (30Amino-1,4-dimethyl-5H-
N-Nitrosomethylethylamine	pyrido[*4,3-b*]indole)
N-Nitrosomethylvinylamine	Trypan blue
N-Nitrosomorpholine	Uracil mustard
N′-Nitrosonornicotine	Urethane

(After IARC, 1987.)

assigned to 2A (*probably carcinogenic*) or 2B (*possibly carcinogenic*) on the basis of epidemiological, experimental and other relevant data.

Group 2A – The agent is *probably* carcinogenic to humans: (Table 7.3) – This category is used when there is limited evidence of carcinogenicity in humans and sufficient evidence of carcinogenicity in experimental animals. Exceptionally, an agent may be classified into this category solely on the basis of limited evidence of carcinogenicity in humans or of sufficient evidence of carcinogenicity in experimental animals strengthened by supporting evidence from other relevant data.

Group 2B – The agent is *possibly* carcinogenic to humans: (Table 7.4) – This category is generally used for agents for which there is limited evidence in humans in the absence of sufficient evidence in experimental animals. It may also be used when there is inadequate evidence of carcinogenicity in humans or when human data are non-existent but where there is sufficient evidence of carcinogenicity in experimental animals. In some instances, an agent for which there is inadequate evidence or no data in humans but limited evidence of carcinogenicity in experimental animals together with supporting evidence from other relevant data may be placed in this group.

Group 3 – The agent is not classifiable as to its carcinogenicity to humans – Agents are placed in this category when they do not fall into any other group. These are summarized in Supplement 7 (IARC, 1987).

Group 4 – The agent is probably not carcinogenic to humans – This category is used for agents for which there is evidence suggesting lack of carcinogenicity in humans together with evidence suggesting lack of carcinogenicity in experimental animals. In some circumstances, agents for which there is inadequate evidence of or no data on carcinogenicity in humans but evidence suggesting lack of carcinogenicity in experimental animals, consistently and strongly supported by a broad range of other relevant data, may be classified in this group.'

Comment   Tables 7.2 – 7.4 summarize IARC's evaluation of the data according to the above criteria. Group 1 (Table 7.2) represents those compounds, occupations and habits which have been identified conclusively as posing a carcinogenic risk to humans. Such factors have usually been identified in the work-place, where relatively high exposures have occurred or with a drug or cultural habit: adequate epidemiological data are usually available. Unfortunately, for few of these is sufficient information available to permit direct extrapolation to low dose responses.

In Groups 2A and 2B (Table 7.3 and 7.4) considerable weight is given to the animal data so that uncertainties remain as to their relevance in humans. Accordingly, there is a measure of subjectivity especially in relation to the terms '*probable*' and '*possible*'. No attempt is made here to address the impact on humans of the compounds listed in Tables 7.3 and

7.4. Where a compound is considered significant for a specific cancer site, it is reviewed in the appropriate section. For the large number of others of unknown activity in humans, the reader is referred to the original IARC monograph or other relevant IARC publications.

7.4 Evaluation of low level chemical risks – some public health considerations

Epidemiological data and dose extrapolation

General agreement exists regarding the need to control or eliminate unnecessary high exposures to humans by chemicals carcinogenic to animals or man. There is, however, controversy as to the degree of risk to human health which may result from very low exposures to potential carcinogens. Public policy requires that some form of scientific technique or judgmental approach be developed to determine whether the conditions can be defined under which such chemical exposures represent a trivial or, conversely, a significant hazard.

In modern states, with good industrial hygiene most occupational exposures to chemical carcinogens should occur at levels far lower than those at which an adverse effect is likely to be detected and ambient exposures are generally much lower (Hemminki & Vainio, 1984). In such circumstances, epidemiological methods are of little help except in setting the upper bounds of a possible effect (Chapter 4).

When dose–response data are available, it may be possible to extrapolate to low doses. But, there are few human carcinogens for which good data on dose–response relationship exist, with such exceptions as tobacco smoking, and possibly alcohol. However, even in situations involving several doses at high levels, simple linear relationships with dose cannot be assumed. For example, the effects of cigarette smoking in humans are related to the square of the dose and the fourth power of the time. Thus, the relative risk at age 60 for a man smoking 20 cigarettes a day for 20 years is about one order of magnitude less than that of a man smoking 10 cigarettes a day for 40 years. For chemicals, doses are usually limited and target cell exposures not available. Half a dozen cancer cases scattered over several dose levels are usually uninformative. Thus, lack of precision does not permit discrimination between linear and non-linear dose–response relationships or confirmation of the existence of a threshold (Day, 1985). Using data from cancer chemotherapeutic trials may, however allow linear extrapolation with caveats (Kaldor *et al.*, 1988).

An IARC working party concluded (IARC, 1982): 'Quantitative estimation of the risk of human cancer, particularly in man, is a difficult task. Many issues complicate the process. Among them are: the long induction-latent period, typically of many years duration between beginning of exposure and appearance of disease; the possible two-stage process of carcinogenicity; the paucity of epidemiological data on most chemical compounds; the mixed nature of most chemical exposures; and the modification of carcinogenic effects not only by other chemical exposures but also by a variety of life-style factors.'

Long-term and short-term assays for carcinogenesis

This is an immense subject which has recently been reviewed by the IARC (Montesano *et al.*, 1986). This report provides an excellent introduction to general concepts and technical approaches. The object of the various tests developed over the last 50 years has been to provide methods whereby chemicals, mixtures and other agents can be surveyed and tested for carcinogenic properties. Thus, such studies may permit not only the identification of the potential carcinogenic compounds used in a work-place where mixed exposures occur, but also the screening of new chemicals for carcinogenicity prior to their commercialization.

Extrapolation from animals to humans

Since 1970, the total number of chemicals actually demonstrated as carcinogenic to humans has remained relatively constant but the list of known animal carcinogens has grown (IARC, 1987). It is accepted that demonstration of carcinogenic activity in animals can qualitatively predict that a potential carcinogenic risk to humans can exist. Further, where there are data for both humans and animals, there is more concordance than is generally recognized in relation to the target organs affected (Table 7.5) and this fact should not be ignored when considering a potential human hazard. However, the mouse hepatoma may be an exception. None the less, attempts to correlate the carcinogenic potency of a chemical in humans based on animal data are controversial. Further useful new data on dose responses in humans, for comparing with animals, are unlikely to become available for many compounds, as modern public health and industrial hygiene practices should ensure control of high exposures to potential carcinogens in developed countries, with the possible exception of drugs used for fatal diseases.

Most identified human carcinogens are also animal carcinogens, with two possible exceptions: ethanol and arsenic. However, the converse is not necessarily true since no satisfactory human data exist for the majority of the chemicals which are carcinogenic to animals. This may be due to the fact that human exposures are usually so low that the risk lies far below the limit of detection, or that there are species differences in susceptibility. Since World War II, testing of chemicals in animals by governments and

Table 7.5. *Target organs in animals for known or probable human carcinogens.*

Exposure	Target organ[a]	
	Human	Animal
Occupational		
Arsenic and arsenic	Skin lung	Limited evidence
compounds	Liver angiosarcoma	Lung
Coal-tar pitches	Skin, lung, bladder (Gastro-intestinal tract leukemia)	Mouse: skin
Mineral oils, untreated and mildly treated	Skin (respiratory tract, bladder, gastrointestinal tract)	Mouse, rabbit, monkey:
Mustard gas	Lung, larynx, pharynx	Mouse: (lung, local)
2-Naphthylamine	Bladder (liver)	Mouse: liver, lung Rat, hamster, dog, primates: bladder
Nickel and nickel compounds	Nasal sinus, lung (larynx)	Mouse, rat, hamster, rabbit: local Rat: lung
Shale-oils	Skin (colon)	Mouse: lung, local Rabbit: local
Soots and extracts	Skin, lung	Mouse: skin, local Rat: lung
Talc containing asbesti-form fibres	Lung (pleura)	Inadequate evidence
Vinyl chloride	Angiosarcoma, lung	Mouse: angiosarcoma, mammary gland, lung Rat: zymbal gland Hamster: liver, skin, forestomach Rabbit; lung, skin
Environmental and Cultural		
Aflatoxins	Liver (lung)	Mouse: liver, lung Rat: liver, kidney; colon Hamster, primates, ducks, fish: liver
Alcoholic beverages	Oral cavity, pharynx, larynx, esophagus, liver (breast)	Inadequate evidence Primates alone show alcoholic hepatitis
Betel quid with tobacco	Oral cavity, (pharynx larynx, esophagus)	Mouse: (skin, local) Hamster: (forestomach, cheek pouch)
Erionite	Pleura, peritoneum	Mouse, rat: pleura, peritoneum
Hepatitis B virus	Liver	Note similar virus in animals produces HCC
Human T-cell leukemia virus	Leukemia	
Ionizing radiation	Leukemia, skin All organs	All organs
Radon and its decay products	Lung	Rat, dog: lung

Table 7.5 (*cont.*)

| Exposure | Target organ[a] | |
	Human	Animal
Tobacco products, smokeless	Oral cavity (pharynx, esophagus)	On skin, but inadequate evidence
Tobacco smoke	Lung, bladder, oral cavity, larynx, pharynx, esophagus, pancreas renal pelvis (stomach, liver, cervix)	Rat, hamster: respiratory tract
UV radiation	Skin	Rodents: skin
Drugs		
Analgesic mixtures containing phenacetin	Renal pelvis/ureter, bladder	Rat: (kidney, renal pelvis liver)
Azathioprine	Lymphoma, skin, mesenchymal tumors, hepatobiliary system	Mouse: (lymphoma) Rat: (lymphoma, Zymbal gland)
N,N-*Bis*(2-chloroethyl)-2-naphthylamine (Chlornaphazine)	Bladder	Mouse: (lung) Rat: (local) Dogs: Not known
1,4-Butanediol dimethanesulphonate (Myleran)	Leukemia	Mouse: (leukemia, lymphoma, ovary)
Chlorambucil	Leukemia	Mouse: lung (ovary, lymphoma) Rat: lymphoma, leukemia
1-(2-Chloroethy)-3(4-methylcyclohexyl)-1-nitrosourea (Methyl-CCNU)	Leukemia	Rat: (lung)
Cyclophosphamide	Bladder, leukemia	Mouse: leukemia, lung, local, mammary gland Rat: bladder, mammary gland, leukemia
Diethystilboestrol	Cervix/vagina, breast, testis (endometrium)	Mouse: cervix/vagina, uterus, mammary gland, ovary, lymphoma Rat: mammary gland, pituitary Hamster: kidney, cervix/vagina, endometrium
Melphalan	Leukemia	Mouse: lymphosarcoma, lung Rat: peritoneum
8-Methoxypsoralen Methoxcalen) plus UV radiation	Skin	Mouse: skin
MOPP and other combined chemotherapy including alkylating agents	Leukemia	No adequate data
Estrogen replacement therapy	Endometrium, breast	As below, for estrogens, steroidal

Table 7.5 (*cont.*)

	Target organ[a]	
Exposure	Human	Animal
Estrogens, non-steroidal	Cervix/vagina, breast, testis (endometrium)	*for diethylstiboestrol*, see above
		for dienestrol Hamster: kidney
		for hexoestrol Hamster: kidney
		for chlorotriansisene No adequate data
Estrogens, steroidal	Endometrium, breast	*for conjugated estrogens* Hamster: (kidney)
		for oestradiol-17-β and esters Mouse: mammary gland, pituitary, uterus, cervix/vagina, testis, lymphoma, bone Rat: mammary gland, pituitary Hamster: kidney Guinea-pig: uterus
		for oestriol Mouse: (mammary gland) Hamster: (kidney)
		for oestrone Mouse: mammary gland Rat: mammary gland, pituitary, adrenal Hamster: kidney
		for ethinyloestradiol Mouse: Pituitary, mammary gland, uterus, cervix/vagina Rat: liver, pituitary, mammary gland Hamster: kidney
		for mestranol Mouse: pituitary, mammary gland Rat: mammary gland
Oral contraceptives, combined	Liver	Similar to above for progestin and oestrogen combinations
Oral contraceptives, sequential	Endometrium	*for dimethisterone in combination with ethinyloestradiol*
	Leukemia	Inadequate evidence
Treosulfan		No data available

[a] *Suspected target organs in parentheses.*
(*After IARC*, 1987.)

industries has become increasingly systematized. The National Toxicological Program (NTP, 1989) in the United States Program represents the largest of these programs but extensive global testing is also carried out by many other bodies including industry. Unfortunately, only a limited number of chemicals can be tested for logistical reasons including costs which are approximately one million dollars per chemical per single test in two species only. This deficiency has led to a search for alternate methods of testing such as short-term screening tests and increasing emphasis on mechanistic studies at the cellular and molecular level. None the less, animal studies remain the backbone of regulations designed to protect humans against hazardous exposures to known or suspected carcinogens.

Short-term tests

In view of the vast number of man-made chemicals and mixtures developed by industry, as well as natural compounds, short-term tests have been developed to screen out those chemicals most likely to be carcinogenic. These tests employ a range of systems (Montesano *et al.*, 1986). They include bacteria, cultured mammalian cells, yeasts, etc. The best known is that of Ames which depends on a mutated bacteria. *The tests in general do not test for carcinogenicity* per se, *but rather attempt to demonstrate biological effects of possible relevance to carcinogenesis*, such as DNA damage. They are used also to distinguish genotoxic and non-genotoxic chemicals (Chapter 6). Specific tests for the latter group are also being sought.

Quantitative risk assessment (QRA)

Due to the need, especially in the United States, to avoid the appearance of bias in promulgating regulations, considerable emphasis has been placed on quantitative risk assessment (QRA). This approach uses biomathematical modelling to calculate the probable degree of a cancer risk to humans from animal experimentation. Such models are usually based on some form of linear response and contain simplistic inferences and assumptions as to the nature and variety of carcinogenic mechanisms involved. Thus, the choice of model and the many variables and variances involved in the assumptions or mechanisms can modify conclusions by several orders of magnitude. Neither the conclusions and/or assumptions can usually be validated.

There is an extensive literature on the many differing models in use. Existing mathematical models include the probit, one hit, Weibull, logit, gamma multi-hit, Armitage–Doll multistage, and a simplified statisticopharmacokinetic approach. Refinements of these models that consider time-to-tumor response include the Hartley–Sielken model (Hartley & Sielken, 1977), National Center for Toxicological Research linear extrapolation procedure (Farmer *et al.*, 1982), as well as a multistage model (Crump *et al.*, 1981).

The probit, logit, and Weibull models describe the characteristics of the study population in terms of its tolerance to the agent. The proportions of the population having tolerances above or below a certain dosage are thus calculated. The distribution of the logarithm of the tolerances is assumed to be normal in the probit model. Cornfield (1977) suggested that the normal distribution may not provide a reliable description of the distribution at values as low as 1 per million. As dose decreases, the probit curve approaches zero more rapidly than curves generated by other models. For practical purposes, many of the existing mathematical models are indistinguishable from each other in their dose–response curves in the experimental dose range, but diverge at very low doses. Care must be taken to give proper weight to background effects.

In practice, a numerical value of the upper bounds of risk is determined, expressed as the number of cancers estimated likely to occur over a lifetime under certain conditions of exposure. This calculation requires extrapolations downward from usually a very limited set of high dose–responses in laboratory studies. Unfortunately, the experimental data available from animals are usually very restricted being often confined to two or even to one very high dose. Pharmacokinetic data are usually lacking. The estimated risk is then compared with an arbitrary standard of safety, such as 1×10^{-6} or 10^{-5} lifetime risk. The latter are too small to measure in practice. Extrapolation, moreover, may not meet assumptions of linear dose–response at low doses. Thus, the very large animal studies to date, such as the ED_{01} with 2-acetylaminofluorene (NCTR/SOT, 1983) have not clarified the response curve in the low dose region. This experiment was consistent with both a linear response in one site and a threshold in another. Even for ionizing radiation, which has been extensively studied, the dose curve at very low levels still remains uncertain but is generally regarded as quadratic linear (Chapter 12). For logistic and sensitivity reasons more accurate experimental data of the ED_{01} type of experiment are unlikely to be available since they would require enormous numbers of animals.

In conclusion, choice of biomathematical model based on animal data and extrapolation to humans, essentially represents a value judgment. Despite their increasing mathematical sophistication, they are unlikely to contribute more objective measurements of very low carcinogenic risks in humans, despite further knowledge of pharmacokinetics and molecular events, since the probability of individual events, even if presumed critical, cannot easily be verified or extrapolated. On the other hand, such models, especially if using pharmacokinetic data and cell kinetics, may be of value in the management of risk and in determining how molecular mechanisms might work. There is, as yet, insufficient information regarding the predictive value of most biomarkers and cytological abnormalities as indicators of metabolic variation or damage to DNA to justify their use quantitatively as surrogates for a neoplastic end-point. For more detailed discussion on modern developments there are a number of reviews (Moolgavkar, 1986*a,b*; Moolgavkar *et al.*, 1988; Krewski *et al.*, 1989; Paustenbach, 1989).

Comment
For further discussion on low-level exposures, the existence of a threshold and the evaluation of negative studies, see Chapter 4, p. 40. The conclusions of a recent workshop are relevant (Doll & Wald, 1985). This group, after reviewing a number of rodent carcinogens for which there was no convincing evidence of a carcinogenic effect in humans, emphasized the importance of scientific judgment in making appropriate control and managerial decisions (Chapter 4).

When controversy arises in regulatory practice regarding an IARC Monograph evaluation, this does not usually imply criticism of the factual data on carcinogenicity or their evaluation. Rather, it reflects the failure to recognize that use of the findings for regulation by public health and governmental officials is complex and necessitates judgment and consideration of the caveats outlined in the preamble to the IARC Monographs.

7.6   Environmental chemical pollutants in human cancer
In addition to ecological considerations, and point source exposures as in an occupation, the public has become increasingly concerned about cancer risks in the general environment due to chemical pollutants, usually man-made, in food, water and air, etc. Such chemicals are usually present in very small quantities and their impact cannot usually be detected by epidemiological techniques.

General industrialization
Attempts have been made to correlate cancer patterns with general industrial development, on the assumption that such industrialization is a surrogate for increased ambient exposure to chemical

pollutants. In general, no consistent relationship has been found to support a causal association in inter-country comparisons (Higginson, 1979). The differences in cancer patterns between Mormons and non-Mormons in urban Utah cannot be attributed to the effect of industrial pollution *per se*. An association of bladder cancer with the presence of the petrochemical industry in New Jersey was later traced to earlier exposures in a single plant manufacturing 2-naphthylamine. Workers in modern states with largely automated technology should be at lower risk than those in less industrialized countries using older and less controlled techniques.

In conclusion, 'industrialization' cannot be regarded as synonymous with chemical exposure and cannot substitute for the determination of actual exposures.

Air pollution

The impact of air-borne carcinogens in or near the work-place, and due to such cultural habits as smoking is unquestionable. However, the role of ambient pollution is more controversial. The impact of ambient carcinogens, especially polynuclear aromatic hydrocarbons, was studied extensively in the 1940s and the early 1950s, especially in North America. Since the role of cigarette smoking was unknown at that time, these early epidemiological studies were generally unsatisfactory. Today there is a general but not absolute consensus that heavy ambient air pollution may have an impact on smokers but probably not significantly so in non-smokers (Cederlöf *et al.*, 1978).

In recent years, indoor air pollution, notably radon, has received attention: this form of pollution may reach quite high levels within certain houses due to their location, the building material used or increased insulation (Chapter 16).

Water pollution

Attempts to determine the impact of chemicals or cancer patterns, notably halogenated methanes in water sources, have been made mostly through the ecological type of epidemiological studies. Results have been equivocal as confounding variables cannot be eliminated (Grisham, 1986). Differences in bladder cancer incidence between populations exposed to water treated by chlorination as compared to other methods have been reported but are not confirmed (Cantor *et al.*, 1987). No convincing relationship has been shown between nitrates in water and gastrointestinal cancer (Chapter 26), and certain data are strongly against an association.

Food contamination
This is discussed in Chapter 12.

Pesticides and fungicides
In view of their widespread use, and the fact that some are animal carcinogens, these have naturally given rise to public concern. Epidemiological studies on ambient exposures, usually based on temporal or geographical correlations have failed to show an impact. No convincing reports of cancer due to residues of modern pesticides have been produced, although an increased risk for benign developmental hemangiomas have been demonstrated in offsprings of Colombian floriculture workers. Some studies on herbicides have suggested a low-level effect, mainly soft tissue sarcoma and non-Hodgkin's lymphoma but the results remain equivocal (see Chapters 37 and 55).

Contamination and waste disposal
Certain carcinogens such as polycyclic aromatic hydrocarbons are found in soil, for example, beside roads or airport runways, probably originating from exhausts. Arsenic and asbestos are contaminants in the ambient environment following the weathering of certain rocks. In the past, it was common practice to dispose of known, or potential, toxic agents including possible carcinogens, with other waste. It was often widely assumed its levels were below those at which an effect was to be anticipated. Further, it was believed that certain tars, etc. including PAHs tended to bind to soil where they would be metabolized by bacteria and would not significantly migrate to air or underlying aquifers. However, in the 1970s as the ecological damage and the possible cancer risks to health that could result from such deposits became apparent, such wastes became a matter of general public concern. This concern was reinforced by the finding that certain waste sites contained highly toxic chemicals, such as dioxin.

Health studies around deposits are fraught with many uncertainties; since it is not always possible to define the exposed population sufficiently to establish an accurate baseline for the presumed health effect (Chapter 4). To date, no convincing cancer hazard has been demonstrated (Grisham, 1986), but such possibilities, due to past uncontrolled exposures, cannot be excluded in the future. Regulations and new manufacturing processes have now led to a significant change in the situation, so that such sites are being cleaned up and better methods of disposal developed, in some countries. Random associations must be carefully examined and the effects of possible confounding variables such as social class or smoking habits critically assessed.

Evaluation of mixtures

It is recognized that many cancers are multifactorial in origin. A number of studies on humans, usually involving tobacco, have shown a synergistic or multiplicative effect with asbestos, alcohol and radon which may be dependent on the strong promoting effect of tobacco smoking. There is thus natural concern regarding the effects of multiple pollutants at small doses acting concurrently in causing human disease (Vainio *et al.*, 1990).

In the USA, the National Research Council concluded that it has not proved possible to identify the effect of individual pollutants in the diet. *In vivo* and *in vitro* experimental studies on multiple carcinogen exposures show both additive and inhibitory effects. Inconsistencies in the effect of additive doses of a mixture of carcinogens which show a lower impact than anticipated has recently been reported (Takayama *et al.*, 1989; Fears *et al.*, 1989). Most ambient human exposures usually occur outside the range at which a detectable impact is likely to occur. Apart from such situations as smoking with its strong promotional element, most human data are consistent with an additive effect. If an effect of the whole cannot be identified, it is improbable that the effect of the part can be identified or is likely to be a significant risk.

7.7 Naturally occurring chemicals

Ames *et al.* (1987) have emphasized the natural world of plants, including vegetable foods, contains a wide range of both genotoxic and non-genotoxic carcinogens, sometimes in considerable quantities (Table 7.6). By extrapolating potency from rodent data, which is somewhat controversial, he has concluded that man-made carcinogens, chemical pollutants, are relatively unimportant in comparison to natural chemical carcinogens in the ambient environment. This view has been challenged by Perera and Boffetta (1988).

7.8 Conclusion

The further role of industrial chemicals in human cancer is discussed in Chapter 8 and under individual sites. Despite major attempts to identify the impact of very low levels of chemical pollutants, such as pesticides, herbicides, colorants, etc, in the ambient environment, little has been demonstrated. Doll and Peto (1981) attribute < 1–5% of cancers to chemical pollutants but, in no individual case, are the data wholly

Table 7.6. *Estimated daily dose of various chemicals from some environmental sources per 70 kg per person.*

Exposure	Chemical
Environmental pollution	
Tap water, 1 liter	Chloroform, 83 μg (US average)
Well water, 1 liter contaminated (worst well in Silicon Valley)	Trichloroethylene, 2800 μg
Well water, 1 liter contaminated, Woburn	Trichloroethylene, 267 μg
	Chloroform, 12 μg
Swimming pool, 1 h (for child)	Tetrachloroethylene, 21 μg
Conventional home air (14 h/day)	Chloroform, 250 μg (av. pool)
	Formaldehyde, 598 μg
Mobile home air (14 h/day)	Benzene, 155 μg
	Formaldehyde, 2.2 mg
Pesticide and other residues	
Daily intake	PCBs, 0.2 μg (US average)
	DDE-DDT, 2.2 μg (US average)
	Ethylene dibromide, 0.42 μg (US average)
Natural pesiticides and dietary toxins	
Bacon, cooked (100 g)	Dimethylnitrosamine, 0.3 μg
	Diethylnitrosamine, 0.1 μg
Sake (250 ml)	Urethane, 43 μg
Comfrey herb tea, 1 cup	Symphytine, 38 μg (750 μg of pyrrolizidine alkaloids)
Peanut butter (32 g; one sandwich)	Aflatoxin 64 ng (US av., 2 ppb)
Dried squid, broiled in gas oven	Dimethylnitrosamine, 7.9 μg
Brown mustard (5 g)	Allyl isothiocyanate, 4.6 mg
Basil (1 g of dried leaf)	Estragole, 3.8 mg
Mushroom, one raw (15 g) (*Agaricus bisporus*)	Mixture of hydrazines, and so forth
Natural root beer (12 oz 354 ml)	Safrole 6.6 mg (now banned)
Beer, before 1979 (12 oz 354 ml)	Dimethylnitrosamine, 1 μg
Beer (12 oz 354 ml)	Ethyl alcohol, 18 ml
Wine (250 ml)	Ethyl alcohol, 30 ml
Comfrey-pepsin tablets (9 daily)	Comfrey root, 2700 mg
	Symphytine, 1.8 mg
Food additives	
Diet Cola (12 oz 354 ml)	Saccharin, 95 mg
Drugs	
Phenacetin	(avg. dose) 300 mg
Metronidazole	(therapeutic dose) 2000 mg
Isoniazid pill	(prophylactic dose) 300 mg
Phenobarbital	one sleeping pill 60 mg
Clofibrate	(avg. daily dose) 2000 mg
Occupational exposure	
Formaldehyde	Workers' average daily intake 6.1 mg
Ethylene dibromide	Workers' daily intake (high exposure) 150 mg

(After Ames *et al.*, 1987.)

convincing as is indicated by the width of their estimates. The impact of *individual* industrial pollutants in the ambient environment, if present, must, in most cases, be exceedingly small in absolute terms.

7.9   References

Ames, B.N., Magaw, R. & Gold, L.S. (1987). Ranking possible carcinogenic hazards. *Science*, **236**, 271–80.

Blair, E.H. & Bowman, C.M. (1983). Control of existing chemicals. In *TSCA's Impact on Society and Chemical Industry*, ed. G.W. Ingle, ACS Symposium Series, No. 213,.

Cantor, K.P., Hoover, R., Hartge, P., Mason, T.J., Silverman, D.T., Altman, R., Austin, D.F., Child, M.A., Key, C.R., Marrett, L.D., Myers, M.H., Narayana, A.S., Levin, L.I., Sullivan, J.W., Swanson, G.M., Thomas, D.B. & West, D.W. (1987). Bladder cancer, drinking water source, and tap water consumption: A case-control study. *J. Natl. Cancer Inst.*, **79**, 1269–79.

Cederlöf, R., Doll, R., Fowler, B. *et al.* (1978). Air pollution and cancer risk assessment methodology and epidemiological evidence. *Environ. Health Perspect.*, **22**, 1–12.

Cornfield, J.C. (1977). Carcinogenic risk assessment. *Science*, **198**, 693–9.

Crump, K.S., Howe, R.B., Masterman, M.D. & Watson, W.W. (1981). *RANK 81: A Fortran Program for Risk Assessment Using Time-to-Occurrence Dose–Response Data.* Prepared for US Department of Health and Human Services, National Institute of Environmental Health Services. Ruston, LA: K.S. Crump and Co.

Day, N.E. (1985). Statistical considerations. In *Interpretation of Negative Epidemiological Evidence for Carcinogenicity*, ed. N.J. Wald & R. Doll, IARC Scientific Publications No. 65, pp. 13–27. Lyon: International Agency for Research on Cancer.

Doll, R. (1985). Interpretation of negative epidemiological evidence for carcinogenicity. Proceedings of a symposium held in Oxford, 4–6 July, 1983. Purpose of symposium. In *Interpretation of Negative Epidemiological Evidence for Carcinogenicity*, ed. N.J. Wald & R. Doll, IARC Scientific Publications No. 65, pp. 3–10. Lyon: International Agency for Research on Cancer.

Doll, R. & Peto, R. (1981). The causes of cancer: quantitative estimates of avoidable risks of cancer in the United States today. *J. Natl. Cancer Inst.*, **66**, 1191–308.

Doll, R. & Wald, N.J. (eds.). (1985). *Interpretation of Negative Epidemiological Evidence for Carcinogenicity*, IARC Scientific Publications No. 65. Lyon: International Agency for Research on Cancer.

EPA (Environmental Protection Agency) (1986). *Guidelines for Carcinogen Risk Assessment.* September 24, 1986, Part II. Federal Register **51**(185), 33992–4003.

Farmer, J.H., Kodell, R.L. & Gaylor, D.W. (1982). Estimation and extrapolation of tumor probabilities from a mouse bioassay with survival/sacrifice components. *Risk Anal.*, **2**, 27–34.

Fears, T.R., Elashoff, R.M. & Schneiderman, M.A. (1989). The statistical analysis of a carcinogen mixture experiment. III. Carcinogens with different target systems, aflatoxin B_1, *N*-butyl-*N*-(-4-hydroxybutyl)nitrosamine, lead acetate, and thiouracil. *Toxicol. Ind. Health*, **5**, 1–23.

Grisham, J.W. (ed.) (1986). *Health Aspects of the Disposal of Waste Chemicals*, A Report of the Executive Scientific Panel. Oxford: Pergamon Press.

Hartley, H.O. & Sielken, R.L., Jr. (1977). Estimation of 'safe doses' in carcinogenic experiments. *J. Environ. Pathol. Toxicol.*, **1**, 241–78.

Hemminki, K. & Vainio, H. (1984). Human exposure to potentially carcinogenic compounds. In *Monitoring Human Exposure to Carcinogenic and Mutagenic Agents*, IARC Scientific Publications No. 59, pp. 37–45, ed. A. Berlin, M. Draper, K. Hemminki, & H. Vainio. Lyon: International Agency for Research on Cancer.

Higginson, J. (1979). Perspectives and future developments in research on environmental carcinogenesis. In *Carcinogens: Identification and Mechanisms of Action*, ed. A.C. Griffin & C.R. Shaw, pp. 187–208. New York: Raven Press.

Higginson, J. (1987). Publication of 'negative' epidemiological studies. *J. Chron. Dis.*, **40**, 371–2.

IARC (1982). *IARC Monographs on the Evaluation of the Carcinogenic Risk of Chemicals to Humans, Some Industrial Chemicals and Dyestuffs*, volume 29, p. 391. Lyon: International Agency for Research on Cancer.

IARC (1987). *Overall Evaluations of Carcinogenicity: An Updating of IARC Monographs Volumes 1 to 42*, IARC Monographs on the Evaluation of Carcinogenic Risks to Humans, Supplement 7. Lyon: International Agency for Research on Cancer.

Kaldor, J.M., Day, N.E. & Hemminki, K. (1988). Quantifying the carcinogenicity of antineoplastic drugs. *Eur. J. Clin. Oncol.* **24**, 703–11.

Krewski, D., Murdoch, D.J. & Withey, J.R. (1989). Recent developments in carcinogenic risk assessment (with discussion). *Health Physics*, **Supplement 1**, 313–26.

Montesano, R., Bartsch, H., Vainio, H., Wilbourn, J. & Yamasaki, H. (eds.) (1986). *Long-Term and Short-Term Assays for Carcinogens: A Critical Appraisal*, IARC Scientific Publications No. 83. Lyon: International Agency for Research on Cancer.

Moolgavkar, S.H. (1986*a*). Carcinogenesis modeling from molecular biology to epidemiology. *Ann. Rev. Public Health*, **66**, 151–69.

Moolgavkar, S.H. (1986*b*). Hormones and multistage carcinogenesis. *Cancer Surveys*, **5**, 635–48.

Moolgavkar, S.H., Dewanji, A. & Venzon, D.J. (1988). A stochastic two-stage model for cancer risk assessment. I: The hazard function and the probability of tumor. *Risk Anal.*, **8**, 383–92.

NCTR/SOT (National Center for Toxicological Research, Society of Toxicology) (1983). A report on the workshop on biological and statistical implications of the ED_{01} study and related data bases. *Fund. Appl. Toxicol.*, **3**, 129–60.

NTP (National Toxicological Program) (1989). *Fiscal Year 1989 Annual Plan*, NTP-89–167, June 1989 Washington: US Department of Health and Human Services, Public Health Service.

Paustenbach, D.J. (ed.) (1989). *The Risk Assessment of Environmental Hazards, A Textbook of Case Studies*. New York: John Wiley & Sons.

Perera, F. & Boffetta, P. (1988). Perspectives of comparing risks of environmental carcinogens. *J. Natl. Cancer Inst.*, **80**, 1282–93.

Takayama, S., Hasegawa, H. & Ohgaki, H. (1989). Combination effects of forty carcinogens administered at low doses to male rats. *Jpn. J. Cancer Res.*, **80**, 732–6.

UAREP, Universities Associated for Research and Education in Pathology, Inc. (1988). Epidemiology of chronic occupational exposure to formaldehyde: Report of the *ad hoc* panel on health aspects of formaldehyde. *Toxicol. Ind. Health*, **4**, 77–90.

Vainio, H., Sorsa, M. & McMichael, A.J. (eds.) (1990). *Complex Mixtures and Cancer Risk*, IARC Scientific Publications No. 104. Lyon: International Agency for Research on Cancer.

8

Occupational factors

L. SIMONATO
University of Padova

8.1 Introduction

Most known human chemical carcinogens were first identified in the work-place generally due to astute clinical observation following the tradition of Percival Pott (Historical introduction). By the early 1970s, most of the major occupational carcinogenic hazards known today had been recognized (McClure & MacMahon, 1980). Since then, although many industrial processes or compounds have been suspected to carry an elevated cancer risk and extensively studied, rarely has the evidence for humans been sufficient to implicate a previously unknown agent. The burden of occupational cancer in industrial states is generally considered as less than 6% (Wynder & Gori, 1977; Higginson & Muir, 1979; Doll & Peto, 1981) (Conclusions). Smaller estimates have been made in Finland (0.5%) (Hemminki & Vainio, 1984), Japan and other countries.

The period since World War II has seen major improvements in industrial hygienic practices in many countries, so that certain hazardous exposures should have been reduced. Thus, risk estimates made in the late 1970s largely reflect exposures prevalent in earlier decades and may be out of date. None the less, the problem of occupational cancer remains important especially in developing countries which offer a unique opportunity for control and prevention. Methodology and limitations in measuring the burden of occupational cancer are discussed in Banbury Report 9 (Peto & Schneiderman, 1981).

The epidemiological methods used for the detection of occupational carcinogens are in principle the same as for any carcinogenic factor (Chapter 3). For more detailed discussion the reader is referred to the many standard monographs such as that of Rom (1983). The present chapter does not discuss methodology in depth nor individual occupational cancers in extenso, as these latter are mentioned under

Table 8.1. *Agents and industrial processes which have been evaluated by the IARC Monographs Program to be carcinogenic to humans. The information on occupational exposures and target organs has been added by the authors.*

	Main potential occupational source(s) of exposure	Main organ(s) on which a carcinogenic effect has been demonstrated
Aluminium production	n.a.	Lung, bladder
4-Aminobiphenyl	Dye manufacture	Bladder
Arsenic and arsenic compounds	Production and use of arsenical insecticides, mining, copper smelting	Skin, lung, liver
Asbestos	Mining, insulation material production and use, textile, shipbuilding and repairing, brake lining and repair	Lung, pleural and peritoneal mesothelioma
Auramine, manufacture of	n.a.	Bladder
Benzene	Rubber industry, shoe industry, petroleum refining	Leukemia
Benzidine	Dye manufacture	Bladder
Bis(chloromethyl)ether and chloromethyl methyl ether (technical grade)	Production	Lung
Chromium compounds, hexavalent	Chromate pigments production and use, chromium plating, chromium alloy production, stainless steel welding	Lung
Coal-tar pitches, coal-tars, PAHs, bitumens	Coal gasification, coal distillation, coke production	Skin, larynx, lung, oral cavity, bladder
Wood dust	Furniture and cabinet-making	Nose
Hematite mining, underground with exposure to radon	n.a.	Lung
Iron and steel founding	n.a.	Lung
Isopropyl alcohol manufacture (strong-acid process)	n.a.	Nose
Magenta, manufacture of	n.a.	Bladder
Mineral oils (untreated and mildly treated)	Mulespinning, metal machining, jute processing	Skin

Table 8.1 (*cont.*)

	Main potential occupational source(s) of exposure	Main organ(s) on which a carcinogenic effect has been demonstrated
Mustard gas (sulphur mustard)	Production	Lung
2-Naphthylamine	Dye manufacture	Bladder
Nickel and nickel compounds	Nickel refining	Nose, lung
Radon	Mining	Lung
	Rubber industry	Leukemia, bladder
Shale-oils	Shale oil industry	Skin
Soots	Chimney sweep	Skin
Talc containing asbestiform fibers	Production and use	Lung, pleural mesothelioma
Vinyl chloride	Production and polymerization	Liver angiosarcoma

individual sites. There are, however, certain general epidemiological issues of relevance to cancers in the work-place.

8.2 Chemicals in the work-place

The IARC monographs are the major source of information on chemical carcinogens and their possible use. Tables 8.1 to 8.3, have been prepared with some modifications from Supplement 7 of the IARC Monographs (IARC, 1987) and other monographs in this series (Chapter 7). Table 8.1 lists those occupations and industrial chemicals evaluated as having sufficient evidence of presenting a carcinogenic risk to humans. Tables 8.2 and 8.3, respectively, list the substances and industrial processes classified by IARC as probably and possibly carcinogenic to humans. They cover chemicals mainly used in industrial settings, thus entailing a potential occupational exposure. Pharmaceutical chemicals are not included, although production workers, and probably medical and nursing personnel, are potentially exposed. These lists are not exhaustive, nor do the tables imply that a carcinogenic effect has been demonstrated in humans.

8.3 Specific epidemiological considerations

Most cohort studies on industrial populations compare the observed number of cases to the numbers to be expected from a national or regional population of similar age and sex composition over the same time period, and the results are presented as SMRs or SIRs (Chapter 2).

Table 8.2. *Agents and industrial processes which have been evaluated by the IARC Monographs Program to be probably carcinogenic to humans. The information on occupational exposure and target organs has been added by the authors.*

	Main potential occupational source(s) of exposure	Main organ(s) on which a carcinogenic effect has been suggested in humans [a]
Acrylonitrile	Production	Lung
Benzidine-based dyes	Production	Bladder
Beryllium and beryllium compounds	Refining	Lung, experimental evidence only
Cadmium and cadmium compounds	Cadmium smelting, batteries production, electroplating, cadmium alloy production	Lung, prostate, kidney
Creosotes	Application as wood preservative	Skin
Diethyl sulphate	Production	Lung
Dimethylcarbamoyl chloride	Production	Experimental evidence only
Dimethyl sulphate	Production	Lung
Epichlorohydrin	Production	Lung
Ethylene dibromide	Production, use as fumigant and resins solvent	Lymphatic and hematopoietic system
Ethylene oxide	Production, use as fumigant and sterilant	Lymphatic and hematopoietic system
Formaldehyde	Production, manufacture of resins and plastics, use as disinfectant, fumigant and preservative	Nose, nasopharynx
Polychlorinated biphenyls	Production, use in flame retardants, plasticizers, pesticides extenders	Skin (melanoma), liver
Propylene oxide	Production, manufacture of polyurethane resins, use as fumigant and solvent	Experimental evidence only
Silica, crystalline	Mining, tunnelling, quarrying, foundry, pottery	Lung

Table 8.2 (*cont.*)

	Main potential occupational source(s) of exposure	Main organ(s) on which a carcinogenic effect has been suggested in humans [a]
Styrene oxide	Production, use in resins	Experimental evidence only
Tris(2,3-dibromopropyl) phosphate	Production, use in flame retardants for textile and plastics	Experimental evidence only
Vinyl bromide	Production, use in manufacture of copolymers, flame retardants and fumigants	

[a] Target organs are not listed for the experimental situation.

In many countries, the occupation at the time of death is recorded on the death certificate, which makes it possible to calculate a proportionate mortality ratio (PMR). For example, lung cancer is proportionately a less common cause of death among farmers and teachers than among metal workers. Such PMRs can be adjusted for possible differences in age-structure between occupational and comparison groups. They are still however, subject to arithmetic bias, as an unusually high or low frequency of another cancer in the occupational group will influence the proportion of the cancer of interest. None the less, they may give rise to useful hypotheses.

If there is information, notably from a census, on the distribution of occupations in the general population-at-risk, it is also possible to calculate observed and expected numbers and compute a standardized mortality rate (SMR), based on a PMR. Probably the best known of such analyses are those of Occupational Mortality published by the Office of Population Censuses and Survey for Great Britain (1978, 1986) (Table 8.4).

Socio-economic considerations (healthy worker effect)

Differences in cancer patterns may be due to direct hazards in the work-place or indirectly reflect the lifestyle and socio-economic composition of the population from which a work force is recruited. In many countries, these may have considerable impact on cancer variations between different work-places.

Table 8.3. *Some agents and industrial processes which have been evaluated by the IARC Monographs Program to be possibly carcinogenic to humans. The information on occupational exposures and target organs has been added by the authors.*

	Main occupational source(s) of potential exposure (production and usage)	Main organ(s) in humans on which a carcinogenic effect has been demonstrated or suggested[a]
Acetaldehyde	Chemical intermediate, food additive, fruit and fish preservative	Experimental evidence
Acetamide	Solvent, plasticizer and chemical intermediate	Experimental evidence
Acrylamide	Production of polyacrylamides for automobiles, crude oil, processing paper and pulp, mineral and concrete, textiles, cosmetic additives	Experimental evidence
Amitrole	Herbicides	Experimental evidence
Aramite	Pesticides	Experimental evidence
Benzyl violet 4B	Dye manufacture	Experimental evidence
1-3-Butadiene	Styrene-butadiene, rubber	Lymphatic, hematopoietic system
Butylated hydroxyanisole (BHA)	Antioxidant in plastic, rubber; food preservative, petroleum additive	Experimental evidence
beta-Butyrolactone	Chemical intermediate	Experimental evidence
Carbon-black extracts	Pigment, reinforcer in rubber industry	Skin, lung, bladder
Carbon tetrachloride	Production of fluorocarbons, solvents, fumigants, pesticides	Liver

Table 8.3 (*cont.*)

	Main occupational source(s) of potential exposure (production and usage)	Main organ(s) in humans on which a carcinogenic effect has been demonstrated or suggested[a]
Ceramic fibers	Insulation	Experimental evidence
alfa-Chlorinated toluenes	Chemical intermediate, pharmaceutical industry	Lung
Chlorophenols and Chorophenoxy herbicides	Insecticides and herbicides	Soft tissue sarcoma, lymphatic and hematopoietic system
4-Chloro-*ortho*-phenylene-diamine *para*-Chloro-*ortho*-toluidine	Dye intermediate and rubber processing agent	Experimental evidence
Citrus Red No. 2	Dye manufacture	Experimental evidence
para-Cresidine	Dye intermediate	Experimental evidence
DDT	Insecticide	Lung
2,3-Diaminoanisole	Hair dye formulation	Experimental evidence
4,4-Diaminodiphenyl ether	Production of resins	Experimental evidence
2,4-Diaminotoluene	Manufacture of toluene-diiso-cyanates, dyes, hair dye formulation	Experimental evidence
para-Dichlorobenzene	Production of 3,4-dichloroaniline for pesticides, toluene-diisocyanates, solvent	Experimental evidence
3,3′-Dichlorobenzidine	Intermediate in pigment production	Experimental evidence
1,2-Dichloroethane	Intermediate in vinyl chloride production, use as soil fumigant and solvent	Experimental evidence

Table 8.3 (*cont.*)

	Main occupational source(s) of potential exposure (production and usage)	Main organ(s) in humans on which a carcinogenic effect has been demonstrated or suggested[a]
Dichloromethane	Aerosols, paint remover, solvents, fumigants	Experimental evidence
Diepoxybutane	Curing of polymers, treatment of paper and textiles	Experimental evidence
Di(2-ethylhexyl)phthalate	Plasticizer, copolymer resins	Experimental evidence
1,2-Diethylhydrazine	Production	Experimental evidence
Diglycidyl resorcinol ether	Manufacture of epoxy resins	Experimental evidence
Dihydrosafrole	Flavouring agent	Experimental evidence
3,3-Dimethoxybenzidine (*ortho*-Dianisidine)	Intermediate in dye manufacture	Experimental evidence
1,1-Dimethylhydrazine	Propellant, vegetation control, chemical intermediate	Experimental evidence
1,4-Dioxane	Solvent and stabilizer in chlorinated solvents	Experimental evidence
Ethyl acrylate	Acrylic polymers for textile, paper, leather industry	Experimental evidence
Ethylenethiourea	Use in manufacture of neoprene rubber	Experimental evidence
Hexachlorobenzene	Use as fungicide	Experimental evidence
Hexachlorocyclohexanes	Use as pesticide	Lung
Hydrazine	Rocket fuels, herbicides, medicinals	Experimental evidence

Table 8.3 (*cont.*)

	Main occupational source(s) of potential exposure (production and usage)	Main organ(s) in humans on which a carcinogenic effect has been demonstrated or suggested[a]
Lead and lead compounds, inorganic	Lead smelting, battery production, additive for motor fuels, pigment	Lung, digestive system, kidney
Man-made mineral fibers (see Chapter 13)	Insulation	Lung
2-Methylaziridine	Intermediate in surface coating resins, paper treatment, oil additive	Experimental evidence
4,4-Methylenedianiline	Intermediate for diisocyanates in manufacture of polyurethane foams, curing agent	Experimental evidence
Mirex	Insecticide	Experimental evidence
Nitrofen (technical-grade)	Herbicide application	Experimental evidence
Oil Orange SS	Coloring agent in varnishes, oils, fats, waxes	Experimental evidence
Polybrominated biphenyls	Flame retardant	Experimental evidence
Ponceau MX	Dye, textile and leather industry	Experimental evidence
Ponceau 3R	Food colorant	Experimental evidence
Potassium bromate	Baking	Experimental evidence
beta-Propiolactone	Intermediate in production of acrylic acid and esters, sterilization	Experimental evidence

Table 8.3 (*cont.*)

	Main occupational source(s) of potential exposure (production and usage)	Main organ(s) in humans on which a carcinogenic effect has been demonstrated or suggested[a]
Sodium *ortho*-phenylphenate	Fungicide and bacterial agent	Experimental evidence
Styrene	Styrene-butadiene rubber, glass reinforced plastics	Lymphatic and hematopoietic system
2,3,7,8-Tetrachlorodi-benzo-*para*-dioxin (TCDD)	Impurity in production and use of chlorophenols	Soft tissue sarcoma lymphatic and hematopoietic system
Tetrachloroethylene	Dry cleaning, metal degreasing, intermediate in fluorocarbon production	Lymphatic and hematopoietic system, urogenital system
Toluene diisocyanate	Polyurethane foams	Experimental evidence
ortho-Toluidine	Intermediate in dye production	Bladder
Urethane	Chemical intermediate in textile industry	Experimental evidence

[a] Target organs are not listed for the experimental situation.

Table 8.4. *Standardized mortality ratio (SMR) by occupation and cancer site in males aged 15–64[a]*.

Occupation	All sites	Esophagus	Stomach	Large intestine	Lung	Lymphomas
Farmers, foresters, fishermen	92	113	97	120	84	112
Miners and quarrymen	120	83	171	111	116	123
Gas, coke, and chemical workers	118	120	150	108	123	97
Woodworkers	107	127	108	84	113	99
Textile workers	97	91	82	135	104	106
Transport workers	120	128	124	103	128	109
Sales workers	89	90	69	105	85	107
Administrators and managers	74	75	65	99	60	102
Armed forces	161	289	114	146	148	109

[a] The national average is considered to be 100.
(After Office of Population Censuses and Surveys, 1978.)

Traditionally, the healthy worker effect is an important confounding phenomenon which may affect interpretation of occupational studies. Thus chronic diseases in employed populations, e.g. rheumatic heart disease may be reduced because those with lesions predisposing to ill health are weeded out during a pre-employment examination. Since cancer usually cannot be diagnosed in the preclinical phase, for practical purposes, the healthy worker effect related to selection at recruitment is minimal.

A further type of healthy worker effect may, however, operate within modern industries with stable work forces. In addition to better working conditions, such workers often tend to lead healthier lives than the general population including on- and off-the-job behavior such as use of tobacco and alcohol. This is reflected in their health experience (Fox & Adelstein *et al.*, 1978; Logan, 1982). Moreover, differences in cancer rates between salaried and hourly employees can often be attributed to differences in lifestyle rather than specific work-place exposures (O'Berg *et al.*, 1987). In San Francisco, the incidence of cancer in Japanese Americans is approximately half that of black Americans and cancer variations in a work-place could reflect ethnic recruitment patterns. In the UK, the impact of immigrants is now becoming detectable in work-force health data. The potential confounding effects of this phenomenon always must be considered when considering variations between occupations. (Chapter 19).

Latent period

Although most known occupational chemicals have induced cancer in less than 20 years, it is necessary to wait at least two decades after first exposure to a carcinogen in the working environment before excluding an effect. It is considered desirable to extend the surveillance period to include retirees, although, to date, no agent has been identified solely through study of retired individuals. Studies over such long periods also provide valuable information on changing work-place conditions and make a useful contribution to evaluating exposure standards. A current epidemiological study is essentially investigating the effects of conditions of 20 years earlier, and does not necessarily reflect the present situation. As industrial hygiene improves, it is probable that latent periods will be longer as carcinogenic effects may be delayed.

'Negative' studies (See Chapter 4)

Many work-place studies, especially large monitoring and sur-veillance studies, show statistically non-significant associations with elevated (or decreased) cancer mortality or morbidity with relative risks (RR) ranging from 1.3 to 1.5 (as well as less than unity). If large numbers of workers are exposed, such risks could be important: on the other hand, they could be random occurring by chance, or be due to some other variable such as lifestyle. Such findings are often difficult to evaluate and interpret in causal terms even for the studies with adequate statistical power and control for potential confounders. Usually a major limitation is poor characterization of exposure. It is also important to exclude a dilution effect and separate workers according to levels of exposure. Latency must be taken into account particularly when interpreting negative results of epidemiological investigations carried out on sub-stances for which exposures have been relatively recent.

8.4   Measurement of exposures
Job description

A major deficiency in evaluating potential chemical or physical carcinogens in the work-place is lack of good exposure data. For many industrial processes, reliable industrial hygiene measurements did not generally become available before the first half of the 1970s. Even today most data apply to groups rather than individuals. In the past, the most commonly used proxies of exposure, such as job titles and/or duration of employment, have often proved too imprecise for drawing definite conclusions. Thus, job titles such as 'plumber' may have little meaning in the absence of more detailed information on the individual's exact activities and work-place environment. Changing patterns of employment over time as well as evolving methods of manufacture, even in the same industry, may also make accurate assessment of occupational exposures by surrogates extremely difficult. The interplay of cultural, social and behavioral factors can easily confound disease associations in occupational settings, especially in the pre-1960 period. In some countries and employments, the work-force may be unstable and mobile.

None the less, in the absence of better data, occupation must often still be used as an indicator of exposure. Employment records can be obtained from a variety of sources including management and union lists, and industrial hygiene measurements (Olsen & Jensen, 1987; Levine & Eisenbud, 1988). Historical estimates of exposure, moreover, may not correlate well with the findings of more accurate objective measurements at the individual level, although they may be of value at the group level. In recent years, the number of people working in large industrial plants of the traditional smoke-stack industries has been considerably reduced with increased automation. On the other hand, unanticipated health effects may be found not only in a wide variety of small plants, but also in service industries, offices, etc where previously unsuspected exposure to a new or old carcinogenic hazard may unexpectedly surface.

Biomarkers

New approaches to measuring exposures are discussed in Chapters 5 and 18. It is now sometimes possible to measure directly chemicals and their metabolites in biological fluids and tissues, e.g. DNA adducts or indirectly by detection of mutagenic activity in the urine, chromosomal aberrations, sister chromatid exchanges (SCE), etc. While there is often controversy as to the biological significance of biomarkers, they may have their greatest potential in measuring exposures (Chapters 5 and 18). However, the application, on a large scale, of these techniques still has to be explored and evaluated, especially as predictors of cancer.

'Sentinel' cancers

Certain cancers may be so distinctive morphologically that they indicate a specific exposure with a high degree of probability. Such tumors have been described as 'sentinel' cancers, and include pleural mesothelioma (Chapter 35) and angiosarcoma (Chapter 29).

Farmers

In industrial states, rural cancer rates have not been so well documented as urban cancer rates, partly because, in the past, diagnostic facilities have been less satisfactory, exposure histories poor and epidemiological studies conflicting. The cancer experience of farmers is of interest, since they have long been regarded as having unusual cancer experience compared to urban dwellers (Burmeister, 1981; Haenzsel *et al.*, 1956).

Rural areas in the USA have tended to show increased incidence of certain tumors of the lymphoid and hematopoietic systems, including multiple myeloma, as well as prostate and colon, but usually no definite cause has been demonstrated. In recent years, the possible role of pesticides or herbicides has received increased attention. Other studies have shown lower incidence of many cancers (Lyon *et al.*, 1976). These issues are discussed further under individual sites.

8.5   Future developments
Monitoring and surveillance

Future legislative developments may require improved monitoring of work-forces for cancer causing exposures. Large plants possess the necessary resources, and lend themselves most readily to the investigation of potential hazards and the use of modern methods for estimating exposure. It is in these plants that new compounds are most likely to be produced. Such plants can provide extensive data regarding the absence of effects, the impact of mixtures, etc.

In this context, the possibility of utilizing new non-invasive techniques to study bio-markers indicative of exposures may prove useful. The identification of a specific exposure as demonstrated by a bio-marker may indicate the need for prudent control independent of whether an effect on health has been demonstrated.

There is a widespread view that exposure to chemical mixtures may be considerably more hazardous than to individual chemicals. Such assumptions have largely been dependent on the interaction of cigarette smoking with alcoholic beverages, radon and asbestos. It is probable that surveillance carried out in work-places may provide useful data in evaluating the likelihood of a carcinogenic effect following exposure to a range of factors. If no effect is seen following exposure to a chemical mixture, it is unlikely that the impact of an individual component will be greater. Unfortunately, most authors in the past have generally ignored the results of epidemiological studies where exposures to a number of agents and mixtures have occurred although such information might provide a useful contribution to the general data base on hazards in the work place.

In England and Wales, a 1% sample of the 1971 census population has been followed in the National Cancer Registry to assess occupational cancer risk and socio-demographic differences in cancer survival (Office of Population Censuses and Surveys, 1990). In some cases, a sample of the total labor force has been examined (Office of Population Censuses and Surveys, 1990).

Changing employment: industrial and developing countries

Production and use of carcinogens has been, or is, in the process of being regulated in many industrialized countries, although exposure limits and control measures are not always consistent.

In many instances, exposure to carcinogens has been decreasing especially in the last 30 years. This change has sometimes been dramatic, exposure levels in the past being sometimes several orders of magnitude higher. Import or production of compounds has been banned and safer substitutes developed and used. This has been reflected by changes in cancer patterns such as the fall in bladder cancer in the rubber industry. On the other hand, for certain types of carcinogens, e.g. asbestos, the continuous presence of unchanged fibers in the lung extends the risk over a prolonged period.

Whereas industrial hygiene may be adequate in large plants, this may not be true in small plants with few workers in many countries. The latter unfortunately are of inadequate size to permit the ready organization of epidemiological studies. More important, in the USA they are for practical purposes not subject to routine surveillance by regulatory bodies. If a reservoir of occupational cancer due to traditional chemical and physical exposures exists it is most probably in this group.

Since the early 1960s, many developing countries have undergone industrialization but often lack the resources or will to control the import or to regulate the use of harmful substances. Toxic products strictly controlled in an industrialized country may be exported to other countries with less control. Further, industrial processes which have been discontinued or strictly regulated in industrialized countries, may continue or be exported elsewhere. At times this may represent differing national priorities in regard to cost/benefits and perceptions of individual cancer risks. Thus, India continues to produce pipes made of asbestos cement since the alternatives are too costly. Similarly, the manufacture of DDT has been continued in both Africa and Asia as necessary for malarial and parasite control.

Women in the work-place

In all countries, women are entering the work-place in increasing numbers. However, to date, studies have been limited (Bond *et al* 1987).

8.6   Conclusion

There has been tremendous increase of epidemiological studies, especially in the United States, on health problems within the work-place. The majority of studies cover a range of conditions and lack a standardized methodology for measuring exposures and confounding variables. Improved standardization and the subsequent publication of such studies, positive *and* negative, would permit evaluation through meta-analytical techniques (Chapter 4).

8.7   References

Bond, G.G., McLaren, E.A., Cartmill, J.B., Wymer, K.T., Lipps, T.E. & Cook, R.R. (1987). Mortality among female employees of a chemical company. *Am. J. Ind. Med.*, **12**, 563–78.

Burmeister, L.F. (1981). Cancer mortality in Iowa farmers, 1971–78. *J. Natl. Cancer Inst.*, **66**, 461–4.

Doll, R. & Peto, J. (1981). *The Causes of Cancer: Quantitative Estimates of Avoidable Risks of Cancer in the Unites States Today*. Oxford: Oxford University Press.

Fox, A.J. & Adelstein, A.M. (1978). Occupational mortality: work or way of life? *J. Epidemiol. Community Health*, **32**, 73–8.

Haenszel, W., Marcus. S.C. & Zimmerer, E.G. (1956). *Cancer Morbidity in Urban and Rural Iowa*, Public Health Monograph No. 37, Public Health Service Publication No. 426. Washington: US Government Printing Office.

Hemminki, K. & Vainio, H. (1984). Human exposure to potentially carcinogenic compounds. In *Monitoring Human Exposure to Carcinogenic and Mutagenic Agents*, IARC Scientific Publications No. 59, ed. A. Berlin, M. Draper, K. Hemminki & H. Vainio, pp. 37–45. Lyon: International Agency for Research on Cancer.

Higginson, J. & Muir, C.S. (1979). Environmental carcinogenesis: misconceptions and limitations to cancer control. *J. Natl. Cancer Inst.*, **63**, 1290–8.

IARC (1987). *IARC Monographs on the evaluation of carcinogenic risks to humans, Suppl 7. Overall Evaluation of Carcinogenicity: An Updating of IARC Monographs, Volumes 1–42.* Lyon: International Agency for Research on Cancer.

Levine, R.J. & Eisenbud, M. (1988). Have we overlooked important cohorts for follow-up studies?: Report of the chemical industry Institute of Toxicology conference of World War II-era industrial health specialists. *J. Occup. Med.*, **30**, 655–60.

Logan, W.P.D. (1982). *Cancer Mortality by Occupation and Social Class 1851–1971*, IARC Scientific Publications No. 36, Studies on Medical and Population Subjects No. 44. Lyon: International Agency for Research on Cancer. London: Her Majesty's Stationery Office.

Lyon, J.L., Klauber, M.R., Gardner, J.W. & Smart, C.R. (1976). Cancer in Utah – risk by religion and place of residence. *Am. J. Epidemiol.*, **104**, 343.

McClure, K.M. & MacMahon, B. (1980). An epidemiologic perspective of environmental carcinogenesis. *Epidemiol. Rev.*, **2**, 19–48.

O'Berg, M.T., Burke, C.A., Chen, J.L., Walrath, J., Pell, S. & Gallie C.R. (1987). Cancer incidence and mortality in the Du Pont Company: An update. *J. Occup. Med.*, **29**, 245–52.

Office of Population Censuses and Surveys (1978). *Occupational Mortality*, The Registrar General's decennial supplement for England and Wales, 1970–72, Series DS no. 1. London: Her Majesty's Stationery Office.

Office of Population Censuses and Surveys (1986). *Occupational Mortality*, The Registrar General's decennial supplement for Great Britain, 1979–80, 1982–3, Series DS no. 6, Part I, Commentary. London: Her Majesty's Stationery Office.

Office of Population Censuses and Surveys (1990). *Longitudinal Study. Socio-demographic Differences in Cancer Survival*, 1971–1983 England and Wales, ed. E. Kogevinas, Series LS no. 5. London: Her Majesty's Stationery Office.

Olsen, J.H. & Jensen, O.M. (1987). Occupation and risk of cancer in Denmark. An analysis of 93,810 cancer cases, 1970–1979. *Scand. J. Work Environ. Health*, **13**, suppl., 1–91.

Peto, R. & Schneiderman, M. (eds.) (1981). *Quantification of Occupational Cancer*, Banbury Report 9. Cold Spring Harbor, NY: Cold Spring Harbor Laboratory.

Rom, W.N. (ed.) (1983). *Environmental and Occupational Medicine*. Boston: Little, Brown and Company.

Wynder, E.L. & Gori, G.B. (1977). Contribution of the environment to cancer incidence: an epidemiologic exercise. *JNCI*, **58**, 825–32.

9

Cultural factors: tobacco

9.1   Introduction

Tobacco, particularly cigarette smoking, accounts for more cancer deaths than all other known factors. Cancers caused by smoking include those of the lung, oral cavity, pharynx, larynx, esophagus, urinary bladder, renal pelvis and pancreas (IARC, 1986). The most important of these is lung cancer. Whether any excess cancers of the stomach, liver, kidney and cervix are attributable to smoking is still uncertain. As the cigarette habit expands, especially in developing countries, tobacco-associated cancer deaths are increasing. Consumption of smokeless tobacco is also growing in several parts of the world, often on the assumption that it is not dangerous. Several studies suggest that side-stream tobacco smoke, which exposes bystanders to other people's tobacco smoke (passive smoking) may constitute a cancer risk (IARC, 1986; O'Neill et al., 1987).

The literature on tobacco cancer issues has been extensively reviewed (IARC, 1985; 1986; 1987; Zaridze & Peto, 1986; O'Neill et al., 1987). The object of the present chapter is to provide a brief introduction to certain general issues, the role of tobacco usage being described in more detail under specific cancer sites.

9.2   History

Although tobacco smoking was quickly regarded as a vice following its introduction in Europe, the carcinogenic properties of tobacco tar were first demonstrated experimentally by Roffo in the late 1920s. However, it was not until the early 1940s that epidemiological evidence appeared from Germany (Müller, 1939) indicating that smoking was a lung carcinogen. Later, following the work of Wynder and Graham (1950) in the US, and Doll and Hill (1950) in the UK, a large number of studies were undertaken which confirmed the causal relationship, not only with lung but which also indicated that other sites could also be affected (IARC, 1986). There was, however, initial resistance in accepting the carcinogenic role of cigarette smoking. First, the habit did not become widespread until after World War I and the long latent period between starting smoking and lung cancer development meant that the lung cancer epidemic was not recognized until the 1950s. Further, in the earlier period, pathologists frequently misdiagnosed lung tumors which were considered rare (Willis, 1948). An important factor was the unwillingness of many experimentally oriented scientists to accept a pleasurable habit as dangerous and to recognize the strength and relevance of epidemiological studies which they tended to disparage. At the Oxford meeting in 1950 (Historical Introduction), the association was doubted by such an astute observer as Clemmesen, who had found no increase in Denmark despite its excellent cancer registry. As further studies appeared and it was realized that the induction period could be over 20 years, the discrepancy between contemporaneous tobacco consumption figures and cancer rates became explicable.

It was not, however, until the report of the Royal College of Physicians in the UK (1962) and later, that of the Surgeon General in the US (1964), that the causal role of tobacco was fully accepted and the issue of tobacco cancer became of concern to public health and legislative bodies. None the less, tobacco sales continued to rise and governments refused to increase taxes. The tobacco industry remained antagonistic, dismissing the epidemiological data as being 'only statistical', and continued advertising in the media, thus succeeding in maintaining doubts among the public regarding the causal association. In the 1960s, the industry began to introduce filter or low-tar cigarettes. Such cigarettes became popular among the general public, who clearly regarded them as less hazardous, although the term 'safer' was never used by the industry which has continued to maintain that cigarettes were not dangerous.

Later, as concern regarding environmental contamination by chemicals increased, there was a tendency to try and transfer blame for the lung cancer increase to air pollution, although the problem had been extensively examined in the 1940s and 1950s. As recently as 1989, a prominent newspaper reported inaccurately that the Environmental Protection Agency (EPA) regarded radon exposure as the number one cause of lung cancer.

Production and use

Tobacco for smoking comes in several forms (IARC, 1986), of which the following are the most important:

(a) Cigarettes, which are very commonly used in Europe and North America, and increasingly elsewhere.

(b) Cigars, all of which are made from air-cured and fermented tobacco, and, while used all over the world, are in decline in many American and European countries. On occasion, as in Thailand, additives may be incorporated.

(c) Pipe tobacco.

(d) Bidi, used extensively in India, contains a relatively small amount of locally grown tobacco, usually sun-dried. The tobacco is usually rolled in the leaf of the temburni tree and sometimes in tobacco leaves. Size may vary considerably. They produce a smaller volume of smoke than cigarettes.

(e) Kreteks are cigarettes that are widely manufactured in Indonesia. 'Stick bruise' is the cigarette grown in Papua, New Guinea and leads to a long large cigarette known as a stick.

(f) Reverse smoking, i.e. With the glowing end of a cigarette inside the mouth results in cancer of the hard palate in parts of India, Venezuela and Sardinia.

There are a variety of other home-made smoking materials prepared from home-grown tobacco in China, Zambia, Pakistan, etc. which have their own characteristics and names and will not be itemized here. As a generalization, any smoke from tobacco-containing products increases the risk of malignancy. The methods of harvesting and curing various types of tobacco differ radically: there is both flue-cured tobacco where individual leaves are cut as they ripen, and air-cured tobacco which is used for cigar filler. In flue-curing, tobacco is dried entirely by artificial heat in such a way to prevent smoke from coming into contact with the leaf; in air-curing, little or no artificial heat is applied. At present, China, the USA, India and Brazil are the leading producers.

Blond and dark tobacco are typically used in Europe and Latin America respectively and appear different in their impact on human cancer (Chapter 33).

Smoking and public health considerations

Although cigarette manufacture began in the mid-nineteenth century, e.g. papirossi in Russia, it was only with their mass production prior to World War I that the habit expanded enormously. Free distribution of cigarettes to soldiers during World War I introduced many to smoking.

The causal association of cigarette smoking with lung cancer was the first example of the power of modern epidemiology to identify a cause of cancer involving the general population, despite the long latent period. Further, it has been a unique example in illustrating the success of public health intervention outside the work-place in preventing the disease.

Estimates of tobacco smoking in different countries generally reveal rising consumption in most countries from the 1920s to the 1960s (IARC, 1986). Thus, from 1923 there was approximately a six-fold increase in the number of cigarettes consumed per adult in Australia and a five-fold increase in Austria. Overall figures, however, disguise very significant changes that have occurred in many countries in recent years. Thus today, the above figures require modification as there have been changes in the sex ratios of smokers. Females have increased smoking, whereas the prevalence has decreased in many groups of males. Further, there are marked age, class and socio-economic differences in the use and discontinuation of the habit. The use of filtered cigarettes has widely increased in many countries, yet those with high-tar yields of 35 to 55 mg per cigarette remain on the market especially in third world countries.

In the United States and the United Kingdom, cigarettes have a greater effect than pipe or cigar tobacco possibly because inhalation of pipe or cigar smoke is less pleasant. However, those who inhale significantly from cigar tobacco have higher lung cancer rates than cigarette smokers.

Active agents in tobacco smoking

Cigarette smoke is a highly complex mixture of chemicals, over 3000 having been identified. Most studies have concentrated on tar and nicotine yields. Generally, changes in cigarette design since 1955 have been reflected in a decline of average tar and nicotine levels. Thus, in the US, as in the UK, the average tar yield has fallen from just under 40 mg per cigarette to about 13 mg of tar.

This chemical complexity has made it difficult to identify any individual agent as the predominant carcinogenic factor. However, considerable progress has been made in identifying the fractions that are most likely to contain the active carcinogens relevant to humans.

An enormous mass of data has now been collected on the chemical compounds present in tobacco (Table 9.1), and the effects of tobacco smoke and tobacco tar on experimental animals (IARC, 1986; O'Neill *et al.*, 1987; Hecht & Hoffman, 1989). Despite difficulties in reproducing

Table 9.1. *Biologically active agents in mainstream smoke*[a]

Smoke constituent	Conc./cigarette	Biological effect[b]
Total particulate matter	15–40 mg	T, HC
Carbon monoxide	10–23 mg	T
Nicotine	1.0–2.5 mg	T
Acetaldehyde	0.5–1.2 mg	CT
Acetone	100–250 μg	CT
NO_x	50–600 μg	T
Formic acid	80–600 μg	CT
Hydrogen cyanide	400–500 μg	CT, T
Catechol	140–500 μg	CoC
Ammonia	50–130 μg	T
Benzene	20–50 μg	HC
Acrolein	50–100 μg	CT
Acrylonitrile	3.5–15.0 μg	C
Phenol	60–140 μg	TP
Formaldehyde	5–100 μg	C
Carbazole	1 μg	C?
2-Nitropropane	0.2–2.2 μg	C
N'-Nitrosonornicotine	120–3700 ng	C
4-(Methylnitrosamino)1-(3-pyridyl)-1-butanone	120–950 ng	C
N'-Nitrosonabasine	120 ng	C?
N-Nitrosodiethanolamine	0–40 ng	C
N-Nitrosophyrrolidine	2–110 ng	C
N-Nitrosodimethylamine	2–180 ng	C
N-Nitrosomethylethylamine	0.1–40 ng	C
N-Nitrosodiethylamine	0.1–28 ng	C
N-Nitrosodi-n-propylamine	0–1 ng	C
N-Nitrosodi-n-butylamine	0–3 ng	C
N-Nitrosopiperidine	0–9 ng	C
N-Nitrosopyrrolidine	2–42 ng	C
Hydrazine	24–43 ng	C
Urethane	20–38 ng	C
Vinyl chloride	1.3–16 ng	HC
Benz[*a*]anthracene	40–50 ng	C
Benzo[*a*]pyrene	10–50 ng	C
5-Methylchrysene	0.6 ng	C
Dibenz[*a,j*]acridine	3–10 ng	C
2-Naphthylamine	4.3–27 ng	HC
4-Aminobiphenyl	2.4–4.6 ng	HC
2-Toluidine	30–160 ng	C
Polonium-210	0.03–1.0 pCi	

[a] Quantitative data refer to non-filter cigarettes.
[b] Abbreviations: T, toxic-agent; HC, human carcinogen; CT, ciliatoxic agent; CoC, co-carcinogen; TP, tumor promoter; C, animal carcinogen.
(After Hoffmann and Wynder, 1986.)

human exposure, considerable data has been obtained on the carcino-genicity of whole smoke in its gaseous phase. Tumors have been produced in a range of animals either through inhalation or by direct painting of cigarette smoke condensate. Tobacco smoke has shown both initiating and promoting activities which are consistent with the epidemiological studies.

Measuring exposure

Early studies relating to lung cancer were based on patient recall of smoking habits. This proved more than adequate in identifying the impact. However, where low levels of exposure, as in passive smoking, are involved, other techniques must be used. Exposure to tobacco smoke can be determined by measuring chemical or biological markers of tobacco smoke constituents or by measuring intake indirectly from butts or puffing patterns. At present, the only acceptable biochemical markers that can distinguish passively exposed non-smokers from non-exposed individuals are measurements of nicotine in urine and saliva and cotinine in urine, saliva and plasma (Chapter 5). There is some evidence that the prevalence of chromosomal aberrations in the blood cells of smokers is a function of the number and the tar yield of cigarettes smoked.

Individual susceptibility

Approximately 80% of the tar inhaled from mainstream cigarettes is deposited in the respiratory tract, the majority in the tracheo-bronchial region. However, there is wide individual variation in the amount of tar deposited dependent on pattern of smoke inhalation and exhalation. Studies of host factors that influence susceptibility show that smokers with lung cancer are of the extensive debrisoquine metabolizer phenotype and also have high levels of aryl-hydrocarbon hydroxylase (AHH) (Chapter 17). However, the impact of such genetically determined differences in lung and bladder cancer as well as other sites has not been fully established.

Interaction with other factors

In evaluating cancer and its relation to tobacco, the importance of mixed exposures should be taken into consideration. Thus, both smoking and alcohol are causes of cancer of the tongue, mouth, pharynx, larynx and cancer of the esophagus. Both act independently but are partly synergistic. Attribution of risk is complicated since many smokers tend also to consume excess alcohol.

There appears to be a definitive synergistic impact of radon and asbestos (Chapter 5).

In contrast, it has also been suggested that smoking may indirectly reduce the incidence of some hormone-dependent cancers, notably of the endometrium, by reducing blood estrogens at menopause, but the 'gain', if any, is trivial compared to the increased risk of lung cancer.

Influence of duration of dose and cessation of smoking

Such relationships have been examined in depth (Peto, 1986). Duration of use is an important consideration when correlating trends in national cigarette consumption, tar per cigarette and cancer incidence in different cultures and at various time periods. In brief, duration of exposure is of greater importance than dose.

If smoking ceases, the annual excess risk remains roughly constant thereafter. This implies that if the annual excess risk after 30 years is about 0.1%, then this annual excess risk may persist indefinitely. This process is not reversed but the risk remains markedly reduced as compared to that of continued smoking. As a practical public health policy, cessation of smoking means that individuals who stop smoking before developing cancer avoid much of the risk.

Cohort effects

As smoking habits among different age-groups vary, reflecting variations in the proportion of persons born at different times who took up the habits, birth cohort analysis of lung cancer incidence and mortality has provided useful information. The original studies by Clemmensen in Denmark clearly identified the impact of cigarette smoking in younger individuals and its impact on cancer induction (IARC, 1986).

Low tar cigarettes

As noted above, substantial reductions in cigarette tar yield have occurred in many countries in recent years due to a combination of public pressure and regulation.

The IARC (1986) working party concluded that:

'(1) Although smokers of "low tar" cigarettes tend to compensate for lower yields of nicotine and perhaps other smoke components, chiefly by changing the manner of smoking, they do not in general compensate fully for lower tar yields.'

'(2) Case-control and cohort studies suggest that prolonged use of non-filter and "high-tar" cigarettes is associated with greater lung cancer risks than prolonged use of filter and "low-tar" cigarettes.'

'(3) In a few countries, in which smoking had been established for many years, a substantial reduction in mortality from lung cancer has been observed in young and middle-aged men, which is greatest in the youngest age groups. This has occurred at a time when the number of cigarettes smoked by young men in these countries has remained approximately constant. No substantial cause (or cofactor) has so far been identified that offers a plausible explanation for the observed magnitude of the reduction of risk for lung cancer, other than changes in cigarette design which include reduction in tar content.'

Passive smoking

In recent years there has been growing concern regarding the dangers of passive smoking and this is discussed under lung (Chapter 34).

Other cancers have been attributed to passive smoking, including the nasal cavity, brain and a number of other sites. In general, findings are difficult to interpret, especially as a very strong association has not been found in smokers (O'Neill *et al.*, 1987). A limited number of studies have found no clear evidence for an association of cancer in children with parental smoking.

Smoking in developing countries

In view of the different times at which tobacco entered the market, there are significant differences in the present distribution of lung cancer and the prevalence of the habit. Although tobacco consumption has fallen by about 1% per annum in developed countries, it is increasing by 1 to 2% in the developing world. It is inevitable that there will be an enormous impact of smoking in third world countries in future decades which is not reflected in existing cancer rates.

9.3 'Smokeless' tobacco

Tobacco can be taken as snuff (both inhaled and chewed), chewed by itself or with a variety of other ingredients, the best known of which is the betel quid. Tobacco in virtually all of these forms is carcinogenic (Chapters 23, 32 and 33) (Table 9.2).

Snuff inhaled

The snuffs currently used for inhalation in Europe and North America, denoted as dry (Scotch) snuff, comprise powdered tobacco and a variety of additives which blenders keep secret.

Hill in 1761 ascribed nasal cancer to heavy snuff inhalation. Brinton *et al.* (1984) in a case-control study found an increased relative risk (RR) of

Table 9.2. *Relative risk (RR) for cancers of oral cavity and pharynx associated with use of snuff and smoking by 196 white women in North Carolina.*

| | | Numbers | |
	RR	Cases	Controls
Snuff only	4.2	79	80
Smoking only	2.9	70	101
Snuff and smoking	3.3	11	14
Neither habit	1.0	36	153

(After Winn *et al.*, 1981.)

3.1 for adenocarcinoma of the nasal cavity and sinuses and of 1.9 for squamous cell carcinoma in snuff users in the USA, but the snuff was 'dipped' (see below) rather than inhaled.

In South Africa, the snuffs used by the Bantu comprise tobacco leaves admixed with the ash of aloes (Liliaceae family), oil, lemon juice and variety of herbs. Keen *et al.*, (1955) obtained a history of prolonged and heavy use of these snuffs in 80% of patients with cancer of the maxillary sinus compared to 34% in persons with other sites of cancer.

Snuff 'dipped'

Snuff 'dipping' is the name given in the Southern USA to the placing of snuff between cheek and gum. The highly alkaline 'wet' snuff so deposited is chewed or sucked. Winn *et al.* (1981) found that females in North Carolina with cancers of tongue, gum, floor of mouth, other mouth, oropharynx, hypopharynx showed considerable excess of risk for snuff dippers (Table 9.2).

Investigations on an unexpectedly high level of oral cancer in females in several southern and eastern states (Mason *et al.*, 1975), showed that many women in the textile industry took snuff as smoking was forbidden.

Chewing tobacco

Tobacco, whether cut from a roll or plug, twist, or in the commoner loose-leaf form, is still chewed in parts of the US and elsewhere (Williams & Horm, 1977). A population based case-control study showed, among men, that use of chewing tobacco and snuff was strongly associated with cancers of the gum and mouth, but not of the lip or tongue.

In recent years, tobacco chewing and snuff-dipping habits have

Table 9.3. *Relative risks, with 95% confidence intervals, for oral leukoplakia associated with use of nass with and without smoking in 1569 men aged 55–69 years in Samarkand region of the Uzbek SSR.*

	Smoking	
	No	Yes
Nass use		
No	1.0	7.8 (4.4–14.2)
Yes	5.6 (3.4–9.5)	11.5 (5.4–24.3)

(After Zaridze *et al.*, 1985.)

increased among high school and college students, especially athletes. Precancerous lesions were found in over 40% (Greer & Poulsen, 1983).

Nass

Use of nass is widespread in Soviet Central Asia, Northern Iran, parts of Pakistan and Afghanistan (Nasswar). Nass is a mixture of variable composition and usually contains tobacco, ash, lime and cotton seed oil. In Afghanistan, cardamom oil and menthol are added.

The habitual use of nass is associated with oral leukoplakia (Zaridze *et al.*, 1985). Relative risks were significantly elevated in nass users and smokers; the combined habits in risk (Table 9.3) seemed to result in an additive effect.

Betel quid

The chewing of betel quid, with or without tobacco, is widespread in the Indian sub-continent, South-East Asia and parts of Oceania. The habit is of great antiquity, tobacco being added form the sixteenth century onwards. The basic quid comprises the leaf of the betel vine (*Piper betle*), sliced or shaved areca nut from the so-called betel palm (*Areca catechu*), and powdered slaked lime to which are added one or more of a wide variety of additives. However, when tobacco (usually of the sun-dried variety) is added to the chew, the risk of oral and, probably oropharyngeal, hypopharyngeal and oesophageal cancer is substantially increased (Orr, 1933; Hirayama, 1966) (Table 9.4).

9.4 Conclusions and public health considerations

Despite clear-cut knowledge of the effects of smoking, and oral use of tobacco for a number of social and economic reasons, comparatively little has been done through governmental regulation to control

Table 9.4. *Relative risk of oral cancer in chewers and non-chewers in the case-control studies.*

Frequency of chewing	Orr (1933)	Hirayama (1966)
Never	1[a]	1
Occasional	5	8
3–5/day	18	15
5+/day	34	18
Sleeps with quid in mouth	200[a]	63

[a] Risk estimate based on two cases

this habit. The greater part of public health measures have been directed towards education and fostering social pressures against smoking. The possibility that the habit could be made safer, through, for example, the reduction of tars, although not favored in North America, is still considered a potential, if less desirable, alternative in Europe for those who must smoke.

The findings are consistent: oral use of smokeless tobacco, whether prepared industrially or by artisanal means, increases the risk of oral cancer (IARC, 1985).

These habits are far from being esoteric curiosities in that they are widely practised by large numbers of people, possibly as many as 400 million, and give rise to an estimated 100,000 and 50,000 cancers each year in males and females respectively (Parkin *et al.*, 1988) (Chapter 23).

The preparation of snuff and chewing tobacco in the USA is on an industrial scale, some 40 million pounds of snuff being produced in 1980. Estimates of the number of current users of smokeless tobacco range from 7 million to 22 million. In the Orient, however, much of the preparation of the betel quid and its components are at the artisan level and production figures are difficult to obtain.

The tobacco companies, faced with lower sales of cigarettes in the developed countries are now, despite clear evidence of the carcinogenicity of the habit, promoting the use of chewing snuff, the product being sold in the form of sachets for oral use (Cameron, 1985). If the sale of these products, which do not carry any health warning, is allowed to continue the toll of periodontal disease and oral cancer will be high.

For control measures to have a chance of success, the motives underlying adoption of a habit should be understood. Much work has been done in this area for smoking, but very little for the oral use of tobacco.

9.5 References

Brinton, L.A., Blot, W.J., Becker, J.A., Winn, D.M., Browder, J.P., Farmer, J.C. & Fraumeni, J.F. (1984). A case-control study of cancers of the nasal sinuses and para-nasal sinuses. *Am. J. Epidemiol.*, **119**, 896–906.

Cameron, D. (1985). Warning against US tobacco sachets. *The Scotsman*, July 26, 1985, Edinburgh.

Doll, R. & Hill, A.B. (1950). Smoking and carcinoma of the lung. *Br. Med. J.*, **ii**, 739.

Greer, R.O. & Poulsen, T.C. (1983). Oral tissue alteration associated with the use of smokeless tobacco by teenagers. Part 2, Clinical Findings. *Oral Surg.*, **56**, 275–84.

Hecht, S.S. & Hoffman, D. (1989). The relevance of tobacco-specific nitrosamines to human cancers. *Cancer Surv.*, **8**, 273–94.

Hoffmann, D. & Wynder, E.L. (1986). Chemical constituents and bioactivity of tobacco smoke. In *Tobacco: A Major International Health Hazard*, IARC Scientific Publications No. 74, ed. D. Zaridze & R. Peto, pp. 145–65. Lyon: International Agency for Research on Cancer.

Hirayama, T. (1966). An epidemiological study of oral and pharyngeal cancer in central and South-East Asia. *Bull. WHO*, **34**, 41–69.

IARC (1985). *IARC Monographs on the Evaluation of Carcinogenic Risk of Chemicals to Humans*, volume 37, Tobacco habits other than smoking; betel-quid and areca-nut chewing; and some related nitrosamines. Lyon: International Agency for Research on Cancer.

IARC (1986). *IARC Monographs on the Evaluation of Carcinogenic Risk of Chemicals to Humans*, Tobacco smoking, volume 38. Lyon: International Agency for Research on Cancer.

IARC (1987). *IARC Monographs on the Evaluation of Carcinogenic Risks to Humans*, Overall evaluations of carcinogenicity: an updating of IARC Monographs volumes 1 to 42, Supplement 7. Lyon: International Agency for Research on Cancer.

Keen, P., De Moor, N.G., Shapiro, M.P. & Cohen, L. (1955). The aetiology of respiratory tract cancer in the South African Bantu. *Br. J. Cancer*, **9**, 538–8.

Mason, T.J., McKay, F.W., Hoover, R., Blot, W.J. & Fraumeni, J. (1975). *Atlas of cancer mortality for US counties*, 1950–1969. DHEW Publication no. (NIH) 75–780. Washington: US Department of Health, Education and Welfare.

Müller, F.H. (1939). Tobacco abuse and carcinoma of the lung. *Z. Krebsforsch*, **49**, 57–85.

O'Neill, I.K., Brunnemann, K.D., Dodet, B. & Hoffmann, D. (eds.) (1987). *Environmental Carcinogens – Methods of Analysis and Exposure Measurement, Passive Smoking.* IARC Scientific Publications No. 81. Lyon: International Agency for Research on Cancer.

Orr, I.M. (1933). Oral cancer in betel nut chewers in Travancore. Its aetiology, pathology and treatment. *Lancet*, **ii**: 575–80.

Parkin, D.M., Läärä, E. & Muir, C.S. (1988). Estimates of the worldwide frequency of sixteen major cancers in 1980. *Int. J. Cancer*, **41**, 184–97.

Peto, R. (1986). Influence of dose and duration of smoking on lung cancer rates. In *Tobacco: A Major International Health Hazard*, IARC Scientific Publications No. 74, ed. D. Zaridze & R. Peto, pp. 23–33. Lyon: International Agency for Research on Cancer.

Royal College of Physicians (1962). *Smoking and Health*, Summary of a Report of The Royal College of Physicians of London on smoking in relation to cancer of the lung and other diseases. London: Pitman Medical Publishing.

Surgeon General (US Department of Health, Education, and Welfare) (1964). *Smoking and Health*. Report of the Advisory Committee to the Surgeon General of the Public Health Service, Public Health Service Publication No. 1103. Washington: US Government Printing Office.

Williams, R.R. & Horm, H.W. (1977). Association of cancer sites with tobacco and alcohol consumption and socio economic status of patients. Interview study from the Third National Cancer Survey. *J. Natl. Cancer Inst.*, **58**, 525–47.

Willis, R.A. (1948). *Pathology of Tumours*. London: Butterworth & Co.

Winn, D.M., Blot, W.J., Shy, C.N., Pickle, L.W., Toledo, A. & Fraumeni, J.F. (1981). Snuff dipping and oral cancer among women in the Southern United States. *New Engl. J. Med.*, **304**, 745–9.

Wynder, E.L. & Graham, E.A. (1950). Tobacco smoking as a possible etiologic factor in bronchogenic carcinoma. *JAMA*, **143**, 329–36.

Zaridze, D. & Peto, R. (eds.) (1986). *Tobacco: A Major International Health Hazard*, IARC Scientific Publications No. 74. Lyon: International Agency for Research on Cancer.

Zaridze, D.G, Kuvshinov, J.P., Matiakin, E., Polakov, B.I., Boyle, P. & Blettner, M. (1985). *Chemoprevention of precancerous lesions of the mouth and oesophagus in Uzbekistan, USSR*. Proceedings of the Fourth Symposium on Epidemiology and Cancer Registries in the Pacific basin, Hawaii, January 16–20, NCI Monograph. Washington: National Cancer Institute.

10

Cultural factors: alcohol

10.1 Introduction

The use of alcoholic beverages goes back thousands of years, and today they are widely consumed in many societies, although certain religious groups prohibit their use. Early societies largely drank natural fermented products from a wide variety of organic materials such as grain, fruit, sap, honey, etc. Beer is brewed by fermenting malted barley and occasionally other cereals to which hops are added. Wine is made by fermenting grape juice. For the fortified wines, such as sherry, distilled spirits are added. Such spirits are made from different sources of starch or sugar – cereals, molasses, sugar beet, grapes, potatoes, cherries and other fruits. The liquid is distilled when the sugar has fermented.

Although abuse of alcoholic beverages has long been associated with physical and social ill-health, it is comparatively recently that concern has become widespread regarding their carcinogenic effects. Only certain general considerations relevant to epidemiology are presented here and reference should be made to a recent IARC (1988) publication for more detailed discussion. Their specific role is further discussed under individual cancer sites. The terms 'alcohol' and 'alcoholic beverages' are often used interchangeably.

10.2 Trends in consumption

In the mid-nineteenth century, the intake of alcoholic beverages was high in most of Europe and North America. But a decline in consumption began at the beginning of the twentieth century, which continued until the period between the two World Wars. This especially involved strong distilled beverages and was most pronounced in North and East Europe, as compared to wine-drinking countries. The last few decades, however, have been a period of increased consumption in developed countries which is most marked in countries which previously had relatively low levels of average consumption. In the past, countries tended to have certain traditional patterns of beverage consumption, but economic changes and living conditions, including large-scale migration, have led to increasing homogenization of patterns. Whereas original production methods in many countries were on a small scale, globally, the production of alcoholic beverages has become widely commercialized. Table 10.1 gives the increase in the production of commercial alcoholic beverages of all types since 1965 (IARC, 1988). The alcohol (ethanol) content of various alcoholic beverages per average drink is given in Table 10.2.

Individual consumption

There are wide variations in the rates of consumption of alcoholic beverages between countries and regions. Estimates of consumption are frequently based on the difference between the quantities produced and imported and the quantities exported and in stock, or on sales for taxation purposes. Neither calculation allows for non-commercial production or tax-free importation by individual travellers. In alcohol-producing countries, consumption is dominated by the type of beverage produced locally which accounts for most of any increase in consumption. In countries where wine is drunk, however, there has also been a marked increase in consumption of beers and spirits, whereas in countries where beer was the preferred drink, consumption of wine and spirits has become more general. Between 1960 and 1981, commercially produced beer, wine and spirits contributed approximately equal amounts to world ethanol consumption. The IARC reports that, with a few exceptions, the total consumption has increased very substantially over 1960 to 1981, and this rise in consumption is also occurring in Asia, Africa and Latin America.

In carrying out ecological studies relating to use of alcoholic beverages, these variations should be taken into consideration, especially the fact that the per capita intake may mean little, as often a relatively small proportion of the total population who are heavy drinkers account for a considerable part of the alcohol consumption. There are also variations between males and females. In the past, females tended to drink less than men, but these differences are decreasing. In certain countries, abstainers form a relatively large group and may be unduly represented in certain regions such as Utah where a large proportion of the population are members of the Church of the Latter Day Saints. Patterns vary between socio-economic classes, between different members of the community ranging from steady drinking at about the same level every day to 'binge' drinking at the

Table 10.1. *Total commercial production of alcoholic beverages* (*beer, wine and spirits*).

	1965		1980	
	Volume[a]	Per Head[b]	Volume[a]	Per Head[b]
Africa	3.1	1.0	3.3	0.7
Asia, excluding Japan	1.1	0.1	4.3	0.2
Japan	2.1	2.1	4.6	4.0
Australia and New Zealand	0.9	6.4	1.9	10.6
Oceania, excluding Australia and New Zealand	0.0	0.0	0.1	2.0
North America	9.6	4.7	19.7	8.1
Latin America and Caribbean	6.1	2.4	6.8	2.4
Europe, excluding the USSR	38.8	8.7	52.7	10.9
USSR	10.3	4.4	15.0	5.6
World	73.8	2.2	110.1	2.5

[a] Million hectoliters of ethanol
[b] Liters of ethanol
(After IARC, 1988.)

Table 10.2. *Approximate ethanol content of various alcoholic beverages per drink.*

	Ethanol content (%)		Average standard glass		Ethanol per drink	
Beverage	Volume	Weight	USA fl oz (ml)	Europe ml	ml	g
Beer	5	4	12 (350)	250	12–17.5	10–14
Wine	12	10	4 (120)	100	12–14.5	10–12
Spirits	40	32	1.5 (45)	35	14–18	11–14.2

(After IARC, 1988.)

weekends or over longer periods. The latter pattern tends to be more common in the lower socio-economic brackets. Such variations must be taken into consideration in any epidemiological study directed to determining the carcinogenic impact of ethanol or individual beverages. This is especially important for an agent where the possibility of threshold exists and where non-genotoxic mechanisms may be involved.

Table 10.3. *Chemical compounds in beer.*

Carbonyl compounds	Nitrogen compounds
Alcohol	Amines and amides, *N*-
Volatile acids	heterocyclic compounds
Hydroxy and oxo acids	Histamine and other non-
Non-volatile (fixed) acids	volatile *N*-heterocyclic
Esters	Aromatic compounds
	Phenols, Aromatic acids

(After IARC, 1988.)

10.3   Chemical composition

The chemical composition of beverages is a vast subject which cannot be adequately discussed here. The subject covers not only components formed during fermentation, but also naturally formed components in micro-quantities as well as pollutants and additives. Ethanol and water are the main ingredients of most alcoholic beverages. Ethanol is present as a consequence of carbohydrate fermentation with yeast but it can be manufactured from ethylene, a petroleum hydrocarbon. In general, the beverage industry has agreed not to use synthetic ethanol, manufactured from ethylene, for the production of alcoholic beverages due to the presence of impurities. Beer, wine and spirits also contain both volatile and non-volatile flavors. Certain flavored alcoholic beverages may have added synthetic substances and ingredients, in addition to natural flavors from herbs and spices. There is an extensive literature on the aroma compounds which are usually present at low levels and of which more than 1300 have been identified. However, the exact compositions of many alcoholic beverages are trade secrets. Tables 10.3 through 10.6 list some of the major group of compounds that are present in drinks including those with potential carcinogenic properties (IARC, 1988).

10.4   Experimental studies

Alcoholic beverages and ethanol have been tested in a number of studies. Many show important limitations, especially in terms of dietary control. In several instances, ethanol was administered orally with a number of carcinogens, notably *N*-nitroso compounds. Ethanol is almost unique due to the discordance between its carcinogenic effect in man and animals, and its carcinogenicity remains to be demonstrated unequivocally in the latter (IARC 1988). Thus, despite its recognized effect on the human liver, studies on the rodent liver are unsatisfactory, since it is impossible to induce alcoholic hepatitis in rodents by ethanol alone, although this can be done in primates. Few of the latter have been followed for long periods,

Table 10.4. *Chemical compounds in wine.*

Carbonyl compounds	Fixed acids
Acetals	Esters
Alcohols	Nitrogen compounds
Di- and trihydric alcohols fused	Amines and some
alcohols and long-chain alcohols	*N*-heterocyclic compounds
	amides
Volatile acids	Terpenic compounds
Hydroxy acids	Phenolic compounds

(After IARC, 1988.)

Table 10.5. *Chemical compounds in spirits.*

Carbonyl compounds	Acids
Aliphatic aldehydes	Aliphatic acids
Unsaturated aldehydes	Aromatic acids
Aliphatic ketones	Esters
Unsaturated monoketones	of aliphatic acids
Diketones	of aromatic acids
Aromatic aldehydes	
Alcohols	Phenolic compounds
Methanol	
Higher alcohols	

(After IARC, 1988.)

Table 10.6. *Additives and contaminants in alcoholic drinks.*

Flavoring additives	Contaminants
Other additives	*N*-nitrosamines
Trace elements	Mycotoxins
	Ethyl carbamate
	(urethane)
	Asbestos
	Arsenic compounds
	pesticides and
	adulterants

(After IARC, 1988.)

so the relevance of this lesion to hepato-carcinogenesis in humans is unclear.

10.5   Studies on human carcinogenicity

The association between alcohol and human cancer has been recognized for many years. It was noted that many cancers of the oral cavity, pharynx, esophagus and larynx, occurred among individuals employed in the beverage industry in countries with high risks for these sites (Clemmesen, 1941). The residents of Normandy in France who are heavy drinkers of Calvados (distilled apple cider) as well as other beverages show an unusually high incidence of esophageal cancer (Tuyns, 1978). Conversely, religious and other groups who do not drink have lower frequencies of these cancers. These groups include Seventh Day Adventists (Phillips *et al.*, 1980), Mormons (Enstrom, 1980), and Temperance Society members (Jensen, 1983), whose habits are significantly different from those of the general population. In certain Muslim countries, the use of alcoholic beverages is prohibited, in others, although less restricted, the overall intake remains very low.

It is customary to standardize comparative beverage studies on amount of ethanol consumed. All such retrospective questionnaires present certain difficulties, notably underestimation of higher levels of intake, and their accuracy is not of a high standard (IARC, 1988). Many early studies, moreover, did not take into consideration the confounding effect of cigarette smoking.

In evaluating the role of alcohol, several types of enquiries have been made: descriptive studies, including geographical and temporal studies; intra-population studies of identifiable groups with known differences in alcohol consumption, as evidenced by previous treatment for alcoholism, cirrhosis; and registries of driving convictions with raised blood alcohol, etc. Such studies have been frequently used to study alcohol consumption in relation to cancers of the larynx and alimentary tract, especially esophagus, or the correlation between liver cirrhosis and alcoholism within a country or between countries. While some studies have shown a positive correlation between per capita intake others have not. Time trends have also been used as have variations in male to female ratios.

The relationship of alcohol and cancer has been examined in a large number of cohort studies such as patients of an Oslo Hospital discharged with a diagnosis of alcoholism. Similar registries have been used from elsewhere in Scandinavia and hospital records have also been utilized in the UK (Dean *et al.*, 1979; Nicholls *et al.*, 1974; Jensen, 1980). Such studies have proved useful in identifying disease associations for groups of very heavy drinkers compared to the general population. Case control studies with individuals being questioned on their past use of different beverages have been carried out on a large-scale and have identified the association with cancers of the oral cavity, larynx, esophagus, liver, stomach, rectum and more recently, and more questionably, breast, as later discussed under individual sites.

Cohort or case-control studies on liver cancer reveal a weak association with alcohol intake. On the other hand, sequential liver biopsies of heavy drinkers have unequivocally demonstrated the pathogenic sequence of alcoholic hepatitis, cirrhosis and cancer. The epidemiological and pathological findings suggest that these lesions depend on heavy drinking, and that there may be a threshold below which toxic effects do not occur. The complementary action of hepatitis viruses needs to be considered in such cases (Chapter 29). These observations contrast the liver with other organs, e.g. esophagus, with high relative risks and where no obvious threshold is observed, and where it has been suggested that alcohol may act as a solvent for carcinogens occurring in tobacco or the diet. In rodents, ethanol has been shown to facilitate the passage of a carcinogenic PAH through the esophageal mucosa. A promoting effect has also been alleged. Ethanol is known to induce a specific form of a cytochrome P450 involved in the metabolism of many carcinogens.

Cancers of the urinary bladder, kidney, ovary, prostate and lymphatic and hemopoietic systems show no association with consumption of alcoholic beverages.

It has been suggested that the numerous chemicals, including carcinogens and promoters which are present in trace amounts in most alcoholic beverages, may be responsible for their carcinogenic activity. Amounts present are generally very small and, to date, there is no supportive epidemiological evidence.

10.6   Conclusion

The IARC (1988) has concluded that there is *sufficient* evidence for the carcinogenicity of ethanol and alcoholic beverages in humans. Thus the occurrence of malignant tumors of the oral cavity, pharynx, larynx, esophagus and liver is causally related to the consumption of alcoholic beverages. Alcoholic beverages have been categorized in IARC Group 1.

Emphasizing the limitations of the animal studies, the IARC concluded that while there is *sufficient* evidence for the carcinogenicity of acetaldehyde, a major metabolite of ethanol, the evidence is *inadequate* on the carcinogenicity of ethanol and alcoholic beverages in experimental animals (IARC, 1988).

10.7   References

Clemmesen, J. (1941). *Cancer and Occupation in Denmark*, 1935–1939. Copenhagen: Nyt Nordisk Forlag.

Dean, G., MacLennan, R., McLoughlin, H. & Shelley, E. (1979). Causes of death of blue-collar workers at a Dublin brewery, 1954–73. *Br. J. Cancer*, **40**, 581–9.

Enstrom, J.E. (1980). Cancer mortality among Mormons in California during 1968–75. *J. Natl. Cancer Inst.*, **65**, 1073–82.

IARC (1988). *IARC Monograph on the Evaluation of Carcinogenic Risks to Humans*, Alcohol drinking, volume 44. Lyon: International Agency for Research on Cancer.

Jensen O. M. (1980). *Cancer morbidity and causes of death among Danish brewery workers*, IARC Non-Serial publication. Lyon:International Agency for Research on Cancer.

Jensen, O.M. (1983). Cancer risk among Danish male Seventh-day Adventists and other temperance society members. *J. Natl. Cancer Inst.*, **70**, 1011–14.

Nicholls, P., Edwards, G. & Kyle, E. (1974). Alcoholics admitted to four hospitals in England. II. General and cause-specific mortality. *Q.J. Stud. Alcohol*, **35**: 841–55.

Phillips, R.L., Garfinkel, L., Kuzma, J.W., Beeson, W.L., Lotz, T. Brin, B. (1980). Mortality among California Seventh-day Adventists for selected cancer sites. *J. Natl. Cancer Inst.*, **65**, 1097–107.

Tuyns, A.J. (1978). *Alcohol et cancer*. IARC Non-Serial publication. Lyon: International Agency for Research on Cancer.

11

Sexual behavior and reproductive factors

A range of factors is considered in this section: sexual behavior has less impact than reproductive habits.

11.1 Sexual behavior and cervical cancer (Chapter 41)

Sexual behavior has been shown to influence cancer risk only at one site: uterine cervix.

Earlier epidemiological studies tended to describe female sexual variables in terms of marital status and reproductive history, whereas more recent studies identify the number of sexual partners and sexual intercourse as the two major risk factors. The latter are highly correlated and few investigations have separated their effects. After adjusting for age at first intercourse, all studies have shown a significant association with the number of sexual partners. Not all, however, after adjusting for sexual partners, have found a significant association with age at first intercourse.

If a major cause of cervical cancer is a sexually transmitted agent, both number of sexual partners and age at first intercourse are surrogate measures of exposure to the agent. The number of partners will reflect the probability for a susceptible woman of having had intercourse with an infected male and age at first intercourse will be a surrogate of age at first exposure. Both measures of exposure are therefore very crude and subject to a considerable degree of misclassification. Their relevance as risk factors will depend on the prevalence of the putative agent in the population. If low, many sexual partners will increase the probability of becoming infected, but if very high, a woman with only one sexual partner could have an increased risk for cervical cancer if the latter has had several partners and accordingly, a high probability of becoming infected (Muñoz & Bosch, 1989).

Only female sexual behavior has hitherto been associated with cervical cancer but recent epidemiological studies indicate that male sexual behavior also influences a woman's risk for cervical cancer (Buckley *et al.*, 1981). Geographic clusters and several studies have suggested the role of male sexual behavior as a determinant of a woman's risk for cervical cancer. Geographical clusters of high rates for both cancers of the cervix and of the penis have been described (Li *et al.*, 1982), increased risk for cervical cancer has been reported both among wives of men with penile cancer (Smith *et al.*, 1980) and among second wives of men previously married to women with cervical cancer (Kessler, 1977). A small case-control study of monogamous women with CIN (cervical intraepithelial neoplasia) lesions showed a eight-fold increased risk for women whose husbands reported having had 15 or more sexual partners outside marriage (Buckley *et al.*, 1981). However, recent results from studies in Latin America suggest that the contribution of male sexual behavior to the risk of cervical cancer in their wives is less than suggested in earlier studies (Brinton *et al.*, 1989).

11.2   Sexual behavior and cancer in men

Sexual behavior *per se* has not been associated with cancers of the testis and of the penis. However, the protective role of circumcision for cancer of the penis and the above observations on cervical cancers suggest that these cancers may share infectious etiological factors.

Although sexual behavior has for long been suspected to be associated with prostate cancer, at present, convincing evidence is lacking. A few studies have shown that patients with prostate cancer had earlier and more frequent sexual activity, also a more frequent history of venereal disease and numerous sexual partners, especially prostitutes, than control patients (Krain, 1974; Schumann *et al.*, 1977). Other studies have shown the contrary (Rotkin, 1977).

11.3   Reproductive factors and cervical cancer (Chapter 41)

Early epidemiological studies revealed associations of cervical cancer with age at first pregnancy and number of pregnancies. Subsequent studies considered these associations as indirect, reflecting, essentially, the association with the key risk factors, such as age at first intercourse and number of sexual partners. Recent studies, however, have shown a significant increased risk for cervical cancer with the number of pregnancies, even after adjusting for possible confounders (La Vecchia *et al.*, 1986; Brinton *et al.*, 1987). It has been postulated that the transient state of immunosuppression which occurs during pregnancy facilitates the oncogenic role of an infectious agent.

11.4 Reproductive factors and breast cancer

Although it is over two centuries since Ramazzini (1743) and later Rigoni-Stern (1842) reported that breast cancer was more common in nuns than in other women, only recently has the effect of the various reproductive factors been adequately studied (Chapter 40).

Age at first birth and parity

While a clear protective effect of early age at first full-term pregnancy has been found in most studies (MacMahon *et al.*, 1970; Boyle, 1988), no such an effect was found however, in a recent cohort study from Norway. The latter showed a strong protective effect with increasing number of pregnancies independently of the age at first birth (Kvale & Heuch, 1987; Kvale *et al.*, 1987). This was also found by Tulinius *et al.* (1978) and Brinton *et al.* (1983).

Recently, evidence suggesting that births after age 35 appear to increase the risk has been reported (Trichopoulos *et al.*, 1983; Kvale & Heuch, 1987).

Menarche and menopause

The association between age at menarche and breast cancer risk is not clear cut. Most recent studies have reported an increased risk with early menarche (Pike *et al.*, 1981; Paul *et al.*, 1986; Yuan *et al.*, 1988) but some earlier studies did not. Apter *et al.* (1989) find that some of the endocrine characteristics of early menarche are preserved into adulthood, suggesting a role for serum estradiol and sex hormone-binding globulin. The association with menopause is more clear. Women with late age at menopause (over 55 years) are at increased risk compared with women who had natural menopause below age 45. Furthermore, women who have had an artificial menopause under 45 years have a significantly reduced risk (Trichopoulos *et al.*, 1972). It has been postulated that women with early menarche and late menopause not only have a longer duration of exposure to estrogens but also may be exposed to higher levels, especially, during the post-menarcheal period (de Waard & Trichopoulos, 1988).

Lactation

Early epidemiological studies did not show significant association between long-term breast feeding and breast cancer risk, when the confounding effect of parity was taken into consideration (Thomas, 1980).

However, re-analysis of earlier studies (Byers *et al.*, 1985) and more recent studies (McTiernan & Thomas, 1986; Tao *et al.*, 1988; Yuan *et al.*, 1988) have shown a protective effect of long-term lactation.

Several, but not all studies, suggested that the above effects are different in pre-menopausal and post-menopausal women.

The mechanism for the effect of these reproductive factors is not clear. Three mathematical models have been proposed to express the value of reproductive factors, menstrual events and body size in predicting age-specific breast cancer incidence rates. The first proposed a two-stage process in which the initiated cells (first stage) would have a proliferative advantage over normal cells (Moolgavkar *et al.*, 1980). The second proposed that breast cancer incidence rates increase in proportion to a power of breast tissue age (Pike *et al.*, 1983), and the third described breast cancer risk based on the timing of childbearing and menstrual events, parity and body mass (Kampert *et al.*, 1988). Recently, it has been postulated that an energy-rich diet during puberty and adolescence, which is associated with early menarche and increased height, enhances the development of precancerous mammary lesions. These are inhibited by subsequent full-term pregnancies (de Waard & Trichopoulos, 1988), the protective effect being inversely related to the age at first full term pregnancy.

11.5   Reproductive factors and endometrial cancer (Chapter 43)

Endometrial cancer shares many similarities with breast cancer. Nulliparity and late menopause increase the risk whereas increasing parity provides increasing degrees of protection (Henderson *et al.*, 1983). However, no association with age at first full-term birth has been described (Kelsey *et al.*, 1982).

11.6   Reproductive factors and ovarian cancer (Chapter 44)

Cancer of the ovary also shares some similarities with cancer of the breast being more frequent in nulliparous women. Increasing parity confers increasing protection (Casagrande *et al.*, 1979). However, no clear association with age at first full-term birth has been reported.

11.7   Conclusion

It is clear that sexual behavior and reproductive habits are associated with changing risks in a number of cancers certain of which are considered to be hormone dependent to varying degrees. Oral con-traception (OC) is a significant component of modern reproductive practices. Their impact and that of individual hormones, on the above cancers has been reviewed (IARC, 1979; Henderson *et al.*, 1988), and are discussed further under individual sites and in Chapter 18.

11.8   References

Apter, D., Reinilä, M. & Vihko, R. (1989). Some endocrine characteristics of early menarche, a risk factor for breast cancer, are preserved into adulthood. *Int. J. Cancer*, **44**, 783–7,

Boyle, P. (1988). Epidemiology of breast cancer. *Baillière's Clin. Oncol.*, **2**, 1–57.

Brinton, L.A., Hoover, R. & Fraumeni, J.F. (1983). Reproductive factors in the aetiology of breast cancer. *Br. J. Cancer*, **47**, 757–62.

Brinton, L.A., Hamman, R.F., Huggins, G.R., Lehman, H.F., Levine, R.S., Mallin, K. & Fraumeni, J.F. (1987). Sexual and reproductive risk factors for invasive squamous cell cervical cancer. *J. Natl. Cancer Inst.*, **79**, 23–30.

Brinton, L.A., Reeves, W.C., Brenes, M.M., Herrero, R., Gaitan, E., Tenorio, F., de Britton, R.C., Garcia, M. & Rawls, W.E. (1989). The male factor in the etiology of cervical cancer among sexually monogamous women. *Int. J. Cancer*, **44**, 199–203.

Buckley, J.D., Doll, R., Harris, R.W.C., Vessey, M.P. & Williams, P.T. (1981). Case-control study of the husbands of women with dysplasia or carcinoma of the cervix uteri. *Lancet*, **ii**, 1010–5.

Byers, T., Graham, T., Rzepka, T. & Marshall, J. (1985). Lactation and breast cancer: evidence for a negative association in premenopausal women. *Am. J. Epidemiol.*, **121**, 664–74.

Casagrande, J.T., Louie, E.W., Pike, M.C., Roy, S., Ross, R.K. & Henderson, B.E. (1979). 'Incessant ovulation' and ovarian cancer. *Lancet*, **ii**,, 170–3.

De Waard, F. & Trichopoulos, D. (1988). A unifying concept of the aetiology of breast cancer. *Int. J. Cancer*, **41**, 666–9.

Henderson, B.E., Casagrande, J.T., Pike, M.C., Mack, T., Rosario, I. & Pike, M.C., Mack, T., Rosario, I. & Puke, A. (1983). The epidemiology of endometrial cancer in young women. *Br. J. Cancer*, **47**, 749–56.

Henderson, B.E., Ross, R. & Bernstein, L. (1988). Estrogens as a cause of human cancer: the Richard and Hinda Rosenthal Foundation award lecture. *Cancer Res.*, **48**, 246–53.

IARC (1979). *IARC Monographs on the Evaluation of the Carcinogenic Risk of Chemicals to Humans*, Sex hormones (II), volume 21. Lyon: International Agency for Research on Cancer.

Kampert, J.B., Whittemore, A.S. & Paffenbarger, R.S. (1988). Combined effect of childbearing, menstrual events and body size on age-specific breast cancer risk. *Am. J. Epidemiol.*, **128**, 962–79.

Kelsey, J.L., LiVolsi, V.A., Holford, T.R., Fisher, D.B., Mostow, E.D., Schwartz, P.E, O'Connor, T. & White, C. (1982). A case-control study of cancer of the endometrium. *Am. J. Epidemiol.*, **116**, 333–42.

Kessler, I.I. (1977). Venereal factors in human cervical cancer. Evidence from marital clusters. *Cancer*, **39**, 1912–19.

Krain, L.S. (1974). Some epidemiologic variables in prostatic carcinoma in California. *Prev. Med.*, **3**, 154–9.

Kvale, G. & Heuch, I. (1987). A prospective study of reproductive factors and breast cancer. II: Age at first and last birth. *Am. J. Epidemiol.*, **126**, 842–50.

Kvale, G, Heuch, I. & Eide, G.E. (1987). A prospective study of reproductive factors and breast cancer. I: Parity. *Am. J. Epidemiol.*, **126**, 831–41.

La Vecchia, C., Franceschi, S., Decarli, A., Fasoli, M., Gentile, A., Parazzini, F. & Regallo, M. (1986). Sexual factors, venereal diseases, and the risk of intraepithelial and invasive cervical neoplasia. *Cancer*, **58**, 935–41.

Li, J., Li, F.P., Blot, W.J., Miller, R.W. & Fraumeni, Jr., J.F. (1982). Correlation between cancers of the uterine cervix and penis in China. *J. Natl. Cancer Inst.*, **69**, 1063–5.

MacMahon, B., Cole, P., Lin, T.M., Lowe, C.R., Mirra, A.P., Ravnihar, B., Salber, E.J., Valaoras, V.G & Yuasa, S. (1970). Age at first birth and cancer of the breast. A summary of an international study. *Bull. World Health Org.*, **43**, 209–21.

McTiernan, A., & Thomas, D.B. (1986). Evidence for a protective effect of lactation on risk of breast cancer in young women. *Am. J. Epidemiol.*, **124**, 353–8.

Moolgavkar, S.H., Day, N.E. & Stevens, R.G. (1980). Two-stage model for carcinogenesis: Epidemiology of breast cancer in females. *J. Natl. Cancer Inst.*, **65**, 559–69.

Muñoz, N. & Bosch, F.X. (1989). Epidemiology of cervical cancer. In: *Human Papillomavirus and Cervical Cancer*, ed. N. Muñoz, F.X. Bosch & O.M. Jensen, IARC Scientific Publication No 94. Lyon: International Agency for Research on Cancer.

Paul, C., Skegg, D.G., Spears, G.F.S. & Kaldor, J.M. (1986). Oral contraceptives and breast cancer: a national study. *Br. Med. J.*, **293**, 723–31.

Pike, M.C., Henderson, B.E., Casagrande, J.T., Rosario, I. & Gray, G.E. (1981). Oral contraceptive use and early abortion as risk factors for breast cancer in young women. *Br. J. Cancer*, **43**, 72–9.

Pike, M.C., Krailo, M.D., Henderson, B.E., Casagrande, J.T. & Hoel, D.G. (1983). 'Hormonal' risk factors, 'breast tissue age' and the age-incidence of breast cancer. *Nature*, **303**, 767–70.

Ramazzini B. (1743). *De Morbis Artificum*. Venezia: Diatriba J. Corona.

Rigoni-Stern, R. (1842). Fatti statistici relativi alla malattie cancerose. *Giornali per Servire al Progressi della Patologia e della Terapeutica*, **2**, 507–17.

Rotkin, D. (1977). Studies on the epidemiology of prostate cancer: expanded sampling. *Cancer Treat. Rep.*, **61**, 173–80.

Schumann, L.M., Mandel, J., Blanchard, C., Bauer, H., Scarlett, J. & McHugh, R. (1977). Epidemiologic study of prostatic cancer. preliminary report. *Cancer Treat. Rep.*, **61**, 181–6.

Smith, P.G., Kinlen, L.J., White, G.C., Adelstein, A.M. & Fox, A.J. (1980). Mortality of wives of men dying with cancer of the penis. Br. J. Cancer, **41**, 422–8.

Tao, S.C., Yu, M.C., Ross, R.K. & Xiu, K.W. (1988). Risk factors for breast cancer in Chinese women in Beijing. *Int. J. Cancer*, **42**, 495–8.

Thomas, D.B. (1980). Epidemiologic and related studies of breast cancer etiology. In: *Reviews in Cancer Epidemiology*, vol. 1, ed. A.M. Lilienfeld. New York: Elsevier North-Holland.

Trichopoulos, D., MacMahon, B. & Cole, P. (1972). Menopause and breast cancer risk. *J. Natl. Cancer Inst.*, **48**, 605–13.

Trichopoulos, D., Hsieh, C.C., MacMahon, B., Lin, T.M., Lowe, C.R., Mirra, A.P., Ravnihar, B., Salber, E.J., Valaoras, V.G & Yuasa, S. (1983). Age at any birth and breast cancer risk. *Int. J. Cancer*, **31**, 701–4.

Tulinius, H., Day, N.E., Johannesson, G., Bjarnason, O. & Gonzales, M. (1978). Reproductive factors and risk for breast cancer in Iceland. *Int. J. Cancer*, **21**, 724–30.

Yuan, J.M., Yu, M.C., Ross, R.K., Gao, Y.T. & Henderson, B.E. (1988). Risk factors for breast cancer in Chinese women in Shanghai. *Cancer Res.*, **48**, 1949–53.

12

Nutritional factors

12.1 Introduction

Since World War II, there has been a marked increase in epidemiological studies on cancer and diet. At first, concern was greatest in relation to potentially toxic chemicals added to the diet, following experimental studies in the 1920s. Such concern motivated much of the deliberations of the joint World Health Organization/Food and Agricultural Organization (WHO/FAO) Committee on food additives and pesticides in the postwar period (WHO, 1958). In the USA, fear of chemical additives culminated in the passage of Public Law 85–929, known as the Delaney Amendment (1958), which banned the use of any carcinogen as a food additive. None the less, the relationship remains controversial. Later research has largely concentrated on the role of macronutrients such as dietary fat, fiber, as well as other normal food constituents.

The National Academy of Sciences (NAS, 1982), after a complete review of the literature available on diet and cancer, reported that:

'The evidence reviewed by the committee suggests that cancers of most major sites are influenced by dietary patterns. However, the committee concluded that the data are not sufficient to quantitate the contribution of diet to the overall cancer risk or to determine the per cent reduction in risk that might be achieved by dietary modifications.'

Despite those caveats, the Academy in its recommendations not only emphasized the role of diet in human cancer but made concrete suggestions as to the benefits to be anticipated from specific changes in eating habits, as did a further report by the Surgeon General (1988).

The effect of diet is discussed further in relation to cancers at specific sites; however, certain general issues and concepts merit consideration, in view of the high proportions of human cancer attributed to diet.(Wynder

& Gori, 1977; Higginson & Muir, 1979; Doll & Peto, 1981; NAS, 1982; Graham, 1983*a,b*; Lowenthal, 1983; Willett & MacMahon, 1984*a,b*).

12.2   Methodological issues in evaluating the role of diet in human cancer

Unlike traditional chemical carcinogens, exposure to food is ubiquitous, so that populations differ only in degree and patterns of exposure to nutrients and foods. These differences, however, may be considerable.

Laboratory studies

It is assumed with some reservations that animal studies of chemical carcinogens may predict qualitatively for humans, especially where there is evidence of common mechanisms and end-points. However, studying the role of dietary factors, the problem is more complex since macro- and micro-nutrients may behave differently, both qualitatively and quantitatively, in humans and in animals. Experimental diets often compare extreme variations of macro- or micro-nutrients at almost toxicological or pharmacological levels. Thus, inappropriate conclusions may be drawn for humans in whom variations are usually within a more modest range. However, data from rodent studies on dietary carcinogens remain important in regulatory procedures. While pigs or primates may be preferable species for certain nutritional studies, they are prohibitively expensive for routine cancer studies.

Dietary assessment in humans

Most cancers suspected to be diet-related are likely to have a multifactorial origin. The human diet is a complex mass of nutrients and chemicals which are notoriously difficult to measure in observational studies (Lyon *et al.*, 1983; Zaridze *et al.*, 1985; Willett *et al.*, 1987). Diet not only varies by season but also from day to day. Previous dietary patterns may bear no relationship to present eating habits and thus may be difficult to measure accurately.

While a single factor may be examined in animals through dietary manipulation, this is rarely possible in humans unless the suspected agent is identifiable and discrete, such as a mycotoxin or an alcoholic beverage. Modification of one component in a diet is associated usually with a change in others. An increase in calories from fat, for instance, usually reflects a reduced percentage of calories from other sources. Further, diet can influence breast cancer risk indirectly by altering the age of menarche or menopause, both of which are risk factors in mammary cancer, as well as possibly directly through amount and type of fat.

12.3 Dietary components affecting carcinogenesis

Individual cancers can be classified according to their suspected relationship to dietary factors. These include:

(a) Cancers for which a defined carcinogenic agent in the diet, such as aflatoxin, is probably involved.

(b) Cancers possibly due to a defined agent, which is formed from non-cancerous dietary precursors, e.g. the formation of *N*-nitroso compounds from secondary amines and nitrites.

(c) Cancers in which the role of diet is almost certainly indirect including the modification, activation or deactivation of a carcinogen; modulation of late stage carcinogenesis; or non-specific enhancing or inhibitory action. Such effects can be mediated through excess or deficiency of a macro- or micro-nutrient or caloric intake. Thus, vitamins are necessary to maintain the normal structure of epithelial tissues. Other dietary components may increase pro-oxidant state and/or decrease anti-oxidant defence, or the level of metabolizing enzymes.

12.4 Defined carcinogens

Ingested carcinogens and modulators

Such agents can be both man-made and natural and cover a spectrum from sodium chloride to complex molecules with a range of biological effects. While a number of man-made food additives or contaminants have been demonstrated to be animal carcinogens, studies in humans have shown no detectable effects for individual chemicals, micro-nutrients, or pollutants (NAS, 1982). This would suggest that levels of exposure are so low as to be of no practical significance, especially if such exposures are considered in relation to the total burden of unavoidable mutagens and naturally occurring carcinogenic initiators or enhancers found in the average diet (Ames, 1983). To date, aflatoxin is the only ingested carcinogenic contaminant for which reasonably strong evidence of an effect in humans is available (Chapter 29). However, the evidence for ochratoxin A, a mycotoxin, in urothelial carcinogenesis (Chapter 49) and bracken fern in digestive cancers is suggestive.

Endogenous carcinogenic formations: N-*nitroso compounds*

N-nitroso compounds are potent carcinogens affecting numerous organ sites in many animal species (NAS, 1981). They may be present in many foodstuffs (O'Neill *et al.*, 1984); their formation offers a plausible hypothesis for the potential role of bacon and smoked foods in gastric cancer. However, currently there is greater interest regarding their endogenous formation. Thus, secondary and tertiary amines, common in many foods, are suspected of interacting with exogenous or endogenous nitrites to form N-nitroso compounds within the stomach or mouth, a reaction inhibited by ascorbic acid (Preussmann & Eisenbrand, 1984). On the other hand, a number of studies on nitrate ingestion and gastric and oesophageal cancer have failed to demonstrate any correlation. These studies have been hampered by the former lack of methods to assess nitrosamine formation *in vivo*. While the hypothesis appears attractive as a cause of some human cancers, notably stomach and oesophagus, it remains speculative (Correa, 1988). Nevertheless, recommendations have been made to reduce the amount of nitrite and nitrate in preserved foods as much as possible, bearing in mind their function in inhibiting the growth of clostridia.

12.5   Macronutrients and calories
Fats

Fats (lipids) have important biological functions, serving as structural components of membranes, as storage and transport forms of metabolic fuel, and as cell-surface components concerned with cell recognition, species-specificity and tissue immunity.

In animals, high fat diets, especially polyunsaturated fats, increase tumor incidence at a number of sites. Most studies suggest that the enhancing effect is on the later stages of carcinogenesis. Although promoting effects of high fat diets have been described for colon cancer in rodents, possibly due to increased bile acid and neutral steroid excretion, it has not been possible to provide rigorous proof of an association in humans.

Despite study of fats and fatty acids in human cancer, there is still uncertainty as to their definitive role. Thus, dietary fat levels not only tend to correlate both with protein intake and other components in affluent societies but are also a concentrated source of calories. The evidence is most persuasive for a role in breast and large bowel cancer but there are inconsistencies which cannot easily be explained (Willett, 1989). Thus the incidence of breast and colorectal cancer in Finland and Denmark is the inverse of that anticipated from fat intake patterns (Jensen *et al.*, 1982). Despite the marked changes in dietary fat intake that have occurred over several decades in the United States, no convincing impact on breast or colon cancer has been produced – in contrast to heart disease.

The NAS report (1982) failed to identify any specific fat component or carbohydrate definitely related to carcinogenesis in humans; but Geboers *et al.* (1985) concluded that a high-fat diet was associated with an increased risk of several cancers, and recommended reduction to 30% of total calories. De Waard (1986) emphasizes that abundant availability of food leads to increased height and weight in many individuals and, in post-adolescence, to obesity. Citing evidence from Japan and Scotland, he concludes that, for the individual, these are more important risk factors than dietary fat. Obesity is frequently related to cancers of the endometrium and gall bladder. Scandinavian data suggest that a high intake of dietary fiber may partly compensate for a high fat intake. It has been suggested that high levels of dietary fat may enhance breast cancer through increased estrogen formation. Post-menopausal women switching from a low fat vegetarian diet to a high fat western diet showed a decrease in luteinizing hormones, FSH (follicle stumulating hormone), and prolactin. The relationship, however, in pre-menopausal women remains to be defined.

No information in humans is available on the effects of artificial fat replacements.

Protein

The role of protein and essential amino acids in experimental carcinogenesis has been of interest for many years, especially in the liver.

In Africa, in the 1940s and 1950s, there was great interest in primary human liver cancer believed to arise from protein-calorie deficiency (kwashiorkor) in childhood; this association was later disproved. Data for other sites are confusing (NAS, 1982) since correlations between cancer and protein intake are confounded by the association with high protein, fat and meat consumption. In view of the five-fold range in protein intake within the USA, Graham (1983c) believes it is inappropriate to extrapolate from average consumption to the few individuals with a specific cancer, as in a correlation study. Few case-control studies adequately cover the problem of early recall and protein intake over prolonged periods.

Carbohydrates

There are two general classes of carbohydrate – monosaccharides, or simple sugars, and complex polysaccharides, subdivided into starch and nonstarch polysaccharides (NSP). The latter may be considered as the equivalent of dietary fiber (Cummings, 1986).

Most experimental studies suggest that, in general, carbohydrates modulate the later stages of carcinogenesis (promotion). To what extent this effect is specific, i.e. related to the type of carbohydrate, or non-specific, as related to caloric intake or obesity, is unclear and both possibilities may be involved since few experiments control the caloric content (Kritchevsky, 1985).

The absence of a clear-cut consensus probably indicates that most scientists believe that the nutritive carbohydrates alone have no specific effect in humans.

The inhibitory effect of fiber has been examined experimentally but is difficult to equate with epidemiological studies, since most laboratory experiments have examined specific or individual carbohydrates, whereas the human studies have focused on fibrous foods.

Cummings (1986) has reviewed the role of non-starch carbohydrate (NSP) in colon cancer and emphasized the inconsistencies in the data as well as the need to examine the chemistry of fiber, especially pentose NSP (Bingham *et al.*, 1985). It is difficult moreover, to ascertain the relevance of physiological studies in the absence of knowledge of the mechanisms of large bowel cancer. Despite over a dozen population studies showing a relationship between large bowel cancer incidence and/or mortality and fiber intake, there is still no general agreement on its protective role. The NAS report (1982) found 'no conclusive evidence' to indicate that dietary fiber, as found in fruits, vegetables, and cereals, asserts a protective effect against colorectal cancer in humans. The Scandinavian data, however, supports an inverse relationship between fiber intake for breast and colorectal cancer. It further suggests that fiber intake may counteract the effect of a high-fat diet at these sites (Jensen *et al.*, 1982). Some studies on populations in dietary transition have suggested a protective effect for a high consumption of cruciferous vegetables and a pre-disposing effect of high ratio of meat to vegetable intake; no consistent trend was noted though for either colon or rectal cancer for fat or fiber intake. However, it is difficult to separate the protective effects of fiber from possible inhibitory factors from the same sources (Section 12.7).

Calories

In the classical experiments of Tannenbaum (1945a, 1945b), the most striking and specific effect on carcinogenesis was through caloric restriction. Few authors, however, including the NAS (1982) report, comment on possible cancer inhibition in humans by low calorie diets. In countries where protein-calorie malnutrition has been prevalent, certain cancers common in affluent societies tend to be rare, notably of the breast, prostate, endometrium and colo-rectum. However, there are numerous confounding variables to be considered. Thus diets high in fat and carbohydrate are also high in calories, and obesity has been associated with cancers of the breast, endometrium and gall bladder. Few analyses take total energy intake into account.

12.6 Micronutrients and food factors
Vitamins
Deficiencies for certain vitamins have been identified as being significant for several experimental tumors, e.g. riboflavin in butter yellow induced liver cancer, but their role in humans is difficult to establish due to confounding variables. Their role is discussed further under individual cancer sites.

Lipotropes
Experimental studies show that lipotropic deficiency (choline, methionine) may cause liver cancer in animals. There is no evidence, however, to suggest that such deficiency is of significance in humans.

Minerals
A number of minerals have been related to carcinogenesis in animals, few of which appear relevant to humans. Thus, there is no evidence that iron overload *per se* which is widespread in southern Africa has had an impact on cancer patterns (Higginson & Oettlé, 1960). The relationship of idiopathic hemochromatosis to liver cancer is probably due to the coexistent cirrhosis. Cancers of the hypopharynx and upper esophagus have been reported in women who suffer from iron and other deficiencies. High calcium intake has been suggested to inhibit colon cancer (Chapter 28).

12.7 Anticarcinogens
Naturally occurring inhibitors have been found in various foods (Ames, 1983; Wattenberg, 1986). They may act through several mechanisms:

(a) Those which prevent the formation of carcinogens exemplified by ascorbic acid which inhibits the endogenous formation of *N*-nitrosocompounds. Although, Willett and MacMahon (1984*a*), in a review of the epidemiological evidence, found little evidence of a protective effect of vitamin C in humans, recent case-control and cohort studies indicate a protective effect (Gey *et al.*, 1987; Buiatti *et al.*, 1990).

(b) Those which prevent carcinogens from reaching or reacting with a critical target site and are classified according to suspected mechanisms. They include inhibition of carcinogen activation, induction of detoxifying enzymes, and scavenging of the reactive forms of carcinogens. For example, anti-oxidants (beta-carotene, vitamins C and E) trap single oxygen and other free radicals.

(c) Those which prevent tumor induction even after exposure to a carcinogen. The most intensively studied agent is beta-carotene (Ziegler *et al.*, 1986). Experimental evidence indicates that it blocks the progression of early gastric cancer to infiltrating tumors in rats (Santamaria & Bianchi, 1989) and several intervention trials on heavy smokers are under way.

Numerous epidemiological studies have consistently found a protective effect of fresh vegetables and fruits which are rich in vitamin C and beta-carotene. These may also contain other inhibiting agents, such as inducers of detoxifying enzymes and selenium, thus complicating definite conclusions (Salonen *et al.*, 1984, 1985).

Conclusion

There is no certainty that any of the above inhibiting agents are important in human disease, but their potential role in chemoprevention is of great interest and, at present, over 40 intervention trials are in progress.

12.8   Other factors modifying dietary carcinogenesis
Beverages

The most important beverages identified with human cancer are those containing ethanol (Chapter 10). A number of hot beverages have been suspected to be associated with human cancer notably tea, coffee and maté. A number of those contain chemical compounds in small quantities, some of which are recognized animal carcinogens or enhancers. There is no convincing evidence that such beverages and the related chemicals play an important role in human cancer with the exception of hot maté (IARC, 1990).

Role of cooking and preservatives

Formerly, there was extensive interest in the formation of carcinogens during cooking, especially in reheated fats. Experimental studies have confirmed the formation of animal carcinogens and mutagens from pyrolized amino acids (Sugimura *et al.*, 1977), as well as polycyclic aromatic hydrocarbons and *N*-nitroso compounds in charcoal foods.

Epidemiological studies to date have failed to demonstrate any convincing relationship between cooking methods and gastro-intestinal cancer. Certain preserved foodstuffs, however, have been associated with a high frequency of gastric cancer in Central Europe, which has been attributed to the formation of *N*-nitroso carcinogens.

In Japan, diets high in sodium chloride are believed to irritate the stomach and are suspected to cause, or to enhance, gastric cancer.

Intestinal flora

There has been interest on the role of diet in modifying the intestinal bacterial flora and possible carcinogen formation (Hill, 1985). Although mutagens of bacterial origin have been observed in human feces, their role is uncertain.

Age

Studies on migrants and religious groups indicate that, for several sites, the impact of dietary factors, if any, has the greatest impact in early life. Thus changes in cancer patterns in migrants, such as a decrease in gastric cancer and increases in cancers of the prostate and breast seen in migrants from Japan to North America, occur slowly over two or three generations. Such changes have been hypothesized to imply that dietary effects are associated either with permanent metabolic changes in the host or modification of early stage carcinogenesis (Chapter 2). In contrast, relatively rapid changes in incidence have been observed in cancer of the colon and rectum in migrants, suggesting some form of enhancing mechanism, e.g. promotion.

If dietary modification at an early age is critical for cancer induction, then dietary changes adopted in adult life may not have significant impact. This may explain, to some extent, why significant temporal changes have not yet been observed for many cancers believed to be diet-related despite the major changes in the American and European dietary patterns that have occurred over the last four decades.

12.9 Conclusion

For most cancers, while a significant role for diet remains plausible, convincing evidence for a specific component is generally lacking. This discussion is elaborated further under specific sites. It is frequently not possible to compare epidemiological studies on diet as very few control for total energy and standard methods of analysis are not yet available.

12.10 References

Ames, B.N. (1983). Dietary carcinogens and anticarcinogens, oxygen radicals and degenerative diseases. *Science*, **221**, 1256–64.

Bingham, S.A., Williams, D.R.R. & Cummings, J.H. (1985). Dietary fibre consumption in Britain: New estimates and their relation to large bowel cancer mortality. *Br. J. Cancer*, **52**, 399–402.

Buiatti, E., Palli, D., Decarli, A., Amadori, D., Avellini, C., Bianchi, S., Bonaguri, C., Cipriani, F., Cocco, P., Giacosa, A., Marubini, E., Minacci, C., Puntoni, R., Russo, A., Vindigni, C., Fraumeni, J.F., Jr. & Blot, W.J. (1990). A case-control study of gastric cancer and diet in Italy: II. Association with nutrients. *Int. J. Cancer*, **45**, 896–901.

Correa, P. (1988). A human model of gastric carcinogenesis. *Cancer Res.*, **48**, 3554–60.

Cummings, J.H. (1986). Dietary carbohydrates and cancer. *Nutr. Cancer*, **8**, 10–4.

Delaney Amendment (1958). Food Additives Amendment of 1958 to the Federal Food, Drug and Cosmetic Act, Public Law 85–929, Sept. 6, 1958.

De Waard, F. (1986). Dietary fat and mammary cancer. *Nutr. Cancer*, **38**, 5–8.

Doll, R. & Peto, R. (1981). The causes of cancer: quantitative estimates of avoidable risks of cancer in the United States today. *J. Natl. Cancer Inst.*, **66**, 1192–308.

Geboers, J. Joossens, J.V. & Carroll, K.K. (1985). Introductory remarks to the consensus statement on provisional dietary guidelines. In *Diet and Human Carcinogenesis*, ed. J.V. Joossens, M.J. Hill & J. Geboers, pp. 337–42. New York: Excerpta Medica.

Gey, K.F., Brubacher, G.B. & Stahelin, H.B. (1987). Plasma levels of antioxidant vitamins in relation to ischemic heart disease and cancer. *Am. J. Clin. Nutr.*, **45**, 1368–77.

Graham, S. (1983a) Results of case-control studies of diet and cancer in Buffalo, New York. *Cancer Res.*[Suppl.], **43**, 2409s-13s.

Graham, S. (1983b). Toward a dietary prevention of cancer. *Epid. Rev.*, **5**, 38–50.

Graham, S. (1983c). Diet and cancer: Epidemiologic aspects. In *Reviews in Cancer Epidemiology*, vol. 2, ed. A.M Lilienfield, pp. 1–45. New York: Elsevier.

Higginson, J. (1963). The geographic pathology of primary liver cancer. *Cancer Res.*, **23**, 1624–33.

Higginson, J. & Muir, C.S. (1979). Environmental carcinogenesis: Misconceptions and Limitations to Cancer Control (guest editorial). *J. Natl. Cancer Inst.*, **63**, 1291–8.

Higginson, J. & Oettlé, A.G. (1960). Cancer incidence in the Bantu and 'Cape Colored' races of South Africa: report of cancer survey in Transvaal (1953–55). *J. Natl. Cancer Inst.*, **24**, 589–671.

Hill, M.J. (1985). Mechanisms of colorectal carcinogenesis. In *Diet and Human Carcinogenesis*, ed. J.V. Joossens, M.J. Hill & J. Geboers, pp. 149–63. New York: Excerpta Medica.

IARC (1990). *IARC Monographs on the Evaluation of Carcinogenic Risks to Humans*. Coffee, tea, maté, methylxanthines (caffeine, theophylline, thiobromine) and Methylglyoxal, volume 51. Lyon: International Agency for Research on Cancer.

Jensen, O.M., MacLennan, R. & Wahrendorf, J. (1982). Diet, bowel function, fecal characteristics, and large bowel cancer in Denmark and Finland. *Nutr. Cancer.*, **4**, 5–19.

Kritchevsky, D. (1985). Dietary fiber and cancer. *Nutr. Cancer*, **6**, 213–9.

Lowenthal, J.P. (ed.) (1983). Workshop conference on nutrition in cancer causation and prevention. *Cancer Res.*[Suppl.], **43**, 2389s-518s.

Lyon, J.L., Gardner, J.W., West, D.W. & Mahoney, A.M. (1983). Methodological issues in epidemiological studies of diet and cancer. *Cancer Res.*[Suppl.], **43**, 2392s-6s.

NAS (Committee on Nitrite and Alternative Curing Agents in Food, National Academy of Sciences) (1981). *The Health Effects of Nitrate, Nitrite, and N-Nitroso Compounds*, Part 1 of a 2-part study by the Committee on Nitrite and Alternative Curing Agents in Food. Washington: National Academy Press.

NAS (Committee on Diet, Nutrition, and Cancer, National Academy of Sciences) (1982). *Diet, Nutrition and Cancer*. Washington: National Academy Press.

O'Neill, I.K., Von Borstel, R.C., Miller, C.T., Long, J. & Bartsch, H. (eds.) (1984). N-*Nitroso Compounds*: *Occurrence, Biological Effects and Relevance to Human Cancer*, Proceedings of the VIIIth International Symposium on *N*-Nitroso Compounds held in Banff, Canada, 5–9 September 1983, IARC Scientific Publications No. 57. Lyon: International Agency for Research on Cancer.

Preussmann, R. & Eisenbrand, G. (1984). Chemical carcinogens. In *Am. Chem. Soc. Monograph No.* 182, pp. 829–68. Washington.

Salonen, J.T., Alfthan, G., Huttunen, J.K. & Puska, P. (1984). Association between serum selenium and risk of cancer. *Am. J. Epidemiol.*, **120**, 342–9.

Salonen, J.T., Salonen, R., Lappeteläinen, R., Mäenpää, P.H., Alfthan, G. & Puska, P. (1985). Risk of cancer in relation to serum concentrations of selenium and vitamins A and E: matched case-control analysis of prospective data. *Br. Med. J.*, **290**, 417–20.

Santamaria, L. & Bianchi, A. (1989). Cancer Chemoprevention by supplemental carotenoids in animals and humans. *Prev. Med.*, **18**, 603–23.

Sugimura, T., Kawachi, T., Nagao, M., Yahagi, T., Seino, Y., Okamoto, T., Shudo, K., Kosuge, T., Tsuji, K., Wakabayashi, K., Iitaka, Y. & Itai, A. (1977). Mutagenic principle(s) in tryptophan and phenylalanine pyrolysis products. *Proc. Jpn. Acad.*, **53**, 58–61.

Surgeon General (1988). *The Surgeon General's Report on Nutrition and Health*, US Department of Health and Human Services, Public Health Service, DHHS (PHS) Publication No. 88–50210. Washington: Government Printing Office.

Tannenbaum, A. (1945a). The dependence of tumor formation on the degree of caloric restriction. *Cancer Res.*, **5**, 609–15.

Tannenbaum, A. (1945b). The dependence of tumor formation on the degree of caloric restriction. *Cancer Res.*, **5**, 616–25.

Wattenberg, L.W. (1986). Micronutrients and other microconstituents. *Nutr. Cancer*, **8**, 22–4.

WHO (World Health Organization) (1958). Procedures for the testing of intentional food additives to establish their safety for use. Second report of the joint FAO/WHO Expert Committee on Food Additives. *WHO Tech. Rep. Ser.*, **144**, 1–19.

Willett, W.C. (1989). The search for the causes of breast and colon cancer. *Nature*, **338**, 389–94.

Willett, W.C. & MacMahon, B. (1984a). Diet and cancer. *N. Engl. J. Med.*, **310**, 633–8.

Willett, W.C. & MacMahon, B. (1984b). Diet and cancer. *N. Engl. J. Med.*, **310**, 697–703.

Willett, W.C., Polk, B.F., Morris, J.S., Stampfer, M.J., Pressel, S., Rosner, B., Taylor, J.O., Schneider, K. & Hames, C.G. (1983). Prediagnostic serum selenium and risk of cancer. *Lancet*, **ii**, 130–4.

Willett, W.C., Stampfer, M.J., Colditz, G.A., Rosner, B.A., Hennekens, C.H. & Speizer, F.E. (1987). Dietary fat and the risk of breast cancer. *N. Engl. J. Med.*, **316**, 22–8.

Wynder, E.L. & Gori, G.B.(1977). Contributions of the environment to cancer incidence: an epidemiologic exercise (guest editorial). *J. Natl. Cancer Inst.*, **58**, 825–32.

Zaridze, D.G., Muir, C.S. & McMichael, A.J. (1985). Diet and cancer: Value of different types of epidemiological studies. In *Diet and Human Carcinogenesis*, ed. J.V. Joossens, M.J. Hill & J. Geboers, pp. 221–33. New York: Excerpta Medica.

Ziegler, R.G., Mason, T.J., Stemhagen, A., Hoover, R., Schoenberg, J.B., Gridley, G., Virgo, P.W. & Fraumeni, J.F., Jr. (1986). Carotenoid intake, vegetables, and the risk of lung cancer among white men in New Jersey. *Am. J. Epidemiol.*, **123**, 1080–93.

13

Physical factors: fiber carcinogenesis (including crystalline silicates)

13.1 Asbestos

Although known in Roman times, it was not until the late nineteenth century that fibrous silicate minerals were found to be commercially useful and were employed widely in fire-proofing and in the reinforcement of cement in construction material. The modern asbestos industry dates from the discovery of large deposits of chrysotile in Canada and Russia (Bogovski *et al.*, 1973). Asbestos fibers are now regarded as representing an important and possibly unique carcinogenic hazard in the ambient environment or work-place and are probably the most important occupational risk ever identified.

13.2 Nature of asbestos

Asbestos is the generic name used for a group of naturally occurring mineral silicate fibers of the serpentine and amphibole series with length/diameter ratios of over 3:1. Government agencies in various countries and industrial groups currently characterize six fibrous silicates as 'asbestos' (Speil & Leineweber, 1969; Mossman & Gee, 1989): the fibrous serpentine mineral chrysotile and the fibrous amphiboles actinolite, amosite, anthophyllite, crocidolite and tremolite. Current usage of the term asbestos is restricted to these specific silicates. Many other minerals with a fibrous crystalline structure occur naturally, but either do not possess the properties of asbestos, such as heat stability, thermal and electrical insulation, the ability to be woven, stability in acids/alkalis, or they do not occur in sufficient concentrations for commercial exploitation. Tremolite is not exploited as an asbestos mineral but is prevalent in many parts of the world as a contaminant of other forms of asbestos and ores.

In 1976, the production of asbestos was over 5 billion kg, and over 3000 uses were identified including asbestos cement sheets and pipes, insulation material, taping compound and floor and ceiling tiles (IARC, 1977). An important use was friction materials such as brakes for automobiles, railroad cars and airplanes. The asbestos content of a product does not indicate its relative health risk, as in many products the fibers are tightly bound to the matrix or are encapsulated. The potential risk arises when the asbestos fibers are set free, e.g. during drilling or sawing of asbestos cement sheets or in their removal.

13.3   Cancer and asbestos

It has long been recognized that asbestos mining and manufacturing cause pneumoconiosis (asbestosis). By the late 1930s the need to reduce exposures was widely accepted. However, the danger in downstream users who were not directly concerned in production or manufacture, e.g. insulators, was not generally appreciated. In the 1940s asbestosis began increasingly to be suspected as possibly inducing carcinoma of the lung, based on autopsy studies. An increase in lung cancer in asbestos workers was confirmed epidemiologically in the mid-1950s by Doll (1955). Later, Wagner and co-workers (1960) demonstrated that pleural mesothelioma could result from low-level exposures to asbestos, even following long latent periods.

At a historic meeting in New York in 1964, a mass of new material was made available, which included reports on cancer risk in secondary industries using asbestos (Selikoff *et al.*, 1965; Gilson, 1965). The need became urgent to determine in which industries hazardous exposures occurred, which type or types of asbestos were responsible for the carcinogenic effect and to clarify dose–responses as a basis for future preventive strategies. An international committee on asbestos and cancer was established in 1964 by the UICC with the objective of developing a global program to coordinate, define and standardize research and clinical activities. In 1966, the International Agency for Research on Cancer (IARC) took over and later expanded the work of the UICC committee to include synthetic fibers.

By the early 1970s it was accepted that this valuable substance, widely used for protecting against fire hazards, etc., could constitute a significant cancer hazard not only in the traditional asbestos industries but also in other environments where an asbestos hazard had previously not been suspected (Selikoff *et al.*, 1973; Bogovski *et al.*, 1973). The considerable new data that became available were summarized in a series of publications (Bogovski *et al.*, 1973; IARC, 1977, 1988; Wagner, 1980). It clearly causes cancer of the lung and more important it acts multiplicatively with cigarette smoking (Selikoff *et al.*, 1968). It is also the major cause of mesothelioma in industrial societies. A number of other cancers have also been associated with asbestos, e.g. larynx, stomach, etc. but the evidence is less strong and is discussed under individual sites (Wagner, 1980; IARC, 1988). For few carcinogens, apart from radiation and tobacco, has the state of knowledge in the scientific community at a specific period of time been so well documented. Such historical developments have been a matter of great importance in courts in the USA where they have become a major legal issue in compensation.

Occupational related exposures
It is now accepted that, in addition to asbestosis, an increased risk of lung cancer and mesothelioma occurs in any occupation or situation where levels of exposure are significantly above background. Such exposures have been found, for example, in ship-building, boiler laggers, insulators, etc. Mesotheliomas have been reported in individuals living in the neighborhood of an industrial source. In some of these, the level of exposure may have been quite considerable due to the contamination of the household by an asbestos worker bringing home contaminated clothes or by dust escaping from a plant within the neighborhood.

Non-occupational exposures
In recent years, concern regarding asbestos exposure has extended to the possibility that its former use in construction today represents an environmental cancer hazard to occupants in public buildings, shops, schools, etc., especially where maintenance has been poor (Mossman & Gee, 1989). This has led to the organization of extensive programs to remove the fiber from such buildings. There is controversy, however, as to whether removal may always be necessary and may not sometimes create a greater risk to the individual worker than if the asbestos were controlled *in situ*.

Asbestos fibers have now been found in the lungs of most individuals in industrial countries where the problem has been studied. It is believed, however, that this background level from multiple sources seems no imminent hazard and is unrelated to background lung cancer or mesothelioma rates. These issues are further discussed in a number of recent reviews (Bignon *et al.*, 1989; Bignon, 1989; Berry *et al.*, 1989; Peto, 1989). There is no convincing evidence of an effect on humans of fibers in water.

13.4   Other fibers and silicates
The IARC (1987) reviewed a number of other fibers and silicates used in industry, such as silica, wollastonite, attapulgite, sepiolite, talc and erionite used in industry. Fibrous minerals, other than asbestos, exist in

Table 13.1. *Minerals and vitreous fibers (excluding asbestos).*

Man-made vitreous fibers
  Glass
  Mineral wool
  Refractory fiber (aluminium silicate)

Synthetic crystalline fibers
  Alumina
  Silicon carbide
  Sodium aluminium carbonate
  Potassium titanate
  Graphite

Natural mineral fibers
  Wollastonite
  Attapulgite
  Sepiolite
  Amphiboles
  Zeolites

(After Leinweber, 1984.)

nature as contaminants of rocks and ores and may be released during mining, milling or processing (Bignon *et al.*, 1989). Talc, for example, may be contaminated with asbestos fibers including tremolite, anthophyllite and chrysolite.

Erionite is a fibrous zeolite, and the general public is exposed incidentally as it is present with other zeolites in some rocks. An unusual ambient exposure to naturally occurring erionite fibers has been demonstrated in Cappadocia in Central Turkey, where air borne fiber levels are unusually high in villages where vastly increased rates of mesothelioma and lung cancer are reported (Bignon *et al.*, 1989; Baris *et al.*, 1987).

Apart from crystalline silica (quartz), for which the evidence for lung cancer was described by IARC as limited in humans and sufficient in animals, other silicates show no convincing evidence of carcinogenicity.

13.5   Man-made mineral fibers (MMMF)

As the risks associated with asbestos exposure became increasingly recognized, intensive efforts were made to find appropriate substitutes, including the so-called man-made mineral fibers (MMMF) (Table 13.1). Today, the usage of MMMF is about equal to that of asbestos. There has been great interest in evaluating the various types of MMMFs since certain types fall within the range of fiber size believed to be dangerous, as exemplified by asbestos. In 1976, a major co-operative study involving European industry, the IARC and WHO was set up to investigate the issue (Simonato *et al.*, 1987). This coincided with a similar study in the USA (Walton & Coppock, 1987). At a meeting to review these studies, it was concluded that, for buccal cavity, pharynx, larynx, bladder and rectum, while increases in mortality and cancer incidence were sometimes observed, they were not large or consistently related to time since exposure. Taking into consideration animal experiments, it was concluded that these increases were irrelevant (IARC, 1988). For mesothelioma, no excesses were found. For lung cancer, an elevation of mortality was found among workers with at least 20 years since first exposure. This was particularly true for the early technological period of rock-wool and slag-wool production, where high levels of exposures could have occurred. This increase could not be explained by tobacco but there were a number of inconsistencies, including the lack of a dose response and the possible influence of such confounding variables as use of arsenic and polycyclic aromatic hydrocarbons. No increased risk was found after the introduction of dust suppressing agents (Simonato *et al.*, 1987).

13.6   Mechanisms of fiber carcinogenesis

Asbestos appears to be a complete carcinogen, possibly with genotoxic activities, but it may also be a promoter. The view that the carcinogenic properties of fiber depend on the chemical nature of the fiber or contamination by other chemicals such as PAHs is no longer held.

Recent research efforts have concentrated on its physical properties. A fiber is defined as a long thin filament of material of high tensile strength and flexibility with a ratio of length to mean width of > 10 to 1 and cross section of < 0.05 mm^2 to < 0.25 mm^2. Fibers are usually divided into respiratory and non-respiratory categories according to their physical parameters (Walton & Coppock, 1987).

Fiber type, fiber size, deposition, dissolution and migration are all factors of importance in determining carcinogenic potential, especially after inhalation. On intra-pleural injection, long thin fibers are the most potent in producing mesothelioma. It is considered that fibers > 8 μm in length and < 0.25 μm in diameter are equally carcinogenic, irrespective of their source. Short fibers from amosite and chrysotile are much less carcinogenic; the latter, penetrating the lung easily, are cleared more quickly. Analysis of lung tissues suggest that fibers of amosite and chrysotile < 5 μm in length may be relatively innocuous. This is a factor of importance in evaluating the asbestos cancer hazard in the non-occupational environment, especially in buildings containing asbestos-based insulation where almost all fibers are $< 5\,\mu\text{m}$ in length (Davis, 1989). For bronchogenic carcinoma, all types of asbestos have been identified as potential causes although chrysotile, due to its more rapid clearance from the lung, may be less hazardous. Erionite is considered highly carcinogenic.

The measurement of asbestos and other fibers in air, tissues, etc., is now dependent on sophisticated methodologies which both identify types of fiber and measure their number (Bignon *et al.*, 1989). Measurements can be made in the whole lung at autopsy to determine the type and degree of the fiber burden and evaluate more objectively the extent of past exposure. Such investigations may complement epidemiological studies. 'Asbestos bodies', sometimes called 'ferruginous' visible on light microscopy are composed of protein, iron, etc. They are present in sputum and tissues of individuals exposed to asbestos at higher levels but do not represent as accurately as other methods the asbestos burden in the lung.

The extensive physical analyses and experimental studies in animals are reviewed fully in a number of publications (Bogovski, 1973; IARC, 1977, 1987, 1988; Bignon *et al.*, 1989).

13.7   Conclusions

The IARC (1987) concluded that 'the studies of the carcinogenic effect of asbestos exposure, including evidence reviewed earlier, show that occupational exposure to chrysotile, amosite and anthophyllite asbestos and to mixtures containing crocidolite results in an increased risk of lung cancer, as does exposure to minerals containing tremolite and actinolite and to tremolitic material mixed with anthophyllite and small amounts of chrysotile. Mesotheliomas have been observed after occupational exposure to crocidolite, amosite, tremolitic material and chrysotile asbestos. Gastrointestinal cancers occurred at an increased incidence in groups occupationally exposed to crocidolite, amosite, chrysotile or mixed fibers containing crocidolite, although not all studies are consistent in this respect. An excess of laryngeal cancer has also been observed in some groups of exposed workers. No clear excess of cancer has been associated with presence of asbestos fibers in drinking water. Mesotheliomas have occurred in individuals living in the neighborhood of asbestos factories and mines and in people living with asbestos workers'.

The problem of asbestos control relates to whether or not there is a level of exposure which, for practical purposes, can be accepted by society as representing a trivial hazard. The political overtones and the polemics surrounding this subject are well documented in a series of recent letters in Science (1990). There is disagreement of views between the USA and that of other countries; the EPA proposes eventually banning asbestos completely whereas the International Labor Organization (ILO) representing over 100 countries suggests that chrysotile can be used with reasonable safety under certain stringent conditions – especially in view of the uncertainty regarding substitutes.

The risk for MMMF seems to be very much less Doll (1989) has stated that the environmental risk may be so small that an informed society would wish to ignore it.

13.8   References

Baris, I., Simonato, L., Artvinli, M., Pooley, F., Saracci, R., Skidmore, J. & Wagner, C. (1987). Epidemiological and environmental evidence of the health effects of exposure to erionite fibres: a four-year study in the Cappadocian region of Turkey. *Int. J. Cancer.*, **39**, 10–17.

Berry, G., Rogers, A.J. & Pooley, F.D. (1989). Mesotheliomas-asbestos exposure and lung burden. In *Non-Occupational Exposure to Mineral Fibres*, ed. J. Bignon, J. Peto & R. Saracci, IARC Scientific Publications No. 90, pp. 486–96. Lyon: International Agency for Research on Cancer.

Bignon, J. (1989). Mineral fibres in the non-occupational environment. In *Non-Occupational Exposure to Mineral Fibres*, ed. J. Bignon, J. Peto & R. Saracci, IARC Scientific Publications No. 90, pp. 3–29. Lyon: International Agency for Research on Cancer.

Bignon, J., Peto, J. & Saracci, R. (eds.) (1989). *Non-occupational Exposure to Mineral Fibres*, IARC Scientific Publications No. 90. Lyon: International Agency for Research on Cancer.

Bogovski, P., Gilson, J.C., Timbrell, V. & Wagner, J.C. (eds.) (1973). *Biological Effects of Asbestos*, Proceedings of a Working Conference held at the International Agency for Research on Cancer, Lyon, France, 2–6 October 1972, IARC Scientific Publications No. 8. Lyon: International Agency for Research on Cancer.

Davis, J.M.G. (1989). Mineral fibre carcinogenesis: experimental data relating to the importance of fibre type, size, deposition, dissolution and migration. In *Non-Occupational Exposure to Mineral Fibres*, IARC Scientific Publications No. 90, ed. J. Bignon, J. Peto & R. Saracci. Lyon: International Agency for Research on Cancer.

Doll, R. (1955). Mortality from lung cancer in asbestos workers. *Br. J. Indust. Med.*, **12**, 81–6.

Doll, R. (1989). Mineral fibres in the non-occupational environment: concluding remarks. In *Non-Occupational Exposure to Mineral Fibres*, ed. J. Bignon, J. Peto & R. Saracci, IARC Scientific Publications No. 90, pp. 511–8. Lyon: International Agency for Research on Cancer.

Gilson, J.C. (1965). Problems and perspectives: The changing hazards of exposure to asbestos. *Ann. NY Acad. Sci.*, **132**, 696–705.

IARC (1977). *IARC Monographs on the Evaluation of Carcinogenic Risk of Chemicals to Man*, Asbestos, volume 14. Lyon: International Agency for Research on Cancer.

IARC (1987). *IARC Monographs on the Evaluation of the Carcinogenic Risk of Chemicals to Humans*, Silica and some silicates, volume 42, Erionite, pp. 225–39. Lyon: International Agency for Research on Cancer.

IARC (1988). *IARC Monographs on the Evaluation of Carcinogenic Risks to Humans*, Man-made mineral fibres and radon, volume 43. Lyon: International Agency for Research on Cancer.

Leineweber, J.P. (1984). Solubility of fibres *in vitro* and *in vivo*. In *Biological Effects of Man-made Mineral Fibres*, vol. 2, pp. 87–102. Copenhagen: World Health Organization.

Mossman, B.T. & Gee, B.L. (1989). Asbestos-related diseases. *N. Engl. J. Med.*, **320**, 1721–30.

Peto, J. (1989). Fibre carcinogenesis and environmental hazards. In *Non-Occupational Exposure to Mineral Fibres*, ed. J. Bignon, J. Peto & R. Saracci, IARC Scientific Publications No. 90, pp. 457–70. Lyon: International Agency for Research on Cancer.

Science (1990). Asbestos carcinogenicity and public policy, letters to editor. *Science*, **248**, 795–802.

Selikoff, I.J., Churg, J. & Hammond, E.C. (1965). The occurrence of asbestosis among insulation workers in the United States. *Ann. NY Acad. Sci.*, **132**, 139–55.

Selikoff, I.J., Hammond, E.C. & Churg, J. (1968). Asbestos exposure, smoking and neoplasia. *JAMA*, **204**, 106–12.

Selikoff, I.J., Hammond, E.C. & Seidman, H. (1973). Cancer risk of insulation workers in the United States. In *Biological Effects of Asbestos*, Proceedings of a Working Conference held at the International Agency for Research on Cancer, Lyon, France, 2–6 October 1972, IARC Scientific Publications No. 8, ed. P. Bogovski, J.C. Gilson, V. Timbrell & J.C. Wagner. Lyon: International Agency for Research on Cancer.

Simonato, L., Fletcher, A.C., Cherrie, J.W., Andersen, A., Bertazzi, P., Charnay, N., Claude, J., Dodgson, J., Esteve, J., Frentzel-Beyme, R., Gardner, M.J., Jensen, O., Olsen, J., Teppo, L., Winkelmann, R., Westerholm, P., Winter, P.D., Zocchetti, C. & Saracci, R. (1987). The International Agency for Research on Cancer historical cohort study of MMMF production workers in seven European countries: Extension of the follow-up. *Ann. Occup. Hyg.*, **31(4B)**, 602- 23.

Speil, S. & Leineweber, J.P. (1969). Asbestos minerals in modern technology. *Environ. Res.*, **2**, 166–208.

Wagner, J.C., Sleggs, C.A. & Marchand, P. (1960). Diffuse pleural mesothelioma and asbestos exposure in the north western Cape Province. *Br. J. Indust. Med.*, **17**, 260–71.

Wagner, J.C. (ed.) (1980). *Biological Effects of Mineral Fibres*, volumes 1 and 2, Proceedings of a Symposium held at the International Agency for Research on Cancer, Lyon, France, 25–27 September 1979. IARC Scientific Publications No. 30. Lyon: International Agency for Research on Cancer.

Walton, W.H. & Coppock, S.M. (eds.) (1987). Man-made mineral fibres in the working environment. *Ann. Occup. Hyg.*, **31(4B)**, 517–834.

14

Physical factors: implants and thermal chronic injury

14.1   Scars and foreign bodies

Epithelial tumors and fibrous scarring

Carcinomas arise in relation to scar formation as observed in schistosomiasis and asbestosis, but it is not clear to what extent the scar formation *per se* actually contributes to these tumors. Several reports suggest that squamous cell carcinoma of the skin may arise as a complication of chronic ulcers, chronic inflammatory skin diseases, burns and scars or even a single injury. Traditionally this complication has been reported mainly in dark-skinned populations from Africa and Asia (Camain *et al.*, 1972; Mulay, 1963), but has also been described in black Americans (Fleming *et al.*, 1975; Keith *et al.*, 1980). Case reports suggest that skin cancer occasionally complicates the scars of chronic skin diseases such as tuberculosis, leprosy, syphilis and discoid lupus (Keith *et al.*, 1980). Both basocellular carcinoma and dermatofibroma have been reported to develop in a smallpox vaccination scar (Ribeiro *et al.*, 1988).

In India, kangri cancer occurs in burn scars in the lower abdomen and thighs of people who use baskets (kangri) containing clay pots with burning charcoal to warm their bodies in winter (Mulay, 1963).

Soft tissue sarcomas (STS)

Foreign bodies

In rodents, the experimental transplant of a membrane, irrespective of its chemical nature, e.g. glass coverslip or plastic sheet, leads frequently to capsule formation followed by a soft tissue sarcoma.

In humans non-degradable foreign bodies, acquired by accident, implanted surgically, or following shrapnel wounds such as occurred in World War I, also lead to chronic tissue reaction with the formation of scar-like capsule. However, only rare isolated sarcomas have been reported.

At present, greatest concern relates to the surgical implantation of a non-degradable plastic or metal to replace human tissues. Although occasional STSs are reported, these arise surprisingly rarely despite the frequency with which such metallic plates or protheses are found implanted in a wide range of organs (Brand, 1982).

A vast number of breast implants comprised of various formulations of plastic have been made over the last 20 years, but cases of associated breast sarcomas remain extraordinarily rare, nor have there been any reports of increased breast cancer (Deapen *et al.*, 1986). Experience from war wounds suggests that 25% of such tumors should occur within 15 years and 50% within 25 years. Although the absence of reports so far is encouraging, it does not mean that such procedures are completely without risk. A soft-tissue sarcoma in a Japanese woman who had such an implant 19 years earlier has been reported recently (Kobayashi *et al.*, 1988). None the less, there seems little doubt that the ease with which such tumors are induced in animals is not reflected in humans.

Miscellaneous cancers

There is now a considerable literature regarding the origin of pulmonary cancers from tuberculous granulomas and cavities. Definitive conclusions are difficult in view of the overwhelming impact of cigarette smoking and the decrease in tuberculous disease (Richardson *et al.*, 1987). Malignant mesothelioma has also been reported to occur in old scars of the pleura, such as chronic empyema or therapeutic pneumothorax (Hillerdal & Berg, 1985). It has been suggested that radial scars of the breast may represent the earliest recognizable stage of tubular cancer and that about 50% of all invasive cancers origin could be traced to a radial scar. However, other studies do not support this view (Linell *et al.*, 1980; Nielsen *et al.*, 1987).

14.2   Physical and chronic thermal injury in esophageal cancer

It has been suspected that physical and thermal chronic irritation of the esophagus may predispose to cancer, but firm evidence has been difficult to obtain (Chapter 25).

Silica fibers and fragments are common contaminants of coarse breads eaten by the high-risk populations of Iran, Transkei and China (Cook-Mozaffari *et al.*, 1979). In the high-risk areas of Henan, China, millet bran from which bread was made was found to contain up to 70% of silica by weight. Silica was also found in the esophageal mucosa surrounding tumors in patients from this area in amounts ten times higher than that found in tissue from a control group from London. It has been postulated that these silica fragments produce trauma and may also be able to stimulate proliferation by lodging in the esophageal mucosa (O'Neill *et al.*, 1986).

Esophageal thermal injury resulting from drinking hot beverages is difficult to study epidemiologically, since interviews do not provide reliable objective data on temperature. However, studies from Japan, Iran, the Soviet Union and Singapore indicate that people from high-risk areas for esophageal cancer tend to drink tea and other beverages at hotter temperatures than people from low-risk areas. Similar differences have been observed between esophageal cancer cases and controls (Day & Muñoz, 1982; Ghadirian, 1987).

Studies in high-risk areas of South America may provide more satisfactory information. Most local people in such areas drink large quantities of a local tea called maté which is drunk very hot through a metal straw. Approximately 20% of the adult population never drink maté. Case-control studies in Uruguay, and Brazil indicate an increased risk of esophageal cancer from maté drinking even after adjusting for alcohol and tobacco (Victora *et al.*, 1987; de Stefani *et al.*, 1990). Further, an endoscopic survey in Southern Brazil suggest that maté drinkers have a higher risk of developing precancerous lesions of the esophagus than non-drinkers (Munøz *et al.*, 1987). There are two mechanisms by which maté drinking could increase the risk of esophageal cancer. First, maté leaves may contain initiating carcinogenic or promoting substances, or, second, chronic thermal injury may increase the susceptibility of the esophagus to carcinogens. Epidemiological studies lend some support to the latter possibility (IARC, 1990).

14.3   References

Brand, K.G. (1982). Cancer associated with asbestosis, schistosomiasis, foreign bodies, and scars. In *Cancer 1. A Comprehensive Treatise. Etiology: Chemical and Physical Carcinogenesis*, ed. F.F. Becker, pp. 661–92. New York: Plenum Press.

Camain, R., Tuyns, A.J., Sarrat, H., Quenum, C. & Kaye, I. (1972). Cutaneous cancer in Dakar. *J. Natl. Cancer Inst.*, **48**, 33–49.

Cook-Mozaffari, P.J., Azordegan, F., Day, N.E., Ressicaud, A., Sabai, C. & Aramesh, B. (1979). Oesophageal studies in the Caspian littoral of Iran: results of a case-control study. *Br. J. Cancer*, **39**, 293–309.

Day, N.E. & Muñoz, N. (1982). Esophagus. In *Cancer Epidemiology and Prevention*, ed. Schottenfeld, D. & Fraumeni, J.F. Jr., pp. 596–623. Philadelphia: Saunders.

Deapen, D.M., Pike, M.C., Casagrande, J.T. & Brody, G.S. (1986). The relationship between breast cancer and augmentation mammaplasty: An epidemiologic study. *Plast. Reconstr. Surg.*, **77**, 361–7.

De Stefani, E., Muñoz, N., Esteve, J., Vasallo, A., Victora C. & Teuchmann S.V. (1990). Maté Drinking, alcohol, tobacco, diet and oesophageal cancer in Uruguay. *Cancer Res.* **50**: 426–31.

Fleming, I.D., Barnawell, J.R., Burlison, P.E. & Rankin, J.S. (1975). Skin cancer in black patients. *Cancer*, **35**, 600–5.

Ghadirian, P. (1987). Thermal irritation and esophageal cancer in Northern Iran. *Cancer*, **60**, 1909–14.

Hillerdal, G. & Berg, J. (1985). Malignant mesothelioma secondary to chronic inflammation and old scars. Two new cases and a review of the literature. *Cancer*, **55**, 1968–72.

IARC (1990). *IARC Monographs on the Evaluation of Carcinogenic Risks to Humans*, Coffee, tea, maté, methylxanthines and methylglyoxal, volume 51. Lyon: International Agency for Research on Cancer.

Keith, W.D., Kelly, A.P., Sumrall, A.J. & Chabra, A. (1980). Squamous cell carcinoma arising in lesions of discoid lypus erythematosus in black persons. *Arch. Dermatol.*, **116**, 315–17.

Kobayashi, S., Iwase, H., Karamatsu, S., Masaoka, A. & Nakamura, T. (1988). A case of stromal sarcoma of the breast occurring after augmentation mammaplasty. *Gan. No Rinsho.*, **34**, 467–72.

Linell, F., Ljungberg, O. & Anderson, I. (1980). Breast carcinoma: Aspects of early stages, progression and related problems. *Acta Pathol. Microbiol. Immunol. Scand. [A]*, (Suppl.) **272**, 1–233.

Mulay, D.M. (1963). Skin cancer in India. *Natl. Cancer Inst. Monogr.*, **10**, 215–23.

Muñoz, N., Victora, C.G., Crespi, M., Saul, C., Braga, N.M., & Correa, P. (1987). Hot maté drinking and precancerous lesions of the oesophagus: an endoscopic survey in Southern Brazil. *Int. J. Cancer*, **39**, 708–9.

Nielsen, M., Christensen, L. & Andersen, J. (1987). Radial scars in women with breast cancer. *Cancer*, **59**, 1019–25.

O'Neill, C., Jordan, P., Bhatt, T. & Newman, R. (1986). Silica and oesophageal cancer. *Ciba Found. Symp.*, **121**, 214–30.

Ribeiro, R., Labareda, J.M. & Garcia e Silva, L. (1988). Basocellular carcinoma in a smallpox vaccination scar [Portuguese]. *Med. Cutan. Ibero. Lat. Am.*, **16**, 137–9.

Richardson, S., Hirsch, A., Ruffie, P. & Bickel, M. (1987). Relationship between tuberculous scar and carcinomas of the lung. *Eur. J. Radiol.*, **7**, 163–4.

Victora, C.G., Muñoz, N., Day, N.E., Barcelos, L.B., Peccin, D.A., & Braga, N.M. (1987). Hot beverages and oesophageal cancer in Southern Brazil: a case-control study. *Int. J. Cancer*, **39**, 710–16.

15

Physical factors: ultraviolet (UV) light

15.1   Introduction

Certain types of ultraviolet (UV) light are strongly carcinogenic. Yet complete avoidance of exposure is almost impossible. Further, ultraviolet light is indispensable, permitting the skin to synthesize vitamin D, complementing that derived from dietary sources.

15.2   Spectrum of ultraviolet light

The UV portion of the electromagnetic spectrum occupies the wavelengths between 200 nm and 400 nm. It is customary to distinguish between UV-C (200–280 nm), UV-B (280–320 nm) and UV-A (320–400 nm), each having different effects on the skin and eye. The shorter the wavelength, the more destructive the radiation.

Ultraviolet light below 295 nm is totally absorbed by the oxygen and ozone of the atmosphere, that between 295 and 329 nm being partially absorbed. The more oblique the sun's rays, the greater thickness of atmosphere which has to be traversed and hence the shorter rays are diffused or absorbed. Considerable amounts of ultraviolet light may be reflected, thus the combination of snow and blue sky may expose the skin to as much UV-B (310 nm) as comes from the sky directly.

15.3   Effects

The amount of UV light reaching the melanocyte varies by wavelength. UV-A penetrates into the dermis, between 1 to 10% reaching the basal layer, a depth practically never reached by UV-C. Heavy skin pigmentation is, of course, protective. Sunburn is maximal about 24 hours after exposure to UV-B, occurring more rapidly than for UV-A. Damage to DNA parallels the erythema (Parrish, 1982). Prolonged exposure to UV-B gives rise to bronzing and a thickening of the epidermis.

The most striking effects, including mutation, on skin are nearly always due to UV-B. The spectrum of UV-B is very close to the absorption spectrum of DNA, and the photons absorbed by the DNA molecule give rise to damage which is normally repaired. When repair mechanisms are absent, as for example, in xeroderma pigmentosum, skin cancers may appear.

White-skinned persons fall into four phototypes as follows:

(a) always burns and does not tan (180 J/min);
(b) burns easily, tans very little (280 J/min);
(c) burns occasionally, tans well (400 J/min);
(d) burns rarely, tans very easily (650 J/min).

The figures given in brackets represent the number of joules/minute required to provoke a minimal erythemal dose by UV light of 297 nm on non-tanned skin.

Prolonged exposure to the sun gives rise to loss of elasticity of the skin, notably for phototypes (a) and (b). This is frequently associated with pigmented spots and solar keratoses which may develop into squamous cell carcinomas. These observations are reproducible in mice.

15.4 Effect of chemicals on photosensitivity

Many substances applied to, or ingested by, the skin substantially augment the skin sensitivity to UV light. These include such drugs as the tetracyclines, sulphonamides and the phenothiazines. The psoralens used for the treatment of psoriasis are effective through induction of photosensitivity. They also, however, enhance the mutagenic and carcinogenic action of ultraviolet light (Stern & Lange, 1988), but are, none the less, incorporated in some sunscreens.

15.5 Artificial light

Although lamps to induce tanning should emit UV-A almost exclusively, none the less, doses of UV-B escape at levels which have been shown to cause mutation in cell culture and cancer in mice. The increasing use of halogen lamps may give rise to considerable exposure around 230 nm: thus a 100 watt halogen source used as an office lamp some 20 cm from the hands over 1000 hours gives rise to a dose of 400 dem, that is about as much as agricultural workers would receive in a year,

Fluorescent lamps do not completely block the UV-B. Despite the report of Beral *et al.* (1982) of an increased risk of malignant melanoma, it is probable that such exposures, perhaps 9 dem a year from using appropriately shielded lamps, are of little significance.

15.6   Ozone

It is believed that global increases in UV exposure at ground level will probably occur over the coming decades due to stratospheric ozone decreases from a number of factors. To evaluate the impact on skin cancer, careful analyses of future levels will be required.

15.7   Further discussion

The effects of exposure to ultraviolet light are considered in further detail with malignant melanoma and the other forms of skin cancer.

15.8   References

Beral, V., Shaw, H., Evans, H. & Milton, G. (1982). Malignant melanoma and exposure to fluorescent lighting at work. *Lancet*, **ii**, 290–3.

Parrish, J.A., Jaenicke, K.F. & Anderson, R.R. (1982). Erythema and melanogenesis action spectra of normal human skin. *Photochem. Photobiol.*, **36**, 187–91.

Stern, R.S. & Lange, R. (and members of the Photothemotherapy Follow-up Study) (1988). Non-melanoma skin cancer occurring in patients treated with pUVA five to ten years after first treatment. *J. Invest. Dermatol.*, **91**, 120–4.

16

Ionizing radiation

ELISABETH CARDIS
International Agency for Research on Cancer

16.1 Introduction

Detrimental effects of exposure to ionizing radiation, including toxicity, burns and tumor induction, became noticeable very early in the history of radiology. Many pioneer radiation researchers died of neoplasms, among them were Thomas Edison's assistant and Marie Curie. This pattern became clear in the 1940s with the observation of a high incidence of leukemia among radiologists. In the 1930s, a high incidence of osteosarcoma was noted among luminous dial painters who were in the habit of licking the point of their paintbrushes, to make them thinner, thus ingesting radium (Rowland *et al.*, 1978). In the 1950s, a high incidence of leukemia was also detected among survivors of the atomic bombings in Hiroshima and Nagasaki (Folley *et al.*, 1952) and among patients treated with X-rays for ankylosing spondylitis (Court Brown & Doll, 1957).

Many animal experiments and epidemiological studies have been carried out since then to elucidate the mechanisms of radiation-induced carcinogenesis (BEIR III, 1980; UNSCEAR, 1977). It is now accepted that ionizing radiation can induce cancer in most tissues, although there are great differences in organ susceptibility. The role of ionizing radiation in human carcinogenesis is probably the best understood and quantified of all exogenous physical and chemical agents (BEIR V, 1989; UNSCEAR, 1988). Available information is based predominantly on studies of large populations receiving high dose exposures of short duration. Uncertainties remain, however, in particular about the magnitude of the risk associated with low dose exposures received over prolonged periods of time, such as those received by large populations in their occupational or residential environment (e.g. domestic radon).

16.2   Biophysical mechanisms of radiation damage

The physics of radiation are fairly well understood but the biological effects are more complicated. The term *ionizing radiation* encompasses both electromagnetic radiation (such as X- and gamma-rays) and subatomic particles (electrons, protons, neutrons, alpha particles). X- and gamma-rays are *indirectly ionizing radiations* in that their energy deposition in the tissues is through secondary electrons. These electrons, as all *directly ionizing radiations*, can damage DNA directly or can interact with water, leading to the formation of hydroxyl radicals that can interact with DNA. Neutrons are another type of *indirectly ionizing radiation*, in that they interact with the nuclei of atoms of the absorber, setting in motion recoil protons and heavy nuclear fragments which cause ionization throughout the tissue. Energy is deposited along the track of the ionizing particles, but the spatial distribution of the ionizing events varies with radiations that have different velocities, charges and masses. X- and gamma-rays are sparsely ionizing, the ionizing events being few and far between, but they can penetrate deeply into the body. Neutrons are densely ionizing. Alpha particles with energies of environmental interest are also very densely ionizing with very short penetration, and can be stopped by the skin layer. The difference in the ionizing pattern of different radiation types is very important since it implies that, for cancer and for biological damage in general, equal levels of exposure do not cause equal effects at least in some organs.

The amount of repair of biological damage varies with the type of radiation and there is little repair following densely ionizing radiation. Repair also varies with the temporal distribution of an exposure. Accordingly, for equal total doses of gamma and X-rays, more of the damage will be repaired for fractionated and protracted exposures than for acute exposures.

The concept of *Quality Factor* (QF), and, in particular, of *Relative Biological Effectiveness* (RBE) of a given radiation, was introduced to unify the notion of biological damage due to radiation. It is defined as the ratio of the dose of a reference radiation and of the radiation of interest required to produce equal biological effects; 250 keV X-rays or ^{60}Co X-rays are usually used as the reference. It is a function of many factors, including dose, temporal pattern of exposure, radiation type, biological system under consideration and specific end-point selected, e.g. cancer of a specific site or degree of cell damage. Energy deposition patterns clearly affect malignant transformation, sparsely ionizing radiation being less efficient than more densely ionizing radiations, although the exact mechanisms are currently unknown.

Estimates of RBEs for cancer have been derived based on results of epidemiological analyses and experiments on animals. The RBE for neutrons is often taken to be in the range of 5–10, depending on the site. However, various regulatory agencies are now considering the possibility of raising their estimate of quality factors for neutrons from 10 to 20; this would imply lowering levels of permitted exposures, especially in reactor environments when the neutron component of the total dose may be important.

16.3 Pertinent animal and *in vitro* experiments

Ionizing radiation can induce biological changes both *in vivo* and *in vitro* in mammalian cells. These changes include loss of proliferative capacity, mutations, chromosome aberrations and neoplastic transformation. Many experiments, mostly since the early 1950s (BEIR III, 1980; UNSCEAR, 1977) have been carried out specifically to elucidate the mechanism of radiation-induced carcinogenesis, by studying the following:

- the difference in radio-sensitivity of tissues and whole animal systems;
- the difference in carcinogenic potential of radiation of varying types;
- dose–response curves: low and high dose ranges;
- the effect of exposure fractionation and dose rate;
- the effect of combined exposures to radiation and other carcinogenic agents.

The most comprehensive experiments were performed on many thousands of mice in the United States (see, for example, those of Ullrich & Storer, 1979*a*, *b*, *c*). However, no simple conclusion can be drawn, even from these very large experiments, since the effects of dose and dose rate are complex and may vary from tissue to tissue. Further, tissue sensitivity and tumor expression may be influenced by hormonal status and by exposure to other carcinogens (chemical, physical or viral).

16.4 Epidemiological studies

The most informative epidemiological studies of radiation carcinogenesis have been carried out on populations exposed to high levels of ionizing radiation, notably the atomic bomb survivors in Hiroshima and Nagasaki, patients treated with radiation for medical

Table 16.1. *Selected examples of radiation-induced cancers.*

Sources of exposure	Exposure circumstances	Type of cancer reported[a]
Explosions of nuclear weapons		
blast	Atomic bombing survivors in Hiroshima and Nagasaki	Leukemia, breast, lung, thyroid, stomach, colon, bladder, multiple myeloma, esophagus, ovary
fall-out	Populations exposed through atmospheric testing, including Marshall Islanders, veterans in the Pacific, general population in Nevada, Utah	Thyroid, (leukemia)
Diagnostic procedures		
X-rays	Children exposed *in utero* (1950–60s)	Leukemia
thorotrast (thorium dioxide)	Cerebral and limb angiography, X-ray of biliary passages (prior to 1951)	Liver, (bone)
fluoroscopic X-rays	Monitoring of lung infection in patients with tuberculosis	Breast cancer in women
Therapeutic procedures		
X-ray	Post-partum mastitis	Breast
X-ray	Ankylosing spondylitis	Leukemia, lung, stomach, esophagus, (kidney, bladder, pancreas)
Cobalt 60 X-ray and others	Treatment for cancer of the cervix	Leukemia, stomach, rectum, bladder, vagina, female genital, lung, buccal cavity, nasopharynx, esophagus
X-ray	Treatment for benign head and neck conditions (enlarged thymus, tinea capitis, etc.)	Thyroid, skin, CNS
Radium 224	Ankylosing spondylitis, bone tuberculosis	Bone sarcoma
Professional exposures		
X-ray	Early radiologists	Skin, leukemia
Radon	Uranium, and hard-rock mines	Lung cancer
X-ray, gamma rays, neutrons, some internal contamination	Nuclear industry	Multiple myeloma, (prostate, leukemia, lung)
Radium isotopes	Radium dial painters	Bone, head sarcoma

[a] Parenthesis indicate a suggestion of increased risk.

reasons and underground miners exposed to radon and its progeny (Table 16.1).

Atomic bomb survivors

Two years after the explosion of the bombs in 1945, the Atomic Bomb Casualty Commission was established, first in Hiroshima then in Nagasaki, to study the medical effects of the bombing. A cohort of close to 120,000 survivors was set up. Personal interviews were conducted to determine the exact location and position of each survivor and estimate their exposure to the radiation (mostly X-rays and neutrons) from the bomb. This cohort is still being systematically followed for cancer mortality and incidence according to levels of exposure. A further subset of 20,000 survivors receives a complete biennial medical examination.

In the first years following the bombing, increases in leukemia mortality were observed among the exposed survivors. Mortality from leukemia, excluding chronic lymphocytic leukemia (CLL), has stayed elevated and has started to decrease only recently. Since 1970, increased mortality from other tumors has been observed, especially tumors of the lung, oesophagus, stomach, colon, bladder, multiple myeloma in adults of both sexes and of breast and ovarian cancer (Shimizu *et al.*, 1988), as well as an increased incidence of thyroid cancer (Prentice *et al.*, 1982).

Although the increases are significant and dose-related, they are not very large in absolute terms. Among the 54,000 survivors exposed to 0.01 Gy (Gray) or more, 4026 deaths by cancer had been observed by 1982. This is approximately 150 (3.4%) more than would have been expected in a non-irradiated control population.

Medically irradiated populations

Several heavily exposed populations have been followed for cancer mortality or incidence. Their exposure history was reconstructed and the magnitude of their risk determined. In the UK, approximately 14,000 patients who received deep X-ray treatment to the spine and sacroiliac region for ankylosing spondylitis between 1935 and 1954 (Darby *et al.*, 1987) have been followed. Mortality from cancer of heavily irradiated sites was generally increased, becoming apparent about 10 years after treatment. Increase in leukemia mortality, which peaked at 3 to 5 years after irradiation and subsequently declined, was also observed; the increase in leukemia risk did not appear to be clearly related to the estimated bone marrow radiation dose.

An international case-control study, including 4188 women who developed second primary cancers and 6880 individual controls, within a cohort of 150,000 patients with cervical cancer who were treated with radiotherapy for cancer of the cervix, has been carried out by Boice *et al.* (1988). Estimated exposures were reconstructed from treatment records and simulations. Although therapeutic doses to the target and neighboring organs were orders of magnitude higher than the doses received by even the most highly exposed atomic bomb survivors, organs at some distance from the primary treatment field received doses closer to the environmental and occupational doses of current public concern. At very high levels of exposure, dose-related increases were observed for rectum, bladder, vagina and all female genital cancers. Increases were also observed for leukemia and stomach at moderate levels of exposure. None was seen for cancer of the breast. Elevated risks were also described for cancers of the lung, buccal cavity, nasopharynx and esophagus in the earlier cohort report (Boice *et al.*, 1985).

Large increases in risk of breast cancer have been observed among female tuberculous patients receiving multiple X-ray fluoroscopies. As in atomic bomb survivors, and in women treated with X-rays for postpartum mastitis, the risk was greater for those exposed at a younger age (10–14) (Miller *et al.*, 1989).

Studies of children irradiated for enlarged thymus and ringworm (Ron *et al.*, 1989; Modan *et al.*, 1989; BEIR V, 1989) have shown increases in thyroid cancer risk even at low dose levels, beginning as early as five years after exposure. An increased risk of brain and breast tumors was also observed. No increases have been observed, however due to radioactive iodine (UNSCEAR, 1988).

Numerous liver tumors, predominantly cholangiocellular carcinoma and hemangiosarcoma, have been observed in patients following exposure to thorotrast (containing thorium dioxide) for radio-diagnostic purposes many years earlier (Van Kaick *et al.*, 1984).

Children irradiated *in utero*

The sensitivity of the embryo to radiation-induced carcinogenesis has been extensively studied. Some studies showed no association; in the two largest studies, however, children whose mothers received diagnostic X-rays during pregnancy in the 1940s and 1950s had a 40–65% increased risk of cancer (Stewart *et al.*, 1956; Monson & MacMahon, 1984). No case of leukemia in children under 10 was reported among atomic bomb survivors exposed *in utero*. However, a large increase in risk of tumors in adults is now being reported (Yoshimoto *et al.*, 1988), although based on a small number of cases. If this increased risk continues, it would imply that those exposed *in utero* are also at a higher risk of cancer in adult life than those exposed after birth.

Miners

The follow-up of miners exposed to radon and its decay products in hard rock mines such as iron, gold and fluorspar, and particularly in uranium mines, currently provides the best available database for the study of cancer risk among populations with protracted exposure to alpha-emitting radiation (UNSCEAR, 1977; BEIR IV, 1988; IARC, 1988). Dose-related increases in risk of lung cancer have been consistently reported in these populations.

16.5   Current problems in radiation carcinogenesis

An increased carcinogenic risk has now been demonstrated consistently in many studies of populations receiving moderate to high doses of ionizing radiation. Problems exist in the assessment of such risks since current projection models are based mostly on the study of populations exposed acutely to high doses (atomic bombs; medical treatment) whose follow-up is still incomplete. Three-quarters of the atomic bomb survivor cohort was still alive in 1982. Today, public concern is mostly directed to the carcinogenic risks following protracted exposures to low doses of ionizing radiation in the ambient and work environment. Models for estimating such risks depend on assumptions for extrapolation from high to low doses, from acute to chronic exposures from one type of radiation to another, and for predicting lifetime risks from an incomplete follow-up. Predictions from these models vary greatly according to the assumptions used.

Although chronic low-dose exposures may not be more carcinogenic than acute high doses, it is important that this risk be quantified to ensure adequate protection standards for populations exposed to low doses.

The exposures of greatest concern include the following.

Workers employed in the nuclear industry

Despite numerous studies carried out to date on such subjects (BEIR V, 1989; UNSCEAR, 1988), there is, overall, little indication of a dose-related increase in all-cancer mortality. The power of most studies is so low that risks, an order of magnitude larger than those on which current radiation protection standards are based, cannot be excluded. Increased risks of multiple myeloma and of prostate cancers have been observed in several studies and need further examination.

Individuals living around nuclear facilities

Since 1983, a number of clusters of childhood leukemia and lymphoma have been reported in populations living near facilities where plutonium is manipulated (BEIR V, 1989; UNSCEAR, 1988). There are doubts about the adequacy of the methods used for identifying and studying some of these clusters; the risks are, moreover, much higher than would be expected based on current knowledge of radiation biology. Some authors have suggested that areas near existing and potential sites of nuclear installations may share unrecognized risk factors other than radiation contamination (Cook-Mozaffari *et al.*, 1989; Kinlen, 1988). In a recent case-control study, however, Gardner *et al.* (1990) have shown that the leukemia and non-Hodgkin's lymphoma increase in the Sellafield area in children is strongly associated with the father's level of occupational radiation exposures prior to conception. This suggests a possible prezygotic effect of radiation. A number of other studies in the UK, USA, Canada and France are currently under way to elucidate the role, if any, which radiation may play in the induction of such cancers.

Exposures due to the Chernobyl accident

Although the cancer risk to populations living in Western Europe and North America is likely to be extremely small, predictions vary by several orders of magnitude (0–10,000 excess deaths by cancer predicted over the next 50 years for the whole of Europe excluding the USSR (Anspaugh *et al.*, 1988)). Long-term follow-ups of populations through cancer registries may provide valuable information about the adequacy of prediction models for such low level exposures, but the evaluation of incidence may prove to be uninformative if the risk is low.

Fall-out from atmospheric weapons testing

A number of studies of military personnel participating in atmospheric weapons tests have been carried out (BEIR V, 1990; Pearce *et al.* 1990). Increases in leukemia risk have been observed among US, UK and New Zealand test participants although levels of external exposures are thought to be too low to explain them. Increases in leukemia and thyroid cancer risk have also been reported among US populations living near the Nuclear Test Site in Nevada (BEIR V).

Exposure from current diagnostic irradiation

Studies of persons exposed to diagnostic X-rays in the 1940s and 1950s have revealed excesses of cancers. Today, exposures are very much reduced, but the cost–benefit of numerous systematic X-rays, for example, during dental examinations, should be assessed carefully (Preston-Martin *et al.*, 1988).

Natural background radiation

Populations have been living in areas of high natural background radiation for millennia: exposure to cosmic rays increases with increasing altitude, as well as with decreasing distance from the poles; the radioactivity in granitic, schistic and sandstone areas is higher than in other areas. Although the problem had been considered earlier in Sweden, public opinion in the USA was alerted in 1984 by reports of several houses with levels of radon and its decay products several orders of magnitude higher than protection standards currently used in occupational environments. Current projection models for risks from residential exposures to radon are based on the experience of miners. Exposure levels in houses are typically much lower than in mines, even in areas of high natural background radiation and in houses built with radon emitting materials. Exposure may be different from that in mines because of such differences as ventilation and breathing rates; the extrapolation models may, therefore, not be adequate. To date, most epidemiological studies of residential radon exposures have shown little or no effect (Axelson *et al.*, 1988; UNSCEAR, 1988). The exposure assessment in these studies is however, difficult, and the power to identify a risk presumed to be small is quite low. Larger studies to estimate residential risk directly are now under way (UNSCEAR, 1988).

16.6   Distribution of sources of exposure

Mean annual exposure, based on the world population, is of the order of 2–3 mSv. More than two-thirds of this exposure is due to natural sources (Table 16.2). These values vary with, among other factors, location and type of housing, altitude and occupation: exposures from natural sources, excluding extreme values, range from 1.5 to 6 mSv.

16.7   Factors modifying radiation risk

Both dose level and duration of exposure are modifiers of carcinogenic risk. Age at exposure also affects subsequent risks, at least for certain types of tumors (BEIR V, 1990), with children being more sensitive than adults to the effects of radiation-induced carcinogenesis.

In addition, other exposures may affect the risk of radiation-induced cancer. The best documented is the enhancing effect of cigarette smoking on lung cancer risk. In atomic bomb survivors, radiation and cigarettes appear to have an additive effect (Prentice *et al.*, 1983), whereas, among

Table 16.2. *Distribution of average annual dose equivalent, internal and external, per person, based on world population by source (in mSv).*[a]

Natural sources		Human-made sources	
Cosmic rays	0.36	Medical diagnostic	0.4–1
Cosmogenic radionuclides	0.015	Medical therapeutic	0.03
Radioactivity of the earth, buildings, food, soil	2.00	Occupational and environmental contamination	0.02[b]
Radioactivity of our own bodies	0.2	Nuclear power production	0.002

[a] 1 Sv (sievert) is the Si unit for measuring effective dose equivalent: the energy deposited in tissue: 1 Sv = 100 rem (ICRU, 1985).
[b] Including fall-out from atmospheric weapons testing.
(After UNSCEAR, 1988.)

uranium miners, the effect is closer to multiplicative (BEIR IV, 1988). This difference is most likely due to differences in patterns of exposure to radiation – being acute for atomic bomb survivors and protracted for uranium miners.

16.8   Conclusions

Ionizing radiation can induce cancer in a range of tissues, even at comparatively low doses. The carcinogenic risk and the latent period between exposure and disease can vary with cancer type, exposure characteristics, age at exposure and tissue sensitivity. Infants and young adults may be more sensitive to induction of leukemia and breast cancer than older individuals.

16.9   Electromagnetic fields

Exposure to extremely low frequency (ELF, 0–300 Hz) electromagnetic fields has recently been suspected of increasing the risk for cancer, especially acute myeloid leukemia. A number of studies of men likely to have been occupationally exposed to ELF fields, have been carried out in different countries, using indirect assessment of exposure. These have shown, with some consistency, increased rates of some 20% for incidence of or mortality from leukemia, and notably 45% for the acute myeloid form (Coleman & Beral, 1988). These results probably indicate a true increase in risk. Studies based on detailed direct assessment of exposure are currently being carried out (IARC *ad hoc* working group, 1990). Preliminary results of one such study among New York telephone workers (Matanoski *et al.*, 1989), based on a small number of individuals, indicate an increased risk of all cancers combined, as well as of leukemia and of lymphoma. These persons were employed in the job categories with the highest measured exposure to electric and magnetic fields. In several studies, leukemia and cancer risk have been examined in both adults and children in relation to residential exposure to ELF fields. The results are less consistent than those of the occupational studies. Increased risks for leukemia were seen among children, but only a few cases were available. The major problems in estimating risks are the ubiquity and the difficulties in measuring the exposure (IARC *ad hoc* working group, 1990).

16.10 References

Anspaugh, L.R., Catlin, R.J. & Goldman, M. (1988). The global impact of the Chernobyl reactor accident. *Science*, **242**, 1513–9.

Axelson, D., Andusso, K., Desai, G. *et al.* (1988). Indoor radon exposure and active and passive smoking in relation to the occurrence of lung cancer. *Scand. J. Work Environ. Health*, **14**, 286–92.

BEIR III (Committee on the Biological Effects of Ionizing Radiation) (1980). *The Effects on Populations of Exposure to Low Levels of Ionizing Radiation*. Washington: National Academy of Sciences.

BEIR IV (Committee on the Biological Effects of Ionizing Radiation) (1988). *Health Risks of Radon and Other Internally Deposited Alpha-Emitters*. Washington: National Academy of Sciences.

BEIR V (Committee on the Biological Effects of Ionizing Radiation) (1990). *Health Effects of Exposure to Low Levels of Ionizing Radiation*. Washington: National Academy of Sciences.

Boice, J.D., Day, N.E., Andusen, A., Brinton, L.A., Brown, R., Choi, N.W. *et al.* (1985). Second cancers following radiation treatment for cervical cancer. An international collaboration among cancer registries. *J. Natl. Cancer Inst.*, **74**, 945–75.

Boice, J.D., Engholm, G. *et al.* (1988). Radiation dose and second cancer risk in patients treated for cancer of the cervix. *Radiat. Res.*, **116**, 3–55.

Coleman M. & Beral V. (1988). A review of epidemiologic studies of the health effects of living near or working with electricity generation and transmission equipment. *Int. J. Epidemiol.*, **17**, 1–3.

Cook-Mozaffari, P., Darby, S. & Doll, R. (1989). Cancer near potential sites of nuclear installations. *Lancet*, **ii**, 1145–7.

Court Brown, W.M. & Doll, R. (1957). *Leukemia and Aplastic Anemia in Patients Irradiated for Ankylosing Spondylitis*. Medical Research Special Report Series No 295. London: HMSO.

Darby, S.C., Doll, R., Gill, S.K. & Smith, P.G. (1987). Long term mortality after a single treatment course with X-rays in patients treated for ankylosing spondylitis. *Br. J. Cancer*, **55**, 179–90.

Folley, H.H., Borges, W. & Yamasaki, T. (1952). Incidence of leukemia in survivors of the atomic bomb in Hiroshima and Nagasaki, Japan. *Am. J. Med.*, **13**, 311–21.

Gardner, M.J., Snee, M.P., Hall, A.J., Powell, C.A. & Terrell, J.D. (1990). Results of case-control study of leukaemia and lymphoma among young people near Sellafield nuclear plant in West Cumbria. *Br. Med. J.*, **300**, 432–9.

IARC *ad hoc* working group (1990). Extremely low frequency electric and magnetic fields and human cancer risks. Prepared by M. Coleman & E. Cardis. *Bioelectromagnetics*, **11**, 91–9.

IARC (1988). *Monographs on the Evaluation of Carcinogenic Risk to Humans*, Man-made mineral fibers and radon, volume 43. Lyon: International Agency for Research on Cancer.

ICRU (1985). *Determination of Dose Equivalents Resulting from External Radiation Sources*.

ICRU Report 39. Bethesda: International Commission on Radiation Units and Measurements.

Kinlen, L. (1988). Evidence for an infective cause of childhood leukemia: comparison of a Scottish New Town with nuclear reprocessing sites in Britain. *Lancet*, **ii**, 1323–6.

Matanoski, G.M., Elliott, E.A. & Breysse, P.N. (1989). Cancer incidence in New York telephone workers. Poster presented at the Annual Review of Research on Biological Effects of 50/60 Hz Electric and Magnetic Fields; November 15, 1989; Portland, Oregon.

Miller, A.B., Howe, G.R., Sherman, J., Lindsey, J., Yaffe, M., Dinner, M.,Risch, H., Preston, D.L. (1989). Mortality from breast cancer after irradiation during fluoroscopic examinations in patients being treated for tuberculosis. *N. Engl. J. Med.*, **321**, 1285–9.

Modan, B., Alfandary, E., Chetrit A., Katz, L. (1989). Increased risk of breast cancer after low-dose irradiation. *Lancet*, **i**, 629–31.

Monson, R.R. & MacMahon, B. (1984). Prenatal X-ray exposure and cancer in children. In *Radiation Carcinogenesis: Epidemiology and Biological Significance*, ed. J.D. Boice & J.F. Fraumeni, pp. 97–106. New York: Raven Press.

Pearce, N., Prior, J., Methren, D., Culling, C., Marshall, S., Auld, J., de Boer, G. & Bethwaite, P. (1990). Follow up of New Zealand participants in British atmospheric nuclear weapons tests in the Pacific. *Br. Med. J.*, **300**, 1161–6.

Prentice, R.L., Kato, H., Yoshimoto, K. & Mason, M.W. (1982). Radiation exposure and thyroid cancer incidence among Hiroshima and Nagasaki residents. *Natl. Cancer Inst. Monogr.*, **62**, 207–12.

Prentice, R.L., Yoshimoto, Y. & Mason, M.W. (1983). Relationship of cigarette smoking and radiation exposure to cancer mortality in Hiroshima and Nagasaki. *J. Natl. Cancer Inst.*, **70**, 611–22.

Preston-Martin, S., Thomas, D.G., White, S.C. & Cohen, D. (1988). Prior exposure to medical and dental X-rays related to tumors of the parotid gland. *J. Natl. Cancer Inst.*, **80**, 943–9.

Ron, E., Modan, B., Preston, D., Alfandary, E., Stavall, M. & Boice, J.D. (1989). Thyroid neoplasia following low-dose radiation in childhood. *Radiation Res.*, **120**, 516–31.

Rowland, R.E., Stehney, A.F. & Lucas, H.F., Jr. (1978). Dose-response relationships for female radium dial workers. *Radiat. Res.*, **76**, 368–83.

Shimizu, Y., Kato, H. & Schull, W.J. (1988). *Life Span Study Report II. Part 2. Cancer Mortality in the Years* 1950–85 *Based on the Recently Revised Doses* (*DS*86), RERF Technical Report 5–88. Hiroshima: RERF.

Stewart, A., Webb, J., Giles, D. & Hewitt, D. (1956). Malignant disease in childhood and diagnostic irradiation *in utero. Lancet*, **ii**, 447.

Ullrich, R.L. & Storer, J.B. (1979*a*). Influence of gamma irradiation on development of neoplastic disease in mice. I. Reticular tissue tumors. *Radiat. Res.*, **80**, 303–16.

Ullrich, R.L. & Storer, J.B. (1979*b*). Influence of gamma irradiation on the development of neoplastic disease in mice. II. Solid tumors. *Radiat. Res.*, **80**, 317–24.

Ullrich, R.L. & Storer, J.B. (1979*c*). Influence of gamma irradiation on the development of neoplastic disease in mice. III. Dose rate effects. *Radiat. Res.*, **80**, 325–42.

UNSCEAR (United Nations Scientific Committee on the Effects of Atomic Radiation) (1988). *Sources, Effects and Risks of Ionizing Radiation*. New York: United Nations.

UNSCEAR (United Nations Scientific Committee on the Effects of Atomic Radiation) (1977). *Sources and Effects of Ionizing Radiation*, 1977 Report. New York: United Nations.

Van Kaick, G., Muth, H., Kaul, A., Immich, H., Liebermann, D., Lorenz, D., Lorenz, W.J., Lührs, H., Scheer, K.E., Wagner, G., Wegener, K. & Wesch, H. (1984). Results of the German thorotrast study. In *Radiation Carcinogenesis: Epidemiology and Biological Significance*, ed. J.D. Boice & J.F. Fraumeni, pp. 253–62. New York: Raven Press.

Yoshimoto, Y., Kato, H. & Schull, W.J. (1988). Risk of cancer among children exposed *in utero* to A-bomb radiations, 1950–84. *Lancet*, **ii**, 665–9.

17

Biological causes

Parasites have been suspected to be causally associated with cancer of the bladder and liver for at least 80 years. A Nobel Prize was awarded to Fibiger for his report in 1913, of a nematode as the cause of gastric cancer in rats, which, unhappily, was later shown to be a misinterpretation of the data.

In contrast, despite the discovery by Rous early this century that viruses could cause neoplasms in animals, systematic work on the possible role of viral agents in human cancer did not begin until mid-century with recognition of the Bittner factor in milk in mammary cancer in mice and the vertical transmission of certain murine leukemias.

17.1   Viruses and cancer
Hepatocellular carcinoma (HCC) (Chapter 29)

Earlier studies linking liver cancer and hepatitis, although suspected since the 1940s, were handicapped by lack of techniques to identify the virus.

The extensive epidemiological and laboratory evidence that has established the presence of a strong and specific association between hepatitis B virus (HBV) and HCC has been reviewed by Szmuness (1978); Blumberg & London (1985); and Muñoz & Bosch (1987). A positive correlation exists in most studies between the incidence or mortality of HCC and the prevalence of HBsAg (hepatitis B surface antigen) carriers. However, there are as yet unexplained exceptions such as Greenland Eskimos with a high prevalence of HBsAg carriers and a low incidence rate of HCC (Melbye *et al.*, 1984). The association is restricted to the chronically active form of HBV infection characterized by the long-term presence of hepatitis B surface antigen (HBsAg) in the serum. Further aspects are discussed in Chapter 29.

Case-control studies in high and low risk populations have shown that the relative risks (RR) associated with HBsAg in the sera range from 10 to 20 in most studies, although some RRs are higher (Prince *et al.*, 1975; Kew *et al.*, 1979; Yeh *et al.*, 1985; Austin *et al.*, 1986; Trichopoulos, 1987). Prospective cohort studies comparing the occurrence of HCC among HBsAg carriers and non-carrier controls, have shown RRs varying from 7 to over 100 (CL) (Beasley *et al.*, 1981; Hall *et al.*, 1985). These latter studies provide unequivocal proof that HBV infection precedes the development of HCC. The specificity of this association is suggested by absence of such an association with other cancers and metastatic liver cancer.

Laboratory investigations showing integration of HBV–DNA in the genome of human HCC cells and liver cell lines support the epidemiological observations. Integration into liver cells itself, however, is probably not sufficient for the development of HCC since it is also found in asymptomatic HBsAg chronic carriers.

A number of animal models have been described. Thus, the woodchuck hepatitis virus (WHV) which resembles human HBV produces a carrier state followed by chronic hepatitis and later finally HCC (Summers, 1981) a sequence closely resembling the pathogenesis in humans.

In conclusion, the strength, specificity and consistency of the association between HCC and HBV in several populations, the fact that infection precedes the development of HCC and the supportive laboratory investigations on HEPADNA viruses, indicate that the association is causal. However, other viruses may be involved such as the recently identified Hepatitis C virus (Bruix *et al.*, 1989) in some cases in Europe and Japan.

Cervical cancer (Chapter 41)

The epidemiology of cervical cancer indicates a possible association with sexually transmitted agents, most likely a virus (Brinton *et al.*, 1987; Muñoz & Bosch, 1989). Herpes simplex virus type 2 (HSV-2), papilloma virus (HPV) and cytomegalovirus (CMV) have been regarded as the most likely candidates (Chapters 11 and 41).

Herpes simplex virus type-2 (HSV-2)

Numerous case-control studies in several geographical areas have shown that neutralizing antibodies to HSV-2 are more frequent among cervical cancer cases than among controls. Interpretation is difficult, since the serological tests did not measure HSV-2 type-specific antibodies but mainly antibodies common to HSV-1 and HSV-2. Sensitive serological tests for antibodies to type-specific glycoproteins of HSV-1 and HSV-2 have been developed only recently and have not yet been applied in large-scale epidemiological studies. Where a type-specific assay was used in a cohort study of 10,000 women in Czechoslovakia the results were apparently negative. However, closer examination did show RRs of 2.3 for *in situ* cancer and 5.2 for invasive cancer (based on 11 and 3 cancers respectively) despite some overmatching (Vonka *et al.*, 1984).

Subsequently, an association has been suggested between the prevalence of HSV-2 infection and the recent increase in cervical intra-epithelial neoplasia (CIN) in Australia (Armstrong *et al.*, 1986). Moreover, the prevalence of HSV-2 antibodies is higher in Greenland than in Denmark, as is cervical cancer (Kjaer *et al.*, 1988). However, laboratory studies do not provide clear-cut molecular, immunological or experimental evidence supporting an oncogenic effect of HSV-2 (Vonka *et al.*, 1987). A 'hit-and-run' effect has been postulated (Galloway & McDougall, 1983) or a synergistic effect with HPV (zur Hausen, 1982, 1986; di Luca *et al.*, 1987). Since HSV-2–DNA–RNA and viral antigens have not been detected consistently in cancer tissue; these results have led to a reduced interest in HSV-2.

Human papilloma virus (HPV)

Today, molecular cloning of HPV–DNA has led to the identification of more than 60 types of HPV which are being studied in cancerous and normal cervical tissues (zur Hausen, 1989). The epidemiological evidence linking HPV to cervical cancer and other genital tumors has been recently reviewed (Muñoz *et al.*, 1988), and covers four types of studies considered below.

Over 30 case reports suggest that HPV 16 and, to a lesser extent, HPV 18 are associated with advanced CIN or invasive carcinoma, while HPV 6 and 11 are more often found in lower grade CIN and condylomata.

In a case-control study from Latin America of 759 women with invasive cervical cancer and 1467 controls, an increased RR was found for HPV ranging from 2.1 to 9.1 according to the intensity of the reaction and for HPV 6/11 (2.1 to 3.9) (Reeves *et al.*, 1989).

Three small cohorts of women with cytological evidence of HPV infection or CIN, in whom the presence of HPV–DNA was assessed by hybridization tests, have been followed. Although inconclusive, two of these studies suggested that progression to more advanced CIN was greater with HPV types 16 or 18 infection than in types 6 or 11 (Campion *et al.*, 1986; Schneider *et al.*, 1987); however, the third study showed that the so-called low risk types, HPV 6 and 11, were present equally frequently in lesions that progressed to carcinoma *in situ* (Syrjanen *et al.*, 1988).

In an ecological study where the prevalence of HPV 6/11 and 16/18 infection in random cervical scrapes from women in Greenland and Denmark was assessed blind by filter *in situ* hybridization, the prevalence of HPV 16/18 was 1.5 times higher in Denmark, although the incidence of cervical cancer is six-fold lower than Greenland, in contrast to HSV 2 infection (Kjaer *et al.*, 1988). Different results were obtained from Recife and Sao Paulo where the cervical cancer rates correlated with HPV prevalence (Villa & Franco, 1989).

Interpretation of these results is, however, extremely difficult. An important caveat in accepting an association between cervical cancer and HPV is the lack of correlation between HPV positivity, the number of sexual partners, and age at first intercourse, which are strong and consistent cervical cancer risk factors (Chapter 41). Further, in most studies, the less accurate filter *in situ* hybridization test was used.

In conclusion, while there is substantial experimental evidence suggesting the oncogenic potential of HPV, including specific patterns of integration and of transcription of HPV genome into the cellular DNA in most invasive cancers, in high degree CIN lesions, and in cell lines derived from cervical cancers and cells transformed *in vitro* by HPV-16 (zur Hausen, 1989), the epidemiological evidence remains limited.

Little information exists on the prevalence and role of other HPV types (31, 33, 35 and 39), which have also been observed occasionally with cervical neoplasia.

Other viruses

A few sero-epidemiological case-control studies and hybridization experiments searching for CMV–DNA in cervical cancer cells have yielded negative or inconclusive results (Muñoz *et al.*, 1975; McDougall *et al.*, 1986).

Burkitt's lymphoma (BL) and nasopharyngeal carcinoma (NPC) (Chapters 24 and 53): Epstein–Barr virus (EBV)

The EB virus is ubiquitous, and about 95% of adults have antibodies, which complicates interpretation of its role in BL and NPC. However, a number of observations support a causal association with these cancers.

Patients with BL and NPC have higher titers of various EBV antibodies than matched controls. The antibody titers increase with NPC mass and decrease with therapy. High antibody titers are found both in the IgA fraction of serum and in nasopharyngeal washings and saliva (Henle & Henle, 1985). In a cohort of 42,000 children followed for seven years in Uganda, the risk of developing BL was greatest among those with high antibody titers, but the number of cases was small (de Thé *et al.*, 1978).

The epithelial cells of NPC and the B cells of BL contain multiple copies of the viral genome (zur Hausen *et al.*, 1970). The EB virus is able to immortalize human B lymphocytes *in vitro* and to induce lympho-proliferative disorders in certain New World monkey species (Henle & Henle, 1985). Further, fatal malignant lymphoproliferation of B lympho-cytes carrying EBV may occur in subjects with genetic or therapeutically induced immunodeficiency (Purtilo, 1981).

The association between BL and EBV, however, is not consistent. In the high-risk areas of Africa, EBV markers (DNA or EBNA) are found in over 90% of tumors while in low-risk areas they are found in only about 15% of the tumors (Henle & Henle, 1985). BL cells from both African and non-African tumors are characterized by specific chromosomal trans-locations, involving the long arm of chromosome 8 carrying the c-*myc* gene, and one of the 3 loci on chromosomes 2, 14 or 22 carrying the heavy or light chain immunoglobin genes. Lenoir and Bornkamm (1987) have suggested that chronic persistent stimulation by holo-endemic malaria leads to a generation of B lymphocytes at high risk of translocations which appear to involve the c-*myc* and the Ig loci. In a few of these B cells infection by EBV occurs and the cells are immortalized. EBV *per se* does not, however, induce these chromosome translocations (Taub *et al.*, 1982).

In conclusion, although evidence suggests that EBV plays a role in the development of African BL and NPC, the virus may be neither necessary nor sufficient for tumor induction. Genetic factors and environmental co-factors have been proposed to play a role in NPC (Chapter 24).

Leukemias: human T-Cell leukemia viruses

Although a viral etiology has long been suspected in certain leukemias, only recently have clusters of adult T-cell leukemias in Japan and some Caribbean islands been demonstrated to be associated with a retrovirus, HTLV-I (Hinuma *et al.*, 1982). The same virus is suspected to be related to cutaneous lymphoma. A hairy cell leukemia has been associated with another retrovirus, HTLV-II.

Human immunodeficiency virus (HIV)

Infection with HIV causing acquired immunodeficiency syndrome (AIDS) has been associated with an increased risk for certain neoplasms. By far the most common cancer seen in AIDS patients is Kaposi's sarcoma, but an increased risk has also been observed for non-Hodgkin's lymphomas particularly of the B-cell type, such as Burkitt's-like lymphomas and lymphomas of the central nervous system (Biggar *et al.*, 1987). Associations with other tumors (Hodgkin's disease, lymphoblastic leukemias, oral and liver cancers and tumors of the testis and urinary tract) have been postulated but not confirmed. It is believed that HIV essentially facilitates the development of these tumors by causing a decrease of cellular immunity, and reactivating certain latent oncogenic viruses. Thus, cytomegalovirus has been suspected to be associated with Kaposi sarcoma and EBV with non-Hodgkin's lymphomas.

17.2   Parasites and cancer

Malaria and Burkitt's lymphoma (BL)

Although Epstein–Barr virus (EBV) is considered to play a causal role in BL in view of its ubiquity, other factors must be invoked to explain the extremely high frequency of BL in tropical Africa and lowland New Guinea. Holoendemic malaria, inducing a considerable increase in the B lymphocyte turnover, may be one of the events leading to the characteristic chromosomal translocation of BL, followed by EBV infection of the B cell carrying the translocation (Lenoir & Bornkamm, 1987). Falciparum malaria has been considered to be the prime co-factor, and the evidence for its association with BL in Africa has been summarized by Morrow (1982) as follows:

(a) A good correlation exists between the geographical distribution of the two diseases and the peak age for prevalence of malaria (3 years) occurs 3–4 years before the peak incidence of BL. The maximum levels of antimalarial antibodies occur at the same time as the peak incidence of BL.

(b) The incidence of BL is lower in urban than in rural areas which is consistent with this hypothesis as is the older age at onset and higher incidence in young adults migrating from non-malarial to malarial areas.

(c) A decline in the incidence of BL in Uganda has been ascribed, in part, to a decline in malaria due to control measures but it has not been confirmed elsewhere (Geser *et al.*, 1989).

Liver flukes and cholangiocarcinoma

An association between cholangiocarcinoma and *Clonorchis sinensis* has been found in Hong Kong, and with *Opisthorchis viverrini* in Thailand and the USSR (Burton, 1982). The evidence is based on the association between geographical distribution of the liver tumors, and flukes (Srivatanakul *et al.*, 1988). Pathologically, the type of liver cancer is highly distinctive and closely related to hyperplastic lesions of the ducts associated with the presence of flukes. Epidemiological evidence has proven more difficult to interpret due to the very high prevalence of infestation with the parasite and problems in measuring clinically the degree of exposure. A recently developed serological test to measure antibodies to *O. viverrini* may overcome this problem. The mechanism of action is unknown, but it is of interest that opisthorchis infestation greatly enhances the carcinogenic effect of dimethylnitrosamine in the hamster bile ducts (Flavell & Lucas, 1982). In high risk areas of Thailand, subjects positive for *O. viverrini* antibody excreted significantly higher levels of *N*-nitrosoproline after ingestion of proline than did negative subjects.

Schistosomiasis and cancer

Schistosoma hematobium and bladder cancer

Although an etiological association between these two conditions has long been recognized, definitive epidemiological evidence has been difficult to obtain. There is a relatively good correlation between the geographical distribution of the two diseases. In endemic areas the great majority of bladder cancers are well differentiated squamous cell carcinomas and schistosomal ova are usually present with an associated cystitis in a small contracted bladder. It has been suggested that a superimposed bacterial infection may lead to endogenous nitrosamine formation. This contrasts with non-endemic areas where most tumors are of the urothelial type (Burton, 1982). Relative risks of up to 15 (with wide confidence intervals) has been estimated (Gelfand *et al.*, 1967). A difficulty in the conduct of case-control studies has been the assessment of exposure among controls since clinical or radiographical measurements markedly under-estimate infestation.

Schistosoma mansoni and *japonicum*

In a case-control study in China, an association between *S. japonicum* and rectal cancer has been shown but none with colon cancer (Xu & Su, 1984). In a subsequent ecological study involving 70 counties in China, a positive correlation was found between the mortality from colorectal cancer and from schistosomiasis (Doll, 1988). Associations between *S. japonicum* and *S. mansoni* and liver cancer have been suspected but not documented (Inaba *et al.*, 1984). From a pathogenetic viewpoint, this sequence is unlikely.

17.3 Bacterial and fungal infections in cancer

Although of great historical interest, such agents have not been shown to be direct etiological factors in any human cancer. However, the possibility that bacteria may induce the formation of carcinogens such as *N*-nitroso compounds in the bladder or promoters such as fecopentanes in the bowel indicate potential indirect mechanisms.

17.4 References

Armstrong, B.K., Allen, O.V., Brennan, B.A., Fruzynski, I.A., de Klerk, N.H., Waters, E.D., Machin, J. & Gollow, M.M. (1986). Time trends in prevalence of cervical abnormality in women attending a sexually transmitted diseases clinic and their relationship to trends in sexual activity and specific infections. *Br. J. Cancer*, **54**, 669–75.

Austin, H., Delzell, E., Grufferman, S., Levine, R., Morrison, A.S., Stolley, P.D. & Cole, P. (1986). A case-control study of hepatocellular carcinoma and the hepatitis B virus, cigarette smoking, and alcohol consumption. *Cancer Res.*, **46**, 962–6

Beasley, Hwang, L.Y. Lin, C.C. & Chien, C.S. (1981). Hepatocellular carcinoma and hepatitis B virus. A prospective study of 22, 707 men in Taiwan. *Lancet*, **ii**, 1129–33.

Biggar, R.J., Herm, J., Goedart J.J. & Melbye, M. (1987). Cancer in a group at risk of acquired immunodeficiency syndrome (AIDS) through 1984. *Am. J. Epidemiol.*, **126**, 578–86.

Blumberg, B.S. & London, W.T. (1985). Hepatitis B virus and prevention of primary cancer of the liver. *J. Natl. Cancer Inst.*, **74**, 267–73.

Brinton, L.A., Hamman, R.F., Huggins, G.R., Lehman, H.F., Levine, R.S., Mallin, K. & Fraumeni, J.F. (1987). Sexual and reproductive risk factors for invasive squamous cell cervical cancer. *J. Natl. Cancer Inst.*, **79**, 2330.

Bruix, J., Barrera, J.M., Calvet, X., Encilla, T., Costa, T., Santoz-Tapias, J.M., Ventura, M., Vall, M., Bruguera, M., Bru, C., Castillo, R. & Rodes, J. (1989). Prevalence of antibodies to hepatitis C virus in Spanish patients with hepato cellular carcinoma and hepatic cirrhosis. *Lancet*, **ii**, 1004–6.

Burton, G.J. (1982). Parasites. In: *Cancer Epidemiology and Prevention*, ed. D. Schottenfeld & J.R. Fraumeni, Jr., pp. 408–18. Philadelphia: Saunders.

Campion, M.J., McCance, D.J., Cuzick, J. & Singer, A. (1986). Progressive potential of mild cervical atypia: prospective cytological, colposcopic and virological study. *Lancet*, **ii**, 237–40.

de Thé, G., Geser, A., Day, N.E., Tukei, P.M., Williams, E.H., Beri, D.P., Smith, P.G., Dean, A.G., Bornkamm, G.W., Feorino, P. & Henle, W. (1978). Epidemiological evidence for a causal relationship between Epstein–Barr virus and Burkitt's lymphoma. *Nature*, **305**, 112–16.

di Luca, D., Rotola, A., Pilotti, S., Monini, P., Caselli, E., Rilke, F. & Cassai, E. (1987). Simultaneous presence of herpes simplex and human papilloma virus sequences in human genital tumours. *Int. J. Cancer*, **40**, 763–8.

Doll, R.(1988). Epidemiology – the prevention of cancer: some recent developments. *J. Cancer Res. Clin. Oncol.*, **114**, 447–58.

Flavell, D.J. & Lucas, S.B. (1982). Potentiation by the human liver fluke *Opisthorchis viverrini* of the carcinogenic action of *N*-nitrosodimethylamine upon the biliary epithelium of the hamster. *Br. J. Cancer*, **46**, 985–9.

Galloway, D.A. & McDougall, J.K. (1983). The oncogenic potential of herpes simplex viruses: evidence for a 'hit-and-run' mechanism. *Nature*, **302**, 21–4.

Gelfand, M., Winberg, R.W. & Castle, W.M. (1967). Relation between carcinoma of the bladder and infestation with *Schistosoma haematobium*. *Lancet*, **i**, 1249–51.

Geser, A., Brubaker, G.R. & Draper, C.C. (1989). Effect of malaria suppression program on the incidence of African Burkitt's lymphoma. *Amer. J. Epid.*, **129**, 140–52.

Hall, A.J., Winter, P.D. & Wright, R. (1985). Mortality of hepatitis B positive blood donors in England and Wales. *Lancet*, **i**, 91–3.

Henle, W. & Henle, G. (1985). Epstein-Barr virus and human malignancies. *Adv. Vir. Oncol.*, **5**, 201–38.

Hinuma, Y., Kamada, H., Chosa, T., Kondo, T., Kohakura, M., Takenaka, T., Kikuchi, M., Ichamaru, M., Yunoki, S., Sato, I., Matsuo, R., Takiuchi, Y., Ushino, H.Z. & Henaka, M. (1982). Antibodies to adult T cell leukemia virus associated antigen (ATLA) in sera from patients with ATL study controls in Japan: a nation wide sero-epidemiologic study. *Int. J. Cancer*, **29**, 631–5.

Inaba, Y., Maruchi, N., Matsuda, M., Yoshihara, N. & Hamamoto, S. (1984). A case-control study on liver cancer with special emphasis on the possible aetiological role of schistosomiasis. *Int. J. Epidemiol.*, **13**, 408–12.

Kew, M.C., Desmyter, J., Bradburne, A.F. & Macnab, G.M. (1979). Hepatitis B virus infection in southern African blacks with hepatocellular cancer. *J. Natl. Cancer Inst.*, **62**, 517–20.

Kjaer, S.K., De Villiers, E.-M., Haugaard, B.J., Christensen, R.B., Reisen, C., Moller, K.A., Poll, P., Jensen, H., Vestergaard, B.F., Lynge, E. & Jensen, O.M. (1988). Human papillomavirus, herpes simplex virus and cervical cancer incidence in Greenland and Denmark. A population-based cross-sectional study. *Int. J. Cancer*, **41**, 518–24.

Lenoir, G. & Bornkamm, G. (1987). Burkitt's lymphoma, a human cancer model for the study of the multistep development of cancer: proposal for a new scenario. *Adv. Vir. Oncol.*, **7**, 173–206.

McDougall, J.K., Beckmann, A.M. & Kiviat, N.B. (1984). Methods for diagnosing papillomavirus infection. In *Papillomaviruses*, Ciba Foundation Symposium No. 120, p. 86.

Melbye, M., Skinhoj, P., Hojgaard Nielsen, N., Vestergaard, B.F., Ebbesen, P., Hart Hansen, J.P. & Biggar, R.J. (1984). Virus-associated cancers in Greenland: frequent hepatitis B virus infection but low primary hepatocellular carcinoma incidence. *J. Natl. Cancer Inst.*, **73**, 1267–2.

Morrow, R.H. (1982). Burkitt's lymphoma. In *Cancer Epidemiology and Prevention*, ed. D. Schottenfeld, & J.F. Fraumeni, Jr., pp. 779–94. Philadelphia: Saunders.

Muñoz, N. & Bosch, F.X. (1987). Epidemiology of hepatocellular carcinoma. In *Neoplasms of the Liver*, ed. K. Okuda & K.G. Ishak, pp. 3–19. Tokyo: Springer.

Muñoz, N. and Bosch, F.X. (1989). Epidemiology of cervical cancer In *Human Papillomavirus and Cervical Cancer*, ed. N. Muñoz, F.X. Bosch, O.M. Jensen, IARC Scientific Publication No. 94, pp. 9–39. Lyon: International Agency for Research on Cancer.

Muñoz, N., Bosch, F.X. & Kaldor, J.M. (1988). Does human papillomavirus cause cervical cancer? The state of the epidemiological evidence. *Br. J. Cancer*, **57**, 1–5.

Muñoz, N., de Thé, G., Aristizabal, N., Yee, C., Rabson, A. & Pearson, G. (1975). Antibodies to herpesviruses in patients with cervical cancer and controls. In *Oncogenesis and Herpesviruses II*, IARC Scientific Publication No. 11, ed. G. de Thé, M.A. Epstein, & H. zur Hausen, pp 45–51. Lyon: International Agency for Research on Cancer.

Prince, A.M., Szmuness, W., Michon, J., Desmaille, J., Diebolt, G., Linhard, J., Quenum, C. & Sankale, M. (1975). A case-control study of the association between primary liver cancer and hepatitis B infection in Senegal. *Int. J. Cancer*, **16**, 376–83.

Purtilo, D.T. (1981). Malignant lymphoproliferative diseases induced by Epstein–Barr virus in immunodeficient patients, including X-linked, cytogenetic and familial syndromes. *Cancer Genet. Cytogenet.*, **4**, 251–68.

Reeves, W.C., Brinton, L.A., Garcia, M., Berens, M.M., Herrero, R., Gatan, E., Tenorio, F., deBritton, R.C. & Rawls, W.E. (1989). Human papillomavirus infection and cervical cancer in Latin America. *N. Engl. J. Med.*, **320**, 1437–41.

Schneider, A., Sawada, E., Gissmann, L. & Shah, K. (1987). Human papillomaviruses in women with a history of abnormal papanicolaou smears and their male partners. *Obst. Gynecol.*, **69**, 554–62.

Srivatanakul, P., Sontipong, S., Chotiwan, P. & Parkin, D.M. (1988). Liver cancer in Thailand: temporal and geographic variations. *Gastroenter. Hepatol.*, **3**, 413–20.

Summers, J. (1981). Three recently described animal virus models for human hepatitis B virus. *Hepatology.*, **1**, 179–83.

Syrjanen, K., Mantyjarvi, R., Saarikoski, S., Vayrynen, M., Syrjanen, S., Pakkinen,S., Yliskoski, M., Saastamoinen, J. & Castren, O. (1988). Factors associated with progression of cervical human papillomavirus (HPV) infections into carcinoma *in situ* during a long-term prospective follow-up. *Br. J. Obstet. Gynecol.*, **95**, 1096–102.

Szmuness, W. (1978). Hepatocellular carcinoma and the hepatitis B virus: evidence for a causal association. *Prog. Med. Virol.*, **24**, 40–69.

Taub, R., Kirsch, I., Morton, C., Lenoir, G., Swan, D., Tronick, S., Aaronson, S. & Leder, P. (1982). Translocation of the c-*myc* gene into the immunoglobulin heavy chain locus in human Burkitt's lymphoma and murine plasmocytoma cells. *Proc. Natl. Acad. Sci. USA*, **79**, 7837–41.

Trichopoulos, D., Day, N.E., Kaklamani, E., Tzonou, A., Muñoz, N., Zavitsanos, X., Koumantaki, Y. & Trichopoulou, A. (1987). Hepatitis B virus, tobacco smoking and ethanol consumption in the etiology of hepatocellular carcinoma. *Int. J. Cancer*, **39**, 45–9.

Villa, L.L. & Franco, M. (1989). Epidemiologic correlates of cervical neoplasia and risk of human papillomavirus injection in asymtomatic women in Brazil. *J. Natl.Cancer Inst.*, **81**, 332–40.

Vonka, V., Kafka, J., Hirsch, I., Zavadova, H., Krcmar, M., Suchankova, A., Rezacova, D., Broucek, J., Press, M., Domorazkova, E., Svoboda, B. Havrankova, A. & Jelinek, J. (1984). Prospective study on the relationship between cervical neoplasia and herpes simplex type-2 virus. II. Herpes simplex type-2 antibody presence in sera taken at enrolment. *Int. J. Cancer*, **33**, 61–6.

Vonka, V., Kafka, J. & Roth, Z. (1987). Herpes simplex type 2 virus and cervical neoplasia. *Adv. Cancer Res.*, **48**, 149–91.

Xu, Z. & Su, D.L. (1984). Schistosoma japonicum and colorectal cancer: An epidemiological study in the People's Republic of China. *Int. J. Cancer*, **34**, 315–18.

Yeh, F.S., Mo, C.C., Luo, S., Henderson, B.E., Tong, M.J. & Yu, M.C. (1985). A serological case-control study of primary hepatocellular carcinoma in Guangxi, China. *Cancer Res.*, **45**, 872–3.

zur Hausen, H. (1982). Human genital cancer: synergism between two virus infections or synergism between a virus infection and initiating events? *Lancet*, **ii**, 1370–2.

zur Hausen, H. (1986). Intracellular surveillance of persisting viral infections. *Lancet*, **ii**, 489–91.

zur Hausen, H., Schulte-Holthausen, H., Klein, G., Henle, W., Henle, G., Clifford, P. & Santesson, L. (1970). EBV DNA in biopsies of Burkitt's tumours and anaplastic carcinomas of the nasopharynx. *Nature*, **228**, 1056–8.

zur Hausen, H. (1989), Papillomavirus in anogenital cancer as a model to understand the role of viruses in Human Cancers. *Cancer Res.*, **49**, 4677–81.

18

Genetic and other host-risk factors

H. BARTSCH
International Agency for Research on Cancer

18.1 Introduction

Cancer results ultimately from an interplay between genetic and environmental factors. Since the genetic background, lifestyle, and the external and internal environment of human populations are highly variable, three categories of cancers caused by different genetic environmental interactions can be delineated.

Heritable cancers which are largely independent of the environment and where genetic variation appears to be the major determinant are characterized by familial aggregation, and usually occur earlier than non-heritable tumors. They may be associated with other phenotypic manifestations such as a characteristic clinical syndrome preceding their appearance. Probably only a minor fraction, 1–2%, of all cancers are of this type.

Cancers produced by environmental agents in genetically predisposed individuals include syndromes involving an elevated risk of a specific cancer when appropriate environmental conditions occur. Some syndromes derive from the presence in the homozygous state of single autosomal recessive genes. However, only for individuals with xeroderma pigmentosum is the specific environmental agent known, notably exposure to ultraviolet light.

Cancers largely induced by environmental agents, for example, lung cancer due to tobacco smoking, bladder cancer due to aromatic amine exposure, were hitherto considered independent of genetic variation. As is true for the majority of malignant neoplasms. Recent studies suggest, however, that several such cancers are modified by inherited host factors and thus also have a genetic component.

Some of the recognized host risk factors that affect cancer causation in man are briefly described in this chapter. The possibilities, which are offered by integrating into epidemiological studies new and highly sensitive laboratory procedures and techniques on molecular genetics, characterizing genetic and acquired host susceptibility in humans, are highlighted. Thus, epidemiologists should have some knowledge of the more important techniques described below.

18.2   Molecular and chromosomal approaches to study
Susceptibility to neoplasia
Recent methodological advances have led to a better und-erstanding of the molecular mechanisms involved in the genesis of a malignant cell. These, in turn, have shed light on the nature of genetic lesions responsible for an increased predisposition to cancer. Such studies include the identification of growth factors and their receptors controlling malignant cell proliferation. In addition, specific cellular genes, a large proportion showing homology to the oncogenes of oncogenic retroviruses, have been isolated. When activated, by point mutation, gene amplification or chromosomal transposition, for example, many such genes have been shown capable of transforming cells. It is now possible to study whether, on a constitutional basis, some individuals carry gene alterations in their normal cells, which may predispose them to cancer. This has become possible because of recent technological advances in the analysis of chromosomes and genes.

Restriction enzyme DNA fragment length analysis of genetic polymorphism (RFLP)
Until recently, genetic predisposition could be assessed only by measuring gene products, e.g. histocompatibility antigens or phenotypic markers. Today, genetic polymorphism at the DNA level can be measured by restriction enzyme digestion and DNA hybridization (White *et al.*, 1983). RFLPs are of two types – site or insertion/deletion polymorphism. In the case of site polymorphism, the recognition site for a given restriction enzyme in a particular region of DNA may appear or disappear as the result of point mutation. In the site-absent genotype, a large fragment instead of two smaller fragments is observed. Conversely, in the site-present genotype, smaller than expected fragments are seen. In the case of insertion/deletion polymorphism, variation in fragment length is the result of insertion or deletion of DNA sequences and can be detected by any restriction endonuclease that possesses recognition sites that tightly span the region of sequence alteration. This approach using RFLPs has already proven helpful in identifying individuals with a genetic predisposition to a variety of diseases, including not only non-insulin-

dependent diabetes mellitus, Huntington's disease, and hemoglobin-opathies but also retinoblastoma (Francomano & Kazazian, 1986). The same molecular approach, using specific DNA probes, for oncogenes and ectopic hormones, for example, is now being studied to determine its potential for identifying persons with a genetic predisposition to other cancers.

Studies of gene function by cell transfer

The function of a gene can often be studied most effectively by introducing it into a different type of cell. A mutated oncogene, for example, isolated from a tumor cell, is transferred to a normal cell to determine whether it can cause malignant transformation. There are several methods for introducing DNA into other animal cells.

Mapping genes on specific chromosomes

Once a gene or gene function has been identified, it is necessary to map its location on a specific chromosome. Such maps may provide clues about which genes are affected by chromosome breaks or other abnormalities. Several methods are available.

Deletion analysis

Congenital abnormalities involving deletion of parts of a chromosome almost invariably lead to severe congenital anomalies. If many individuals with a particular abnormality and chromosomal deletion are available for study, one can define precisely the location of a specific gene. This method has limited resolution since each band in a chromosome contains three million base pairs of DNA on average.

Linkage analysis

If two genes are close together on a chromosome, they tend to be inherited as a single unit. Although any two genes on a single chromosome can segregate through the phenomenon of meiotic recombination, the closer they are together the less likely that separation will occur during meiosis. The distance between genes in a linkage map is expressed in recombination units or centiMorgans.

Somatic cell hybridization

Useful methods for mapping genes involve somatic cell hybrids, such as fusion of a rodent (mouse) cell and a human cell. The resultant hybrid usually expresses most of the genes expressed by the two parent lines. If a series of subclones are derived from an original hybrid cell line after the period of maximum chromosome loss, the cells in these clones will contain close to a full complement of mouse chromosomes for example, and a random samples of human chromosomes. By correlating the presence of the gene (as determined by southern blot, for example) with the chromosomes present in the hybrids, it is possible to identify the human chromosome on which the gene is located.

Whole cell hybridization seldom answers questions about the relationship between tumor suppression and chromosomal deletions because many chromosomes from both parents are introduced into the hybrid cells. The development of the microcell hybridization technique allows the transfer of a single chromosome into a recipient cell. Thus human chromosomes from a normal cell can be introduced into a tumor cell line and their effect on tumorigenic potential determined.

Tumor suppressor genes

Studies on retinoblastoma (see below) were the first to lead to the definition and identification of a new class of genes in humans which protect against cancer. This new class of human recessive cancer genes with 'suppressor' functions are termed tumor suppressor genes. Today, the presence of specific chromosomal deletions in many other human cancers, e.g. osteogenic sarcoma, Wilms' tumor, renal cell carcinoma, small lung carcinoma, neuroblastoma, bladder carcinoma, colon cancer and breast cancer, suggests the loss of suppressor genes at specific chromosomal regions, and emphasizes the need to isolate genes lost during tumor development. By studying the effects of normal human chromosomes introduced into cancer cells using microcell hybridization techniques, it is now possible to identify which chromosomes contain tumor suppressor genes. Using smaller chromosomal fragments, these genes can be localized in specific regions, following which tumor suppressor genes may be isolated by techniques similar to those used in the cloning of the Rb-1 locus (Stanbridge *et al.*, 1983; Weissman *et al.*, 1987).

18.3   Inherited disorders associated with an increased risk of cancer

These disorders can be divided into three groups (Mulvihill, 1976): constitutional chromosomal abnormalities (gain or loss of chromosomal material); single gene locus disorders; polygenic disorders (multifactorial predisposition).

Constitutional chromosome anomalies

In Down's syndrome, trisomy 21 is associated with mongolism and with an 18-fold increased risk of leukemia. Males affected by Klinefelter's syndrome, characterized in males by the presence of extra X chromosomes, have a 20-fold increased risk of breast cancer. The mechanisms underlying the increased cancer risk has not been identified for either syndrome; hormonal factors are, however, suspected to play a role in the latter.

'Single gene' disorders

This group of heterogeneous disorders involves subjects in which cancer occurs as a sole feature, or as a rare complication in association with other developmental anomalies.

Familial adenomatous polyposis (FAP)

Several syndromes which are characterized by polyps of the gastrointestinal tract have been defined. FAP (or familial polyposis coli) and Gardner syndrome are the two most important. They are inherited as autosomal dominant traits with high penetrance but variable expression. At the age of 40 about half of patients with the mutant gene have large bowel cancer, by the age of 70, nearly all. The molecular defects associated with such conditions have only recently been investigated (Bodmer *et al.*, 1987; Solomon *et al.*, 1987; Vogelstein *et al.*, 1988).

Studies, using highly polymorphic probes, have searched for allele loss in sporadic tumors as compared to normal tissue from the same FAP individual. A substantial portion of sporadic colorectal tumors were found to become homo- or hemizygous at specific chromosomal regions implying that the FAP gene becomes recessive in a relatively high proportion of colorectal carcinomas.

Multiple neuroendocrine neoplasia (MEN) syndromes

Three neoplastic syndromes affecting neuroendocrine cells, all inherited in an autosomal dominant manner, are known. MEN type 1 involves mainly the parathyroid, pituitary and pancreatic islets (Ponder, 1984). The tumor cells may be functional and produce specific hormones. MEN type 2a corresponds to familial association among medullary carcinoma of the thyroid, pheochromocytoma, and, less frequently, parathyroid adenoma. MEN type 2b differs from MEN-2 in that all the patients have mucosal neuromas and/or intestinal ganglioneuromas. MEN type 2a has been shown to be genetically linked to a locus near the centromere of chromosome 10. The availability of polymorphic DNA probes for the region permits the use of restriction fragment-length polymorphisms to identify new carriers of the gene for this cancer syndrome (Sobol *et al.*, 1989).

Hamartomatous disorders

Neurofibromatosis (von Recklinghausen disease) is characterized by the presence of multiple skin nodules (hamartomas) which histologically are neurofibromas. The incidence of the disease is estimated to be 1 in 3000 in the USA, and 10 to 15% of neurofibromatosis patients will develop malignant changes. It appears that inheritance of a single gene which has now been identified results in a phenotypic abnormality which, although not in itself cancerous, may be associated with the development of malignant neoplasms.

Hereditary neoplasms associated with cytogenetic anomalies

Retinoblastoma (Rb) arises from embryonal cells and its incidence is about 5 per 100,000 children born in the USA. It is not accompanied by any clinically recognizable syndrome before the tumor appears (Knudson, 1971, 1985). About 40% of retinoblastomas are hereditary. In patients with inherited susceptibility, tumors are frequently multiple and bilateral. They develop earlier than in sporadic cases, and the risk of developing second primary retinoblastomas is elevated. The locus for hereditary Rb (Rb1) has been assigned to chromosomal region 13q14 (deleted in the susceptible individuals) (Nove *et al.*, 1979), and the risk of retinoblastoma is increased by a factor of 100,000 in 'carriers'. The Rb1 locus has been cloned (Friend *et al.*, 1986; Lee *et al.*, 1987). Knudson proposed a model, now confirmed, in which the hereditary form of the cancer resulted from at least two events: a germinal mutation affecting all cells of the body, and a second somatic mutation affecting one or a small number of retinal cells. Two events should also occur for the sporadic cancers to develop, but both must occur in the same somatic cell. Recent DNA-sequencing techniques have been described that can distinguish hereditary from non-hereditary retinoblastoma and thus can be used in risk estimation and genetic counselling (Yandell *et al.*, 1989). Molecular studies have also demonstrated that, although the mode of inheritance of retinoblastoma appears to be as an autosomal dominant, it is a recessive mutation which is inherited and the appearance of malignancy is the consequence of chromosomal changes in the retinoblasts resulting in homozygosity or hemizygosity for the altered allele (Hansen & Cavenee, 1987). Thus recessive mutations appear to be important contributing factors in oncogenesis (one normal allele is adequate to protect against cancer).

Wilms' tumor is a kidney tumor of childhood, and occurs in both a heritable and a non-heritable form; the heritable form is frequently bilateral. The Wilms' tumor locus is known to be located on the short arm of chromosome 11. A mechanism of tumorigenesis similar to that observed for retinoblastoma has been identified. Thus several investigators by using RFLP, have observed a reduction to homozygosity in many loci on the short arm of chromosome 11. Thus, the Wilms' tumor gene is probably a recessive mutation, and both alleles must become mutant for the malignant phenotype to be expressed (Koufos *et al.*, 1984).

Loss of heterozygosity may also be the key common mechanism for other embryonal tumors such as hepatoblastoma and rhabdomyosarcoma. Whether such a mechanism applies to other childhood embryonal tumors, e.g. neuroblastoma, or to other adult cancers such as medullary cancer of the thyroid, or renal cell carcinoma associated with a constitutional t(3,8) translocation is now being tested by comparing the genotype of tumors and non-malignant cells of the patients using DNA markers.

Functional anomalies

This group includes four syndromes related to chromosomal instability, increased radiosensitivity and impairment of DNA repair mechanism, which predispose to cancer. These are inherited as autosomal recessive traits.

Ataxia telangiectasia (AT)

This is characterized by progressive cerebellar ataxia, impaired immunity and hypersensitivity to ionizing radiation and certain chemicals. Such individuals have an increased cancer rate, mainly lymphoid neoplasms. The molecular anomaly may be a defect in the processing of DNA. The incidence of the homozygote has been estimated to be about 1 per 100,000 live births (Bridges *et al.*, 1985). Therefore about 1 to 2% of the general population are carriers of the AT gene in the heterozygous state. Swift *et al.* (1971) has suggested that AT heterozygotes who appear to be normal members of the population may be cancer prone, but this is unproven.

Bloom's Syndrome (BS)

This is characterized by growth retardation, a telangiectasic erythrematous rash on the face, and increased risk of leukemia and lymphoma and other solid tumors (German *et al.*, 1979). The characteristic anomaly of BS is a tendency for homologous chromosome interchanges associated with increased sister chromatid exchanges. Cells of such patients are defective in DNA ligase I activity.

Fanconi's anemia

In this, skeletal and visceral malformations are associated with bone-marrow failure. An increased risk of leukemia and squamous cell cancer in such patients has been linked with an increased risk of chromosomal aberration by DNA probably by cross-linking agents (German, 1972).

Xeroderma pigmentosum (XP)

These patients have in common an impairment of their capacity to repair ultraviolet-induced DNA lesions. As a consequence, their risk of developing cancer of the exposed skin is very high. However, there is no spontaneous increase in chromosomal or chromatid fragility in this syndrome (Robbins, 1978). Heterozygotes for XP genes have not been reported as having an increased risk to cancer. In XP the radiosensitivity has been shown to be associated in most cases with defects of excision repair of bases in DNA of the skin damaged by UV irradiation.

Chromosome abnormalities are associated with many types of tumors. Some, such as the rearrangements of Burkitt's lymphoma and the Philadelphia chromosome of chronic myelogenous leukemia, involve breakage of chromosomes close to known oncogenes. Others involve amplification of genes or addition or deletion of chromosomal material. Analysis of common abnormalities may give clues to the sites of genes that are involved in cancer causation and progression. These observations have led to the suggestion that such fragile sites, both common and rare, may play a significant role in the chromosomal translocations and other genetic rearrangements involved in human oncogene activation. Accordingly, environmental exposures to genotoxic agents, such as tobacco smoke, may increase the probability of developing specific tumors in individuals whose genomes harbor fragile sites at particular locations (Yunis & Soreng, 1984). Although epidemiological and family studies have not yet confirmed this thesis, it warrants further exploration, as do current efforts to understand the molecular mechanisms underlying the fragile site phenomenon (Nowell & Croce, 1988).

Multifactorial inheritance – familial clustering

If no clear-cut Mendelian segregation is observed, one way of assessing whether an inherited component contributes to a disease is the demonstration of an increased risk among the relatives of affected individuals. Familial clustering of breast cancer, has been well documented (Anderson, 1977). However, with the exception of some rare 'cancer family syndromes', e.g. Li–Fraumeni syndrome, there is no formal proof of the genetic basis of familial segregation of breast cancer cases. The proof will require identification of genetic markers associated with this cancer, at present an area of intensive study.

Some geographical differences in cancer incidence provide evidence for racial or ethnic differences in cancer susceptibility due to multifactorial predisposition. For example, Ewing's sarcoma is almost absent in black populations. A genetic determinant of this cancer could include inherited cancer resistance.

18.4   Pharmacogenetic variation and cancer risk

The majority of human cancers are thought to have a large environmental component in their induction (Higginson, 1968; Doll & Peto, 1981). Among the chemicals causing cancer in humans, so far identified (IARC, 1987), 80–90% have been shown to react with DNA and cause genotoxic effects (Bartsch & Malaveille, 1989). Most of these carcinogens must be converted into DNA-reactive intermediates (electrophiles) through metabolic activation reactions by host enzymes, that are in part under genetic control. This observation has provided a unified framework for understanding the mechanism of action of numerous structurally unrelated carcinogenic chemicals (Miller & Miller, 1981). The most important group of drug-metabolizing enzymes is the cytochrome P450 family (Gonzalez *et al.*, 1987) which catalyze different oxidative reactions with most endogenous and exogenous substances. Conjugation enzymes catalyze the linkage of various endogenous groups, e.g. glucuronic acid, sulphate and glutathione, with the xenobiotics often leading to detoxification. Thus, the balance between activating and detoxifying (inactivating) reactions determines the level of reactive intermediates in the cell, and their availability to undergo covalent binding with DNA.

Individual differences in the metabolism of carcinogens are due to three types of interdependent factors. Thus, the final adverse biological effect (toxicity, cancer) is determined by the dose of the carcinogens, the genetic background of the exposed person and the acquired features of the host.

Circumstantial evidence for the existence of subjects at higher risk for cancer because of differences in carcinogen metabolizing enzymes (pharmacogenetic variants) can be summarized as follows.

Experiments on inbred mouse strains show that the carcinogenic and genotoxic effects of certain polycyclic aromatic hydrocarbons are determined, largely by the genetic make-up of the animals in the so-called Ah-locus (Nebert *et al.*, 1982).

As the human population is genetically heterogeneous, a consistent observation has been that carcinogen metabolizing enzymes as well as the amounts of the resulting carcinogen-DNA adducts vary widely among individual subjects and tissues, by up to two orders of magnitude (Harris *et al.*, 1984).

Pharmacogenetic variants in the human population exist. There are certain subjects who have a particular sensitivity to the adverse biological effects of specific drugs, indicating genetically controlled variations in the levels of the enzymes involved in their metabolism (detoxification). The difference between pharmacogenetic disorders and 'inborn errors of metabolism' lies in the fact that the former is covert and may only be detected when the individual is challenged with the particular drug that will cause the side effects (Kalow, 1987).

Lastly, of the more than five dozen human pharmacogenetic differences so far described, three polymorphisms show an apparent association with malignancy: (a) acetylation, (b) debrisoquine 4-hydroxylation (and related drugs) and (c) the Ah-locus. The latter two involve differences in the expression of one or more cytochrome P450 genes (Gonzales *et al.*, 1987; Kalow, 1987).

The slow acetylator phenotype among chemical dye workers exhibits an increased risk of bladder cancer (Cartwright *et al.*, 1982; Hein, 1988). Recent studies also suggest that the rapid acetylator phenotype is more likely to develop colorectal cancer (Hein, 1988); the extensive debrisoquine metabolizer phenotype has been reported to have a disproportionally higher risk of lung cancer among cigarette smokers (Ayesh *et al.*, 1984; Caporaso *et al.*, 1989), and cancer of the liver (Idle *et al.*, 1981). Finally, individuals of high AHH (aryl hydrocarbon hydroxylase, benzo(*a*)pyrene as a substrate) inducibility in lymphocytes have been suspected of exhibiting an increased risk of cigarette smoke-induced bronchogenic carcinoma (Kellermann *et al.*, 1973; Kouri *et al.*, 1982). This was confirmed in a case-control study, using surgical lung tissue specimens, where it was shown that cigarette smokers who have inducible pulmonary Ah-locus associated enzymes (cytochrome P450 IA (CYPIA)) are at a higher risk of developing lung cancer than the non-inducible phenotype (Petruzzelli *et al.*, 1988).

Once the carcinogen becomes bound to DNA, the adduct must be removed by enzymatic repair mechanisms, if permanent damage is to be prevented. In human tissues these repair enzymes, e.g. O^6-alkyl-DNA-alkyltransferase and uracil DNA glycosylase, display individual variation (Setlow, 1983; Harris *et al.*, 1984), for which the underlying reasons remain largely unknown (Myrnes *et al.*, 1983; Pegg *et al.*, 1982). Except for XP and UV-light, genetically controlled variations of DNA repair enzymes have not yet been linked to an increased cancer risk in carcinogen-exposed humans.

With the increasing knowledge about the molecular mechanisms of pharmacogenetic disorders, and the availability of new methods for the selective and non-invasive determination in humans of metabolic phenotypes and genotypes, the following questions are now being addressed. How large are the genetic versus environmental contributions to individual cancer risk? How great is the genetic variability between individuals? This approach continues to require the integration of laboratory methods into epidemiological studies (Perera & Weinstein, 1982; Bartsch & Armstrong, 1982; Higginson, 1968, 1988).

18.5   Endogenous formation of carcinogenic agents
Reactive oxygen species

During normal metabolic processes in the body reactive intermediates are continuously generated, e.g. epoxides, peroxides, hydroxylamines, N-oxides and other labile oxygenated intermediates as well as reactive oxygen species, such as superoxide anion, singlet oxygen, hydroxyl radical and hydrogen peroxide (Ames, 1983). As a consequence, mammals have developed cellular defence systems (e.g. detoxifying enzymes, free radical scavenging proteins and low molecular weight compounds, antioxidants) that control the levels of such reactive intermediates. However, under certain conditions, often linked to nutritional imbalances or pathological alterations, it has been speculated that an increased pro-oxidant state, i.e. an increased amount of active oxygen species (superoxide anion, hydrogen peroxide, hydroxyl radical), may be related to the development of some cancers (Cerutti, 1985; Del Maestro, 1980). Further, some tumor-promoting agents produce reactive oxygen species, while inhibitors of tumor promotion have anti-oxidant properties. The pro-oxidant state can also be induced by a variety of agents such as carcinogens (chemicals and ionizing radiation), tumor promoters and high fat diet. Active oxygen species and free radicals initiate lipid peroxidation (LPO) and cause damage to cell membranes resulting in the loss of membrane polyunsaturated fatty acids, increased diene conjugation, formation of other lipid peroxidation products and cholesterol oxidation. Accordingly, due to the relative stability of its products, LPO is used as a method to monitor cellular damage caused by free radical and active oxygen species.

In humans, LPO has not been directly linked to cancer development, although it has been related to lung diseases (Dillard *et al.*, 1978; Taylor *et al.*, 1986). However, there is some evidence that vitamins A and E may have protective functions in some cancers, for example, among smokers: as pointed out in Chapter 9 such situations are difficult to analyze due to the other confounding variables. In colonic tumors, elevated malondialdehyde levels have been found as compared to healthy tissue.

The little attention that has been paid so far in human studies to the simultaneous measurement of the anti-oxidant status and of other defense mechanisms that control reactive oxygen species may explain the controversies regarding the role of diets in certain cancers, e.g. fat intake in relation to colon and breast cancer (Riboli, 1987; Willett *et al.*, 1987; Boyle, 1988). Several cross-sectional studies in breast and colon cancer cases are in progress to study the role of the pro-oxidant state, as related to dietary factors and variations in the body's anti-oxidant defense.

N-Nitroso compounds

Another example of carcinogens that can also be formed in the human body are nitroso compounds (NOC). In addition to exposure to preformed NOC, a versatile class of animal carcinogens, humans are exposed to a wide range of nitrogen-containing compounds and nitrosating agents, which can react *in vivo* to form *N*-nitroso compounds (National Research Council, 1981). Nitrite, nitrate and nitrosating agents can also be synthesized endogenously in reactions mediated by bacteria and activated macrophages (Marletta, 1988).

A sensitive procedure to quantitative human exposure to endogenous *N*-nitroso compounds has been developed (Ohshima & Bartsch, 1981). It is based on the excretion of *N*-nitrosoproline (NPRO) and other *N*-nitrosamino acids in the urine. These are measured as an index of endogenous nitrosation, following ingestion of administered precursors. The NPRO test has been applied to human subjects in clinical and epidemiological studies, and its kinetics and the role of dietary modifiers of endogenous nitrosation have been investigated (Bartsch *et al.*, 1989).

In most subjects at high risk for cancers of the stomach, esophagus, oral cavity and urinary bladder, higher exposures to endogenous NOC were found on testing, but individual exposures were greatly affected by modifiers in the diet or disease state. Vitamin C efficiently lowered the body burden of intragastrically formed NOC. The results point to an etiological role of NOC in these human cancers and possible explanation of the protective effects of fruits and vegetables (sources of vitamin C) described for several neoplasms (Mirvish, 1983).

The process of endogenous nitrosation in humans, however, is highly complex, and influenced by environmental and host factors. Thus the simple determination of nitrate and nitrite in body fluids is insufficient to assess *in vivo* nitrosation in man; this requires individual monitoring, rather than measurement of precursor intake, in evaluating the association of endogenous formation of NOC with cancer at specific sites in future studies.

18.6   Hormonal patterns and immunological risk factors
Hormones
         Epidemiological evidence strongly implicates a number of hormones as, at the very least, permissive for the development of several types of human tumors (Armstrong, 1982). However, despite extensive research, the mechanism of action and relevance of hormonal markers of risk for such endocrine associated cancers, as breast, endometrium, prostate and ovary are not yet fully understood.

Hormones exert their effects on target cells by binding to specific receptors which interact with the genome to cause alterations in gene expression. The influence of the hormone–receptor complex on transcription of DNA may lead to induction of tumors and may facilitate their growth in endocrine-responsive tissues such as breast, endometrium, and prostate. Water-soluble hormones tend to bind to receptors on the cell surface leading to a sequence of intracellular events involving phosphorylation of proteins. There are similarities between the effects of these latter hormones and the products of activated oncogenes.

         Blood estradiol and estrone levels
         Carcinoma of the endometrium has been found in clinical association with obesity, diabetes, and nulliparity. This association probably reflects the summation of a series of endocrine changes each of which may predispose to high levels of free estrogen (Nisker *et al.*, 1980). Indeed, women with endometrial cancer have higher blood levels of estrone and estradiol than controls (Benjamin & Deutsch, 1976; Carlström *et al.*, 1979; Judd *et al.*, 1980). Thus, obesity is also associated with increased conversion of androstenedione into these estrogenic hormones and with reduced plasma levels of sex-hormone-binding globulin, which increases the percentage of free estradiol in the blood.

The incidence of breast cancer in women is weakly associated with the number of years of ovarian function as manifested by years of active menstruation, with later age at first pregnancy, and perhaps with the prolonged administration of estrogens in certain forms of contraceptive pills. The finding by Apter *et al* (1989) that some of the endocrine characteristics of early menarche – a risk factor for breast cancer – are preserved into adulthood, suggest a causal role for serum estradiol and sex-hormone-binding globulin. The women with breast cancer seem to be exposed to elevated levels of biologically active estradiol (England *et al.*, 1974). Non-protein bound estradiol levels were significantly raised in both pre- and post-menopausal women with breast cancer (Moore *et al.*, 1982; Reed *et al.*, 1983).

Androgens and progesterone

Prostatic cancer in men appears to depend on the presence of potent androgens such as testosterone. Evidence for this requirement is provided by the absence of prostate cancer in eunuchoid men and by the low incidence of prostatic cancer in patients with cirrhosis. Higher serum testosterone levels have been recorded in patients with prostate cancer than in controls (Ghanadian *et al.*, 1979), which was confirmed among US blacks but not among African blacks (Ahluwalia *et al.*, 1981). Endocrine measurements for many years have been made on some 10,000 normal women living in the Island of Guernsey (Bulbrook *et al.*, 1971). A subnormal excretion of a urinary androgen metabolite (etiocholanolone) was significantly associated with a two-fold increase in risk of breast cancer in pre-menopausal women.

Prolactin

As shown in experiments in animals, oestrogen might sometimes act indirectly through elevation of the serum levels of the pituitary hormone, prolactin. Most of the several case-control studies of pre-menopausal women with breast cancer found higher levels of prolactin in the patients than in the controls (e.g. Malarkey *et al.*, 1977). In a prospective study, however, no significant differences were detected among pre-menopausal women, though the prolactin levels were significantly elevated among post-menopausal women with breast cancer (Kwa *et al.*, 1981). Care, however, has to be taken to measure prolactin at the appropriate time of day.

Immunological factors

The etiology of cancer has been suspected of being related to the impairment of immuno-surveillance. Because immune impairment can be a consequence of the disease, it cannot be studied by the case-control approach. Studies of individuals with certain diseases that affect immune function and of groups treated with immunosuppressive drugs provide some evidence on the subject.

Immunosuppressive drugs in transplant recipients

The incidence of non-Hodgkin's lymphomas, squamous cell cancer of the skin, Kaposi's sarcoma, primary liver cancer and melanoma is increased in transplant recipients treated with immunosuppressive drugs (Hoover & Fraumeni, 1973; Kinlen *et al.*, 1979; Penn, 1982). The increases amounted to about 45-fold for non-Hodgkin's lymphoma and to over 25-fold for squamous cell skin cancer (Kinlen *et al.*, 1983). The increase of Kaposi's sarcoma is more than 100-fold compared to that in the general population (excluding AIDS patients) (Penn, 1982).

Immunosuppressive drugs in patients without transplants

Patients without transplants treated with immunosuppressive drugs appear to experience increases, though of a lower magnitude, of the same malignancies that are increased in transplant patients. Relative risks of over 10-fold for non-Hodgkin's lymphoma and five-fold for squamous cell carcinoma of the skin were recorded (Kinlen, 1982).

Chronic renal failure

Patients with chronic renal failure (a group who show immune impairment) have an increased incidence of non-Hodgkin's lymphoma in the absence of immunosuppressive therapy (Kinlen *et al.*, 1980; Slifkin *et al.*, 1977).

Genetically determined immunodeficiency disorders

Large numbers of cases of non-Hodgkin's lymphoma in rare genetically determined immunodeficiency disorders such as ataxia telangiectasia and the Wiskott–Aldrich syndrome, are indicative of increased risks (Filipovitch *et al.*, 1980). A study of patients with common variable immunodeficiency found a 30-fold increase of lymphomas (Kinlen *et al.*, 1985).

Acquired immune deficiency syndrome (AIDS)

Patients with AIDS show a greatly increased incidence of Kaposi's sarcoma amounting to much more than 100-fold. Cerebral non-Hodgkin's lymphoma is also increased in these patients.

Blood groups

ABO blood groups

Individuals with blood group A have a slightly increased risk of stomach cancer, ranging from 2%–8%. The excess of blood group A largely occurs in subjects with the diffuse type of gastric cancer (Correa & Haenszel, 1982).

HLA antigens

Patients with Hodgkin's disease show an increased frequency of HLA antigen A1 (Amiel, 1967; Dausset *et al.*, 1982). An excess of antigens A2 and Sin-2 (BW46) has been reported and later confirmed in association with nasopharyngeal carcinoma in Chinese from south China (Simons *et al.*, 1975).

18.7   Future perspectives: molecular cancer epidemiology

Although significant progress has been made, there are still major gaps in our understanding of the remaining causes of human cancers and of the fundamental mechanisms involved in the multistage carcinogenic process. Several concepts and methods have already emerged that provide new approaches to identifying environmental carcinogens and host factors.

Conventional approaches in cancer epidemiology are seriously limited for definitively establishing cause-and-effect relationships. In addition, such approaches are largely retrospective rather than predictive. At the same time, although animal bioassays and newly developed short-term tests are extremely useful, there is a paucity of information on how the results obtained from these studies can be extrapolated to humans (Weinstein, 1981).

The solution to this problem is not simple repetition of the same studies, but the development of an entirely different type of approach, which combines epidemiological methods with laboratory techniques that can measure specific and meaningful biochemical parameters in human tissues and biological fluids, now generally referred to as 'molecular epidemiology' (Perera & Weinstein, 1982). A variety of highly sensitive, specific and reproducible laboratory procedures are now available (Bartsch *et al.*, 1988) that can be used to assess in humans specific factors related to genetic and acquired host susceptibility, metabolism and tissue levels of carcinogens, levels of covalent adducts formed between exogenous and endogenous carcinogens and cellular macromolecules and markers of early cellular responses to exposure to carcinogens.

Progress made in the understanding of the mechanisms of multistage carcinogenesis has led to the development of further markers that can be used in epidemiological studies, for example, levels of growth factors in biological fluids, their receptors in biopsy samples, and alterations in the expression of regulation of oncogenes/cell cycle genes and tumor suppressor genes. Finally, new techniques in molecular genetics have provided probes for assaying the role of such specific host genes in the origin of human cancers. In this way, in future, markers or genes associated with inheritability of susceptibility to common cancers will be identified and new ways of early detection diagnosis and treatment as well as genetic counselling might prove possible.

18.8   References

Ahluwalia, B., Jackson, M.A., Jones, G.W., Williams, A.O., Rao, M.S. & Rajguru, S. (1981). Blood hormone profiles in prostate cancer patients in high-risk and low-risk populations. *Cancer*, **48**, 2267–73.

England, P.C., Skinner, L.G., Cottrell, K.M. & Selwood, R.A. (1974). Serum estradiol 17 B in women with benign and malignant breast disease. *Br. J. Cancer*, **30**, 571–6.

Filipovich, A.H., Spector, B.D. & Kersey, J. (1980). Immunodeficiency in humans as a risk factor in the development of malignancy. *Prev. Med.*, **9**, 252–9.

Francomano, C. & Kazazian, H.H., Jr (1986). DNA analysis in genetic disorders. *Ann. Rev. Med.*, **37**, 377–95.

Friend, S.H., Bernards, R., Rogel, S., Weinberg, R.A., Rapaport, J.M., Albert, D.M. & Dryja, T.P. (1986). A human DNA segment with properties of the gene that predisposes to retinoblastoma and osteosarcoma. *Nature*, **323**, 643–6.

German, J. (1972). Genes which increase chromosomal instability in somatic cells and predispose to cancer. In *Progress in Medical Genetics*, ed. A.G. Steinberg & A.G. Bearn, volume VIII, pp. 61–101. New York: Grune & Stratton.

German, J., Bloom, D. & Passarge, E. (1979). Bloom's syndrome VII. Progress Report for 1978. *Clin. Genet.*, **15**, 361–7.

Ghanadian, R., Puah, K.M. & O'Donoghue, E.P.M. (1979). Serum testosterone and dihydrotestosterone in carcinoma of the prostate. *Br. J. Cancer*, **39**, 696–9.

Gonzalez, F.J., Jaiswal, A.K. & Nebert, D.W. (1987). P450 Genes: Evolution, regulation and relationship to human cancer. In *Cold Spring Harbor Symposia on Quantitative Biology: Molecular Biology of* Homo sapiens, volume 51, pp. 879–90. Cold Spring Harbor: Cold Spring Harbor Laboratory.

Hansen, M.F. & Cavenee, W.K. (1987). Genetics of cancer predisposition. *Cancer Res.*, **47**, 5518–27.

Harris, C.C., Vähäkangas, K., Trump, B.F. & Autrup, H. (1984). Interindividual variation in carcinogen activation and DNA repair. In *Genetic Predisposition in Responses to Chemical Exposures*. Banbury Report 16, ed. G. Omenn, pp. 145–54. Cold Spring Harbor: Cold Spring Harbor Laboratory.

Hein, D.W. (1988). Acetylator genotype and arylamine-induced carcinogenesis. *Biochem. et Biophys. Acta*, **948**, 37–66.

Higginson, J. (1968). Present trends in cancer epidemiology. *Proc. Can. Cancer Conf.*, **8**, 40–75.

Higginson, J. (1988). Changing concepts in cancer prevention: limitations and implication for future research in environmental carcinogenesis. *Cancer Res.*, **48**, 1381–9.

Hoover, R. & Fraumeni, J.F. (1973). Risk of cancer in renal transplant recipients. *Lancet*, **ii**, 55–7.

IARC (1987). *IARC Monographs on the Evaluation of Carcinogenic Risks to Humans*, Supplement No. 7, Overall evaluations of carcinogenicity: an updating of IARC monographs volumes 1–42, Lyon: International Agency for Research on Cancer.

Idle, J.R., Mahgoub, A., Sloan, T.P., Smith, R.L., Mbanefo, C.O. & Babanunmi, E.A. (1981). Some observations on the oxidation phenotype status of Nigerian patients presenting with cancer. *Cancer Lett.*, **11**, 331–8.

Judd, H.L., Davidson, B.J., Frumar, A.M., Shamonki, I.M., Lagasse, L.D. & Ballon, S.C. (1980). Serum androgens and estrogens in postmenopausal women with and without endometrial cancer. *Am. J. Obstet. Gynecol.*, **136**, 859–71.

Kalow, W. (1987). Genetic variation in the human hepatic cytochrome P-450 system. *Eur. J. Clin. Pharmacol.*, **31**, 633–41.

Kellerman, G., Shaw, C.R. & Luyten-Kellermann, M. (1973). Arylhydrocarbon hydroxylase inducibility and bronchiogenic carcinoma. *N. Engl. J. Med.*, **289**, 934–7.

Kinlen, L., Doll, R. & Peto, J. (1983). The incidence of tumors in human transplant recipients. *Transplantation Procs.*, **15.**, 1039–42.

Kinlen, L.J. (1982). Immunosuppressive therapy and cancer. *Cancer Surveys*, **1**, 565–83.

Kinlen, L.J., Eastwood, J.B., Kerr, D.N.S., Moorhead, J.F., Olivier, D.O., Robinson, B.H.B., De Wardener, H.E. & Wing, A.J. (1980). A study of cancer in dialysis patients. *Br. Med. J.*, **280**, 1401–3.

Kinlen, L.J., Sheil, A.G.R., Peto, J. & Doll, R. (1979). A collaborative UK–Australian study of cancer in patients with immunosuppressive drugs. *Br. Med. J.*, **ii**, 1461–6.

Kinlen, L.J., Webster, A.D.B., Bird, A.G., Haile, R., Peto, J., Soothill, J.F. & Thompson, R.A. (1985). Prospective study of cancer in patients with hypogammaglobulinaemia. *Lancet*, **i**, 263–5.

Knudson, A.G. (1985). Hereditary cancer, oncogenes, and antioncogenes, *Cancer Res.*, **45**, 1437–43.

Knudson, A.G. (1971). Mutation and cancer. A statistical study of retinoblastoma. *Proc. Natl. Acad. Sci. USA*, **68**, 820–3.

Koufos, A., Hansen, M.F., Lampkin, B.C., Workman, M.L., Copeland, N.G., Jenkins, N.A. & Cavenee, W.K. (1984). Loss of alleles at loci on human chromosomes 11 during genesis of Wilms' tumour. *Nature*, **309**, 170–2.

Kouri, R.E., McKinney, C.E., Slomiany, D.J., Snodgrass, D.R., Wray, N.P. & McLemore, T.L. (1982). Positive correlation between high aryl hydrocarbon hydroxylase activity and primary lung cancer as analyzed in cryopreserved lymphocytes. *Cancer Res.*, **42**, 5030–7.

Kwa, H.G., Cleton, F., Wang, D.Y., Bulbrook, R.D., Bulstrode, J.C., Hayward, J.L., Millis, R.R. & Cuzick, J. (1981). A prospective study of plasma prolactin levels and subsequent risk of breast cancer. *Int. J. Cancer*, **28**, 673–6.

Lee, W.-H., Bookstein, R., Hong, F., Young, L.-H., Shew, J.-Y. & Lee, E.Y.H.P. (1987). Human retinoblastoma susceptibility gene: cloning, identification and sequence. *Science*, **235**, 1394–9.

Malarkey, S.B., Schroeder, L.L., Stevens, V.C., James, A.G. & Lanese, R.R. (1977). Disordered nocturnal prolactin regulation in women with breast cancer. *Cancer Res.*, **37**, 4650–4.

Marletta, M.A. (1988). Mammalian synthesis of nitrite, nitrate, nitric oxide and *N*-nitrosating agents. *Chemical Res. Toxicol.*, **1**, 249–57.

Miller, E.C. & Miller, J.A. (1981). Mechanisms of chemical carcinogenesis. *Cancer*, **47**, 1055–64.

Mirvish, S.S. (1983). The etiology of gastric cancer. Intragastric nitrosamide formation and other theories. *J. Natl. Cancer Inst.*, **71**, 629–47.

Moore, J.W., Clark, G.M.G., Bulbrook, R.D., Hayward, J.L., Murai, J.T., Hammond, G.L. & Siiteri, P.K. (1982). Serum concentrations of total and non-protein bound oestradiol in patients with breast cancer and in normal controls. *Int. J. Cancer*, **29**, 17–21.

Mulvihill, J.J. (1976). Host factors in human lung tumors: An example of ecogenetics in oncology. *J. Natl. Cancer Inst.*, **57**, 3–7.

Myrnes, B., Giercksky, K.-E. & Krokan, H. (1983). Interindividual variation in the activity of O^6-methyl guanine–DNA methyltransferase and uracil–DNA glycosylase in human organs. *Carcinogenesis*, **4**, 1565–8.

National Research Council (1981). *The Health Effects of Nitrate, Nitrite and N-Nitroso Compounds*. Part I. Washington: National Academy Press.

Nebert, D.W., Negishi, M., Lang, M.A., Hjelmeland, L.M. & Eisen, H.J. (1982). The Ah locus, a multigene family necessary for survival in a chemically adverse environment: comparison with the immune system. *Adv. Genet.*, **21**, 1–52.

Nisker, J.A., Hammond, G.L., Davidson, B.J., Frumar, A.M., Takaki, N.K., Judd, H.L. &

Siiteri, P.K. (1980). Serum sex-hormone-binding globulin capacity and the percentage of free estradiol in postmenopausal women with and without endometral carcinoma. A new biochemical basis for the association between obesity and endometrial carcinoma. *Am. J. Obstet. Gynecol.* **138**, 637–42.

Nove, J., Little, J.B., Weichselbaum, R.R. *et al.* (1979). Retinoblastoma, chromosome 13, and *in vitro* cellular radiosensitivity. *Cytogenet. Cell. Genet.*, **24**, 176–84.

Nowell, P.C. & Croce, C.M. (1988). Chromosomal approaches to oncogenes and oncogenesis. *FASEB J.*, **2**, 3054–60.

Ohshima, H. & Bartsch, H. (1981). Quantitative estimation of endogenous nitrosation in humans by monitoring *N*-nitrosoproline excreted in the urine. *Cancer Res.*, **41**, 3658–62.

Pegg, A.E., Roberfroid, M., von Bahr, C., Foote, R.S., Mitra, S., Brésil, H., Likhachev, A. & Montesano, R. (1982). Removal of O^6-methylguanine from DNA by human liver fractions. *Proc. Natl. Acad. Sci. USA*, **79**, 5162–5.

Penn, I. (1982). The occurrence of cancer in immune deficiencies. *Current Problems in Cancer*, **6**, 1–64.

Perera, F.P. & Weinstein, I.B. (1982). Molecular epidemiology and carcinogen–DNA adduct detection: new approaches to studies of human cancer causation. *J. Chron. Dis.*, **35**, 581–600.

Petruzzelli, S., Camus, A.-M., Carrozzi, L., Ghelarducci, L., Rindi, M., Menconi, G., Angeletti, C.A., Ahotupa, M., Hietanen, E., Aitio, A., Saracci, R., Bartsch, H. & Giuntini, C. (1988). Long-lasting effects of tobacco smoking on pulmonary drug-metabolizing enzymes: a case-control study on lung cancer patients. *Cancer Res.*, **48**, 4695–700.

Ponder, B.A.J. (1984). Role of genetic and familial factors. In *Risk Factors and Multiple Cancer*, ed. B.A. Stoll, pp. 177–204. London: Wiley.

Reed, M.J., Cheng, R.W., Noel, C.T., Dudley, H.A.F. & James, V.H.T. (1983). Plasma levels of estrone, estrone sulfate, and estradiol and the percentage of unbound estradiol in postmenopausal women with and without breast disease. *Cancer Res.*, **43**, 3940–3.

Riboli, E. (1987). Epidemiology of colorectal cancer and diet. In *Causation and Prevention of Colorectal Cancer*, ed. J. Faivre & M.J. Hill, pp. 49–60. Amsterdam: Elsevier Science Publishers B.V.

Robbins, J.H. (1978). Significance of repair of human DNA: Evidence from studies of xeroderma pigmentosum. *J. Natl. Cancer Inst.*, **61**, 645–56.

Setlow, R.B. (1983). Variations in DNA repair among humans. In *Human Carcinogenesis*, ed. C.C. Harris & H. Autrup, pp. 231–54. New York: Academic Press.

Simons, M.J., Wee, G.B., Chan, S.H., Shanmugaratnam, K., Day, N.E. & De-Thé, G. (1975). Probable identification of an HLA second locus antigen associated with high risk of nasopharyngeal carcinoma. *Lancet*, **i**, 142–3.

Slifkin, R.F., Goldberg, J., Neff, M.S., Baez, A., Mattoo, N. & Gupta, S. (1977). Malignancy in end-stage renal disease. *Trans. Am. Soc. Art. Int. Org.*, **23**, 34–9.

Sobol, E., Narod, S.A., Nakamura, Y., Boneu, A., Calmettes, C., Chadenas, D., Charpentier, G., Chatal, J.F., Dupond, J.L., Delepine, N., Deslisle, M.J., Gardet, P., Godefroy, E., Guillausseau, P.J., Guillausseau-Scholer, C., Houdent, C., Lalay, J.D., Mace, G., Parmentier, C., Soubrier, F., Tourniaire, J., & Lenoir, G.M. (1989). The screening for multiple endocrine neoplasia type 2A by DNA polymorphism analysis. *N. Engl. J. Med.*, **321**, 996–1001.

Solomon, E., Voss, R., Hall, V., Bodmer, W.F., Jass, J.R., Jeffreys, A.J., Lucibello, F.C., Patel, I. & Rider, S.H. (1987). Chromosome 5 allele loss in human colorectal carcinomas. *Nature*, **328**, 616–19.

Stanbridge, E.J., Der, C.J., Doersen, C., Nishimi, R.Y., Peehl, D.M., Weissmann, B.E. & Wilkinson, J.E. (1983). Human cell hybrids: analysis of transformation and tumori-genicity. *Science*, **215**, 252–9.

Swift, M., Zimmerman, D. & McDonough, E.R. (1971). Squamous cell carcinoma in Fanconi's anaemia. *J. Am. Med. Assn.*, **216**, 325–6.

Taylor, J.C., Madison, R. & Kosinska, D. (1986). Is antioxidant deficiency related to chronic obstructive pulmonary disease? *Am. Rev. Resp. Dis.*, **134**, 285–9.

Vogelstein, B., Fearon, E.R., Hamilton, S.R., Kern, S.E., Preisinger, A.C., Leppert, M., Nakamura, Y., White, R., Smits, A.M.M. & Bos, J.L. (1988). Genetic alterations during colorectal-tumor development. *N. Engl. J. Med.*, **319**, 525–32.

Weinstein, I.B. (1981). Current concepts and controversies in chemical carcinogenesis. *J. Supramol. Struct. Cell Biochem.*, **17**, 99–120.

Weissmann, B.E., Saxon, P.J., Pasquale, S.R., Jones, G.R., Geiser, A.G. & Stanbridge, E.J. (1987). Introduction of a normal human chromosome 11 into a Wilms' tumor cell line controls its tumorigenic expression. *Science*, **236**, 175–80.

White, R., Barker, D., Holm, T., Berkowitz, J., Leppert, M., Cavenee, W., Leach, R. and Drayna, D. (1983). Approaches to linkage analysis in the human. In *Recombinant DNA Applications to Human Disease*, Banbury Report No. 14, ed. C.T. Caskey & R.L. White, pp. 235–250. Cold Spring Harbor: Cold Spring Harbor Laboratories.

Willett, W.C., Stampfen, M.J., Colditz, G.A., Rosner, B.A., Hennekens, C.H. & Speizer, F.E. (1987). Dietary fat and the risk of breast cancer. *N. Engl. J. Med.*, **316**, 22–8.

Yandell, D.W. (1989). Oncogenic point mutations in the human retinoblastoma gene: their application to genetic counseling. *N. Engl. J. Med.*, **321**, 1689–95.

Yunis, J.J. & Soreng, A.L. (1984). Constitutive fragile sites and cancer. *Science*, **226**, 1199–204.

19

Socio-economic factors

19.1   Introduction

The pioneering studies on occupational mortality of the Registrar General for England and Wales, which began in 1851, have consistently shown differences in mortality between occupational groups (Logan, 1982), including from 1891 onwards, cancer. The question arises whether these differences are due in whole or in part to carcinogenic factors in the work-place.

19.2   Occupational cancer: The Registrar General reports

To assess whether risk of cancer and other diseases is concentrated in one or more strata of society, the various occupational groups in England and Wales have been assigned to one of five social classes on the basis of income, education, etc. This resulted in relatively homogeneous classes. The professions are in social class I; unskilled laborers in social class V. In practice, six divisions are used. Social class III (skilled workers) is divided into those following manual (III M) and non-manual (III N) occupations. The mortality by social class for selected cancer sites is given in Table 19.1. In general, persons belonging to the non-manual social class III are more comparable to social classes I and II, whereas the pattern of risk in skilled manual workers tends to be closer to that of social classes IV and V. The mortality patterns of the retired (65–74) are more or less the same as those of the employed (15–64).

There are striking excesses for oesophagus, stomach, cervix uteri and lung cancer in social classes IV and V whereas the contrary is true for cancer of the testis. No significant gradient is seen for the colon. While mortality from malignant melanoma of the skin is greater in social class I, the converse is true for the other forms of skin cancer. This finding is

Table 19.1. *Standardized mortality ratios (SMR) by social class and cancer site for males aged 15–64 in England and Wales.*

	Total deaths	SMR by social class					
		I	II	IIIN	IIIM	IV	V
All malignant neoplasms (140–209)							
Malignant neoplasms of:							
buccal cavity and pharynx (140–149)	1,021	116	87	104	94	104	163
oesophagus (150)	1,913	81	86	85	108	113	139
stomach (151)	7,724	50	66	79	118	125	147
intestine except rectum (152, 153)	4,360	105	100	105	106	101	109
rectum and rectosigmoid junction (154)	2,989	84	90	103	114	106	108
pancreas (157)	3,206	103	97	105	110	101	104
larynx (161)	660	65	65	81	102	132	194
trachea, bronchus and lung (162)	31,983	53	68	84	118	123	143
skin (172, 173)	718	118	117	107	96	90	113
male breast (174)	75	236	85	114	108	78	121
prostate (185)	1,438	91	89	99	115	106	115
bladder (188)	2,261	79	83	91	120	105	115
other unspecified urinary organs (189)	1,383	101	103	112	103	102	110
brain (191)	2,306	108	101	111	105	100	92
Leukemia (205–207)	2,035	113	100	107	101	104	95
Other neoplasms of lymphatic and hematopoietic tissue (200–209 remainder of)	3,412	123	101	105	103	106	96

(After Registrar General, 1978.)

consistent with current information on habits relating to sunlight exposure among the professional classes.

For some occupations with a raised mortality, an explanation on the basis of work-related exposures to known chemical and physical carcinogens is not obvious. For some, such as bartenders, the excess risk lies largely with the oesophagus and, more recently, the lung. These increases are almost certainly linked to the ready availability of alcohol and tobacco for such individuals (Chapter 8).

When the diverse occupations within the same social class were compared, the risks for many cancer sites were remarkably close (Table 19.2). This table suggests that the excess observed compared with the national average lay not so much in direct exposures to hazards in the work-place, but rather that the exposures were associated with the social

Table 19.2. *Standardized mortality ratios from all cancers in males aged 15–64, adjusted for social class.*

Occupation	Non-adjusted[a]	Adjusted[b]
Farmers, foresters, fishermen	92	92
Miners, quarrymen	120	105
Gas, coke and chemical workers	118	102
Woodworkers	107	95
Clothing workers	97	86
Transport workers	120	106
Sales workers	89	104
Administrators and managers	74	94
Armed forces	161	—

[a] The non-adjusted ratios compare mortality with that of the total population, considered to be 100.
[b] The adjusted ratios compare mortality for people within the same social group (mean 100) and are therefore a more accurate indication of the effects of occupation *per se*.
(After Registrar General, 1978.)

group from which the higher risk occupations were recruited. The excesses and deficits of lung cancer found in several occupations broadly correlated with smoking habits. A low proportion of current smokers (33%) and a very low lung cancer SMR (32) were found in qualified medical practitioners, whereas coach and bus drivers, who smoked 28% more than the national average, had an SMR for lung cancer of 125.

Fox and Adelstein (1978) concluded that at-work exposures were likely to account for, at most, 18% of cancer in males aged 15–64. They stressed the need to examine all aspects of the environment in studying cancer differences in socio-economic groups, including such personal habits as diet. These non-occupational, socio-economic differences have existed for many years and have proven difficult to evaluate and control. Thus, although the mortality from gastric cancer has fallen steadily in England and Wales since 1921, over the years the ratio of mortality between the various social classes has remained virtually constant. Careful analysis of different social groups will often demonstrate the presence of risk factors known to be associated with specific sites. Thus, the professional classes and working wives tend to defer their first pregnancy, hence they have a higher breast cancer rate. The association of excess drinking and smoking with poverty and social deprivation is well recognized. The difference which may be found between salaried and non-salaried employees is often a guide to the epidemiologist that socio-economic factors may be involved. In conclusion, it is still sad to note that poverty *per se*, especially in industrial states tends to be associated with higher cancer levels. This is illustrated by the increased frequency in blacks in the USA compared to other ethnic groups which often reflects less satisfactory lifestyle conditions.

Lynge and Thygesen (1990) have recently reported on the cancer patterns related to occupation and social status in a large cohort (2.8 million) aged 20–64 years, in 1970, within Denmark. The study was made by linkage of individual records from the 1970 census, the Central Population Register death certificates and cancer registration. This methodology would appear to offer a useful approach to evaluating both social and occupational factors. Table 19.3 summarizes their findings in males and shows a two-fold difference between the highest and lowest category. These differences are discussed by site and socio-economic group in their report. In general, the variations are not as marked as in the UK data. In their studies, farmers showed unusually low cancer rates for most sites.

19.3   Religious groups

The extreme rarity of penile cancer in Jewish males and the low level of cervix uteri cancer in Jewish females (around 4) has long been known, phenomena ascribed to early ritual circumcision of the male. In India, both cervix and penile cancer are commoner in Hindu than in Muslim populations, possibly for the same reason. Within the United States, both Seventh Day Adventists who follow an ovo-lacto-vegetarian diet and Mormons, who do not, have less alcohol and tobacco related forms of cancer (habits which both groups eschew), but also less cancer of the large bowel and breast. There is little difference in urban and rural Mormon populations in contrast to non-Mormons (Table 19.4). The Amish have low cervix uteri cancer rates as have the Hutterites in Canada. These differences in cancer risks are believed to reflect lifestyle factors, including diet, of those who follow the precepts of their religion. Jensen (1983) has recently reported how closely the patterns of cancer in total abstainers in Denmark approach to those of Seventh Day Adventists.

19.4   Ethnic groups

As pointed out in Chapter 2, differences found in cancer patterns by ethnic group, apart from skin, are largely believed to result from environmental causes, although the role of genetic factors cannot be ruled

Table 19.3. *Relative risks for the overall cancer incidence and mortality of the Danish men in the socio-economic groups with more than 50 cancer cases (all economically active men = 1.00).*

	Relative risk	
	Cancer incidence	Cancer mortality
Unskilled worker, shipping/fishing	1.28	1.26
Skilled worker, other building	1.15	1.20
Skilled worker, other industries	1.15	1.20
Salaried employees IV	1.12	1.15
Skilled workers, metal industry	1.11	1.18
Self-employed, other industries II	1.10	1.10
Unskilled workers, cleaning	1.09	1.15
Salaried employees III	1.08	1.02
Unskilled workers, transport	1.08	1.14
Self-employed, other industries I	1.06	0.98
Self-employed, other industries III	1.04	1.08
Skilled workers, wood industry	1.03	1.02
Unskilled workers, manufacture	1.02	1.05
Salaried employees II	0.97	0.82
Unskilled workers, building	0.96	0.99
Self-employed, other agriculture	0.92	0.82
Salaried employees I	0.92	0.78
Unskilled workers, agriculture	0.77	0.80
Self-employed, farm II	0.69	0.64
Self-employed, farm I	0.68	0.64
All economically active	1.00	1.00

(After Lynge & Thygesen, 1990.)

Table 19.4. *Standardized incidence ratios[a] for selected sites in Utah (1969–1971) by religion and residence.*

	Mormons		Non-Mormons	
Cancer site (sex)	Urban	Rural	Urban	Rural
All (M)	73	72	115	76
Tobacco-related (M)	44	43	106	59
Colon (M)	67	49	104	54
Lung (M)	37	39	96	54
Breast (F)	84	74	121	97
Cervix (F)	54	60	120	111

[a] These ratios compare risk in the various sites with the general population of Utah, regarded as equalling 100.
(After Lyon *et al.*, 1980.)

out. Gradual changes in risk following migration and in the offspring of migrants usually reflect a different socio-economic level and lifestyle.

19.5   Conclusion

Much of the differences in cancer risk between occupational groups may be due to lifestyle and dietary factors, and such differences should not be ignored in the evaluation of cancer patterns among work forces.

None the less, such observations in no way reduce the need to identify occupational physico-chemical hazards since their control may be relatively straightforward through appropriate measures to control exposure (Chapter 8).

19.6   References

Fox, A.J. & Adelstein, A.M. (1978). Occupational mortality 1970–72: Work or way of life? *J. Epidemiol. Comm. Health.*, **32**, 73–8.

Jensen, O.M. (1983). Cancer risk among Danish male Seventh Day Adventists and other temperance society members. *J. Nat. Cancer Inst.*, **70**, 1011–14.

Logan, W.P.D. (1982). *Cancer Mortality by Occupation and Social Class, 1851–1971*, IARC Scientific Publications No. 36, Studies on Medical and Population Subjects No. 44. A joint publication of the Government Statistical Service and the International Agency for Research on Cancer, Office of Population Censuses and Surveys. London: Her Majesty's Stationery Office.

Lynge, E. & Thygesen, L. (1990). Occupational cancer in Denmark: Cancer incidence in the 1970 census population. *Scand. J. Work Environ. Health*, **16** Suppl 2, 1–35.

Lyon, J.L., Gardner, J.W. & West, D.W. (1980). Cancer risk and life-style: Cancer among Mormons from 1967–1975. In *Cancer Risk in Defined Populations. Banbury Report*, **4**, 3–30.

Registrar General (1978). *Occupational Mortality* 1970–1972, The Registrar General's decennial supplement for England and Wales, 1970–72, Series DS no. 1, Office of Population Censuses and Surveys. London: Her Majesty's Stationery Office.

Part III

Legal and ethical considerations

20

Legal and regulatory issues in cancer epidemiology

20.1   Introduction

In recent years, epidemiological evidence has become of increased importance in the law courts, notably in the United States, in relation to regulatory and toxic tort cases in a number of health related areas (Barnard, 1989). Accordingly, the epidemiologist may be called upon to explain the nature and limitations of studies on human disease and their causes, including the relation between environment and cancer. Such issues have become the subject of considerable legal controversy since epidemiological opinions can seldom be absolute and often contain inherent uncertainties (Huber, 1985; Thomas, 1983).

Certain issues of specific concern to the cancer epidemiologist are outlined briefly in this chapter, largely in terms of experience in the United States. The reader is referred to the reviews of Black and Lillienfeld (1984) and Schwartzbauer & Shindell (1988) for more in depth discussion.

Regulatory issues

Over the last half century, an important aspect of public health policy has been directed to reducing the cancer burden through regulatory control of potential chemical carcinogens present in the work-place or the ambient environment. In many industrial countries in Europe, recommended or compulsory standards and regulations are established by relevant ministries and/or health officials and, more recently, the European Economic Community (EEC). In the USA, such regulations are usually put forward by agencies such as the FDA, EPA, and OSHA which rely on data from various disciplines including epidemiology. In addition, other non-health issues may be taken into consideration such as technical feasibility.

In addition, epidemiological opinion may also be sought when proposed standards are challenged in the courts as frequently happens in the USA during the first stages of regulation. Such challenges are brought by an affected industry in support of arguments, for example, of insufficient evidence of probable harm, or by special interest groups alleging delayed implementation or requesting stricter controls or bans.

Toxic tort cases

In one category of tort action related to cancer, an individual or group of individuals claim compensatory and sometimes punitive damages on the grounds that a specific cancer has been caused following exposure to a known or a suspected carcinogen, as in the work-place or due to proximity to a toxic waste disposal dump. Action is taken against the agent or individual believed responsible for the exposure. Individuals as well as employers and industries may be held responsible.

Another variant of tort cases is related to product liability. Such actions arise from the concept that an individual is responsible for any harm to another which results from his wilful action or negligence, even indirectly. Formerly, manufacturers used to shelter behind the principle of *caveat emptor* in the case of merchandise. Today, the concept of product liability has been extended widely. Thus, it includes the sale and use of a product if the manufacturer could reasonably have been expected to be aware that such use could possibly constitute a hazard. Again, compensation and punitive damages may be involved.

The epidemiologist may be requested to give his opinion both on the probability of a human cancer risk following such exposures, and also on the date at which sufficient evidence existed that the defendant could reasonably have regarded his product as constituting a risk.

20.2   Toxic tort litigation and epidemiological evidence
Strength of the evidence

Toxic tort litigation raises questions about the application of common law to the evaluation of evidence on causation and the implications of epidemiological proof.

The underlying premise in such actions is that a toxic tort plaintiff has the burden of proving each element of his case, including causation. The problem of latency and the frequent absence of an identifiable factor make the situation more difficult in toxic tort cases relating to cancer than for an acute toxic episode. Such issues may go back many years, such as the causation of a recent cancer by an old trauma or irritation, for which contemporary evidence is rarely available. Schwartzbauer and Shindell (1988) point out that epidemiology is the only scientific discipline that deals with the integrated use of statistics and biological science to identify and establish the causes of disease in humans. Thus, the appropriate use of an epidemiological standard can provide courts with a rational and consistent means of evaluating evidence. In the absence of any identifiable exposure, the issues of causation are often complex and require resolution by expert witnesses. The latter may use a range of disciplines in addition to epidemiology including clinical, experimental and statistical data.

In establishing causation based on epidemiological data Black and Lillienfeld (1984) refer to what can be described as 'the more likely than not test', that is, a test that will meet the need for substantive evidence based on the understanding of the methods of epidemiology. The above authors have reviewed the application of different descriptive and analytical epidemiology approaches to various situations. On relative risk, they point out that the stronger the association between the factor and disease, the greater the certainty of the observed relative risk. When a relative risk of ten or more is observed, one can be reasonably certain of a causal relationship providing the number of cases is sufficient, but such occurrences are not common. Many cancers have a multifactorial etiology which cannot be ignored in trying to specify the role of individual factors.

These authors conclude that toxic tort plaintiffs should be held to the same requirements as plaintiffs in most other tort actions, and be required to produce evidence sufficient to establish that the factor at issue is 'more likely than not' to cause cancer. At present in the USA, the courts do not regard animal data as necessarily predictive of human harm. Thus, claims of alleged potential harm based on animal data alone are not considered justification for claiming damages, thus increasing the emphasis on epidemiological methods and data.

They also discuss the distinction between the data supporting a regulatory standard for possible toxic carcinogens and that used in determining tort liability. They point out that the former requires far less convincing proof than would be satisfactory to epidemiologists. As a result, the regulatory agencies employ methods that would not meet the test of epidemiological sufficiency, often using limited animal studies, even if unsupported by human data. While this may be appropriate for regulations, it should not carry over to tort cases.

20.3 The epidemiologist as an expert witnesses

In giving expert testimony the role of the epidemiologist is that of a scientific expert who must give an objective opinion on technical matters free from personal and outside bias. This evidence can be based on his own knowledge or his evaluation of the work of others. As yet, no court has determined the formal qualifications necessary for a competent witness to offer expert testimony about epidemiology. In general, a witness need only have such knowledge, skill, experience, training or education as to make it appear that his opinion will probably aid the trial in its search for truth. A medical degree is not required to be an epidemiologist and many physicians lack qualifications in epidemiology.

The epidemiologist may be involved in several types of cases. Thus, he may be required to give his opinion as an expert on the cause of a cancer in an individual, who is alleged to have been exposed to a particular toxic substance. In such circumstance, he will be required to explain the epidemiological evidence that such a chemical compound probably does, or does not, induce cancer in humans and the scientific background to his conclusions. Thus, he must instruct the court on the meaning of probabilities and their significance and the weight of the scientific evidence as he sees it. In some cases the issues may be relatively simple. He may need to explain the distinction between the statement that '85% of all lung cancers are probably due to cigarette smoking' from 'a particular lung cancer in an individual has an 85% chance of being due to smoking'. Thus, this latter statement might be misleading in the case of a smoker heavily exposed to asbestos dust. Since smoking and asbestos have a possible multiplicative effect, both are major causes and the attributable risk due to asbestos may be of the same order as tobacco. In this instance, his conclusion as to cause will largely depend on proof of significant previous asbestos exposure and he must explain his reasoning to the jury.

In rare instances the type of tumor produced by a factor may be so characteristic (a 'sentinel' tumor) that a reasonable judgment can be expressed without much difficulty, as with mesothelioma due to asbestos, or angiosarcoma due to vinyl chloride or thorotrast.

A more difficult situation arises when a common tumor or a cluster of cancers is perceived by an individual or group as being the result of exposure to toxic waste or some other low-level environmental exposure. The epidemiological data are usually negative or uninformative, and positive results may be random or due to confounding.

An individual may have developed a tumor such as a leukemia or lymphoma in a situation where some level of an isolated and doubtful exposure can be identified. There is no way in which the epidemiologist can carry out a study on a single individual. Further, the epidemiological data available almost always relate to much higher exposures in defined populations, very different from those that are being examined in the courts. The literature available may be negative or inconclusive, based on studies with an inadequate number of subjects. The demonstration of a cluster of cancers near a dump-site may be accepted as a fact but this does not necessarily permit any definitive conclusions regarding its cause without additional information.

In many cases, due to the insensitivity of the epidemiological method the epidemiologist must often admit that he cannot absolutely exclude the probability of a hazard, even if he believes that none is present. Such deficiencies in methodology and the need to use a weight of the evidence approach must be explained to the jury. In such cases, reasoning may permit a rational decision on the triviality or the significance of a suspected risk.

One of the most significant cases of this type occurred in Scotland (Muir, 1983) and was brought by a special interest group related to the claimed carcinogenic impact of water fluoridated for dental purposes. This long lawsuit resulted in the court deciding, on the weight of the evidence, that fluoride caused no harm. The views of epidemiologists were of great value in determining the decision in the court.

A further example illustrating etiological uncertitudes and the different conclusions drawn by different legal bodies, relates to the use of herbicides contaminated with dioxin during the Vietnam war where potential harm to veterans was alleged. One case was heard in Australia before a Royal Commission, and a second before a general court in the USA. The epidemiological data which had been collected on veterans in America and elsewhere showed no conclusive evidence of a carcinogenic or other health effects, in contrast to the animal data. In Australia, the Commission, presided over by a judge, concluded that the veterans had not been harmed, and no awards were made (Royal Commission, 1985). In contrast, in the USA, a settlement was agreed between the various manufacturers and the courts to pay compensation to all veterans although harm had not been demonstrated (Schuck, 1986). The epidemiological data were largely ignored in the judgment so that, in fact, everyone was being compensated for a theoretical but unproven risk.

The courts and expert evidence

There is increasing awareness on the part of trial and appellate judges that they must have greater control in the area of expert testimony. It has been emphasized that juries are increasingly being asked to make difficult decisions about highly complicated etiological issues of science and medicine. Many of these complexities are difficult to explain to juries who are ill qualified to assess the technical problems of interpreting complicated concepts. Accordingly, the latter will largely rely on its instincts as to the credibility of the various technical witnesses which at times may lead to irrational decisions as seen from a scientific viewpoint. This had led to a search especially in the USA for alternate procedures outside the courts for solving such complex issues, such as 'a science court'.

None the less, in courts where a large number of similar cases have been seen, certain guidelines for their solution have begun to develop and the epidemiologist should be aware of the pertinent legal literature.

A tort study group in the USA concludes that findings on causation should be based on credible scientific and medical evidence, not on opinions (Austrian, 1989). It was considered that one of the most pernicious developments in tort law has been the extent to which findings on causation have been based on printed opinions outside the mainstream of scientific or medical consensus. Jasanoff (1989) has developed this theme, and pointed out that scientific evidence is interpreted differently in the court than in the laboratory, but emphasized that the collective opinions of experts can be influential.

20.4   Regulation and the concept of risk

In recent years, there has been increasing discussion on the role of epidemiology in defining the concept of risk. According to Barnard (1989), five general concepts have arisen in the USA from the interactions of law and science. These include safe level; significant risk; acceptable risk; *de minimis* risk; and negligible risk. These terms have been developed and defined by the courts and regulatory agencies. In the regulatory context, the objective is to evaluate scientific data and to present an estimate of the probability that potential for population harm could occur. Utilizing quantitative risk assessment (QRA) this is often calculated as a probability of less than 10^{-6} or 10^{-5}. Such low levels of risk cannot be confirmed or rejected by epidemiological techniques (Chapter 4).

In the case of potential dangers associated with a particular product or degree of risk, the federal rules of evidence permit expert witnesses to describe the scientific methodology involved and place on the courts the burden of determining its relevance and conformity with the general scientific consensus.

Where a regulatory body is involved, as in the USA, animal data may frequently be relied on to set a regulation. This contrasts with the area of product liability in which the courts have concluded that *in vitro* and *in vivo* studies of this kind on a chemical, either singly or in combination, are not capable of proving causation in human beings in the face of contradictory epidemiological evidence.

Safety

It is impossible to discuss here the major implications involved in legal decisions on safety, an area constantly changing. Further, there may be different viewpoints expressed by the lower and the upper courts. OSHA has contended that there is no absolutely 'safe' level for a carcinogen and therefore the burden to show a safe level rests on industry. The Supreme Court, in relation to potential hazards in the work-place, stated 'that safe is not the equivalent of risk-free.... Similarly, a work-place can hardly be considered unsafe unless it threatens workers with a significant risk of harm' (Austrian, 1989).

Significant risk

Significant risk is difficult to measure and might not mean the same to the epidemiologist and to the courts. In the USA, it was concluded that decisions by the agencies on relation to safety and significance should depend on judgment based not only on scientific data but also on consideration of which risks are acceptable in the world where we live. These criteria require that a regulation be supported by substantial evidence and that there is a significant risk of harm. In such a context, the epidemiologist, especially working within the occupational milieu, has an important role.

Acceptable risk

The use of this term is generic. In its broad application it is basically judgmental, depending on scientific data and what society will accept. Thus, the role of the epidemiologist is to make available a sound, statistical and scientific evaluation in characterizing the risk, but the societal aspects may lie outside his competence.

De minimis risk

This term has been discussed elsewhere (Chapter 7). As pointed out, the epidemiologist can contribute little as most human studies have been at levels of exposure at which no detectable effect could be expected. However, a series of well-designed negative studies may, at times, be useful in supporting a decision that a risk is to be regarded as *de minimis* or trivial, by a regulatory body or the courts. Recently, Congress has attacked the concept of *de minimis* risk as used by the FDA in relation to food additives.

Negligible risk

In the USA, the National Academy of Sciences has proposed a concept of negligible risk as an interpretive device to describe very low risks but without any numerical attachments. It is chiefly used in relation to pesticides in food stuffs and agricultural processes in parallel with the application of *de minimis* risks. At the time of writing, Congress is considering such legislation.

20.5   Conclusions

There are many legal areas relating to public health where epidemiological data may be important, whether the data demonstrate a detectable or no convincing evidence of an effect.

The major criteria for an epidemiologist as an expert witness in relation to an individual risk require that he makes it clear that he is dealing in probabilities using his best judgment based on his own interpretation of the weight of the evidence. Further, difficult although it sometimes may be, he must not identify with either plaintiff or defendant in expressing his opinion. In the USA, it is illegal for an expert to be paid on a contingency basis.

20.6   References

Austrian, M.L. (1989). Expert evidence in toxic tort litigation. *For the Defense*, February, 17–22.

Barnard, R.C. (1989). Some regulatory definitions of risk: Interaction of science and legal principles. *Regul. Toxicol. Pharmacol.*, in press.

Black, B. & Lillienfeld, D.E. (1984). Epidemiologic proof in toxic tort litigation. *Fordham Law Rev.*, **52**, 732–85.

Huber, P. (1985). Safety and the second best: the hazards of public risk management in the courts. *Columbia Law Rev.*, **85**, 277–337.

Jasanoff, S. (1989). Science on the witness stand. *Issues in Science and Technology*, Fall, 80–7.

Muir, C.S. (1983). Cancer epidemiology: past, present and future. *Prog. Clin. Biol. Res.*, **132A**, 71–105.

Royal Commission (Royal Commission on the Use and Effects of Chemical Agents on Australian Personnel in Vietnam) (1985). *Final Report July* 1985. Volume 8: Conclusions, Recommendations and Epilogue. Canberra: Australian Government Publishing Service.

Schwartzbauer, E.J. & Shindell, S. (1988). Cancer and the adjudicative process: The interface of environmental protection and toxic tort law. *Am. J. Law Med.*, **XIV**, 1–76.

Schuck, P.H. (1986). *Agent Orange on Trial: Mass Toxic Disasters in the Courts*. Cambridge, MA: Belknap Press of Harvard University Press

Thomas, W.A. (ed.) (1983). *Symposium on Science and the Rules of Legal Procedure*, sponsored by National Conference of Lawyers and Scientists, a joint organization of the American Bar Association and the American Association for the Advancement of Science. 101 Federal Rules Decisions, 599.

21

Ethical responsibilities of the epidemiologist

21.1   Ethical considerations in cancer epidemiology

Today the subject of bioethics has become part of formal training in all health professions (Kieffer, 1978). In earlier years, the majority of epidemiologists were physicians and governed by the constraints of medical ethics as based on the Hippocratic oath. Although research on human subjects is common to many branches of medicine, concern regarding the individual subject and the protection of his rights in such studies is of comparatively recent origin, as illustrated by the Nuremberg Code and the Declaration of Helsinki (1976).

There is currently no formal code *per se* for epidemiologists practising their discipline. As epidemiology has expanded, however, and become a profession in its own right, practised by scientists of varying disciplinary backgrounds, a number of issues specifically relevant to epidemiology have arisen. These include the responsibility of the epidemiologist towards the subjects in a study, his responsibility to the community at large, and his communication of the results of his studies either to the subjects involved or to the public (Soskolne, 1989). While these issues are not fundamentally different from those facing the physician, they have certain features which differentiate them from the usual problems facing the practising doctor.

21.2   Issues in epidemiology

Essentially, the task of the epidemiologist is to advance knowledge by the identification of the determinants of disease with a view to benefiting the community, and, indirectly, the individual. Thus, his investigations are either undertaken for general research ends or to provide data for public health purposes such as the presence or absence of an environmental cancer hazard in a community. His subjects are not patients in the sense that he is directly responsible for treatment so that malpractice problems, etc, do not enter into his experience. On the other hand, he is responsible for ensuring that the subjects of his study either individually and collectively do not suffer unnecessary physical or mental discomfort and harm as a result of his investigations. The use of an invasive technique to measure some parameter for a study is not acceptable if it carries a significant risk to the individual unless it can be shown unequivocally that a comparable benefit to that individual may be anticipated (Jonsen, 1978).

Informed consent

If an epidemiological enquiry requires the active participation of human subjects, informed consent is required. This ensures that the individual comprehends the aims, nature and benefits of the proposed investigation. The epidemiologist must be certain that participation is voluntary and not through the pressure of third parties who may require the information for other reasons. For example, an employer might commission an epidemiological study of a group of individuals without ensuring that they are aware of the nature of the project and its rationale. In some cultures, informed consent is not given by the individual but rather at the village or comparable level after discussion by village elders or other equivalent representatives.

There are situations where data must be obtained from sources collated for other purposes, e.g. large-scale research requiring use of national statistics. In such circumstances, the individual subjects would not need to be contacted for their consent, provided that the anonymity of the data is guarded. If there is any doubt of the nature of a study and there is any question of invasion of privacy, it is advisable to have it reviewed by competent colleagues to ensure that the study meets acceptable ethical and scientific standards. Indeed, in some countries, this is mandatory.

Guarding privacy

In recent years the preservation of privacy has become an area of concern. On the one hand, application of restrictive regulations to publicly collected data by national or state authorities has led to the refusal to make this information available to reputable epidemiologists to carry out desirable research. In several western European countries, it is difficult if not impossible to ascertain the cause of death for members of a cohort study. In France, the death certificate is a confidential document. Inability to match death certificates against cancer registry holdings means that an invaluable source of data quality control and the means to calculate survival are lost. The requirement in the Federal Republic of Germany that the cancer patient had to give consent for his case to be included in the cancer registry in effect destroyed the value of the regulation permitting registration. Many of those demanding complete privacy are also those who wish a risk-free environment but seem unwilling to allow the studies that would assist in evaluating potential cancer risks.

Particular care is needed when dealing with confidential data which may be detrimental to the individual and yet be necessary in developing appropriate public health responses. An example is the relationship between AIDS and Kaposi's hemangiosarcoma in the USA, where, at present, the confidentiality of infection with the AIDS virus is determined by the individual concerned. Thus, access to a patient's medical records remains a matter of continuing discussion (Strasser *et al.*, 1987). Some of the information sought by the epidemiologist may be very personal. Failure to examine the susceptibilities of individuals within the culture in which they are being examined may lead to unnecessary mental stress. The epidemiologist as a health professional has clear responsibilities to guard the confidentiality of his research material, e.g. questionnaires. In modern society, with concern for the role of environment, it is desirable to ensure that the privacy of the individual be safeguarded, but not to the extent that the generation of data necessary to protect the community cannot be carried out.

Peer review

Peer review, while not obligatory, is useful not only to ensure that a study is well designed and gives due consideration to the individuals concerned but also to provide protection to the researcher against later accusations of bad faith, incompetence, etc., as well as the institute which he represents. A peer review group should be satisfied as to the scientific and other pertinent credentials of the analyst who is undertaking the study. It should also assure itself that the reasons for carrying out the study are sound, that it is carefully planned and of adequate size to meet its overall objectives, and that the necessary steps have been taken to guard individual confidentiality and to assure publication within reasonable time.

Informing the patient and the public

The medical profession has long been concerned with communication to the individual patient. Today, the health professional has an acknowledged responsibility to make relevant information available to patients, colleagues, and, under certain circumstances, to the public

(AMA, 1980). Although existing codes govern the conduct of physicians and their associates in medical research and in clinical procedures requiring informed consent, the ethical guides for the communication of the existence of potential health risks have not been defined. The withholding of pertinent information or the provision of unqualified, incomplete or uncertain data may be detrimental to the individual and/or the community. Thus, in addition to possible legal questions, this situation raises medical and ethical concerns in a variety of settings regarding the epidemiologist's role in communicating information to the public.

In Europe, such situations were governed originally by learned societies which laid down strict criteria for public communication. Prior to the 1950s, the General Medical Council in the UK did not permit a doctor to be identified, when commenting on an issue in the press. The rationale was to prevent exaggerated claims by incompetent individuals or by physicians as a means of advertising their skills. This attitude changed as concern about environmental and health issues has become more prevalent and has been accompanied with a gradual loss of faith in the credibility of public health officials and other authorities in some countries (Soskolne, 1989). These changes in public attitudes, associated with strong pressures to know everything, have placed the individual epidemiologist in a difficult position.

Where benefits and risks can be identified and measured and consequent effective public action taken, the epidemiologist has little problem in lending his expertise to addressing the public issues, for example, reduction of cigarette smoking as a method of preventing lung cancer.

However, he may face difficulties in deciding on the acceptability and disclosure of risks in the following circumstances: 1) the inadequacy of measurement of a risk; 2) the absence of alternatives to continued risk exposure or the potentially greater dangers from alternative risks; and 3) the lack of any medical treatment. Pochin (1982) has written 'in medicine, the proper review of risk and of benefit, and the assurance that overall benefit is obtained with minimized risk, can never be a simple matter of knowing the probabilities and doing the arithmetic.... In any particular case the risk may be judged to be trivial, but what means that word trivial? Or it may be judged to be so large that it outweighs the expected benefit, but is it then truly large in a quantitative sense, or is it only a conspicuous and perhaps unfamiliar type of risk which seems to be large?'.

The need to know: protecting the individual

In the past, it was considered good medical practice to conceal a serious diagnosis, such as cancer, from the patient, because of the physician's knowledge of the patient and his particular circumstances. The rationale for not divulging all the facts to the patient was the view that distressful news may be detrimental. 'In much wisdom is much grief: and he that increase the knowledge increaseth sorrow.' (Ecclesiastes, i, 18). Now, societal and legal pressures are pushing for full disclosure of all relevant medical details to every patient (and possibly subject in an epidemiological study), no matter how tenuous the relationship with disease or exposure (Senate Bill S.79, 1987).

In such cases, the principle should be accepted that the potential risk of harm should be very low unless a compensating benefit can be offered. Thus, it might be considered unethical to inform an individual, simply to satisfy idle curiosity or a regulation, that he possesses some physiological abnormality of uncertain or predictive value. Examples include an unevaluated biomarker, such as an occasional chromosomal abnormality, which may pose only a trivial or non-existent risk to his health. Where there may be some conflict of interest between the public interest and the individual, the individual's rights would appear to be primary (Royal College of Physicians, 1982). In such cases, the epidemiologist must act judiciously (use common sense) and ponder the consequences of his decisions for the direct or indirect well-being of an individual.

The possibility that ethical and legal requirements may conflict is increasing and this issue requires more consideration than is possible in this chapter.

Obligation to society

The epidemiologist often assumes that his research will improve public health and provide benefits to society. He must however, avoid the very real danger of unduly magnifying the significance of his work and presenting uncertain data without caveats (Brennan, 1977). Conversely, the decision to down-play a possible risk when there is the possibility of public over-reaction or when the results have major socio-economic or health implications is extraordinarily difficult.

These considerations require that he communicates his results with care and judgment. None the less, no matter how much the epidemiologist tries to suppress his personal values, there may be reasonable and honest differences of opinion in the interpretation of data and its significance amongst trained epidemiologists. These occur in any field of science.

The reports of an epidemiologist should be governed by the results of the scientific research he presents. His associates or employer should not be taken into consideration in evaluating data as this introduces external bias. He should not permit any external body to modify his interpretation of the data, or delay the publication of his reports without compelling reasons (AOMA, 1976). In general, controversial situations should not arise if care is taken in terms of publication and presentation to meet standard scientific norms, and colleagues have been consulted adequately (Mathis, 1982).

21.3   References

AMA (1980). American Medical Association principles of medical ethics. *Am. Med. News,* August 1/8, 9.

Brennan, M.J. (1977). Truth versus data. *Med. Pediatr. Oncol.,* **3**, 199–205.

AOMA (American Occupational Medicine Association) (1976). Code of ethical conduct for physicians providing occupational-medical services. *J. Occup. Med.,* **18**.

Declaration of Helsinki (1976). Recommendations guiding medical doctors in biomedical research involving human subjects. Adopted by the 18th World Medical Assembly, Helsinki, Finland, 1964, and revised by the 29th World Medical Assembly, Tokyo, 1975. *J. Irish Med. Ass.* **69**, 74–5.

Jonsen, A.R. (1978). Do no harm. *Ann. Int. Med.,* **88**, 827–32.

Kieffer, G.H. (1978). *Bioethics: A Textbook of Issues,* pp. 434–6. Reading, MA: Addison-Wesley Publishing Co.

Mathis, J.F. (1982). An industrial scientist's perspective on scientific peer review. *Fundam. Appl. Toxicol.,* **2**, 280–2.

Pochin, E. (1982). Risk and medical ethics. *J. Med. Ethics,* **8**, 180–4.

Royal College of Physicians, Faculty of Occupational Medicine (1982). *Guideline on Ethics for Occupational Physicians,* 2nd edition, pp. 2–5. London: Royal College of Physicians.

Senate Bill S.79. (1987). High risk occupational disease notification and prevention act of 1987. Introduced by Senator Metzenbaum, January, 1987.

Soskolne, C.L. (1989). Epidemiology: Question of science, ethics, morality, and law. *Am. J. Epidemiol.,* **129**, 1–8.

Strasser, T., Jeanneret, O. & Raymond, L. (1987). Ethical aspects of prevention trials. In *Ethical Dilemmas in Health Promotion,* ed. S. Doxiadis, pp. 183–94. New York: John Wiley & Sons.

Part IV

Introduction: total and specific site epidemiology

Guidelines for chapters 22 – 57

Chapter 22 addresses the overall incidence of cancer. The following chapters, 23–57, summarize information in a fairly standard manner on the descriptive epidemiology and etiological factors for the principal cancer sites. The discussion for each site is subdivided into sections to preserve uniformity in presentation. On occasion, a section may be omitted for lack of data – in that event the layout given below is none the less maintained.

Introduction

A general statement on the major feature(s) of cancer at this site.

Histology, classification and diagnosis

Outlines information on pathogenesis, histological classification, and diagnosis and their relevance to epidemiological and etiological evaluation.

Descriptive epidemiology

This section summarizes the major features of the epidemiology of the cancer in question. It supplements the material in Appendix 1 at the end of the book and the summarizing histogram for each chapter. Incidence figures, age-adjusted to the 'world' standard population are given as average annual rates per 10^5 with the (exception of Chapter 58 where they are present in rates per 10^6). Normally the words 'average annual age adjusted per 10^5' are omitted.

The histogram covers a group of 'standard' populations representative of the major geographical regions in the world. All centers chosen have reliable cancer registries of many years standing.

(a) The registry of Detroit (USA) is used to represent typical cancer patterns in the white and black populations of the United States;
(b) the Birmingham Cancer Registry (UK) is typical of a mixed rural and industrial population in England;
(c) Norway is a nordic country with little heavy industry;
(d) the registry in Slovenia (Yugoslavia) represents a largely rural population of Eastern Europe;
(e) The prefecture of Miyagi in North East Japan has a mixed economy;
(f) Cali (Colombia) represents an industrial Latin American city with a large number of recent rural migrants;
(g) the registry of the city state of Singapore covers a population of largely south Chinese origin, with access to a high level of medical services;
(h) Bombay represents a large urban complex in west central India;
(i) Israel covers Jewish populations of diverse origins.

In addition, the histograms also include the populations with the highest rates recorded in Volume V of *Cancer Incidence in Five Continents* (Muir *et al.*, 1987) (see Fig. 23 for example). The lowest recorded rates are not given for many sites since these are frequently based on less than ten cases per million person years. When a rate is less than 0.05 no value is given. More extensive incidence data are given in Appendix I. Comments may be made on urban/rural and ethnic differences. While the major emphasis is on incidence, mortality and relative frequency data may be quoted. Age and sex distribution are usually only discussed when pertinent to etiological evaluation as are temporal changes.

Etiological inferences

This section describes etiological inferences which may be suggested by the descriptive data (Chapter 2).

Known and suspected causes

This section summarizes the views of the authors as determined from available descriptive and analytical epidemiological material. If possible, a distinction is made between causative associations and situations where the evidence is suggestive, but not completely conclusive. Thus, further studies may be indicated. Anecdotal or speculative associations are generally not discussed unless pertinent to public health policies.

The authors have tried to avoid details of individual epidemiological studies in discussion of individual sites unless required for interpretation or to indicate current uncertainties. Thus, for the liver and cervix, there is more discussion of the analytical epidemiological data compared to other sites. Acceptance of the conclusions of a study imply that the study is regarded as adequately executed, meets acceptable biostatistical criteria, and that consideration has been given to possible biases and confounding variables.

Relevant laboratory studies

Relevant laboratory studies are limited since it is impossible to evaluate with any adequacy the enormous data available. Discussion is largely confined to studies that may be relevant to the human situation. Many developments in molecular biological techniques are insufficiently developed to provide adequate understanding of their role in field investigations. The brief statements made indicate the types of studies that may be of value, and are further discussed in Chapter 5.

Attributable risks

Where a factor has been identified as important, an attempt will be made where possible to approximate the proportion of cancers attributable to that risk.

Conclusions

Conclusions regarding etiological factors and their significance in relation to potential prevention strategies are briefly reviewed.

Bibliography

Cancer Epidemiology and Prevention (Schottenfeld & Fraumeni, 1982) covers adequately the literature prior to 1982. Accordingly, references are for the most part limited to recent reviews or key articles. Descriptive epidemiological data are summarized from the various volumes of *Cancer Incidence in Five Continents* (Doll *et al.*, 1966, 1970; Waterhouse *et al.*, 1976, 1982; Muir *et al.*, 1987) (see Chapter 2). The greater part of the incidence data presented here are contained in the most recent volume. A review of cancer in developing countries has recently been published (Parkin, 1986). For statements on the burden of cancer the estimates made by Parkin *et al.* (1988) are used. For many cultural, chemical and occupational causes, the IARC Monographs provide adequate coverage of the relevant literature.

References

Doll, R., Payne, P. & Waterhouse, J. (eds.) (1966). *Cancer Incidence in Five Continents*, Volume I, A technical report, UICC. Berlin: Springer Verlag.

Doll, R., Muir, C. & Waterhouse, J. (eds.) (1970). *Cancer Incidence in Five Continents*, Volume II. Geneva: UICC.

Muir, C., Waterhouse, J., Mack, T., Powell, J. & Whelan, S. (eds.) (1987). *Cancer Incidence in Five Continents*, Volume V, IARC Scientific Publication No. 88. Lyon: International Agency for Research on Cancer.

Parkin, D.M. (ed.) (1986). *Cancer Occurrence in Developing Countries*, IARC Scientific Publications No. 75. Lyon: International Agency for Research on Cancer.

Parkin, D.M., Läärä, E. & Muir, C.S. (1988). Estimates of the worldwide frequency of sixteen major cancers in 1980. *Int. J. Cancer*, **41**, 184–97.

Schottenfeld, D. & Fraumeni, J.F., Jr. (eds.) (1982). *Cancer Epidemiology and Prevention*. Philadelphia: W.B. Saunders Company.

Waterhouse, J., Muir, C.S., Correa, P. & Powell, J. (eds.) (1976). *Cancer Incidence in Five Continents*, Volume III, IARC Scientific Publications No. 15. Lyon: International Agency for Research on Cancer.

Waterhouse, J., Muir, C., Shanmugaratnam, K. & Powell, J. (eds.) (1982). *Cancer Incidence in Five Continents*, Volume IV, IARC Scientific Publications No. 42. Lyon: International Agency for Research on Cancer.

Overall cancer incidence

22.1   Global cancer burden

The existence of differing patterns of cancer occurrence throughout the world has been known for many years, as perusal of the
fascinating monograph published in 1915 by Hoffman, the actuary to the
Prudential Assurance Company reveals. It was not, however, until 1984
that estimates (based on the year 1975) were made, not only of the global
cancer burden but also for each of the 24 demographic regions recognized
by the United Nations (UNO, 1986). This was later updated by Parkin *et
al.* (1988), who estimated the global total of new cancers to be 6.35 million.
This number was almost exactly divided between the sexes and between
developed and developing countries, although two-thirds of the world
population dwells in the latter.

The 'top ten' cancers are given in Table 22.1. Unfortunately, these
figures are essentially estimates, since they are not uniformly collected,
being derived from various sources. The latter include incidence figures
from cancer registries, and incidence estimates extrapolated from
mortality. For large areas of the world, numbers are based on relative
frequency data, mostly obtained from the monograph *Cancer Occurrence
in Developing Countries* (Parkin, 1986). Regrettably, the calculation of
age-specific and age-standardized incidence rates, which provide a
measure of the difference in risk between populations was not possible.
The methods used, notably for the developing countries, are discussed in
the original papers.

Despite the caveats, the information probably reflects reasonably well
the relative burden and site pattern for most regions, a few of which have
been selected for graphic presentation by bar diagrams (Figures
22.1–22.8). The numbers within the bars give the estimated number of
incident cases in thousands. It is worth noting that the first five ranking

Table 22.1. *Estimates of most frequent cancers worldwide, 1980.*

	Males		Females		Both sexes	
	Number[a]	%	Number[a]	%	Number[a]	%
1. Lung	513.6	15.8	1. Breast	572.1	18.4	1. Stomach	669.4	10.5
2. Stomach	408.8	12.6	2. Cervix	465.6	15.0	2. Lung	660.5	10.4
3. Colon/rectum	286.2	8.8	3. Colon/rectum	285.9	9.2	3. Breast	572.1	9.0
4. Mouth/pharynx	257.3	7.9	4. Stomach	260.6	8.4	4. Colon/rectum	572.1	9.0
5. Prostate	235.8	7.3	5. Corpus uteri	148.8	4.8	5. Cervix	465.6	7.3
6. Esophagus	202.1	6.2	6. Lung	146.9	4.7	6. Mouth/pharynx	378.5	6.0
7. Liver	171.7	5.3	7. Ovary	137.6	4.4	7. Esophagus	310.4	4.9
8. Bladder	167.7	5.2	8. Mouth/pharynx	121.2	3.9	8. Liver	251.2	4.0
9. Lymphoma	139.9	4.3	9. Esophagus	108.2	3.5	9. Lymphoma	237.9	3.7
10. Leukemia	106.9	3.3	10. Lymphoma	98.0	3.2	10. Prostate	235.8	3.7
11. —	—	—	11. —	—	—	11. Bladder	219.4	3.5
12. —	—	—	12. —	—	—	12. Leukemia	188.2	3.0

[a] in thousands
(After Parkin *et al.*, 1988.)

Fig. 22.1 This figure shows that the commonest global malignancy in males by far is lung cancer, as is breast cancer in females. However, when both sexes are combined, stomach cancer, although declining (Chapter 26), is the most important. The high proportion of mouth/pharynx cancer in males reflects the frequency of this cancer in a large area of the Indian subcontinent.

THE WORLD

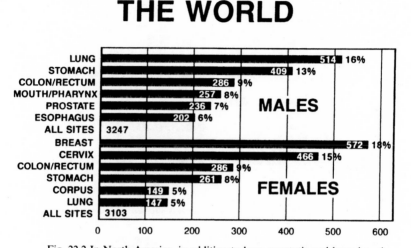

Fig. 22.2 In North America, in addition to lung, prostatic and large bowel cancers in males, are also very important tumours. Whereas in females, breast and colon are still more frequent than lung.

NORTHERN AMERICA

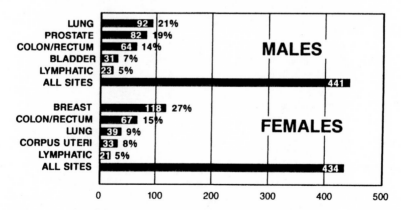

cancers accounted for about 60% of all forms of malignancy in each of the regions depicted. The age-adjusted incidence rates are not given, but such data are presented for selected regions of the world in individual chapters, and in Appendix 1.

These numbers can be used to estimate the cancer burden in terms of the

Fig. 22.3 In Western Europe, stomach cancers are among the first five ranking sites in both sexes.

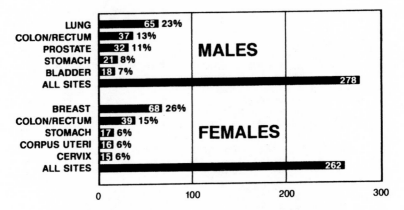

Fig. 22.4 In Eastern Europe, the pattern is substantially the same as in Western Europe.

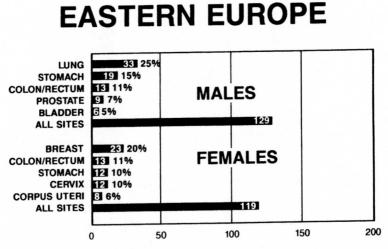

number of persons to be diagnosed and treated, which by the year 2010 will probably be of the order of 10 million. This may be an underestimate, since it would imply only an increase of 1.5% per annum since 1980.

22.2   Cancer – all sites

Since the term cancer covers a range of neoplastic diseases with differing biological characteristics and causes, data should be presented for individual cancers when making comparisons for these to have any

Fig. 22.5 In Japan, the overwhelming preponderance of stomach cancer in both sexes is apparent.

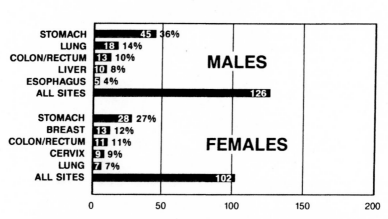

JAPAN

Fig. 22.6 In China, stomach, esophageal and liver cancer predominate in males, whereas cervix cancer is most common in females. Breast remains relatively low (6%) and does not appear in the first five ranking sites.

CHINA

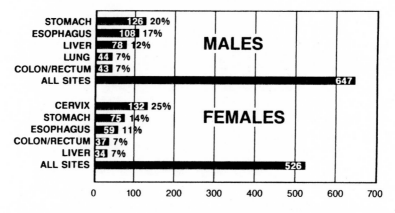

biological meaning. None the less, it is not infrequent to group all forms of cancer together under the heading 'All sites' in describing the disease in general terms. As some cancer registries do not collect information on non-melanoma skin cancer (ICD 173), such comparisons are often made for 'All Sites but 173' (Fig. 22.9).

The highest rate (All Sites but 173) in males is found in the black population of Detroit (400), the lowest in the Kuwaiti population of

Fig. 22.7 In Southern Asia, cancers of the mouth and pharynx occupy first place in males and third in females.

SOUTHERN ASIA

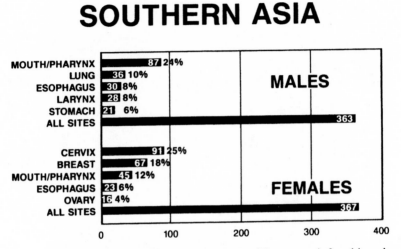

Fig. 22.8 In Western Africa a preponderance of liver cancer is found in males, also very high levels of malignant lymphoma, e.g. Burkitt's lymphoma. In females, cervix is the commonest form of cancer.

WESTERN AFRICA

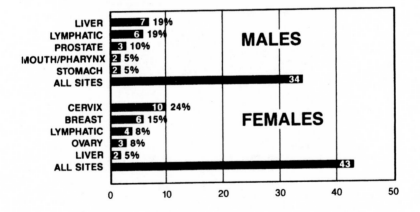

Kuwait (72). Given the very high level of medical services available in Kuwait, the difference is not likely to be artefactual (Appendix 1, Table 1.2).

In comparing populations, it should be noted that the term 'all sites' may conceal large differences in the level of the constituent cancers in

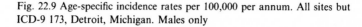

Fig. 22.9 Age-specific incidence rates per 100,000 per annum. All sites but ICD-9 173, Detroit, Michigan. Males only

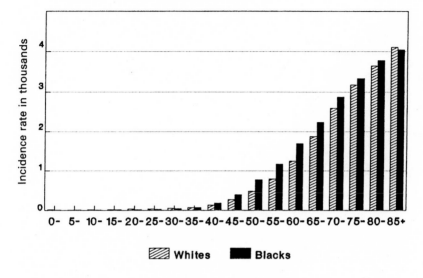

different countries and populations. Differences in 'all sites' cannot be regarded as representing the influence of general ambient carcinogens. Thus, much of the major differences, such as those between the low-risk American Japanese (M 189.0: F 176.5) and the high-risk black populations (M 389.4: F 249.2) living in the same city, San Francisco, are probably partly or largely attributable to nutrition, alcohol and smoking, which influence individual cancer sites.

Estimates of 'all sites' are used for planning health services: even then changes in incidence of specific cancer sites and current methods of treatment must be taken into account when estimating needs.

22.3   References

Parkin, D.M. (ed.) (1986). *Cancer Occurrence in Developing Countries*, IARC Scientific Publications No. 75. Lyon: International Agency for Research on Cancer.

Parkin, D.M., Läärä, E. & Muir C.S. (1988). Estimates of the worldwide frequency of sixteen major cancers in 1980. *Int. J. Cancer*, **41**, 184–97.

UNO (United Nations Organization) (1986). *Demographic Indicators of Countries. Estimates and Projections as Assessed in* 1984. New York: United Nations Organization.

Part V

Buccal cavity

Lip, oral cavity and pharynx

ICD-9 140, 141, 144, 145, 146, 148 and 149
(also salivary glands ICD-9 142)

23.1   Introduction

Cancer of the oral cavity and pharynx is the fourth most common cancer in males and the eighth most common in females on a worldwide basis. Their incidence varies significantly in different countries. As a group, those cancers are relatively rare in northern Europe, but are common in the Latin countries of Europe and in the Indian subcontinent. The nasopharynx (ICD-9 147) is considered in Chapter 24; the salivary glands (ICD-9 142) at the end of this chapter.

23.2   Histology, classification and diagnosis

These cancers are predominantly squamous carcinomas. They are frequently preceded by leukoplakia, notably in the mouth. Numerous histological types of salivary glands cancer are described. The most frequent is pleomorphic adenoma of which most occur in the parotid gland. While initially benign, it has a tendency to recur and a proportion eventually become malignant.

23.3   Descriptive epidemiology
Incidence and time trends
Lip

Fairly high rates are seen in some fair-skinned populations, notably in Canada, where rates are generally above 5. The highest are in Newfoundland (15.1) and Saskatchewan (12.3) (Fig. 23.1). Rates above 10 are seen in rural Rumania, southern Ireland, Queensland, Australia and Sicily. Most rates, however, are less than 5 and in Asia rates range from nil to 0.1. In Israel the incidence is close to that seen in Europe.

Fig. 23.1 Incidence rates around 1980: Lip (ICD-9 140).

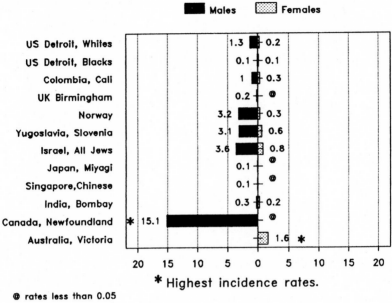

██ Males   ▦ Females

US Detroit, Whites	1.3	0.2
US Detroit, Blacks	0.1	0.1
Colombia, Cali	1	0.3
UK Birmingham	0.2	@
Norway	3.2	0.3
Yugoslavia, Slovenia	3.1	0.6
Israel, All Jews	3.6	0.8
Japan, Miyagi	0.1	@
Singapore, Chinese	0.1	@
India, Bombay	0.3	0.2
Canada, Newfoundland	✱ 15.1	@
Australia, Victoria		1.6 ✱

20 15 10 5 0 5 10 15 20

✱ Highest incidence rates.

@ rates less than 0.05

(after Muir *et al.*, 1987)

Tongue

Rates are high in India (Bombay 9.4; Nagpur 8.3), and in males in certain parts of France (7 to 8 in Doubs, Bas-Rhin, Calvados) (Fig. 23.2). Elsewhere, rates are generally below 2.

Oral Cavity

Cancers of the mouth, gums, and floor of mouth are relatively uncommon. However, considerable geographical differences may be seen, high rates occurring against a background of generally low incidence (less than 2). The highest rates are seen in females in Bangalore (India 15.7) and in males in Bas-Rhin (France 13.5) (Fig. 23.3). A few communities have rates around 10 (black males in Connecticut, Pacific Island Polynesians in New Zealand and in Madras).

Oropharynx

In most populations, these cancers are rare, with rates less than unity. In Caribbean and Latin populations, rates range from 2 to 5, being greatest in Martinique (8.4). Indian rates are similar. In the United States,

Fig. 23.2 Incidence rates around 1980: Tongue (ICD-9 141).

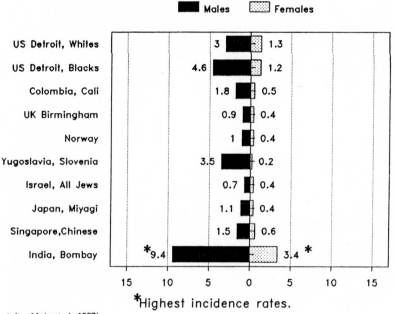

(after Muir *et al.*, 1987)

Fig. 23.3 Incidence rates around 1980: Mouth (ICD-9 143–5).

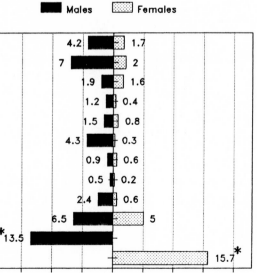

(after Muir *et al.*, 1987)

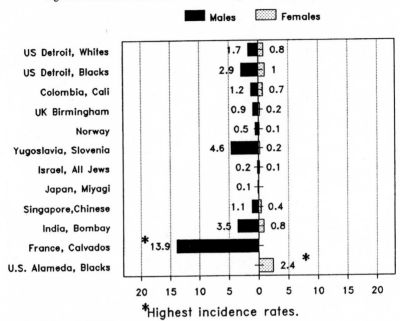

Fig. 23.4 Incidence rates around 1980: Oropharynx (ICD-9 146).

(after Muir *et al.*, 1987)

rates in blacks tend to be double those in whites, in both sexes. In French males, rates range from 6.3 in Isere to 14.5 in urban Calvados (Fig. 23.4).

Hypopharynx

The incidence of this cancer is comparable to the oropharynx, except in India, where it is twice as frequent in both sexes (Fig. 23.5).

Age and sex distribution

For all the above sites, the incidence increases with age. Lip and tongue cancers are very rare in females, except in Bombay (2.4). For oral cavity, male : female ratios are usually very high, but values of 0.3 and 0.8 are seen in Bangalore and Madras in India. The ratios vary considerably for hypopharyngeal cancer, being very high in France but near unity in the UK.

23.4   Etiological inferences

The geographical distribution is consistent with the view that in whites in North America, Europe and Australia the incidence of lip cancer correlates with skin cancer incidence and sunlight exposure. For other

Fig. 23.5 Incidence rates around 1980: Hypopharynx (ICD-9 148).

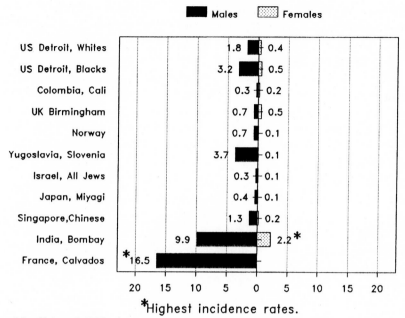

(after Muir *et al.*, 1987)

sites, the data are consistent with local cultural habits, notably use of tobacco in some form and/or alcohol.

23.5 Known and suspected causes
Sunlight

The lip is exposed to the same factors which influence cancer of the skin, notably ultra-violet light, hence the higher risk in outdoor occupations such as farming and fishing.

Tobacco

Tobacco use in several forms is probably the most important single etiological factor. Cancer of the lip and the smoking of clay or metal pipes have long been linked. Oral cancer is also consistently more common among smokers, especially of cigars and pipes (Wynder *et al.*, 1957). Risk is further increased by heavy consumption of alcohol. The oral use of snuff has been associated with carcinoma of the gingiva and buccal mucosa.

Some of the world's highest rates for oral and pharyngeal cancer are found in India and parts of Asia (Hirayama, 1966; Muir & Kirk, 1960; Bhide *et al.*, 1984). Tobacco chewing, often described as 'betel chewing', is very common. The product is sold as 'pan', a mixture of sun-cured tobacco, areca-nut shavings, slaked lime and various additives wrapped in the leaf of the betel vine. This quid is placed between cheek and gum and may remain in place for up to an hour. Certain habitués sleep with the quid in place. In Bihar, 'khaini', a mixture of powdered Indian tobacco and lime is placed in the gingivo-buccal fold where it is left to dissolve. This habit is essentially similar to 'snuff-dipping' in the United States. Cancer subsequently arises in the habitual site of placement of the quid. In Soviet Central Asia and parts of Afghanistan, oral cancer appears due to the chewing of tobacco as 'nass', a combination of tobacco leaf, wood ash, lime, cotton and sesame oil.

There are many other forms of tobacco usage associated with oral cancer (Muir & Zaridze, 1986). Although the composition of these quids shows considerable regional and individual variation, all have strong carcinogenic activities. A number of other lesions have been associated with betel quid chewing, including leukoplakia, and sub-mucous fibrosis in the oral cavity. These are now, in general, regarded as precancerous lesions and indicators of later malignancy.

Smoking of 'bidi', a small cigarette comprising sun-dried tobacco wrapped in the leaf of the temburni tree, has been associated with cancers of the tonsil, esophagus, hypopharynx and base of tongue. Cancer of the palate may follow reverse smoking, i.e. with the burning end of the cheroot in the mouth, a habit not only of Andhra in India but also in Sardinia, Venezuela and Panama.

Alcohol

Excessive alcohol consumption has been associated with cancer of the oral cavity, oro- and hypopharynx, larynx and esophagus. As heavy drinkers also frequently smoke heavily, separation of the effects of alcohol and tobacco is not always easy. A significant increase in both hypopharyngeal and esophageal cancers has been shown due to alcohol alone (Tuyns et al., 1988).

Nutritional deficiencies

The possible predisposing role of malnutrition and vitamin deficiencies has proved difficult to establish in the presence of strong carcinogenic factors, although case control studies have shown lower levels of vitamin A and B in oral cancer cases than controls. A protective effect of vegetables has been reported from India (Notani & Jayant, 1987).

An unusual condition known as Plummer-Vinson or Patterson Kelly Syndrome, associated with tumors of the post-cricoid region and upper alimentary tract, was formerly common in Scandinavia. It is believed due to long-standing iron and multivitamin deficiency (Mahboubi & Sayed, 1982). Intervention studies using beta-carotene suggest a beneficial effect on oral leukoplakia in some high risk groups.

Occupational factors

The association of outdoor occupations with lip cancer in farmers and in fishermen is well known. In addition, a number of occupations have reported a higher than expected rate of oral cancer, as in asbestos, steel, metal and textile mill workers. In most studies, however, the influence of tobacco and alcohol has not been excluded.

Radiation

Bone cancers arising in the mandible were early reported in watch dial painters using radium-containing luminous paint and only incidentally involved the mouth.

Miscellaneous

The link between syphilis and cancer of dorsum of the tongue has a long history, but probably reflects greater use of alcohol and tobacco by such patients. The role of poor dentition remains obscure. Mouthwashes are unrelated to oral cancer. A relation with human papilloma virus, especially types 6, 11 and 16 and with Herpes simplex virus type I, has been suggested but not confirmed (Maitland *et al.*, 1987).

Etiological factors have recently been extensively reviewed by Boyle *et al.*, (1990).

23.6   Relevant laboratory studies

Nair *et* al. (1987) has shown that nitroso-nornicotines in tobacco and the alkaloid, arecoline, which is the principal stimulant in the areca nut, can be nitrosated giving rise to compounds carcinogenic to experimental animals. Carcinogenic agents are also present in snuff.

23.7   Attributable risks

Reanalysis of the 1966 data of Hirayama (1966) for those chewing the betel quid (with and without tobacco) by smoking habit, shows that the attributable risk for oral cancer in males was 6.7% for smokers alone, 22% for chewing betel without tobacco, 50% for smoking chewers of tobaccoless betel quids, 89% for chewers of tobacco containing quids and 92% for smokers who chewed tobacco containing quids. In countries where the incidence of the buccal cavity and pharyngeal cancer is high, it is likely that 90% are due to some form of the tobacco habit or to the combined action of tobacco smoke and alcohol.

23.8   Conclusions

Although these sites pose differing problems for therapy, these cancers show common etiological factors which, in terms of prevention, are underestimated when the sites are considered separately (See Chapter 9). The betel quid, with or without tobacco, has a role in Asian society which goes beyond its diaphoretic and stimulatory properties and will probably prove as difficult to control as has tobacco and alcohol use elsewhere. The increasing use and promotion of 'smokeless' tobacco both in the United States and elsewhere is a matter for concern.

Salivary glands

Despite their proximity, these cancers show no relationship to tumors of the buccal cavity. There are some geographical differences in site distribution. Other than ionizing radiation, the causes are unknown.

23.9   References

Bhide, S.V., Shah, A.S., Nair, J. & Nagarajrao, D. (1984). Epidemiological and experimental studies on tobacco-related oral cancer in India. In N-*Nitroso Compounds: Occurrence, Biological Effects and Relevance to Human Cancer*, IARC Scientific Publications No. 57, ed. I.K. O'Neill, R.C. von Borstel, C.T. Miller, J. Long & H. Bartsch, pp. 851–7. Lyon: International Agency for Research on Cancer.

Boyle, P., Zheng, T., MacFarlane, G.T., McGinn, R., Maisonneuve, P., La Vecchia, C. & Scully, C. (1990). Recent advances in the etiology and epidemiology of head and neck cancer. *Current Opinion in Oncology*, **2**, 539–45.

Hirayama, T. (1966). An epidemiological study of oral and pharyngeal cancer in Central and Southeast Asia. *Bull WHO*, **34**, 41–69.

Mahboubi, E. & Sayed, G.M. (1982). Oral cavity and pharynx. In *Cancer Epidemiology and Prevention*, ed. D. Schottenfeld & J.F. Fraumeni, Jr., pp. 583–95. Philadelphia: W. B. Saunders.

Maitland, N.J., Cox, M.F., Lynas, C., Prime, S.S., Meanwell, C.A. & Scully, C. (1987). Detection of human papillomavirus DNA in biopsies of human oral tissue. *Br. J. Cancer*, **56**, 245–50.

Muir, C.S. & Kirk, R. (1960). Betel, tobacco and cancer of the mouth. *Br. J. Cancer*, **14**, 598–608.

Muir, C.S. & Zaridze, D.G. (1986). Smokeless tobacco and cancer: An overview. In *Tobacco. A Major International Health Hazard*, IARC Scientific Publications No. 74, ed. D.G. Zaridze & Peto, R., pp. 35–44. Lyon: International Agency for Research on Cancer.

Muir, C., Waterhouse, J., Mack, T., Powell, J. & Whelan, S. (eds.) (1987). *Cancer Incidence in Five Continents*, Volume V, IARC Scientific Publication No. 88. Lyon: International Agency for Research on Cancer.

Nair, J., Nair U.J., Ohshima, S.V., Bhide & Bartsch, H. (1987). Endogenous nitrosation in the oral cavity of chewers while chewing betel quid with or without tobacco. In *The Relevance of* N-*Nitroso Compounds to Human Cancer: Exposures & Mechanisms*, ed. H. Bartsch, I. O'Neill & R. Schulte-Hermann, IARC Scientific Publications No. 84, pp. 465–84. Lyon: International Agency for Research on Cancer.

Notani, P.N. & Jayant, K. (1987). Role of diet in upper aerodigestive tract cancers. *Nutr. Cancer*, **10**, 103–13.

Tuyns, A.J., Esteve, J., Raymond, L., Berrino, F., Benhamou, E., Blanchet, F., Boffetta, P., Crosignani, P., del Moral, A., Lehmann, W., Merletti, F., Pequignot, G., Riboli, E., Sancho-Garnier, H., Terracini, B., Zubiri, A. & Zubiri, L. (1988). Cancer of the larynx/hypopharynx, tobacco and alcohol: IARC international case-control study in Turin and Varese (Italy), Zaragoza and Navarra (Spain), Geneva (Switzerland) and Calvados (France). *Int. J. Cancer*, **41**, 483–91.

Wynder, E.L., Bross, I.D.J. & Feldman, R.M. (1957). A study of the etiological factors in cancer of the mouth. *Cancer*, **10**, 1300–23.

24

Nasopharynx (NPC)

ICD-9 147

24.1 Introduction

Tumors of the nasopharynx (NPC) differ in histology, racial distribution and etiology from other cancers in the mouth and pharynx.

24.2 Histology, classification and diagnosis

NPC tumors are predominantly of squamous epithelial origin, but show varying degrees of aggregation of the tumor cells and infiltration by lymphocytes, resulting in subclassifications, which appear without etiological significance. Malignant lymphomas occasionally arise in the nasopharynx. A rare nasopharyngeal fibroadenomatous polyp is reported in children.

24.3 Descriptive epidemiology

Incidence

NPC is rare in most countries, with incidence rates well under unity, but occurs with high frequency in parts of China and Southeast Asia (Fig. 24.1). High incidence rates (over 10) are also found in migrant Chinese communities such as in Singapore, Hawaii and California. There are considerable variations in rates in the various Chinese language groups in Singapore (Table 24.1), where this is the most frequent cancer in males aged 15 to 34 years. Rates comparable to those in Singapore Chinese have been recorded in Inuit populations of mongoloid origin in Canada, Alaska and Greenland. Moderate rates, in the 3 to 10 range, have been reported in Malta, and parts of Northern Africa, especially Tunisia, Algeria and Sudan.

Age and sex distribution

In Singapore Chinese, cases appear from about 20 years of age, reach a peak around 40, and then level off. In North African populations,

Table 24.1. *Age-standardized incidence rates for nasopharyngeal cancer in principal Singapore chinese dialect groups, by sex, 1968–1982.*

Group	Male	Female
Hokkien	16.6	6.3
Teochex	17.4	6.4
Cantonese	29.9	11.4
Hainanese	16.5	6.5
Hakka	14.5	5.4

(After Lee *et al.*, 1988.)

Fig. 24.1 Incidence rates around 1980: Nasopharynx (ICD-9 147).

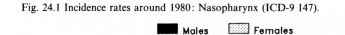

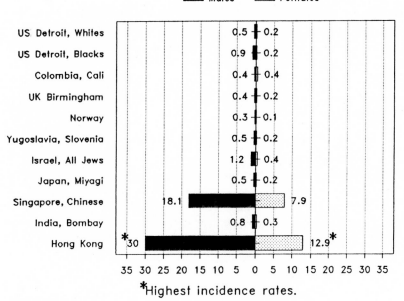

*Highest incidence rates.

(after Muir *et al.*, 1987)

a few cases appear before 15 years of age. In most countries, there is a two- to threefold male excess.

24.4 Etiological inferences
Ethnic factors

These have been reviewed by Shanmugaratnam and Muir (1967) and de-Thé *et al.*, (1973). The highest incidence of NPC is observed in southern Chinese populations, both in mainland China and elsewhere.

This has led to the view that in such cancers there is a significant genetic component in Chinese communities or in individuals with Chinese ancestries, in addition to some environmental factors. Thus, in Thailand, the frequency in persons of mixed Thai and Chinese blood is approximately midway between that of Thais and pure blood Chinese. In general, the frequency in non-Chinese Mongoloid groups, i.e. Thai, Singapore Malay or Indonesians, is lower than in the Chinese. The caucasian Indian and Pakistani populations of Singapore have the same frequency as the Swedes. The risk among southern Chinese varies (Table 24.1). The boat people of Hong Kong have a higher risk than other Cantonese groups, whereas, in Singapore, the Teochew who come from other parts of the Guandong province have a somewhat lesser risk. While the migrant Chinese in Southeast Asia have carried with them, to a considerable degree, the customs and foods of China, there are now increasing numbers of second generation Chinese notably in California who have become more or less westernized. In the United States, while NPC risks among US born Chinese are considerably higher than in US whites, they are lower than in China. In contrast, in Singapore, the risk in Singapore-born Chinese is over 20% greater than for those born in China, in both sexes (Lee *et al.*, 1988).

There appears to be no convincing correlation between NPC and sinonasal cancer.

24.5   Known and suspected causes
Genetic factors

In addition to the ethnic factors described above, occasional high risk families have been described. The early literature has been reviewed by Ho (1972) and Shanmugaratnam (1982). An association with HLA antigen profile has been demonstrated.

Epstein–Barr Virus (EBV)

The evidence for a role of EB virus is discussed in depth in Chapter 17. Patients with NPC have higher titers of antibodies against EBV-related antigens than normal individuals or other head and neck cancer patients. Moreover, EB viral genomes and EBV specific nuclear antigens have been found within epithelial cells of tumors, thus providing evidence for a potential oncogenic role. However, the possibility that the virus is a passenger is not completely excluded. The EBV hypothesis does not exclude a co-carcinogenic role with other agents.

Inhaled substances

The possibility that NPC is associated with inhaled gases e.g. formaldehyde, or particles has been examined (UAREP, 1987), but the results are unconvincing. For most factors with carcinogenic activity in the rest of the respiratory system, e.g. lung, reports of NPC are absent. No convincing relationship to NPC has been observed in tobacco users (Mabuchi *et al.*, 1985). Similarly, the causal role of a cloudy or dusty environment as reported in Africa and China remain unproven (Ho, 1972).

Diet and salted fish

The demonstration in Hong Kong of a possible role for Cantonese salted fish for this tumor provides the most convincing causal hypothesis in recent times (Huang *et al.*, 1978; Yu *et al.*, 1985, 1986). Such fish, which are a common component of the Chinese diet introduced at weaning, have a high level of secondary amines. The latter are believed to interact with nitrite salts used as preservatives, with the formation of *N*-nitroso compounds possibly organotrophic for the nasopharynx. The epidemiological evidence is becoming increasingly convincing with the demonstration of a dose-effect reproduced in Hong Kong, China and Malaysia, and the hypothesis is biologically plausible (Yu *et al.*, 1988, 1989*a*; Lancet, 1989), but the responsible active agent(s) have not been identified. The association has also been studied in Tunisia and Greenland. Other preserved foods reported to have an increased risk are fermented fish sauce, salted shrimp paste, moldy bean curd and two kinds of preserved plums.

24.6   Relevant laboratory studies

Although many nasal chemical carcinogens have been identified (Chapter 32), tumors of the nasopharynx are rare in rodents. Yu *et al.* (1989*b*) induced malignant nasal cavity tumors in rats fed salted fish. The most plausible candidates are systemic carcinogens, such as the asymmetric dialkyl nitrosamines. The role of EB virus as a necessary inducing factor has no counterpart in experimental studies.

The HLA (human leukocyte antigen) system has been extensively explored. The haplotype A2-B Sin 2 carries a two-fold excess risk, although this accounts for only about 25% of the risk (B Sin 2 is now named BW46). Another HLA pattern, a deficit of BW17, carries a survival advantage for those with an established cancer. It is probable that the HLA genes are closely linked to NPC susceptibility genes (de Thé *et al.*, 1989).

24.7   Attributable risks
The data do not permit conclusions.

24.8   Conclusions
There is growing evidence for the role of diet, but while the association with EBV virus is well documented, its role is still not clarified. No recommendations for prevention are as yet available.

24.9   References

Anon. (1989). Salted fish and nasopharyngeal carcinoma (editorial). *Lancet*, **ii**, 840–2.

de-Thé, G., Ablashi D.V., Liabeuf A., & Mourali, N. (1973). Nasopharyngeal carcinoma (NPC) VI: Presence of an EBV nuclear antigen in fresh tumor biopsies – preliminary results. *Biomedicine*, **19**, 349–352.

de-Thé, G., Ho, J.H.C. & Muir, C.S. (1989). Nasopharyngeal carcinoma. In *Viral Infections of Humans: Epidemiology and Control*, ed. A.S. Evans, pp. 737–767. New York: Plenum.

Ho, J.H.C. (1972). Nasopharyngeal carcinoma (NPC). *Adv. Cancer Res.*, **15**, 547–82.

Huang, D. P., Saw, D., Teoh, T.B. & Ho, J.H.C. (1978). Carcinoma of the nasal and paranasal regions in rats fed with Cantonese salted marine fish. In *Nasopharyngeal Carcinoma: Etiology and Control*, IARC Scientific Publications No. 20, ed. G. de-Thé & Y. Ito, pp. 315–28. Lyon: International Agency for Research on Cancer.

Lee, H.P., Day, N.E. & Shanmugaratnam, K. (eds.) (1988). *Trends in Cancer Incidence in Singapore* 1968–1982, IARC Scientific Publications No. 91. Lyon: International Agency for Research on Cancer.

Mabuchi, K., Bross, D.S. & Kessler, I.I. (1985). Cigarette smoking and nasopharyngeal carcinoma. *Cancer*, **55**, 2874–6.

Muir, C., Waterhouse, J., Mack, T., Powell, J. & Whelan, S. (eds.) (1987). *Cancer Incidence in Five Continents*, Volume V, IARC Scientific Publication No. 88. Lyon: International Agency for Research on Cancer.

Shanmugaratnam, K. & Muir C.S. (1967). Nasopharyngeal carcinoma: origin and structure. In *Cancer of the Nasopharynx*, UICC Monograph Series 1, ed. C.S. Muir & K. Shanmugaratnam, pp. 153–62. Copenhagen: Mucksgaard.

Shanmugaratnam, K. (1982). Nasopharynx. In *Cancer Epidemiology and Prevention*, ed. D. Schottenfeld & J.F. Fraumeni, Jr., pp. 536–53. Philadelphia: W.B. Saunders.

UAREP (Universities Associated for Research and Education in Pathology, Inc.) (1987). Epidemiology of chronic occupational exposure to formaldehyde: report of the *ad hoc* panel on health aspects of formaldehyde. *Tox. Ind. Health*, **4**, 77–90.

Yu, M.C., Ho, J.H.C., Henderson, B.E. & Armstrong, R.W. (1985). Epidemiology of nasopharyngeal carcinoma in Malaysia and Hong Kong. *Natl. Cancer Inst. Monog.*, **69**, 203–7.

Yu, M.C., Ho, J.H.C., Lai, S.-H. & Henderson, B.E. (1986). Cantonese-style salted fish as a cause of nasopharyngeal carcinoma: report of a case-control study in Hong Kong. *Cancer Res.*, **46**, 956–61.

Yu, M.C., Mo, C.-C., Chong, W.-X., Yeh, F.-S. & Henderson, B.E. (1988). Preserved foods and nasopharyngeal carcinoma: A case-control study in Guangxi, China. *Cancer Res.*, **48**, 1954–9.

Yu, M.C., Huang, D.P. & Henderson, B.E. (1989a). Diet and carcinogenesis: a case-control study in Guangzhou, China. *Int. J. Cancer*, **43**, 1077–82.

Yu, M.C., Nichols, P.W., Zou, X.N., Estes, J. & Henderson, B.E. (1989b). Induction of malignant nasal cavity tumors in Wistar rats fed Chinese salted fish. *Br. J. Cancer*, **60**, 198–201.

Part VI

Digestive system

25

Esophagus

ICD-9 150

25.1 Introduction

In 1980 this was the sixth most common cancer in the world, occupying fourth place in developing and fifteenth in developed countries. There are remarkable inter- and intra-country variations in incidence related to environmental factors.

25.2 Histology, classification and precancerous lesions

The common histological type is squamous cell carcinoma accounting for 80–90% of all tumors. Adenocarcinoma is relatively uncommon (10–20%). Approximately half of the former occur in the middle third of the esophagus, whereas the majority of adenocarcinomas arise in the lower third, being associated with glandular metaplasia (Barrett's esophagus) and reflux esophagitis. Endoscopic surveys in populations at high risk for esophageal cancer in Iran and China (Muñoz et al., 1982, Crespi et al., 1984) and experiments in primates (Adamson et al., 1977) suggest that chronic esophagitis is followed by epithelial atrophy and dysplasia. Such lesions are much more common in high than in low incidence areas.

25.3 Descriptive epidemiology
Incidence

Figure 25.1 summarizes the global picture, but, due to marked regional differences, reference should be made to reports from individual countries (Day & Muñoz, 1982). The highest incidence and mortality rates (sometimes exceeding 100) are found in the so-called 'Asian esophageal cancer belt' which stretches from European Russia and Turkey to Eastern

Fig. 25.1 Incidence rates around 1980: Esophagus (ICD-9 150).

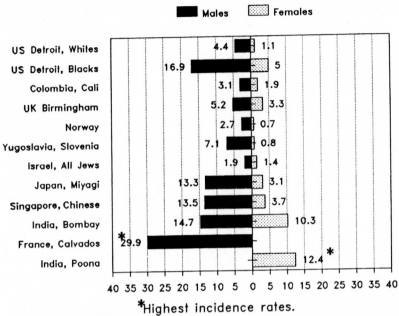

■ Males   ▨ Females

	Males	Females
US Detroit, Whites	4.4	1.1
US Detroit, Blacks	16.9	5
Colombia, Cali	3.1	1.9
UK Birmingham	5.2	3.3
Norway	2.7	0.7
Yugoslavia, Slovenia	7.1	0.8
Israel, All Jews	1.9	1.4
Japan, Miyagi	13.3	3.1
Singapore, Chinese	13.5	3.7
India, Bombay	14.7	10.3
France, Calvados	*29.9	
India, Poona		12.4 *

40 35 30 25 20 15 10 5 0 5 10 15 20 25 30 35 40

*Highest incidence rates.

(after Muir *et al.*, 1987)

China. It includes the Soviet republics of Turkmenistan, Kazakhstan and Azerbaijan and Northern Siberia, the Turkoman desert in Northeast Iran and Afghanistan, and several provinces in China including Xinjiang, Henan, Hebei and the eastern coast of northern Jiangsu province, North Sichuan, South Fujian and northeastern Guangdong (Fig. 25.2). Very high rates (over 40) are found in certain black communities of Southern Africa including the Transkei and Zimbabwe. Localized areas of increase are found in western Kenya and southern Malawi, but the tumor is rare in north and west Africa (Day & Muñoz, 1982).

In North America, the rate in blacks is 3–4 times higher than in whites. Clusters of high rates (over 15) occur in the Caribbean Islands of Puerto Rico, Jamaica and Martinique, and in an area covering Southern Brazil, Uruguay and Northeast Argentina. In Europe, the highest rates (30) are found in France (Normandy, Brittany and Bas-Rhin) (Figure 25.3). In Asia, high rates are observed among Chinese from Shanghai, Hong Kong and Singapore and in some areas of India and Japan.

Time trends

In the 'Asian esophageal cancer belt' this tumor appears to have been common for many centuries and the rates seem stable (Lu *et al.*,

Fig. 25.2 Incidence rates, standardized to the world population, of esophageal cancer among males in Central Asia.

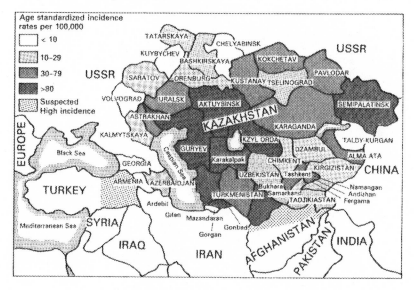

1985). In the black population of South Africa, a slight increasing trend has been reported (Jaskiewicz *et al.*, 1987). In contrast, dramatic increases in squamous carcinoma have been observed in the last two decades among blacks in the United States. The rates for whites are relatively stable (Blot & Fraumeni, 1987; Bang *et al.*, 1988), but an increase in adenocarcinoma has been reported among men (Yang & Davis, 1988). A moderate increase in Italian men has been ascribed to alcohol consumption (La Rosa *et al.*, 1988).

Age and sex distribution

The age-specific incidence rates increase rapidly with age. A clear male predominance is seen in America and Europe with sex ratios reaching 20 in the high-risk areas of France. On the other hand, in the high-risk Asian belt, as the incidence rises the proportional excess in males decreases with even a female excess in some areas.

25.4 Etiological inferences

The large difference in incidence within short distances and the sharp incidence changes over time suggest a major role for exogenous factors. Sex ratios indicate that exposure to causal factors is greater in

Fig. 25.3 The mortality from cancer of the esophagus in the nine countries of the European Economic Community in the 1970's. The distribution of the age-standardized mortality rates is given in the histogram at the lower left of the diagram. The figure 6 (males) and 2 (females) above the histogram indicates that in 6 regions, rates were above 25 (males) and in 2 above 6 (females). In males the concentration of risk in France, particularly in the North and West, contrasts with the pattern in females where the highest levels (although lower than in males) were found in Scotland and Ireland.

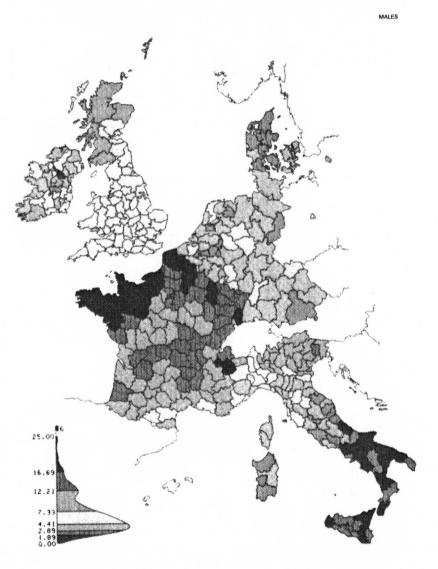

MALES

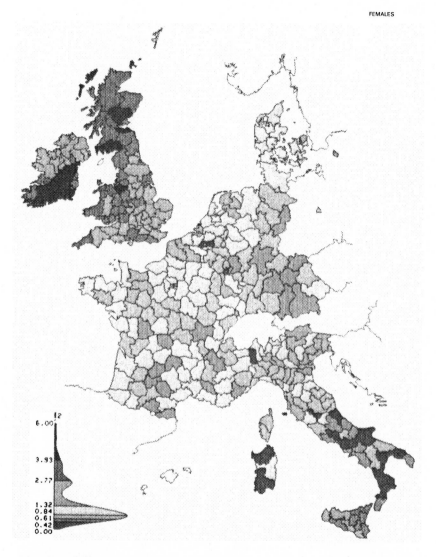

FEMALES

males than females in America and Europe but similar in both sexes in the high risk Asian populations. Correlation studies indicate that the etiological agents are not the same in all countries.

25.5   Known and suspected causes

Cancers of the esophagus can be classified into those predominantly due to alcohol and tobacco use and those due to other factors.

Table 25.1. *Relative risks for esophageal cancer according to daily amounts of tobacco and alcohol consumed.*

Alcohol consumption (g/day)	Tobacco consumption (g/day)			
	0–9	10–19	20–29	⩾ 30
0–40	1.0	3.4	3.2	3.0
41–80	7.3	8.4	8.8	35.0
81–120	11.8	13.6	12.6	83.0
⩾ 121	49.6	65.9	137.6	155.6

(After IARC, 1986*b*.)

Familial and hereditary factors

The small number of esophageal cancers associated with tylosis are due to a single autosomal gene with dominant effect. The high rates in the Asian belt are restricted to people of Turkish or Mongol origin, in contrast to local populations of Caucasian origin. Studies for genetic markers in these populations have so far been negative (Day & Muñoz, 1982).

Alcohol and tobacco-related esophageal cancer

In North and South America, Europe and South Africa, numerous case-control studies have identified alcohol and tobacco as the major risk factors (Day & Muñoz, 1982). A dose–response relationship has been found with alcohol and cigarettes, also the duration of the habit. There is evidence that alcohol and tobacco interact in a multiplicative fashion (Table 25.1) (Tuyns *et al.*, 1977; Victora *et al.*, 1987; Yu *et al.*, 1988; Segal *et al.*, 1989). Contrary to early emphasis on spirits, recent studies suggest that the association is essentially with the amount of ethanol consumed rather than the type of beverage. Studies in Denmark and South Africa have shown an increased risk of esophageal cancer with heavy beer intake (Adelhardt *et al.*, 1985; Segal *et al.*, 1989).

The risk attributable to ethanol alone, however, has been difficult to evaluate as most drinkers also smoke cigarettes. In the Calvados population in France, risk increased steadily with the amount of alcohol consumed among non-smoking subjects (Tuyns, 1983).

Some studies indicate a possibly higher risk among smokers of pipes and hand-rolled cigarettes than among smokers of commercial cigarettes (Tuyns & Estève, 1983; Segal *et al.*, 1989). Risks are higher for smokers of high-tar as compared to middle or low-tar cigarettes in Italy (La Vecchia *et al.*, 1986). In Uruguay, smoking of black tobacco cigarettes carries a 3-fold increase in risk compared to blond tobacco cigarettes (de Stefani *et al.*, 1989). Those observations suggest that the swallowing of smoke condensates may be important, alcohol acting as a solvent.

Non-alcohol and tobacco related esophageal cancer

No satisfactory explanation is available regarding the etiology of esophageal cancer occurring in the Asian belt. The extensive studies conducted by the IARC in Iran (Day & Muñoz, 1982) and recent studies in China (Li *et al.*, 1989) show that alcohol and tobacco play a minor role in these populations. In Iran, opium smoking and chewing of opium pipe scrapings which are highly mutagenic may be a major determinant of oesophageal cancer risk (Ghadirian *et al.*, 1985). Although in China *N*-nitroso compounds have been considered as the leading etiological candidates in view of their importance in experimental esophageal carcinogenesis, convincing evidence of their involvement in humans is still lacking (Lu *et al.*, 1986). A recent case control study in Linxian, China including over 1000 cases and 2000 controls did not confirm etiological hypotheses involving the consumption of pickled vegetables, moldy foods and nitrates (Li *et al.*, 1989).

Nutritional factors (Chapter 12)

In esophageal cancer whether related or not to tobacco and alcohol, a diet poor in fresh vegetables, fruit and dairy products has been a common denominator (Day & Muñoz, 1982; Victora *et al.*, 1987). Such a diet is low in vitamins A, C and riboflavin which are believed to maintain the integrity of the esophageal mucosa.

In the high-risk populations of Iran and China such vitamin deficiencies have been linked to the high prevalence of precancerous lesions. A double blind, randomized trial in Huixian, China, however, did not reveal any change in such lesions, apart from prevalence of micronuclei in individuals receiving supplementary vitamins over a period of a year, as compared to controls receiving a placebo (Muñoz *et al.*, 1985; 1987). Subsequent analysis indicated that the absence of an effect may be explained by increases in vitamin levels in the placebo group arising from unanticipated dietary improvements from other sources (Wahrendorf *et al.*, 1988).

Esophageal cancer has been reported in the Plummer Vinson syndrome which is associated with iron and vitamin deficiency and which was very common in Scandanavia.

Physical and thermal chronic injury (Chapter 14)

There is some evidence indicating that drinking very hot beverages or eating coarse food or foodstuffs containing silica fibers increases the risk of developing esophageal cancer.

Miscellaneous

Occupation

Risks in barmen and commercial travellers are associated with lifestyle. Studies in Sweden have identified vulcanization workers and chimney sweeps as groups at high risk (Norell *et al.*, 1983). Long-term occupational exposure to metal dust, especially beryllium, has been reported to increase the risk in the lower third, after adjustment for alcohol, tobacco and other risk factors (Yu *et al.*, 1988).

Other suspected agents include radiation, asbestos, and ingestion of bracken fern (IARC, 1986*a*). A role for human papillomaviruses has been suggested, analogous to studies in bovines, but has not been confirmed.

25.6   Relevant laboratory studies

While the evidence indicates that alcoholic beverages cause human cancer, extensive laboratory studies (Mandard *et al.*, 1981; IARC, 1988) have failed to show that ethanol is carcinogenic *per se* to animals.

The opium pyrolysates suspected to play a role in Iran are highly mutagenic, transform cells in culture, and are also carcinogenic for mice and hamsters (Friesen *et al.*, 1985).

Since certain *N*-nitroso-compounds induce experimental esophageal cancer readily, laboratory assays to detect exposure to nitrosamines at the cellular level have been developed based on DNA and protein adducts (Chapter 5). Pilot studies indicate that some of these adducts (O^6-methylguanine) are present at higher levels in the esophageal mucosa of individuals from high-risk populations in China than in low-risk populations from Europe (Umbenhauer *et al.*, 1985). However, extensive epidemiological studies have not yet been done as these assays require relatively large amounts of esophageal tissue. Amplification or over expression of growth factor/receptor genes *erb* B and *hst* has been found in esophageal tumors but their etiological implications remain unknown (Hollstein *et al.*, 1988).

25.7   Attributable risks

Alcohol and tobacco account for about 80–90% of esophageal cancer in North and South America, Europe, and Japan but a very small proportion of cases in the Asian belt. In South Africa and India, tobacco is probably more important than alcohol. Smoking and chewing of opium pyrolysates may be the main cause in Iran, but the determinants of the high risk in China and other populations of the Asian belt remain to be identified.

25.8   Conclusions

Where alcohol, tobacco and poor nutrition are responsible for the great majority of esophageal cancer appropriate control would reduce the incidence of the disease.

25.9   References

Adamson, R.H., Krolikowski, F.J., Correa, P., Sieber, S.M. & Dalgard, D.W. (1977). Carcinogenicity of 1-methyl-1-nitrosourea in non-human primates. *J. Natl. Cancer Inst.*, **59**, 415–22.

Adelhardt, M., Möller Jensen, O. & Sand Hansen, H. (1985). Cancer of the larynx, pharynx and oesophagus in relation to alcohol and tobacco consumption among Danish brewery workers. *Dan. Med. Bull.*, **32**, 119–23.

Bang, K.M., White, J.E., Ganse, B.L. & Leffall, L.D. (1988). Evaluation of recent trends in cancer mortality and incidence among blacks. *Cancer*, **61**, 1255–61.

Blot, W.J. & Fraumeni, J.F. (1987). Trends in esophageal cancer mortality among US blacks and whites. *Am. J. Public Health*, **77**, 296–8.

Crespi, M., Muñoz, N., Grassi, A., Qiong, S., Jin, W.K. & Jien, L.J. (1984). Precursor lesions of oesophageal cancer in a low-risk population in China: Comparison with high-risk populations. *Int. J. Cancer*, **34**, 599–602.

Day, N.E., & Muñoz, N. (1982). Esophagus. In *Cancer Epidemiology and Prevention*, Schottenfeld, D. & Fraumeni, J.F. eds, pp.526–623. Philadelphia: Saunders.

de Stefani, E., Muñoz, N. & Estève, J., Vasallo, A., Victora, C. & Teuchmann, S. (1990). Maté drinking, alcohol, tobacco, diet and oesophageal cancer in Uruguay: A case-control study. *Cancer Res.* **50**, 426–31.

Friesen, M., O'Neill, I.K., Malaveille, C., Garren, L., Hautefeuille, A., Cabral, J.R., Galendo, D., Lasne, C., Sala, M., Chouroulinkov, I., Mohr, U., Turusov, V. & Day, N.E. (1985). Characterization and identification of 6 mutagens in opium pyrolysates implicated in oesophageal cancer in Iran. *Mutat. Res.*, **150**, 177–91.

Ghadirian, P., Stein, G.F., Gorodetzky, C., Roberfroid, M.B., Mahon, G.A,T., Bartsch, H. & Day, N.E. (1985). Oesophageal cancer studies in the Caspian littoral of Iran: some residual results, including opium use as a risk factor. *Int. J. Cancer*, **35**, 593–7.

Hollstein, M., Bos, J., Galiana, C., Mandard, A.M., Yamasaki, H., & Montesano, R. (1988). Mutation and amplification of cellular oncogenes in human esophageal cancer. *Proc. Ann. Meet. Am. Assn. Cancer Res.* **29**, A1034.

IARC (1986a). *IARC Monographs on the Evaluation of the Carcinogenic Risk of Chemicals to Humans*, Some naturally occurring and synthetic food components, furocoumarins and ultraviolet radiation, volume 40. Lyon: International Agency for Research on Cancer.

IARC (1986b). *IARC Monographs on the Evaluation of the Carcinogenic Risk of Chemicals to Humans*, Tobacco Smoking, volume 38. Lyon: International Agency for Research on Cancer.

IARC, 1988. *IARC Monographs on the Evaluation of Carcinogenic Risks to Humans*, Alcohol drinking, volume 44. Lyon: International Agency for Research on Cancer.

Jaskiewicz, K., Marasas, W.F. & van der Walt, F.E. (1987). Oesophageal and other main cancer patterns in four districts of Transkei 1981–1984. *S. Afr. Med. J.*, **72**, 27–30.

La Rosa, F., Cresci, A., Orpianesi, C., Saltalamacchia, G., & Mastrandrea, V. (1988).

Esophageal cancer mortality: relationship with alcohol intake and cigarette smoking in Italy. *Eur. J. Epidemiol.*, **4**, 93–8.

La Vecchia, C., Liati, P., Decarli, A., Negrello, I. & Franceschi, S. (1986). Tar yields of cigarettes and risk of oesophageal cancer. *Cancer*, **38**, 381–5.

Li, J.Y., Ershow, A.G., Chen, Z.J., Wacholder, S., Li, G.Y., Guo, W., Li, B. & Blot, W.J. (1989). A case-control study of the oesophagus and gastric cardia in Linxian. *Int. J. Cancer* **43**, 755–61.

Lu, S.H., Montesano, R., Zhang, M.S., Feng, L., Luo, F.J., Chui, S.X., Umbenhauer, D., Saffhill, R. & Rajewsky, M.F. (1986). Relevance of *N*-nitrosamines to oesophageal cancer in China. *J. Cell. Physiol.* (Suppl.), **4**, 51–8.

Lu, J.B., Yang, W.X., Liu, J.M., Li, Y.S. & Qin, Y.M. (1985) Trends in morbidity and mortality for oesophageal cancer in Linxian County. *Int. J. Cancer*, **36**, 643–5.

Mandard, A.M., Marnay, J., Helie, H., Tuyns, A.J. & Le Talaer, J.Y. (1981). Absence of effect of ethanol and apple brandy on the upper digestive tract and esophagus of the wistar rat. *Bull. Cancer (Paris)*, **68**, 49–58.

Muir, C., Waterhouse, J., Mack, T., Powell, J. & Whelan, S. (eds.) (1987). *Cancer Incidence in Five Continents*, volume V, IARC Scientific Publication No. 88. Lyon: International Agency for Research on Cancer.

Muñoz, N., Crespi, M., Grassi, A., Qing, W.G., Qiong, S. & Cai, L.Z. (1982). Precursor lesions of oesophageal cancer in high-risk populations in Iran and China. *Lancet*, **i**, 876–9.

Muñoz, N., Wahrendorf, J., Lu J. B., Crespi, M., Thurnham, D.I., Day, N.E., Zhang C.Y., Zheng H.J., Li, B., Li, W.Y., Lin, G.L., Lan, X.Z., Correa, P., Grassi, A., O'Conor, G.T. & Bosch, X. (1985). No effect of riboflavine, retinol and zinc on prevalence of precancerous lesions of oesophagus: a randomized double-blind intervention study in a high-risk population of China. *Lancet*, **ii**, 111–4.

Muñoz, N., Hayashi, M., Lu, J.B., Wahrendorf, J., Crespi, M. & Bosch, F.X. (1987). The effect of riboflavin, retinol and zinc on micronuclei of buccal mucosa and of oesophagus: a randomized double-blind intervention study in China. *J. Natl. Cancer Inst.*, **79**, 687–91.

Norell, S., Lipping, H., Ahlbom, A. & Osterblom, L. (1983). Oesophageal cancer and vulcanisation work. *Lancet*, **i**, 462–3.

Segal, I., Reinach, S.G. & de Beer, M. (1989). Factors associated with oesophageal cancer in Soweto, South Africa. *Br. J. Cancer*, **58**, 681–6.

Tuyns, A.J., Péquignot, G. & Jensen, O.M. (1977). Le cancer de l'oesophage en Ille-et-Vilaine en fonction des niveaux de consommation d'alcool et de tabac. Des risques qui se multiplient. *Bull. Cancer*, **64**, 45–60.

Tuyns, A.J. & Estève, J. (1983). Pipe, commercial and hand-rolled cigarette smoking in oesophageal cancer. *Int. J. Cancer*, **12**, 110–13.

Tuyns, A.J. (1983). Oesophageal cancer in non-smoking drinkers and in non-drinking smokers. *Int. J. Cancer*, **32**, 443–4.

Umbenhauer, D., Wild, C.P., Montesano, R., Saffhill, R., Boyle, J.M., Huh, N., Kirstein, U., Thomale, J., Rajewsky, M.F. & Lu, S.H. (1985). O^6-Methyldexyguanosine in oesophageal DNA among individuals at high risk of oesophageal cancer. *Int. J. Cancer*, **36**, 661–5.

Victora, C.G., Muñoz, N., Day, N.E., Barcelos, L.B., Peccin, D.A. & Braga, N.M. (1987). Hot beverages and oesophageal cancer in Southern Brazil: a case-control study. *Int. J. Cancer*, **39**, 710–16.

Wahrendorf, J., Muñoz, N., Lu, J.B., Thurnham, D.I., Crespi, M. & Bosch, F.X. (1988). Blood, retinol and zinc riboflavin status in relation to precancerous lesions of the esophagus: findings from a vitamin intervention trial in the People's Republic of China. *Cancer Res.*, **48**, 2280–3.

Yang, P.C. & Davis, S. (1988). Incidence of cancer of the oesophagus in the US by histologic type. *Cancer*, **61**, 612–17.

Yu, M.C., Garabrant, D.H., Peters, J.M. & Mack, T.M. (1988). Tobacco, alcohol, diet, occupation and carcinoma of the oesophagus. *Cancer Res.*, **48**, 3843–8.

26

Stomach

ICD-9 151

26.1 Introduction

Large differences in incidence exist worldwide. Although stomach cancer rates have been steadily decreasing in most populations over the last 4–5 decades, none the less, it still remains the most frequent cancer in the world (Parkin *et al.*, 1988). Many hypotheses have been proposed to explain this general decline, but the causes remain essentially unknown.

26.2 Histology, classification and diagnosis

Two main histological types of stomach cancer, which differ not only in morphology but also in their epidemiological characteristics, have been described (Lauren, 1965). The *intestinal* or *expanding* adenocarcinoma is characterized by the tendency to form glandular structures resembling the colonic mucosa and has often, grossly, a polypoid appearance. It is more prevalent in males and older age groups. The *diffuse* or *infiltrative* type of adenocarcinoma is characterized by lack of cellular cohesiveness and diffuse infiltration of the gastric wall. It is equally frequent in males and females. It is relatively more frequent in younger age-groups, and has a worse prognosis than the intestinal type.

In populations with high or intermediate rates, the intestinal type of cancer predominates, but the diffuse type is more common in populations with low rates (Muñoz, 1988).

The following precursor lesions have been postulated for the intestinal type but none is recognized for the diffuse type.

Superficial gastritis (the earliest precursor lesion) is characterized by focal necrosis with regenerative hyperplasia mainly affecting the neck of the glands.

Chronic atrophic gastritis (CAG), the next stage, is characterized by loss of normal gastric glands which are partly replaced by connective tissue or

Fig. 26.1 Incidence rates around 1980: Stomach (ICD-9 151).

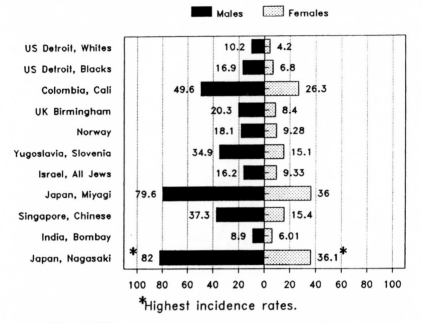

(after Muir *et al.*, 1987)

by intestinal metaplasia. At least two types of intestinal metaplasia with probably different malignant potential have been characterized histologically and histochemically. The initial stage of metaplasia, often associated with benign gastric lesions is called type I, (complete or small intestine type). The advanced stage type III, (incomplete or colonic type) is frequently associated with gastric carcinoma, and is considered a dysplastic lesion (Filipe, 1988).

In Colombia and Costa Rica, the prevalence of chronic atrophic gastritis and intestinal metaplasia is greater in the high-risk than in the low-risk areas for gastric cancer.

Pernicious anemia, and the post-gastrectomy state which are associated with gastritis also show an increased risk of stomach cancer.

26.3   Descriptive epidemiology (Fig. 26.1)
Incidence
Due to its high lethality, death rates have until recently approximated incidence rates.

The highest incidence rates (over 50) are found in Japan and China. Rates are also high in Costa Rica, Colombia, Chile, Peru, Ecuador and Brazil. Intermediate rates (15–25) are observed in Switzerland, France,

Fig. 26.2 Trends in age-adjusted death rates for malignant neoplasm of the stomach from 1960–1987 in certain countries.

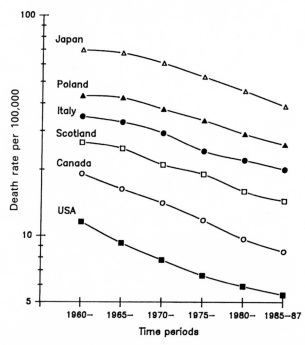

Scotland, Denmark and Norway. In Europe, relatively high rates (25–40) are found in most Scandinavian and Eastern European countries, in some regions of England, Germany, north Italy and Yugoslavia, Austria, Spain and Portugal. The low rates are observed in Caucasian populations of North America (10–15), and in India, and in most African and Middle-East countries, and in Bolivia, Paraguay and Panama. Low rates are seen in Greece and in southern coastal regions of Yugoslavia and Italy.

Urban–rural distribution

Recent data do not show consistent differences in risk between urban and rural populations. In Colombia and Costa Rica with large differences in cancer risk within relatively small areas, most high-risk groups are from rural areas with a predominance of the intestinal type.

Time trends

A steady decline in stomach cancer rates has occurred in many countries during this century. Figure 26.2 taken from Kurihara *et al.* (1984) shows the mortality trends for certain countries for the periods

Fig. 26.3 Time trends in standardized gastric cancer death rates per 100,000 in Norway, by sex.

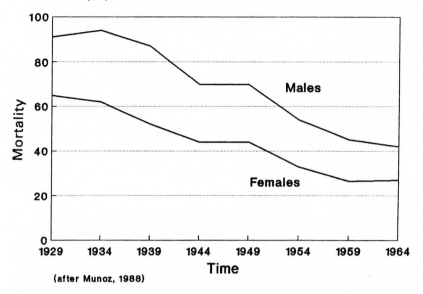

(after Munoz, 1988)

1960–87. The decline is apparent in both sexes, but in high-risk countries such as Japan, Chile and Portugal the decline occurred later than in the United States and Europe. In Norway mortality rates started to decline in 1930, levelled off following the 1940–45 war and resumed their decline in 1951 (Fig. 26.3). This decline was mainly due to a decrease in the intestinal type of stomach cancer (Muñoz & Asvall, 1971).

Migrants born in high-risk countries retain their high risk when they move to the low-risk environment of the USA but their US-born offspring show rates closer to those of the adopted country. The intestinal type of stomach cancer predominates in migrants from high-risk populations and the decline is essentially in this type (Muñoz, 1988). Similar findings have been reported from Japan (Hanai *et al.*, 1982), Finland (Sipponen *et al.*, 1987) and from Italy (Amorosi *et al.*, 1988).

Age and sex

Stomach cancer is extremely rare below the age of 30, thereafter it increases rapidly in both males and females. The risk for intestinal type rises faster with age than the risk for the diffuse type, both in high- and low-risk populations (Correa *et al.*, 1973).

In general, there is a two- to three-fold excess of stomach cancer in males. Below 30 years the sex ratio is closer to one, it then increases to a maximum in age-groups 55 to 59 and thereafter declines. The peak at 55 to 59 years is explained by the earlier rise in the intestinal type in males than in females (Muñoz, 1988).

Social class differences

An inverse socio-economic gradient has been observed in most populations, the rates in lower socio-economic groups being two to three times higher than in more affluent classes.

26.4   Etiological inferences

The continuous decline of the stomach cancer rates over the last five decades, the large differences in incidence among populations and the results of migrant studies suggest a predominant role for external environmental factors generally believed to be dietary. Although higher rates are found in lower socio-economic groups in most countries, attempts to correlate the incidence of stomach cancer internationally by such criteria are inconsistent, and low rates are found in both poor and rich states. Migrant populations provide clear evidence that risk factors operating in early life determine the future risk of developing stomach cancer.

26.5   Known and suspected causes
Genetic factors

Family aggregation studies in general show that close relatives of stomach cancer patients have a 2–3 fold higher risk than controls. This could be due to genetic factors or to sharing the same environment. There is evidence that blood type A is associated with a higher risk of stomach cancer, specially of the diffuse type (Correa *et al.*, 1973). In Japan, patients with diffuse type of stomach cancer have more often a positive family history than those with intestinal type. Recent studies in a high-risk Colombian population indicate, in addition to environmental factors, that a recessive autosomal gene with penetrance dependent on age and mother's CAG status determines the risk of developing chronic atrophic gastritis (Bonney *et al.*, 1986).

Dietary factors (see Chapter 12)

For many years, diet has been regarded as probably the most important etiological factor and several hypotheses have been advanced.

These include not only natural carcinogens or carcinogenic precursors in the food, but also chemical additives, contaminants, or pollutants. Indirectly, diet is postulated to effect gastric cancer through a lack of dietary inhibitors or through a modulating role of macronutrients. The final carcinogenic potential of a diet probably represents the complex interaction of foods which have a variety of enhancing and inhibitory properties.

Carcinogenic precursors

The use of smoked foods was originally associated with stomach cancer in Iceland (Dungal, 1961). Later, case-control and cohort studies suggest that a high intake of smoked, salted and fried foods and the frequent ingestion of complex carbohydrates and starchy foods increase the risk of developing stomach cancer (Higginson, 1966; Nomura, 1982; Joosens & Kesteloot, 1988; La Vecchia *et al.*, 1987). In Japan and the United States, studies suggest that a higher risk is associated with Japanese-style dietary habits which are characterized by a high intake of dried or salty fish, pickled vegetables and rice (Haenszel *et al.*, 1972; Kato *et al.*, 1987; Hirayama, 1988). A protective effect of high intake of dairy products (Muñoz & Asvall, 1971) has been suggested but the most consistent finding has been the protection conferred by fresh fruits and vegetables, possibly due to anti-oxidants (Buiatti *et al.*, 1989, Graham *et al.*, 1990, Hirayama, 1988).

Several hypotheses have been proposed to interpret these dietary associations of which the most extensively studied has been the role of *N*-nitroso compounds (Bartsch *et al.*, 1989). Such compounds are formed in the stomach from precursors present in food. It has been postulated that normally they do not effect the gastric mucosa, unless the mucous barrier is damaged by irritants, such as salted foods. This would result in chronic atrophic gastritis (CAG), intestinal metaplasia and later gastric cancer. Although there is some experimental and indirect epidemiological support, definitive proof is lacking (Ohshima *et al.*, 1988) (Chapter 12).

Food additives and contaminants

In most industrialized countries there is no significant relationship between the food additives currently in use and cancer of the stomach. In fact consumption of industrially processed diets tend to be associated with a lower incidence of this cancer, which has been attributed to increased use of anti-oxidants and refrigeration and decrease in the use of nitrites and salt. Such an hypothesis is consistent with the results of a number of animal experiments.

Miscellaneous

Alcohol

Although a relationship between alcoholic beverages and gastric carcinoma has been reported from Japan, other studies have failed to demonstrate such a link.

Tobacco

Many years ago, an association between smoking and cancer of the cardia was reported and recent studies from Japan and China are supportive (Li *et al.*, 1989; Hirayama, 1988). No association has been found by others.

Soils and trace elements

A relationship between trace elements in soil and gastric cancer has been described but the evidence is conflicting.

Bacteria

Spiral bacterium *Helicobacter pylori* (formerly *Campylobacter*) which colonize the gastric mucosa in humans and animals is strongly implicated in the etiology of acute and chronic gastritis but its role in stomach cancer is unknown.

Gastrectomy

Studies in Scandinavian countries (Arnthorsson *et al.*, 1988) and in the UK (Caygill *et al.*, 1986) suggest that the risk of stomach cancer increases subsequent to gastric resection for non-malignant diseases, especially after 20 years.

Other factors

In some cases radiation has been identified as a cause, also asbestos. The evidence for the latter is not convincing and may be due to diagnostic artifact. Earlier mortality studies showed a frequent relationship with dusty occupations which may represent confounding by other lifestyle factors.

26.6   Relevant laboratory studies

It has been shown that salt, bile acids, aspirin, alcohol and nitrite enhance gastric carcinogenesis in rats. On the other hand, butylated hydroxyanisole (BHA), selenium and difluoromethylornithine (DFMO) inhibit gastric carcinogenesis (Newberne *et al.*, 1987). Early studies on the glandular stomach in rodents using carcinogens, e.g. PAH, were essentially negative. However, cancer of the glandular stomach can now be produced readily in rodents with oral *N*-nitroso compounds, e.g. *N*-Methyl-*N*-Nitro-*N*-nitroso guanidine (NNNG). The relevance of such compounds to human cancer is uncertain.

Although reliable methods to assess the potential to form *N*-nitroso compounds endogenously have been developed in recent years, so far they have been of little help in clearly identifying the role of these compounds in human gastric carcinogenesis. The recent development of sensitive and specific methods to detect DNA alkylation adducts and oxidative DNA damage may help in assessing exposure to various carcinogenic substances in epidemiological studies (Bartsch *et al.*, 1989).

A few studies have shown that the gastric mucosa of patients with precancerous lesions and with stomach cancer express various oncogene products and a transforming gene has been identified (Sakamoto *et al.*, 1987).

26.7   Attributable risks

Although there is evidence indicating that dietary factors are involved in the development of stomach cancer, knowledge of the role of individual components is insufficient to quantify the degree of risk. The number of cancers due to other factors, such as radiation, etc., is very small.

26.8   Conclusions

Large differences in incidence among populations and a dramatic decline over the last five decades in most populations, are the outstanding epidemiological characteristics of stomach cancer. These findings have long suggested a predominant role for exogenous factors, especially diet, but its role remains to be established.

The recommendation of dietary changes in the direction suggested by epidemiological observations (avoidance or decrease of salty and smoked food and increase of fresh vegetables and fruits) is in agreement with general recommendations for a healthy diet, but the actual impact of these dietary changes especially if made in adult life on the incidence of stomach cancer cannot be stated with certainty.

26.9 References

Amorosi, A., Bianchi, S., Buiatti, E., Cipriani, F., Palli, D. & Zampi, G. (1988). Gastric cancer in a high-risk area in Italy. Histologic patterns according to Lauren's classification. *Cancer*, **62**, 2191–6.

Arnthorsson, G., Tulinius, H. & Egilsson, V. (1988). Gastric cancer after gastrectomy. *Int. J. Cancer*, **42**, 365–7.

Bartsch, H., Ohshima, H., Pignatelli, B. & Calmels, S. (1989). Human exposure to endogenous *N*-nitroso compounds: quantitative estimates in subjects at high risk for cancer of the oral cavity, oesophagus, stomach and urinary bladder. *Cancer Surv.*, **8**, 335–62.

Bonney, G.E., Elston, R.C., Correa, P., Haenszel, W., Zavala, D.E., Zarama, G., Collazos, T. & Cuello, C. (1986). Genetic etiology of gastric carcinoma: I. Chronic atrophic gastritis. *Genetic Epidemiol.*, **3**, 213–24.

Buiatti, E., Palli, D., Decarli, A., Amadori, D., Avellini, C., Bianchi, S., Biserni, R., Cipriani, F., Cocco, P., Giacosa, A., Marubini, E., Puntoni, R., Vindigni, C., Fraumeni, J. & Blot, W. (1989). A case-control study of gastric cancer and diet in Italy. *Int. J. Cancer*, **44**, 611–16.

Caygill, C.P.J., Hill, M.J., Kirkham, J.S. & Northfield, T.C. (1986). Mortality from gastric cancer following gastric surgery for peptic ulcer. *Lancet*, **i**, 929–31.

Correa, P., Sasano, N., Stemmermann, G.N. & Haenszel, W. (1973). Pathology of gastric carcinoma in Japanese populations: comparisons between Miyagi prefecture, Japan, and Hawaii. *J. Natl. Cancer Inst.*, **51**, 1449–59.

Dungal, H. (1961). The special problem of cancer of the stomach in Iceland. *J. Am. Med. Assn.*, **178**, 789–98.

Filipe, M.I. (1988). Intestinal metaplasia in the histogenesis of gastric carcinoma. In *Gastric Carcinogenesis*, ed. P.I. Reed & M.J. Hill, pp. 19–28. Amsterdam: Elsevier Science Publishers.

Graham, S., Haughey, B., Marshall, J., Brasure, J., Zielezny, M., Freudenheim, J., West, D., Nolan, J. & Wilkinson, G. (1990). Diet in the epidemiology of gastric cancer. *Nutr. Cancer*, **13**, 19–34.

Haenszel, W., Kurihara, M., Segi, M. & Lee, R.K.C. (1972). Stomach cancer among Japanese in Hawaii. *J. Natl. Cancer Inst.*, **49**, 969–88.

Hanai, A., Fujimoto, I. & Taniguchi, H. (1982). Trends of stomach cancer incidence and histological types in Osaka. In *Trends in Cancer Incidence: Causes and Practical Implications*, ed. K. Magnus, pp. 143–54. New York: Hemisphere Publ. Corp.

Higginson, J. (1966). Etiological factors in gastro-intestinal cancer in man. *J. Natl. Cancer Inst.*, **37**, 527–45.

Hirayama, T. (1988). Actions suggested by gastric cancer epidemiological studies in Japan. In *Gastric Carcinogenesis*, ed. P.I. Reed & M.J. Hill, pp. 209–27. Amsterdam: Elsevier Science Publishers.

Joosens, J.V. & Kesteloot, H. (1988). Salt and stomach cancer. In *Gastric Carcinogenesis*, ed. P.I. Reed & M.J. Hill, pp. 105–26. Amsterdam: Elsevier Science Publishers.

Kato, I., Tominaga, S. & Kuroishi, T. (1987). Per capita food/nutrients intake and mortality from gastrointestinal cancers in Japan. *Jpn. J. Cancer Res.*, **78**, 453–9.

Kurihara, M., Aoki, K. & Tominaga, S. (eds.) (1984). *Cancer Mortality Statistics in the World*. Nagoya: University of Nagoya Press.

La Vecchia, C., Negri, E., Decarli, A., D'Avanzo, B. & Franceschi, S. (1987). A case-control of diet and gastric cancer in Northern Italy. *Int. J. Cancer*, **40**, 484–98.

Lauren, P. (1965). The two histological main types of gastric carcinoma. Diffuse and so-called intestinal type. *Acta Pathol. Microbiol. Scand.*, **64**, 31–49.

Li, J.Y., Ershow, A.G., Chen, Z.J., Wacholder, S., Li, G.Y., Guo, W., Li, B. & Blot, W.J. (1989). A case-control of oesophageal and gastric cardia in Linxian. *Int. J. Cancer* (in press)

Muir, C., Waterhouse, J., Mack, T., Powell, J. & Whelan, S. (eds.) (1987). *Cancer Incidence in Five Continents*, volume V, IARC Scientific Publication No. 88. Lyon: International Agency for Research on Cancer.

Muñoz, N. (1988). Descriptive epidemiology of stomach cancer. In *Gastric Carcinogenesis*, ed. P.I. Reed & M.J. Hill, pp. 51–69. Amsterdam: Elsevier Science Publishers.

Muñoz, N. & Asvall, J.E. (1971). Time trends of intestinal and diffuse types of gastric cancer in Norway. *Int. J. Cancer*, **8**, 144–57.

Newberne, P.M., Charnlay, G., Adams, K., Cantor, M., Suphakarn, V., Roth, D. & Schrager, T.F. (1987). Gastric carcinogenesis: a model for the identification of risk factors. *Cancer Lett.*, **38**, 149–63.

Nomura, A. (1982). Stomach. In *Cancer Epidemiology and Prevention*, ed D. Schottenfeld & J.F. Fraumeni, Jr., pp.624–37. Philadelphia: W.B. Saunders.

Ohshima, H., Pignatelli, B., Malaveille, C., Friesen, M., Calmels, S., Shuker, D., Muñoz, N. & Bartsch, H. (1988). Markers of intragastric nitrosamine formation and resulting DNA damage. In *Gastric Carcinogenesis*, ed. P.I. Reed & M.J. Hill, pp. 175–85. Amsterdam: Elsevier Science Publishers.

Parkin, D.M., Läärä, E. & Muir, C.S. (1988). Estimates of the worldwide frequency of 16 major cancers in 1980. *Int. J. Cancer*, **41**, 184–7.

Sakamoto, H., Joshida, T., Miyagawa, K. & Terada, M. (1987). A novel transforming gene from human stomach cancer. *Gan To kagaku Ryoho*, **14**, 2147–51.

Sipponen, P., Jarrei, O., Kekki, M. & Siurala, M. (1987). Decreased incidence of intestinal and diffuse types of gastric cancer in Finland during a 20-year period. *Scand. J. Gastroenterol.*, **22**, 805–71.

27

Small intestine

ICD-9 152

27.1 Introduction

Tumors of the small intestine are uncommon in all parts of the world and comprise a number of different histological types.

27.2 Histology, classification and diagnosis

Four major types of neoplasms are found. The most common are adenocarcinomas which comprise about half of all small intestinal cancers. Second in frequency are carcinoids (argentaffinoma). Lymphomas of different types also occur, many being previously described as lymphosarcoma and reticulum cell sarcoma. Certain B cell sarcomas that occur in the Mediterranean area are regarded as showing similarities to Burkitt's lymphoma (Chapter 53). Rare sarcomas e.g. leiomyosarcoma, are observed.

27.3 Descriptive epidemiology

Incidence and time trends

The incidence of small intestinal cancer is very low, most rates being less than unity (Fig. 27.1). In view of their rarity, time trends are uninformative.

Age and sex distribution

Most of the tumors occur after the age of 50 with the exception of Mediterranean lymphoma which tend to be more frequent in children. There is a modest male excess in incidence.

27.4 Known and suspected causes

Very little has been added to our knowledge of these cancers since the review of Lightdale *et al.* (1982).

Fig. 27.1 Incidence rates around 1980: Small intestine (ICD-9 152).

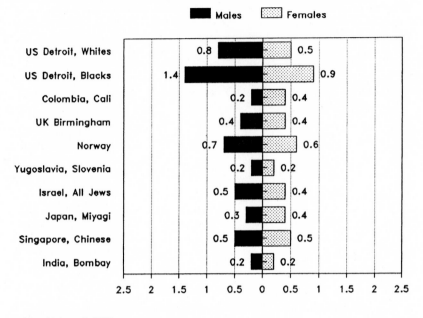

(after Muir *et al.*, 1987)

Adenocarcinoma

These tumors are highly lethal. Their causes are essentially unknown but they have been shown to be more common in regional enteritis and in Peutz–Jeghers syndrome. Some rare cases may be associated with familial polyposis coli.

Carcinoid (argentaffinoma)

Carcinoid, the second most frequent small bowel cancer, occurs in the appendix where it may be found incidentally at surgery or autopsy. These tumors can be both benign and malignant and tend to grow very slowly. Large metastasizing carcinoids may secrete serotonin giving rise to a defined clinical syndrome.

Lymphomas

Malignant lymphomas are of several types. The Mediterranean lymphoma, which occurs commonly in comparatively young people, may be primary in nature since it is most frequent in the upper part of the small intestines. These tumors may produce incomplete immunoglobulin alpha chains and are not dissimilar histologically to Burkitt's lymphoma. Among the risk factors suggested are parasites, immuno-deficiency states and celiac disease. Only for the latter is the evidence reasonably supportive.

27.5   Laboratory studies

Although small intestinal adenocarcinomas can be produced relatively easily in rodents by feeding polycyclic hydrocarbons, there is little evidence that the latter are relevant to the human disease.

27.6   Conclusions

Tumors of the small intestine are rare and their etiology remains unknown.

27.7   References

Lightdale, C.J., Koepsell, T.D. & Sherlock, P. (1982). Small intestine. In *Cancer Epidemiology and Prevention*, ed. D. Schottenfeld & J.F. Fraumeni, Jr., pp. 692–702. Philadelphia: W.B. Saunders.

Muir, C., Waterhouse, J., Mack, T., Powell, J. & Whelan, S. (eds.) (1987). *Cancer Incidence in Five Continents*, volume V, IARC Scientific Publication No. 88. Lyon: International Agency for Research on Cancer.

28

Large intestine: colon and rectum

ICD-9 153–154

28.1 Introduction

While cancers of the colon and rectum show some differences in their geographic and temporal distribution, it is usual to discuss them together in terms of causation.

28.2 Histology, classification and diagnosis

Epithelial tumors of the colorectum are adenocarcinomas. In many patients, such cancers are frequently associated with benign polyps and adenomas as well as dysplastic mucosal lesions which are believed to be precancerous (Ponz de Leon *et al.*, 1987).

Geographic differences have been observed in the distribution by sub-site (Schottenfeld & Winawer, 1982). Unfortunately, the anatomical boundary around the recto-sigmoid (which for international classification purposes is assigned to the rectum), is variable and the terms sigmoid and recto-sigmoid are often used interchangeably by clinicians. De Jong *et al.*, (1972) concluded, however, that this made little difference to incidence rates. Non-epithelial tumors are discussed in Chapter 37.

28.3 Descriptive epidemiology
Incidence

For colon cancer, the highest male incidence rates are in the white population of Connecticut, USA (34.1). The highest female rate (29.0) is in the black population of Detroit (Fig. 28.1). Rates, in the range of 15 to 20, are observed in Canada and much of western Europe. In western Europe, the incidence tends to be more than twice that east of the Elbe River. In Asia and Latin America, rates are low to intermediate (10 to 15). Within Israel, the rates in Jews born in Europe or America (21.1 in males and 17.7 in females) are substantially greater than those born in Africa or

Fig. 28.1 Incidence rates around 1980: Colon (ICD-9 153).

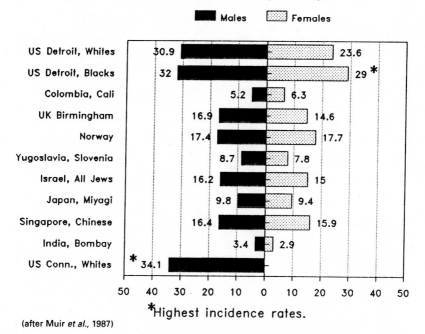

Males   Females

US Detroit, Whites	30.9 ... 23.6
US Detroit, Blacks	32 ... 29 *
Colombia, Cali	5.2 ... 6.3
UK Birmingham	16.9 ... 14.6
Norway	17.4 ... 17.7
Yugoslavia, Slovenia	8.7 ... 7.8
Israel, All Jews	16.2 ... 15
Japan, Miyagi	9.8 ... 9.4
Singapore, Chinese	16.4 ... 15.9
India, Bombay	3.4 ... 2.9
US Conn., Whites	* 34.1

50 40 30 20 10 0 10 20 30 40 50

*Highest incidence rates.

(after Muir *et al.*, 1987)

Asia (9.3 and 13.3), or in Israel (13.0 and 14.2). In the non-Jewish population, rates are very low, slightly under 5 in both sexes. In contrast to rates in Japan (around 12 in both sexes), Japanese in the San Francisco Bay Area (31), and in Hawaii (34) have rates similar to whites. US Chinese have rates about three times greater than those in Shanghai with intermediate levels of risk in Hong Kong and Singapore Chinese.

It has been suggested that differences between the developed and developing countries are due to more tumors clustering around the recto-sigmoid in the former, the incidence of cecum and ascending colon cancer being much the same everywhere. However, the ratios of sigmoid/colon/cecum and ascending colon are higher in low incidence countries such as Japan.

Although incidence and mortality rates are usually lower, the geographical distribution of rectal cancer shows many similarities to the colon (Fig. 28.2).

Time trends

In countries with previously high rates, temporal changes in rates have been relatively small, contrasting with countries with low rates where greater increases have occurred especially in the rectum. The rates for

Fig. 28.2 Incidence rates around 1980: Rectum (ICD-9 154).

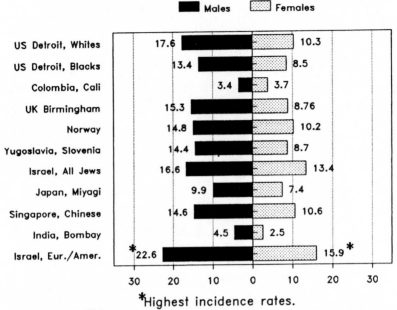

*Highest incidence rates.

(after Muir *et al.*, 1987)

colon cancer in blacks in the USA have increased and are now close to those for whites in some areas (in Detroit, the rates are higher). Incidence and mortality are relatively similar in trend. Doll (1989) has described decreases for mortality in the under 45 group in the UK which he believes reflect changes in both incidence and efficacy of therapy.

Age and sex distribution

In contrast to colon cancer which is slightly commoner in females before 60 years, the sex ratio for cancers of the rectum is usually 1.5 to 2.

28.4   Etiological inferences

Geographical, temporal and migrant studies strongly suggest the role of environmental agents which may modulate cancer induction even in adult life. Polish and Japanese migrants to the United States have shown substantial increases in mortality from large bowel (mainly colon) cancer. As the risk in non-migrant compatriots did not change it is assumed that the new environment was responsible. It is speculated that initiation had already occurred before migration, and the increase was largely due to modulating dietary factors. The more rapid rise in rectal than in colon cancer among Japanese migrants is also consistent with this theory. In Florida, retirees from the northeast United States show a decrease in rates.

It is not established that rectal and colonic cancers are caused by the same etiological agents. Although the similarity of incidence patterns suggests some common causal factors, differences in sex ratio would indicate that other stimuli are involved. Wynder (1987) and others believe that the recto-sigmoid approximates to the colon more closely than the rectum. Jensen *et al.* (1980) and Mellemgaard *et al.* (1989) found that the mortality of colon cancer in spouses was that of the general population in both Sweden and Denmark. Thus, married life with presumably a common diet was alone not the only determining factor.

28.5 Known or suspected causes

The early literature has been reviewed by Schottenfeld and Winawer (1982).

Familial and hereditary factors
Familial adenomatous polyposis coli (FAP)

This is a hereditary condition associated with multiple polyps in the large intestine in several family members. These show a high frequency of malignant transformation (see Chapter 18). An increase has also been reported in patients with angio telangiectasia.

There may also be some hereditary susceptibility involved in isolated polyps but this is less well defined. Macklin (1960) found familial clustering in colonic cancer, which she believed was polygenic. Reviewing 670 persons in 34 kindreds, Cannon-Albright *et al.* (1988) concluded that the data supported dominant inheritance of susceptibility to colorectal adenomas and associated colorectal cancers, with a gene frequency of 19%. In this model, adenomas and colorectal cancers occurred only in genetically susceptible persons, although the results were barely statistically significant. It was concluded that genetic and environmental factors are involved in the formation and transformation of polyps.

Geographical studies on population susceptibility have not yet been made.

Individual susceptibility (Chapter 18)
Bodmer *et al.* (1987), localized the gene for familial adenomatous polyposis on chromosome 5. Fearon *et al.* (1990) have shown that allelic deletions involving chromosome 18q occur in more than 70 percent of colorectal cancers and are thought to signal the existence of a tumor suppressor gene in the affected region. A case can be made for the role of

both activation of the oncogene (albeit early in progression) and inactivation of multiple tumor suppression genes (Stanbridge, 1990).

Vogelstein *et al.* (1988) have evaluated four genetic alterations involved in the progression of colorectal neoplasia. Their results were consistent with the mutational activation of an oncogene coupled with the loss of several suppressor genes, which correlate with progression, and such genes have been identified. In conclusion, the evidence would suggest that most tumors occur in a specific but considerable segment of the population which possesses increased susceptibility. Such observations are consistent with the hypothesis that genetic and environmental factors interact in the formation and transformation of polyps and add to the complexity of interpreting epidemiological studies on diet.

Diet (Chapter 12)

Although cancers of the colon and rectum are almost certainly due to environmental factors of which the most important is believed to be diet, published investigations have not produced any wholly convincing hypothesis. There are numerous epidemiological studies attempting to link large bowel cancers to dietary or food components. Unfortunately, diets and foods high in fiber and vegetables, for example, are closely correlated and are usually low in fat, thus complicating evaluation of individual components. The NAS/NRC (1982) concluded that there is no evidence linking colorectal cancers to ingested carcinogens, with the possible exception of beer.

Three major dietary hypotheses have been proposed:

  (a) a causal association with fat,
  (b) a protective effect of dietary fiber; and
  (c) a protective effect of vegetables.

Fat

While the NAS report emphasized the association between colon cancer and total dietary fat, for which meat intake is sometimes used as a surrogate, other studies, especially in Scandinavia, have failed to confirm this association (Jensen, 1985). Enstrom (1975) describes inconsistencies in correlating colon cancer incidence trends with per capita beef intake in the United States and such a hypothesis cannot explain the lower frequency of these cancers in both Seventh Day Adventists (vegetarians) and Mormons (meat-eaters). A correlation has been suggested between colon cancer mortality and coronary heart disease for both of which fat is regarded as a risk factor, as in Hawaii. However, although coronary heart disease has fallen markedly, and major long-term changes in quantity and character of fat intake have taken place in the United States and Australia over the last 15 years, no concurrent changes have occurred in colon or rectal cancer incidence. Other observations also show inconsistencies (Jensen *et al.*, 1985; Willett & MacMahon, 1984*a*, *b*).

Fiber

The term 'fiber' covers a variety of non-starch polysaccharides with different physiological properties. The pentose fraction is believed to be the protective non-nutritive carbohydrate component (Cummings *et al.*, 1978), but this remains to be confirmed (Chapter 12). In Africa, the inverse relationship between dietary fiber intake and colorectal cancer (Higginson & Oettlé, 1960; Burkitt, 1971) has long been assumed. However, Walker *et al.* (1986), in a comparative study of different races in South Africa found that a low incidence of colon cancer was more associated with low fecal pH than dietary fiber suggesting that components of diet other than fiber affected cancer incidence.

Studies in Denmark and Finland, countries of contrasting large bowel cancer incidence, examining the dietary habits of a sample of rural and urban populations in both countries, concluded that fiber was protective by diluting the fat-derived bile acids in bulkier stools. Transit time was not different in these populations (IARC, 1977, 1982).

Vegetables

There is some evidence of a protective effect, especially for cruciferous vegetables such as cabbage, cauliflower and broccoli (Chapter 12). Due to confounding however, their role has proven difficult to investigate since diets high in fiber also contain certain inhibitors and vitamins.

Other dietary factors

No convincing relationship has been shown with protein intake. Potter and McMichael (1986) showed an increased risk with protein and caloric intake confined to those consuming a low fiber diet, especially women. Graham *et al.* (1988) have also emphasized a possible role of high calories. A reported inverse relationship between low serum cholesterol levels prior to cancer development and increased large intestine cancer remains unconvincing (McMichael *et al.*, 1984).

Micronutrients

Slattery *et al.* (1988) suggest that a high calcium intake may be protective against colon cancer through reducing exposure of the bowel to fats and bile acids. Decreased colonic cell proliferation has been described with supplementary calcium in familial colon cancer and in multiple polyposis (Lipkin *et al.*, 1989). This theory is consistent with reports of a protective effect of high doses of vitamin D. The administration of various other vitamins has been described as inversely related to colorectal cancer, but the evidence remains unconvincing (Wu *et al.*, 1987).

Alcohol
The evidence for a role of alcoholic beverages is inconsistent (Wu *et al.*, 1987) but heavy beer intake may be related to rectal cancer (Jensen, 1985; Kune *et al.*, 1987).

Socio-economic and occupational factors
Many studies show a higher incidence in upper income and groups. Most occupational studies show no consistent patterns, but increases in some sedentary occupations have been reported (Demers *et al.*, 1985), which probably reflect dietary and socio-economic conditions (Gerhardsson *et al.*, 1986).

Inflammatory bowel disease
Colorectal cancer is increased nearly 20-fold among individuals with long standing ulcerative colitis (Gyde *et al.*, 1988). Crohn's disease has also been associated with increased susceptibility.

Miscellaneous
The protective effect of early age of first pregnancy (Howe *et al.*, 1985) exogenous hormones (Furner *et al.*, 1989) and exercise (Gerhardsson *et al.*, 1986), remains to be confirmed.

Other tumors
Lymphomas on the large intestines rarely occur in Europe. In the Middle East, however, they are found especially in children and show similarities to Burkitt's lymphoma (Chapter 53).

28.6   Relevant laboratory studies
Animal studies
Intestinal adenocarcinoma has been reduced by such chemicals as hydrazine in rodents. While the morphogenesis appears similar, most tested compounds are unlikely to be relevant to humans. However, such models have been used to demonstrate the modulating effects of bile salts, fats, fiber, etc. (Chester *et al.*, 1986; Reddy *et al.*, 1977; Minoura *et al.*,

1988; Weisburger & Wynder, 1987). Theoretically, a number of chemicals could be converted in the bowel to carcinogens or modulators through bacterial action (Hill, 1985). Fecal mutagens, known as fecapentaenes have been identified, but their role in humans remains uncertain (Schiffman *et al.*, 1989).

28.7 Attributable risks

No meaningful estimates can be made in the absence of defined causes. However, Wahrendorf (1987) has calculated that dietary modifications could lead to a 15% – 20% reduction in incidence. FAP and other hereditary factors probably account for less than 2% of all tumors. The impact of genetic susceptibility needs more accurate delineation but could affect up to 50% of the population.

28.8 Conclusions

Geographical differences and the rapid change in risk in migrants strongly support a major role for environmental factors of which diet would appear the most logical. Dietary components, however, have proved difficult to define due to their complexity. The current advice – to reduce dietary fat intake, (particularly animal fat) and increase fiber intake through fresh fruit and vegetables, is not based on strong data but is considered unlikely to be harmful.

The implication for prevention following the demonstration of a large susceptible subgroup in the population remains to be evaluated and complicates the analysis of case-history studies.

28.9 References

Bodmer, W.F., Bailey, C.J., Bodmer, J., Bussey, H.J., Ellis, A., Gorman, P., Lucibello, F.C., Murday, V.A., Rider, S.H., Scambler, P. *et al.* (1987). Localization of the gene for familial adenomatous polyposis on chromosome 5. *Nature*, **328**, 614–16.

Burkitt, D.P. (1971). Epidemiology of cancer of the colon and rectum. *Cancer*, **28**, 3–13.

Cannon-Albright, L.A., Skolnick, M.H., Bishop, T., Lee, R.G. & Burt, R.W. (1988). Common inheritance of susceptibility to colonic adenomatous polyps and associated colorectal cancers. *N. Engl. J. Med.*, **319**, 533–7.

Chester, J.F., Gaissert, H.A., Ross, J.S., Malt, R.A. & Weitzman, S.A. (1986). Augmentation of 1,2-dimethylhydrazine-induced colon cancer by experimental colitis in mice: Role of dietary vitamin A. *J. Natl. Cancer Inst.*, **76**, 939–42.

Cummings, J.H., Southgate, D.A.T., Branch, W., Houston, H., Jenkins, D.J. & James, W.P. (1978). Colonic response to dietary fibre from carrot, cabbage, apple, bran and guar gum. *Lancet*, **i**, 5–8.

de Jong, U.W., Day, N.E., Muir, C.S., Barclay, T.H.C., Bras, G., Foster, F.H., Jussawalla, D.J., Kurihara, M., Linden, G., Martinez, I., Payne, P.M., Pedersen, E., Ringertz, N. & Shanmugaratnam, T. (1972). The distribution of cancer within the large bowel. *Int. J. Cancer*, **10**, 463–77.

Demers, R.Y., Demers, P., Hoar, S.K. & Deighton, K. (1985). Prevalence of colorectal polyps among Michigan pattern and model makers. *J. Occup. Med.*, **27**, 809–12.

Doll, R. (1989). Progress against cancer: Are we winning the war? *Acta Oncol.*, **28**, 611–21.

Enstrom, J.E. (1975). Colorectal cancer and consumption of beef and fat. *Br. J. Cancer*, **23**, 432–9.

Fearon, E.R., Cho, K.R., Nigro, J.M., Kern, S.E., Simons, J.W., Ruppert, J.M., Hamilton, S.R., Preisinger, A.C., Thomas, G., Kinzler, K.W. & Vogelstein, B. (1990). Identification of a chromosome 18q gene that is altered in colorectal cancers. *Science*, **247**, 49–56.

Furner, S.E., Davis, F.G., Nelson, R.L. & Haenszel, W. (1989). A case-control study of large bowel cancer and hormone exposure in women. *Cancer Res.*, **49**, 4936–40.

Gerhardsson, M., Norell, S.E., Kiviranta, H., Pedersen, N.L. & Ahlbom, A. (1986). Sedentary jobs and colon cancer. *Am. J. Epidemiol.*, **123**, 775–80.

Graham, S., Marshall, J., Haughey, B., Mittelman, A., Swanson, M., Zielezny, M., Byers, T., Wilkinson, G. & West D. (1988). Dietary epidemiology of cancer of the colon in Western New York. *Am. J. Epidemiol.*, **128**, 490–503.

Gyde, S.N., Prior, P., Allan, R.N., Stevens, A., Jewell, D.P., Truelove, S.C., Lofberg, R., Brostrom, O. & Hellers, G. (1988). Colorectal cancer in ulcerative colitis: A cohort study of primary referrals from three centres. *Gut*, **29**, 206–17.

Higginson, J. & Oettlé, A.G. (1960). Cancer incidence in the Bantu and 'Cape Colored' races of South Africa: Report of a cancer survey in the Transvaal (1953–55). *J. Natl. Cancer Inst.*, **24**, 589–671.

Hill, M.J. (1985). Mechanisms of colorectal carcinogenesis. In *Diet and Human Carcinogenesis*, ed. J.V. Joossens, M.J. Hill & J Geboers, pp. 149–63. Amsterdam: Elsevier Science Publishers BV.

Howe, G.R., Craib, K.J. & Miller, A.B. (1985). Age at first pregnancy and risk of colorectal cancer: A case-control study. *J. Natl. Cancer Inst.*, **74**, 1155–9.

IARC Intestinal Microecology Group (1977). Dietary fibre, transit time, faecal bacteria, steroids and colon cancer in two Scandinavian populations. *Lancet*, **ii**, 207–11.

IARC (1982). Report of the 2nd IARC international collaborative study on diet and large bowel cancer in Denmark and Finland. *Nutr. Cancer*, **4**.

Jensen, O.M., Bolander, A.M., Sigtryggsson, P., Vercelli, M., Nguyen-Dinh, X. & MacLennan, R. (1980). Large bowel cancer in married couples in Sweden. *Lancet*, **i**, 1161–3.

Jensen, O.M. (1985). The role of diet in colorectal cancer. In *Diet and Human Carcinogenesis*, ed. J.V. Joossens, M.J. Hill & J Geboers. Amsterdam: Elsevier Science Publishers BV.

Kune, S., Kune, G.A. & Watson, L.F. (1987). Case-control study of alcoholic beverages as etiological factors: The Melbourne Colorectal Cancer Study. *Nutr. Cancer*, **9**, 43–56.

Lipkin, M. Friedman, E., Winawer, S.J. & Newmark, H. (1989). Colonic epithelial cell proliferation in responders and non-responders to supplemental dietary calcium. *Cancer Res.*, **248-54**.

Macklin, M.T. (1960). Inheritance of cancer of the stomach and large intestine in man. *J. Natl. Cancer Inst.*, **24**, 551–71.

McMichael, A.J., Jensen, O.M., Parkin, D.M. & Zaridze, D.G. (1984). Dietary and endogenous cholesterol and human cancer. *Epid. Reviews*, **6**, 192–216.

Mellemgaard, A., Jensen, O.M. & Lynge, E. (1989). Cancer incidence among spouses of patients with colorectal cancer. *Int. J. Cancer*, **44**, 225–8.

Minoura, T., Takata, T., Sakaguchi, M., Takada, H., Yamamura, M., Hioki, K. & Yamamoto, M. (1988). Effect of dietary eicosapentaenoic acid on azoxymethane-induced colon carcinogenesis in rats. *Cancer Res.*, **48**, 4790–4.

Muir, C., Waterhouse, J., Mack, T., Powell, J. & Whelan, S. (eds.) (1987). *Cancer Incidence in Five Continents*, volume V, IARC Scientific Publication No. 88. Lyon: International Agency for Research on Cancer.

NAS/NRC Committee on Diet, Nutrition, and Cancer (1982). *Diet, Nutrition and Cancer*. National Research Council, National Academy of Sciences Washington: National Academy Press.

Ponz de Leon, M., Antonioli, Al, Ascari, A., Zanghieri, G. & Sacchetti, C. (1987). Incidence and familial occurrence of colorectal cancer and polyps in a health-care district of Northern Italy. *Cancer*, **60**, 2848–59.

Potter, J.D. & McMichael, A.J. (1986). Diet and cancer of the colon and rectum: A case-control study. *J. Natl. Cancer Inst.*, **76**, 557–69.

Reddy, B.S., Watanabe, K., Weisburger, J.H. & Wynder, E.L. (1977). Promoting effect of bile acids in colon carcinogenesis in germfree and conventional F344 rats. *Cancer Res.*, **37**, 3238–42.

Schiffman, M.H., Van Tassell, R.L., Robinson, A., Smith, L., Daniel, J., Hoover, R.N., Weil, R., Rosenthal, J., Nair, P.P., Schwartz, S., Pettigrew, H., Curiale, S., Batist, G., Block, G. & Wilkins, T.D. (1989). Case-control study of colorectal cancer and fecapentane excretion. *Cancer Res.*, **49**, 1322–6.

Schottenfeld, D. & Winawer, S.J. (1982). Large intestine. In *Cancer Epidemiology and Prevention*, ed. D. Schottenfeld & J.F. Fraumeni, Jr., pp. 703–27. Philadelphia: W.B. Saunders.

Slattery, M., Sorenson, A.W. & Ford, M.H. (1988). Dietary calcium intake as a mitigating factor in colon cancer. *Am. J. Epidemiol.*, **128**, 504–14.

Stanbridge, E.J. (1990). Identifying tumor suppressor genes in human colorectal cancer. *Science*, **247**, 12–13.

Vogelstein, B., Fearon, E.R., Hamilton, S.R., Kern, S.E., Preisinger, A.C., Leppert, M., Nakamura, Y., White, R., Smits, A.M.M. & Bos, J.L. (1988). Genetic alterations during colorectal-tumor development. *N. Engl. J. Med.*, **319**, 525–32.

Wahrendorf, J. (1987). An estimate of the proportion of colo-rectal and stomach cancers which might be prevented by certain changes in dietary habits. *Int. J. Cancer*, **40**, 625–8.

Walker, A.R.P., Walker, B.F. & Walker, A.J. (1986). Faecal pH, dietary fibre intake, and proneness to colon cancer in four South African populations. *Br. J. Cancer*, **53**, 489–95.

Weisburger, J.H. & Wynder, E.L. (1987). Etiology of colorectal cancer with emphasis on mechanism of action and prevention. *Import. Adv. Oncol.*, 197–220.

Willett, W.C. & MacMahon, B. (1984a). Diet and cancer. *N. Engl. J. Med.*, **310**, 633–8.

Willett, W.C. & MacMahon, B. (1984b). Diet and cancer. *N. Engl. J. Med.*, **310**, 697–703.

Wu, A.H., Paganini-Hill, A., Ross, R.K. & Henderson, B.E. (1987). Alcohol, physical activity and other risk factors for colorectal cancer: A prospective study. *Br. J. Cancer*, **55**, 687–94.

Wynder, E.L. (1987). Amount and type of fat/fiber in nutritional carcinogenesis. *Prev. Med.*, **16**, 451–9.

29

Liver

ICD-9 155

29.1   Introduction

Liver cancer is the eighth most common cancer in the world, and is particularly frequent in certain regions of Africa, China, Japan and East Asia. Unless otherwise specified, the following discussion relates to tumors of the liver cells (hepatocellular carcinoma).

29.2   Histology, classification and diagnosis

In considering the etiology of primary cancer of the liver, three major types may be considered:

Hepatocellular carcinoma (HCC) is by far the most common type, arising directly from liver cells. There are several histological subtypes which do not appear of etiological significance. A rare type of solitary hepatoma (both benign and malignant) arises in an apparently undamaged liver. HCC is frequently associated with severe liver damage and cirrhosis, especially in Africa. Liver cirrhosis may be considered as a premalignant condition; the risk, however, varies with type and cause of the cirrhosis being much higher in African macro-nodular cirrhosis.

Cholangiocarcinoma or tumors of the intra-hepatic bile ducts form less than 10% of liver tumors in industrial countries. They are, however, common in South East Asia where they are usually associated with certain parasites.

Miscellaneous tumors arising from the endothelial cells, connective tissue or reticular cell elements of the liver, e.g. angiosarcomas and rare embryonal cancers (hepatoblastoma).

29.3   Descriptive epidemiology

Incidence

The highest rates for liver cancer occur in Sub-Saharan Africa (Table 29.1). In the 1950s, rates of over 100 in males were reported from

Table 29.1. *Age-adjusted incidence rates of liver cancer in Africa.*

	Males	Females
Mozambique, Laurenço Marques	112.9	30.8
Zimbabwe, Bulawayo	64.6	25.4
South Africa – Natal – Black	28.4	6.9
Indian	9.5	3.8
– Cape – Bantu	26.3	8.4
– Colored	1.5	0.7
– White	1.2	0.6
Gambia	33.0	13.0
Senegal, Dakar	25.6	9.0
Nigeria, Ibadan	15.4	3.2
Swaziland	10.5	3.0
Tanzania – Kilimanjaro	9.2	1.6
Algeria	1.6	1.4

(After Muñoz and Bosch, 1987.)

Mozambique (Doll *et al.*, 1966). High rates (over 20) are also observed in China, Japan and other countries of South East Asia and in some Melanesian populations. Modest increases in migrants from these countries to North America are found. Intermediate rates are found in certain regions of eastern and southern Europe, such as Rumania, Switzerland, Spain, Greece and blacks in the USA, and low rates (below 5) in caucasian populations in North and Latin America, the rest of Europe, Australia, North Africa (Figure 29.1) (Muñoz & Bosch, 1987).

Age distribution

In both high and low risk populations, the rates increase progressively with age with a tendency to level off in the older age groups. In the high-incidence areas, the rates commence to increase after 20 years of age, and reach a high by 40 years but in the low-risk areas the rise occurs much later, usually after 40 years.

Sex distribution

Males are more prone to develop liver cancer than females especially in high-risk populations. However, solitary hepatomas are equally common in females.

Time trends

In the past, liver cancer rates were highly influenced by classification and diagnostic errors, especially in countries with low incidence. This complicates interpretation of time trends. Muñoz and

Fig. 29.1 Incidence rates around 1980: Liver (ICD-9 155).

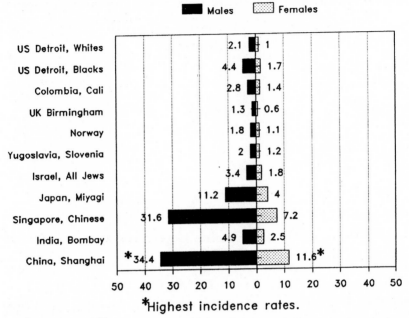

(after Muir *et al.*, 1987)

Bosch (1987) have reviewed incidence data from 73 populations; all except 3 were at low risk. In 13 a significant increasing trend in males was found, two registries showed a decline and the remaining 58 showed no clear trend.

In sub-saharan Africa, available data suggest that a decline in the liver cancer rates is occurring. Van Rensburg *et al.* (1985) reported a decrease of over 40% in liver cancer in Mozambique between 1968 and 1975.

29.4   Etiological inferences

The wide geographical and temporal variations in incidence strongly suggest a major role of environmental factors. The age and sex distribution indicate that the relevant exposures occur earlier in life in the high-risk populations and that males are more susceptible or more intensely exposed than females. Clinical and pathological differences between HCC and associated cirrhotic lesions in Africa and Asia as compared to North America and Europe are consistent with hypotheses predominately implicating viruses in the former and alcohol in the latter.

Hepatic hemangiosarcoma is regarded as a 'sentinel' tumor for certain carcinogens (see below).

Table 29.2. *Case-control studies on HBsAg and HCC.*

Study population	Number of subjects		Relative risk for HBsAg+ with 95% CI	Attributable risk (%)
	HCC	Controls		
High-risk areas				
Senegal	165	328	12.4 (7.7–19.3)	56.3
South Africa	289	213	12.6 (7.7–20.1)	56.7
Hong Kong	107	107	21.3 (10.1–45.9)	78.5
People's Republic of China	50	50	17.0 (4.3–99.4)	77.9
Philippines	104	841	10.83 (5.3–20.9)	63.9
Intermediate risk area:				
Greece	194	451	10.7 (6.8–16.6)	41.6
Low-risk area				
USA	34	38	48.4 (1.5–∞)	4.5
USA	86	161	28.6 (10.0–∞)	2.7

(After Muñoz and Bosch, 1987)

29.5 Known and suspected causes

A number of factors have been causally associated with hepatocellular carcinoma.

Viruses

Hepatitis B Virus (HBV) (Chapter 17).

In 1940, workers in West Africa first suggested that the cirrhosis in which liver cancer arose was due to viral hepatitis. Additional reports appeared in the European and North American literature (Higginson, 1963). The subsequent identification of markers specific for hepatitis B virus (HBV) placed such studies on a more objective basis (Nishioka, 1985; Blumberg & London, 1985; Popper *et al.*, 1987; Muñoz & Bosch, 1987).

At the global level there is a strong positive correlation between the incidence and mortality from HCC and the prevalence of HBsAg carriers (Chapter 17). However, correlation studies cannot properly adjust for other confounding variables, and no temporal relationship can be established between exposure and disease when both factors are assessed cross-sectionally.

Case control studies in high- and low-risk populations have shown that the relative risk associated with the presence of HBsAg in serum is markedly increased (Table 29.2).

Cohort studies comparing the occurrence of HCC among HBsAg carriers with that of a non-carrier control population or with HCC rates

Table 29.3. *Relative risk (RR) for primary liver cancer demonstrated in selected cohort studies on HBsAg carriers.*

Study population	Cohort		HCC risk	
	Total	HBsAg+	RR (95% CI)	Attributable risk (%)
Taiwan	22,707	3454	104.0 (51–212)	93.9
Japan	32,177	496	10.4 (5.0–19.1)	12.7
Japan, Osaka	—	8646	6.6 (4.0–10.2)	10.1[a]
USA, New York	—	6850	9.7 (2.0–28.3)	1.0[b]
England and Wales	—	3934	42.0 (14.0–100.0)	4.0[b]

[a] Assuming a prevalence rate of HGsAg in the general population of 2.0%.
[b] Assuming a prevalence rate of HGsAg in the general population of 0.1%.
(After Muñoz and Bosch, 1987.)

in the general population have yielded relative risks ranging from 7 to 100 (Table 29.3). These prospective cohort studies provide unequivocal evidence that the HBV infection precedes the development of HCC (Beasley *et al.*, 1981). The consistency of the findings and the size of the relative risk strongly indicate that the association is causal. Pathological studies are also consistent with such a relationship (Obata *et al.*, 1980; Paterson *et al.*, 1985).

Accordingly, several intervention studies and public health programs aimed at preventing HBV infection have been initiated (GHIS, 1987). The objective is to demonstrate that HBV vaccination of newborns in high-risk countries could prevent the occurrence of HCC in later life. In planning such campaigns account should be taken that perinatal transmission of HBV is higher in certain countries such as Japan and Taiwan than in others, e.g. African countries.

Only a small fraction of HBsAg carriers eventually develop HCC, and a certain proportion of HCCs are not associated with HBV. Thus, while HBV is probably the second most important human carcinogen so far identified after tobacco smoking, it is neither a sufficient nor a necessary cause of HCC. Other factors possibly necessary for the induction of HCC are discussed below.

Hepatitis C virus (HCV)

The recent development of specific markers for HCV (formerly called non-A – non-B hepatitis) has given further possibilities to explore the viral etiology of HCC specially in low-risk populations where HBV only accounts for about 10% of HCC. Preliminary studies indicate that antibodies to HCV are present in about 60–70% of patients with HCC and other chronic liver diseases and in less than 10% of healthy subjects from Italy and Spain (Bruix *et al.*, 1989; Colombo *et al.*, 1989).

Mycotoxins: aflatoxin (AF) (also see supplement)

Aflatoxins are mycotoxins elaborated by the fungi *Aspergillus flavus* and *Aspergillus parasiticus*. AF is hepatocarcinogenic in many animal species, including primates. AFB_1 is the most potent of the four major types (Busby & Wogan, 1984). The evidence for humans (Bosch & Muñoz, 1988) is less strong, being based largely on correlation studies at the population level. Methods now available for assessing exposure at the individual level have not yet been applied to large-scale epidemiological studies. Human exposure can occur following ingestion of contaminated food or of products derived from animals that have consumed AF-contaminated feeds. The main sources of AF in most countries are peanuts, peanut derivatives and corn. Although, under appropriate conditions, any foodstuff could host the growth of the mold and the production of toxins. Table 29.4 summarizes the findings of the five most comparable correlation studies. Although the techniques used to estimate AF exposure and HCC incidence rates varied from study to study, the overall correlation is highly significant.

Only two case-control studies have been reported. In the Philippines, relative risks of 17.0 and 13.9 (p < 0.05) were reported for individuals classified as having a 'very heavy' or 'moderately heavy' mean intake of AF, as compared to those with a lower intake. The effect of AF was higher among heavy alcohol consumers (RR = 35.5), and a dose–response was demonstrated (Bulatao-Jayme *et al.*, 1982). No adjustment was made for HBV status. In contrast, a study conducted in Hong Kong, showed no effect of aflatoxin as estimated from the degree of consumption of corn and beans, the two major local sources (Lam *et al.*, 1982).

Combined effect of HBV and aflatoxin

The possibility of a two-stage mechanism in liver cancer has been long suspected (Higginson, 1956). However, the current impossibility of measuring chronic exposure to aflatoxin at the individual level is the major obstacle in the evaluation of the combined effect of HBV and aflatoxin (see pp. 57). Van Rensburg *et al.* (1985), in a study in Mozambique and Transkei, observed that the prevalence of HBsAg carriers was low to intermediate in regions where the rate of HCC was extremely high. They also noted that gold miners, whose diet changed after moving to South Africa for work, experience a reduction in HCC risk within a year. They

Table 29.4. *Correlation studies on human exposure to aflatoxin B1 and HCC incidence.*

Country	Incidence rate of HCC in males over 15 ys. (per 10^5/year)	Aflatoxin B1 (ng/kg body wt/day)
Kenya		
High altitude	3.11	4.88
Middle altitude	10.80	7.84
Low altitude	12.92	14.81
Swaziland I		
Highveld	7.02	8.34
Middleveld	14.79	14.43
Lumbobo	18.65	19.89
Lowveld	26.65	53.34
Highveld	4.39	14.3
Middleveld	10.62	40.0
Lumbobo	11.07	32.9
Lowveld	23.02	127.1
Swaziland II		
Transkei	9.1	16.5
Mozambique		
Massinga	9.3	38.6
Manhica-Magude	12.1	20.3
Inharrime	17.8	86.9
Inhambane	21.8	77.7
Zavala	28.8	183.7
Morrumbene	29.1	87.7
Homoine-Maxixe	47.9	131.4
Panda	60.7	
Thailand		
Songkhla	2.0	5.6
Ratburi	6.0	31.48

(After Muñoz and Bosch, 1987.)

concluded that the HBsAg carrier state was an indicator of initiation, and that aflatoxin was responsible for late-stage or promoting effects. In Swaziland, a joint study by IARC/FAO/UNEP in 1982 measured aflatoxin exposure and the prevalence of HBsAg carriers. A positive correlation was found between the minimal incidence rates in males and estimates of aflatoxin exposure based on diet and crop samples. A positive correlation was also found with the prevalence of HBsAg carriers. Multivariate analysis of the joint effect indicated that aflatoxin was the most important determinant of the geographical variation of HCC in Swaziland (Peers *et al.*, 1987).

Table 29.5. *Joint effects of HBsAg, alcohol and cigarette smoking on risk for HCC.*

Reference	Cases/Controls	Factor	RR (95% CI)
Lam et al. (1982)	107/107 of which 19/88 (HBsAg-)	HBsAg	21.3 (10.1–45.9)
		Smoking (> 50 yrs)	8.2 (1.5–91.9)
		Smoking (all ages)	3.3 (1.0–13.4)
		Alcohol	1.6[a]
Austin *et al.* (1986)	67/63	HBsAg (in males)	— (3.8–infinity)
		Alcohol (in males)	3.3[a]
Trichopoulos *et al.* (1987)	194/456 of which 104/456 (HBsAg-)	HBsAg	13.7 (8.0–23.5)
		Smoking	
		20–30 cigs/day	2.4[a]
		+30 cigs/day	7.3[a]
Yu *et al.* (1983)	78/78	Hepatitis	13.0 (2.2–272.4)
		Alcohol	4.2 (1.3–13.8)
		Smoking	2.6 (1.0–6.7)
		Smoking (alcohol ≥ 80 g/day)	14.0 (1.7–113.9)

[a] Adjusted by age, sex and either smoking or alcohol.
(After Bosch and Muñoz, 1988.)

Alcohol

Chronic alcohol abuse and alcoholic cirrhosis have long been suspected as a cause of HCC. A review (IARC, 1988) of available case-control and cohort studies concluded that six of the ten case-control studies showed significant association at the two- to three-fold level between alcohol consumption and primary liver cancer. The combined results of the ten cohort studies showed a significant 50% increase in risk. A later case-control study in the United States yielded similar results (Yu *et al.*, 1988). Most studies showing a positive association with alcohol have been conducted in western countries, while those showing no association have been carried out in high-risk areas of Asia (Lam *et al.*, 1982; Tu *et al.*, 1987) and in Greece (Trichopoulos *et al.*, 1987) (Table 29.5). However, alcohol may be becoming a more important cause of liver disease in Africa and Asia than 30 years ago (Paterson *et al.*, 1985). Caution is necessary, however, in interpreting these results since adjustment for potential confounders such as HBV infection has often not been made and the diagnostic unreliability of HCC (based on death certificates) in most cohort studies is well known.

Cirrhosis and hepatocellular carcinoma

The association between cirrhosis and HCC has long been recognized but not clearly understood. No correlation has been observed between the mortality from HCC and cirrhosis in different geographical areas. The highest death rates for cirrhosis are observed in Chile, Mexico, Portugal, France, Puerto Rico, Italy, Ireland, and Austria, which have low rates for HCC; lower death rates for cirrhosis are reported in Thailand, Hong Kong, and Greece, which have relatively high rates for HCC. Histological type of liver cancer was not considered.

Cirrhosis of different etiology and morphological types shows variations in neoplastic potential, cancer arising more frequently in the macro-nodular than micronodular form. The former is more frequent in Africa and Southeast Asia, high-incidence areas for HCC, and tends to be subclinical, cancer being the first sign of illness. The micronodular type is prevalent in the low-risk areas of Europe and the USA and is often of alcoholic etiology. HCC is usually a late sequela arising several years after the diagnosis of cirrhosis (Muñoz & Bosch, 1987).

The critical question remains whether the same agents that cause cirrhosis also cause HCC, and/or whether the nodular hyperplasia associated with cirrhosis can lead to HCC *per se*. In Senegal, 60% of cases of HCC that were positive for HBsAg arose in non-cirrhotic livers and the association was similar for HCC with and without cirrhosis (Prince *et al.*, 1975). However, Trichopoulos *et al.* (1987) found a stronger association between HBV and HCC cirrhotic patients (RR,31) than among non-cirrhotic patients (RR, 7), and findings in Japan were similar (Obata *et al.*, 1980). Cirrhosis, therefore, is not always a necessary event. It is believed that HBV can both initiate the carcinogenic process, and also act as a late-stage carcinogen (enhancer) through the liver cell hyperplasia associated with cirrhosis. Nodular hyperplasia in alcoholic cirrhosis is a usual precursor of liver HCC, however, an increased risk for HCC in alcoholics in the absence of cirrhosis has been reported (Lieber *et al.*, 1979). It has been suggested that HBV could be the ultimate cause of HCC in patients with alcoholic liver disease without HBsAG in the serum but with HBV–DNA integrated in the liver cells (Brechot *et al.*, 1982). This is unlikely since HBV–DNA integration is common only in HCC patients with HBsAg in the serum (Tabor, 1989).

In the above context, the absence of fully developed cirrhosis does not necessarily imply that the non-cancerous liver is normal and, in Africa, most non-cirrhotic livers associated with HCC show evidence of damage consistent with viral origin.

Tobacco smoking

An association between tobacco smoking and HbsAg negative HCC has been reported (Trichopoulos *et al.*, 1987). In populations who are heavy cigarette smokers the secular trend of HCC has not paralleled smoking trends. The IARC monograph (1986) concluded that there was insufficient evidence to regard this association as causal.

Oral contraceptives

The occurrence of benign liver adenomas and occasional HCCs among oral contraceptive (OC) users is well known. Five recent case-control studies have reported a significantly increased risk for HCC among women who had used OCs for eight years or more with a modest dose–response relationship (Henderson *et al.*, 1983; Neuberger *et al.*, 1986; Forman *et al.*, 1986; Palmer *et al.*, 1989; La Vecchia *et al.*, 1989) Numbers, however, were small. The increased risk was also present among HBsAg-negative HCC cases. A recent multinational case-control study shows no evidence that short-term use of oral contraceptives enhanced the risk of liver cancer, but no adjustment was made for HBV and smoking (WHO, 1989).

An analysis of the time trends in mortality from liver cancer in the UK showed a small but consistent increase in young women, but a similar trend was not found for other countries with similar patterns of oral contraceptives use (Forman *et al.*, 1983).

Occupation

Despite widespread exposure of large populations, in the work-place or elsewhere, to a range of experimental hepato-carcinogens, hepatomas of the type so common in rodents are strikingly rare. Despite widespread use of pesticides, such as DDT known to produce hepatomas in mice, no concomitant increase in human liver cancer has been found in Western countries or in Asia. In a recent cohort study of workers exposed to aflatoxin in companies processing livestock feed in Denmark, a two- to three-fold increase in risk for cancer of the liver and of the biliary tract was reported (Olsen *et al.*, 1988) but adjustment for potential confounders was not done.

Parasites

No parasites have been associated with HCC but see cholangiocarcinoma and Chapter 17.

Miscellaneous

HCC has been associated with a number of hereditary metabolic diseases including hereditary tyrosinemia, homozygous alpha 1 antitrypsin deficiency, familial hemochromatosis. Also with schistosomiasis, but the evidence is not convincing. A recent follow-up study suggested that patients with HBV-associated chronic liver disease with higher serum ferritin levels are slightly more likely to develop HCC than those with lower levels (Hann *et al.*, 1989), but no relationship has been found between HCC and African siderosis (Higginson, 1963).

Childhood neoplasms

The majority of childhood neoplasms in the liver occur in very early life and are described as embryonal hepatoblastomas, the cause of which is unknown. A few adult type HCCs have been reported, for which the causes are also unknown.

Cholangiocarcinoma

Cholangiocarcinomas are very rare in North America and Europe. However, it is the most common form of liver cancer found in Southern China and Northeast Thailand, where it has been associated with heavy infestation by *Clonorchis sinensis* and *Opisthorchis viverrini* primarily in the intra-hepatic bile ducts. Infestation usually results from the consumption of uncooked fish (Bhamarapravati & Virranuvatti, 1966) (Chapter 17).

Hepatic Angiosarcoma (HAS)

This is a rare tumor. It has been associated with exposures to thorotrast, inorganic arsenic, and vinyl chloride (Falk, 1988). Approximately four per year were found in the United States in large populations covered by the SEER program between 1973–86, the rate being relatively stable.

Thorotrast was originally introduced as a radiographical contrast medium for carotid angiography and liver-spleen scans in the 1930s and 1940s. Tumors related to vinyl chloride monomer exposure seem to have fallen following introduction of appropriate regulations.

A number of experimental carcinogens, also known to cause HAS, include nitrosamines, urethane, hydrazines, azoxymethane, and lasiocarpine. None has been identified as significant carcinogens in humans. The senecio alkaloids have been studied in depth, since human exposure was considerable in some countries, e.g. Jamaica. A few individual cases have been reported in humans related to other factors but chance association seems probable.

29.6 Relevant laboratory investigations

The identification and characterization of the various serological markers of HBV (HBsAg, anti-HBs, anti-HBc, HBeAg, anti-HBe) and of HBV–DNA have made possible a thorough investigation of the role of HBV in HCC. Laboratory assays to measure aflatoxin metabolites and adducts in various body fluids have been developed and offer potential to assess aflatoxin exposure at the individual level. Such assays, however, measure rather recent exposure. Therefore, it is necessary to rely on repeated measurements of such markers in any prospective study directed to elucidating the role of aflatoxin in human liver cancer (Wild *et al.*, 1990). Recent experimental work (De Flora *et al.*, 1989), however, tends to support a multifactorial origin for HCCs in woodchuck hepatitis. This virus (WHV) turns on specific wood chuck P450 enzymes involved in metabolizing carcinogens, including those that activate aflatoxin. An enhancing activity between alcohol and *N*-nitroso compounds has been described (Porta *et al.*, 1985).

At present, the relevance of spontaneous mouse hepatomas to humans is uncertain, especially those attributed to latent retrovirus. Mouse hepatomas are produced by a wide range of chemicals, the majority of which have not been demonstrated as significant in human liver carcinogeneses, the oral contraceptive induced solitary hepatoma excepted.

29.7 Attributable risks

Epidemiological data indicate that HBV accounts for 50–90% of HCC in high-risk populations and for 1–10% in low-risk countries (Tables 29.2 and 29.3). Aflatoxin exposure probably plays an important role in the high-risk areas of Africa and Southeast Asia and a marginal role in low-risk areas in America and Europe; however, it is not yet possible to quantify this risk. HCV might turn out to be one of the most important risk factors for HCC in low-risk populations. Alcohol probably plays a major role in America and Europe and may be becoming more important in developing countries of Africa and Asia. Tobacco smoking and oral contraceptives may also make some relatively insignificant contribution to the risk of developing HCC. *Clonorchis sinensis* and *Opisthorchis viverrini* are the main determinants of the high incidence of cholangiocarcinoma in Asia.

29.8   Conclusions

At present, preventive strategies are directed to control aflatoxin exposures, occasional occupational hazards, and avoiding excessive use of alcohol beverages. Mass vaccination against HBV of newborn babies in high-risk populations and vaccination of groups at high-risk for HBV in low-risk populations is being evaluated. Control of parasites has been highly effective in SE Asia for cholangiocarcinoma.

29.9   References

Austin, H., Delzell, E., Grufferman, S., Levine, R., Morrison, A.S., Stolley, P.D. & Cole, P. (1986). A case-control study of hepatocellular carcinoma and the hepatitis B virus, cigarette smoking, and alcohol consumption. *Cancer Res.*, **46**, 962–6.

Beasley, R.P., Linn, C.C., Hwan, L.Y. & Chien, C.S. (1981). Hepatocellular carcinoma and hepatitis B virus: a prospective study of 22,707 men in Taiwan. *Lancet*, **ii**, 1129–33.

Bhamarapravati, N. & Virranuvatti, V. (1966). Liver diseases in Thailand. An analysis of liver biopsies. *Am. J. Gastroenterol.*, **45**, 267–75.

Blumberg, B.S. & London, W.T. (1985). Hepatitis B virus and prevention of primary cancer of the liver. *J. Natl. Cancer Inst.*, **74**, 267–73.

Bosch, F.X. & Muñoz, N. (1988). Prospects for epidemiological studies on hepatocellular cancer as a model for assessing viral and chemical interactions. In *Methods for Detecting DNA Damaging Agents in Humans: Applications in Cancer Epidemiology and Prevention*, IARC Scientific Publications No. 89, ed. H. Bartsch, K. Hemminki & I.K. O'Neill, pp. 427–38. Lyon: International Agency for Research on Cancer.

Brechot, C., Nalpas, B., Courouce, A.M., Duhamel, G., Callard, P., Carnot, F., Tiollais, P. & Bethelot, P. (1982). Evidence that hepatitis B virus has a role in liver-cell carcinoma in alcoholic liver disease. *N. Engl. J. Med.*, **306**, 1384–7.

Bruix, J., Barrera, J.M., Calvet, X., Ercilla, G., Costa, J., Sanchez-Tapias, J.M., Ventura, M., Vall, M., Bruguera, M., Bru, C., Castillo, R. & Rodes, J. (1989). Prevalence of antibodies to hepatitis C virus in Spanish patients with hepatocellular carcinoma and hepatic cirrhosis. *Lancet*, **ii**, 1004–6.

Bulatao-Jayme, J., Almero, E.M., Castro, C.A., Jardeleza, T.R. & Salamat, L.A. (1982). A case-control dietary study of primary liver cancer risk from aflatoxin exposure. *Int. J. Epidemiol.*, **11**, 112–19.

Busby, W.F. & Wogan, G.N. (1984). Aflatoxins. In *Aflatoxins in Chemical Carcinogenesis*, ed. C.E. Searle, 2nd edn., pp. 945–1136. Washington: American Chemical Society.

Colombo, M., Kuo, G., Choo, Q.L., Donato, M.F., Del Ninno, E., Tommassini, M.A., Dioguardi, N. & Houghton, M. (1989). Prevalence of antibodies to hepatitis C virus in Italian patients with hepatocellular carcinoma. *Lancet*, **ii**, 1006–8.

De Flora, S., Hietanen, E., Bartsch, H., Camoirano, A., Izzotti, A., Bagnasco, M. & Millman, I. (1989). Enhanced metabolic activation of chemical hepatocarcinogens in woodchucks infected with hepatitis B virus. *Carcinogenesis*, **10**, 1099–106.

Doll, R., Payne, P. & Waterhouse, J. (eds.) (1966). *Cancer Incidence in Five Continents*, Volume I, A Technical Report, UICC, International Union Against Cancer. Berlin: Springer Verlag.

Falk, H. (1988). Vinyl chloride-induced hepatic angiosarcoma. In *Unusual Occurrences as Clues to Cancer Etiology*, Proceedings of the 18th International Symposium of The Princess Takamatsu Cancer Research Fund, ed. R.W. Miller, S. Watanabe, J.F. Fraumeni, Jr., T. Sugimura, S. Takayama & H. Sugano. Tokyo: Japan Scientific Societies Press.

Forman, D., Doll, R. & Peto, R. (1983). Trends in mortality from carcinoma of the liver and the use of oral contraceptives. *Br. J. Cancer*, **48**, 349–54.

Forman, D., Vincent, T.J. & Doll, R. (1986). Cancer of the liver and the use of oral contraceptives. *Br. Med. J.*, **292**, 1357–61.

GHIS (Gambia Hepatitis Study Group) (1987). The Gambia Hepatitis Study Group (1987). *Cancer Res.*, **47**, 5782–7.

Hann, H-W.L, Kim, C.Y., London, W.T. & Blumberg, B. (1989). Increased serum ferritin in chronic liver disease: a risk factor for primary hepatocellular carcinoma. *Int. J. Cancer*, **43**, 376–9.

Henderson, B.E., Preston-Martin, S., Edmondson, H.A., Peters, R.L. & Pike, M.C. (1983). Hepatocellular carcinoma and oral contraceptives. *Br. J. Cancer*, **48**, 437–40.

Higginson, J. (1956). Primary carcinoma of the liver in Africa. *Br. J. Cancer*, **10**, 609–22.

Higginson, J. (1963). The geographical pathology of primary liver cancer. *Cancer Res.*, **23**, 1624–33.

Hino, O., Kitagawa, T. & Sugano, H. (1985). Relationship between serum and histochemical markers for hepatitis B virus and rate of viral integration in hepatocellular carcinomas in Japan. *Int. J. Cancer*, **35**, 5–10.

IARC (1986). *IARC Monographs on the Evaluation of the Carcinogenic Risk of Chemicals to Humans*, Tobacco smoking, volume 38. Lyon: International Agency for Research on Cancer.

IARC (1988). *Alcohol Drinking*, vol. 44, pp. 207–14, 255. Lyon: International Agency for Research on Cancer.

Lam, K.C., Yu, M.C., Leung, J.W.C. & Henderson, B.E. (1982). Hepatitis B virus and cigarette smoking: risk factors for hepatocellular carcinoma in Hong Kong. *Cancer Res.*, **42**, 5246–8.

La Vecchia, C., Negri, E. & Parazzini, F. (1989). Oral contraceptives and primary liver cancer. *Br. J. Cancer*, **59**, 460–1.

Lieber, C.S., Seitz, H.K., Garro, A.J. & Worner, T.M. (1979). Alcohol-related diseases and carcinogenesis. *Cancer*, **39**, 2863–6.

Muir, C., Waterhouse, J., Mack, T., Powell, J. & Whelan, S. (eds.) (1987). *Cancer Incidence in Five Continents*, Volume V, IARC Scientific Publication No. 88. Lyon: International Agency for Research on Cancer.

Muñoz, N. & Bosch, F.X. (1987). Epidemiology of hepatocellular carcinoma. In *Neoplasms of the Liver*, Okuda, K. & Purchase, I.F., eds., pp. 3–19. Tokyo: Springer.

Neuberger, J., Forman, D., Doll, R. & Williams, R. (1986). Oral contraceptives and hepatocellular carcinoma. *Br. Med. J.*, **292**, 1355–7.

Nishioka, K. (1985). Hepatitis B virus and hepatocellular carcinoma: postulates for an etiological relationship. *Adv. Viral Oncol.*, **5**, 173–99.

Obata, H., Hayashi, N., Motoike, Y., Hisamutsu, I., Okuda, H., Koibayashi, S. & Nishioka, K. (1980). A prospective study on the development of hepatocellular carcinoma from liver cirrhosis with persistent hepatitis B virus infection. *Int. J. Cancer*, **25**, 741–7.

Olsen, J.H., Dragsted, L. & Autrup, H. (1988). Cancer risk and occupational exposure to aflatoxin in Denmark. *Br. J. Cancer*, **58**, 392–6.

Palmer, J.R., Rosenberg, L., Kaufman, D.W., Warshauer, M.E., Stolley, P. & Shapiro, S. (1989). Oral contraceptive use and liver cancer. *Am. J. Epidemiol.*, **130**, 878–82.

Paterson, A.C., Kew, M.C., Herman, A.A.B., Becker, P.J., Hodkinson, J., Isaacson, C. (1985). Liver morphology in Southern African blacks with hepatocellular carcinoma: a study within the urban environment. *Hepatology*, **5**, 72–8.

Peers, F., Bosch, X., Kaldor, J., Linsell, A. & Pluijmen, M. (1987). Aflatoxin exposure, hepatitis B virus infection and liver cancer in Swaziland. *Int. J. Cancer*, **39**, 545–53.

Popper, H., Shafritz, D.A. & Hoofnagle, J.H. (1987). Relation of the hepatitis B virus carrier state to hepatocellular carcinoma. *Hepatology*, **7**, 764–72.

Porta, E.A., Markell, N. & Dorado, R.D. (1985). Chronic alcoholism enhances hepatocarcinogenicity of diethylnitrosamine in rats fed a marginally methyl-deficient diet. *Hepatology*, **5**, 1120–5.

Prince, A.M., Szmuness, W., Michon, J., Desmaille, J., Diebolt, G., Linhard, J., Quenum, C. & Sankale, M. (1975). A case-control study of the association between primary liver cancer and hepatitis B infection in Senegal. *Int. J. Cancer*, **16**, 376–83.

310 *Digestive system*

Tabor, E. (1989). Hepatocellular carcinoma: Possible etiologies in patients without serologic evidence of hepatitis B virus infection. *J. Med. Virol.*, **27**, 1–6.

Trichopoulos, D., Day, N.E., Kaklamani, E., Tzonou, A., Muoz, N., Zavitsanos, X., Koumantaki, Y. & Trichopoulou, A. (1987). Hepatitis B virus, tobacco smoking and ethanol consumption in the etiology of hepatocellular carcinoma. *Int. J. Cancer*, **39**, 45–9.

Tu, J.T., Gao, R.N., Zhjjang, D.H., Gu, B.C., Xu, G.X., Gang, R.K., Pan, J.P., Yu, H., Huang, Y.L. & Zhou, X.H. (1987). Risk factors of primary liver cancer in the high prevalence area Chongming County: Results from a 5-year follow-up. In *Cancer of the Liver, Esophagus, and Nasopharynx*, ed. G. Wagner & Y.H. Zhang, pp. 19–26. New York: Springer-Verlag.

Van Rensburg, S.J., Cook-Mozafarri, P., van Schalkwyk, D.J., van der Watt, J.J., Vincent, T.J. & Purchase, I.F. (1985). Hepatocellular carcinoma and dietary aflatoxin in Mozambique and Transkei. *Br. J. Cancer*, **51**, 713–26.

WHO (1989). Combined oral contraceptives and liver cancer. World Health Organization collaborative study of neoplasia and steroid contraceptives. *Int. J. Cancer*, **43**, 254–9.

Wild, C.P., Jiang, Y.-Z., Sabbioni, G., Chapot, B. & Montesano, R. (1990). Evaluation of methods for quantitation of aflatoxin–albumin adducts and their application to human exposure assessment. *Cancer Res.*, **50**, 245–51.

Yu, M.C., Mack, T., Hanisch, R., Peters, R.L., Henderson, B.E. & Pike, M.C. (1983). Hepatitis, alcohol consumption, cigarette smoking, and hepatocellular carcinoma in Los Angeles. *Cancer Res.*, **43**, 6077–9.

Yu, H., Harris, R.E., Kabat, G., & Wynder, E.L. (1988). Cigarette smoking, alcohol consumption and primary liver cancer: A case-control study in the USA. *Int. J. Cancer*, **42**, 325–8.

30

Gall bladder and extrahepatic biliary ducts

ICD-9 156

30.1   Introduction

Cancers of the biliary tract include the gall bladder and the extrahepatic bile ducts. They are relatively rare, representing about 1% of all cancers, but in some regions unusual high frequencies may be found.

30.2   Histology, classification and diagnosis

Gall bladder tumors are predominantly adenocarcinomas, although squamous cell and undifferentiated carcinomas can occur. Tumors of the common bile duct may be difficult to distinguish clinically from tumors of the head of the pancreas. These tumors have a poor prognosis so that mortality rates reflect incidence fairly accurately. There is evidence that chronic cholecystitis with epithelial changes, often associated with gall stones, ranging from hyperplasia to atypical hyperplasia and dysplasia, may be precancerous.

30.3   Descriptive epidemiology
Incidence and time trends

Relatively high rates (over 5) are seen among the American Indians, in Japan and in some Latin American and Eastern European countries (Fig. 30.1). The ratio of gall bladder to other biliary cancers in industrial countries is approximately 3:1.

Sex distribution

In general, the rates of gall bladder cancer are higher in females than in males, while those of extrahepatic bile ducts are higher in males. The female predominance in gall bladder cancer is particularly noticeable in high incidence areas.

Fig. 30.1 Incidence rates around 1980: Gall bladder, etc. (ICD-9 156).

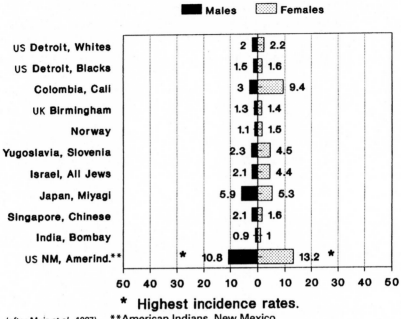

■ Males   ▦ Females

	Males	Females
US **Detroit, Whites**	2	2.2
US **Detroit, Blacks**	1.5	1.6
Colombia, Cali	3	9.4
UK Birmingham	1.3	1.4
Norway	1.1	1.5
Yugoslavia, Slovenia	2.3	4.5
Israel, All Jews	2.1	4.4
Japan, Miyagi	5.9	5.3
Singapore, Chinese	2.1	1.6
India, Bombay	0.9	1
US **NM, Amerind.****	* 10.8	13.2 *

50 40 30 20 10 0 10 20 30 40 50

* **Highest incidence rates.**

(after Muir *et al.*, 1987)   **American Indians, New Mexico

Age distribution

The age-specific incidence rates increase progressively with age in both sexes from the third decade. Time trends, however, are difficult to interpret because of changes in the ICD classification and regional variations in chole cystectomy.

30.4   Etiological inferences

Geographical and racial distribution strongly suggest that tumors of the gall bladder have an ethnic predisposition probably related to metabolic factors associated with gall bladder disease.

30.5   Known and suspected causes
Gallstones and related metabolic factors

While the basic cause is unknown, there is widespread agreement that gall bladder disease and stone formation are potential risk factors (Fraumeni & Kantor, 1982; Nervi *et al.*, 1988). The risk associated with gallstones has been estimated in three ethnic groups from a case-control study using autopsied subjects. The relative risk for US blacks and whites was: males, 2.8 and 6.9 respectively, and 4.5 and 4.3 in females. It was 20.9 for American Indians (Lowenfels *et al.*, 1985). A three-fold increase in the incidence of gallbladder cancer has been reported in a cohort of 2583 white patients from the USA with previously diagnosed gallstones.

Several risk factors have been identified for gall stones which include race, sex, parity, obesity and hormonal changes but the precise metabolic defects are not yet understood. Thus, individuals predisposed to stones have bile in which cholesterol is supersaturated to which biliary stasis may contribute. Bile salts may be converted to carcinogenic compounds through bacterial degradation which gives rise to a plausible causal hypothesis.

Other risk factors include administration of clofibrate, exogenous estrogens (Yen *et al.*, 1987), gastrointestinal disorders, and hemolytic disease, etc., which affect metabolism and stone formation. Overnutrition is also probably a factor.

Chronic infection

It is possible that chronic cholecystitis per se may also predispose to gall bladder cancer. Thus, a four- to six-fold increase in risk has been reported in chronic carriers of *Salmonella typhi* (Mellemgaard, 1988).

Parasites

In certain Asian countries, carcinomas of the bile ducts are associated with infestation by liver flukes (*Clonorchis sinensis, Opisthorchis viverrini*), but the majority of the tumors are intrahepatic.

Other causes

A number of cases have been associated with certain occupations, such as the rubber and textile industries, metal and possibly asbestos workers (Malker *et al.*, 1986). Whereas some of these associations may possibly be explicable on terms of exogenous chemicals, at present the evidence is inconclusive.

An excess risk has also been reported in a cohort of patients with peptic ulcers, who had undergone gastric surgery (Caygill *et al.*, 1988), and in patients with ulcerative colitis.

30.6   Relevant laboratory studies

These are, in general, metabolic studies related to gall stone formation and the carcinogenicity of bile components.

30.7   Attributable risks

It has been estimated that approximately 30% of gall bladder cancer in blacks is related to gallstones while the respective figures for whites and Indians are 50% and 90% (Lowenfels *et al.*, 1985).

30.8   Conclusions

Carcinomas of the gall bladder, and, to a lesser extent the extra-hepatic bile duct, can be regarded as late sequelae of the common biliary tract diseases which have both ethnic and inherited components.

30.9   References

Caygill, C., Hill, M., Kirkham, J. & Northfield, T.C. (1988). Increase risk of biliary tract cancer following gastric surgery. *Br. J. Cancer*, **57**, 434–6.

Fraumeni, J.F. & Kantor, A.F. (1982). Biliary tract. In *Cancer Epidemiology and Prevention*, ed. D. Schottenfeld & J.F. Fraumeni, Jr., pp. 683–91, Philadelphia: W. B. Saunders.

Lowenfels, A.B., Lindstrom, C.G., Conway, M.J. & Hastings, P.R. (1985). Gallstones and risk of gallbladder cancer. *J. Natl. Cancer Inst.*, **75**, 77–80.

Malker, H.S., McLaughlin, J.K., Malker, B.K.; Stone, B.J., Weiner, J.A., Ericsson, J.L. & Blot, W.J. (1986). Biliary tract cancer and occupation in Sweden. In *Br. J. Ind. Med.* **43**, 257–62.

Mellemgaard, A. (1988). Risk of hepatobiliary cancer in carriers of *Salmonella typhi*. *J. Natl. Cancer Inst.*, **80**, 288.

Muir, C., Waterhouse, J., Mack, T., Powell, J. & Whelan, S. (eds.) (1987). *Cancer Incidence in Five Continents*, Volume V, IARC Scientific Publication No. 88. Lyon: International Agency for Research on Cancer.

Nervi, F., Duarte, I., Gmez, Rodrguez, Del Pino, G., Ferrerio, O., Covarrubias, C., Valdivieso, V., Torres, M.I. & Urzúa, A. (1988). Frequency of gallbladder cancer in Chile, A high-risk area. *Int. J. Cancer*, **41**, 657–60.

Yen, S., Hsieh, C.C. & MacMahon, B. (1987). Extrahepatic bile duct cancer and smoking, beverage consumption, past medical history, and oral-contraceptive use. *Cancer*, **59**, 2112–16.

31

Pancreas

ICD-9 157

31.1 Introduction

Adenocarcinoma of the pancreas is the fifteenth most common cancer in the world, and is more frequent in developed, than in developing, countries. Tobacco is the most important etiological factor so far identified.

31.2 Histology, classification and diagnosis

Tumors of the pancreas can be divided into common adenocarcinomas and infrequent islet cell tumors of the endocrine pancreas. Many pancreatic tumors were formerly attributed to the gastro-intestinal tract or the liver, which may partly explain the reported incidence rise since 1950.

31.3 Descriptive epidemiology
Incidence

The incidence and distribution of adenocarcinomas has been reviewed by Mack (1982). Geographic variations are not as great as for other gastrointestinal cancers. Among males, high rates (over 10) are seen in American blacks, Maoris in New Zealand, and in some European countries; intermediate rates (over 4) in whites in North America, the rest of Europe, Australia, Japan, China, Israel and in most South American countries; and low rates (less than 4) in Africa, India and some South American countries (Figure 31.1). (The rate in male Koreans in Los Angeles is based on 11 cases.) In the USA, rates are higher in blacks than in whites, but are relatively low in Seventh Day Adventists and Mormons. A consistent association with social class has not been observed. Higher frequencies in urban than in rural areas may be a diagnostic artefact.

Fig. 31.1 Incidence rates around 1980: Pancreas (ICD-9 157).

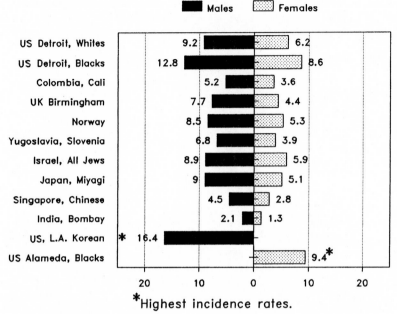

(after Muir *et al.*, 1987)

Age and sex distribution

Such tumors are slightly more frequent in males than in females, with sex ratios ranging from 1.1 to 2.5. Rates increase steadily with age starting in the third decade. An increase in incidence and mortality has been observed in most populations, partly due to better diagnosis.

31.4   Etiological inferences

The modest geographic variations have been uninformative as to cause. Convincing correlations in incidence with other sites are not observed. An increased mortality reported in American Jews has not been explained. The lower rates in Seventh Day Adventists and Mormons suggest a role for lifestyle factors.

31.5   Known and suspected causes

Discussion will be limited to adenocarcinomas as little is known regarding the etiology of islet cell tumors.

Tobacco smoking

A UK study (Cuzick & Babiker, 1989) estimated a risk ratio of 4.4 for cigarette smokers of more than 20 cigarettes per day relative to non-smokers, with a significant dose–response after controlling for potential confounders. Cohort studies and most case-control studies in North America, Europe, Norway and Japan have also shown an increased risk for pancreatic cancer among cigarette smokers. The IARC monograph (1986) concluded that smoking is an important cause of pancreatic cancer.

Alcohol drinking

The IARC monograph (1988) concluded that alcohol drinking is unlikely to be causally related.

Diabetes mellitus

An association with diabetes has long been suspected but is difficult to study. An increased risk however, was found in diabetics even after exclusion of cases occurring within a year of the diagnosis of cancer (Whittemore *et al.*, 1983; Hiatt *et al.*, 1988). Cuzick and Babiker (1989) found a four-fold increase in risk.

Coffee drinking

A postulated association between coffee drinking and pancreatic cancer has not been subsequently confirmed (Wynder *et al.*, 1986; Jensen, 1986; Cuzick & Babiker, 1989; Clavel *et al.*, 1989; Boyle *et al.*, 1989; IARC, 1990).

Diet

Early studies suggested an increased risk related to excess intake of some sources of fats and animal protein (Mack, 1982; Armstrong, 1982). Subsequent studies have shown a positive association with fried and grilled meat, and margarine, pork and dairy products, and a protective effect associated with the frequent consumption of fruits and vegetables (Gold *et al.*, 1985; Falk *et al.*, 1988; Norell *et al.*, 1986a). While the possibility of confounding variables cannot be excluded, these findings are consistent with those in Seventh Day Adventists (Mills *et al.*, 1988).

Occupation

While numerous occupations, including those involving exposure to petroleum products and paint thinners (Norell *et al.*, 1986b), have been reported as associated with a moderate increase in risk, no obvious common exposure has been detected (Mack, 1982). A reported increase in Scandinavian chemists was not found in the United Kingdom.

Miscellaneous causes

Attempts to link this tumor to chronic pancreatitis have been unsuccessful. While positive associations have been found after gastrectomy and cholecystectomy (Hyvarinen *et al.*, 1987) and an inverse association with allergies, no meaningful pathogenic mechanisms can be demonstrated.

31.6   Relevant laboratory studies

Tumors of the pancreas can be induced in experimental animals by tobacco-specific nitrosamines. Ninety percent of pancreatic cancers have an activated *ras* oncogene. The type of mutations are similar to those in the lung and different to those in the colon, suggesting etiological similarities to the former, such as a possible role of tobacco. Although viruses produce pancreatic cancer in rodents, such studies have not proven informative in relation to human cancer.

31.7   Attributable risks

Approximately 20–40% of pancreatic cancer in males and 10–20% in females can be attributed to smoking. The contribution of dietary factors, previous diabetes mellitus and other suspected factors, if existent, cannot be quantified at present.

31.8   Conclusions

Cigarette smoking is, today, the most important known risk factor for pancreatic cancer. Further research is still needed to clarify the roles of dietary and other factors.

31.9   References

Armstrong, B. (1982). Endocrine factors in human carcinogenesis. In *Host Factors in Human Carcinogenesis*, IARC Scientific Publication No. 39, ed. H. Bartsch, B. Armstrong & W. Davis, pp. 193–221. Lyon: International Agency for Research on Cancer.

Boyle, P., Hsieh, C.C., Maisonneuve, P., La Vecchia, C., Macyarlone, G.J., Walker, A.M. & Trichopoulos, D. (1989). Epidemiology of pancreas cancer. *Int. J. Pancreatol.*, **5**, 327–46.

Clavel, F., Benhamou, E., Auquier, A., Tarayre, M. & Flamant, R. (1989). Coffee, alcohol, smoking and cancer of the pancreas: A case-control study. *Int. J. Cancer*, **43**, 17–21.

Cuzick, J. & Babiker, A.G. (1989). Pancreatic cancer, alcohol, diabetes mellitus and gall-bladder disease. *Int. J. Cancer*: **43**, 415–21.

Falk, R.T., Pickle, L.W., Fontham, E.T., Correa, P. & Fraumeni, J.F. (1988). Life-style risk factors for pancreatic cancer in Louisiana: a case-control study. *Am. J. Epidemiol.*, **128**, 324-36.

Gold, E.B., Gordis, L., Diener, M.D., Seltser, R., Boitnott, J.K., Bynum, T.E. & Hutcheon, D.F. (1985). Diet and other risk factors for cancer of the pancreas. *Cancer*, **55**, 460–7.

Hiatt, R.A., Klatsky, A.L. & Armstrong, M.A. (1988). Pancreatic cancer, blood glucose and beverage consumption. *Int. J. Cancer*, **41**, 794–97.

Hyvarinen, H. & Partanen, S. (1987). Association of cholecystectomy with abdominal cancers. *Hepatogastroenterology*, **34**, 280–4.

IARC (1990). *IARC Monographs on the Evaluation of Carcinogenic Risks to Humans*, Coffee, tea, maté, methylxanthines (caffeine, theophylline, thiobromine) and Methylglyoxal, volume 51. Lyon: International Agency for Research on Cancer. In press.

IARC (1988). *IARC Monograph on the Evaluation of Carcinogenic Risks to Humans*, Alcohol drinking, volume 44, pp. 215–22, 256. Lyon: International Agency for Research on Cancer.

IARC (1986). *IARC Monographs on the Evaluation of the Carcinogenic Risk of Chemicals to Humans*, Tobacco smoking, volume 38, pp. 279–84, 313. Lyon: International Agency for Research on Cancer.

Jensen, O.M. (1986). Coffee and cancer. In *Genetic Toxicology of the Diet*, pp. 287–97. New York: Alan R. Liss, Inc.

Mack, T.M. (1982). Pancreas. In *Cancer Epidemiology and Prevention*, ed. D. Schottenfeld & J.F. Fraumeni, Jr., pp. 638–67. Philadelphia: W.B. Saunders.

Mills, P.K., Beeson, L., Abbey, D.E., Fraser, G.E. & Phillips, R.L. (1988). Dietary habits and past medical history as related to fatal pancreas cancer risk among Adventists. *Cancer*, **61**, 2578–85.

Muir, C., Waterhouse, J., Mack, T., Powell, J. & Whelan, S. (eds.) (1987). *Cancer Incidence in Five Continents*, volume V, IARC Scientific Publication No. 88. Lyon: International Agency for Research on Cancer.

Norell, S.E., Ahlbom, A., Erwald, R., Jacobson, G., Lindberg-Navier, I., Olin, R., Tornberg, B. & Wiechel, K.L. (1986a). Diet and pancreatic cancer: A case-control study. *Am. J. Epidemiol.*, **124**, 894–902.

Norell, S., Ahlbom, A., Olin, R., Erwald, R., Jacobson, G., Lindberg-Navier, I. & Wiechel, K.L. (1986b). Occupational factors and pancreatic cancer. *Br. J. Ind. Med.*, **43**, 775–8.

Whittemore, A.S., Paffenbarger, R.S., Jr., Anderson, K. & Halpern, J. (1983). Early precursors of pancreatic cancer in college men. *J. Chron. Dis.*, **36**, 251–6.

Wynder, E.L., Dieck, G.S. & Hall, N.E. (1986). Case-control study of decaffeinated coffee consumption and pancreatic cancer. *Cancer Res.*, **46**, 5360–3.

Part VII

Respiratory system

32

Sinonasal

ICD-9 160

32.1   Introduction

Cancers of the nose and paranasal sinuses (SNC) are relatively rare, usually constituting less than 1% of all cancers. Although often grouped together, there are biological and etiological differences between sinonasal and other tumors of the respiratory tract, including those of the nasopharynx (NPC) (Chapter 24). Cancers of the middle ear are extremely rare.

32.2   Histology, classification and diagnosis

Cancers of this ICD site can be divided into those of the nasal cavity and the much commoner tumors of the paranasal sinuses: the former are predominantly squamous carcinomas, the latter adeno-carcinomas. Epithelial dysplasia has been reported in a high risk group (Boysen, *et al*, 1986).

32.3   Descriptive epidemiology

Incidence rates tend to be less than 1 in males in most populations, those for females about 0.5. Rates around 1.7 in males have been observed consistently in Japan; the highest rates recorded are in the non-Kuwaiti residents of Kuwait (see Fig. 32.1). Due to their rarity, time trends are difficult to assess, but the incidence seems to be falling in Japan.

32.4   Etiological inferences

Except for the demonstration of clusters related to occupation, due to rarity and lack of geographical variations, the descriptive data are relatively uninformative.

32.5   Known and suspected causes
Occupation

The most important causes are related to occupation.

Fig. 32.1 Incidence rates around 1980: Nose, sinuses (ICD-9 160).

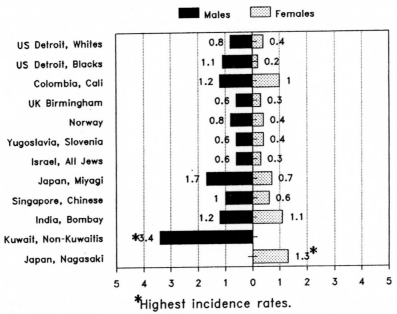

*Highest incidence rates.

(after Muir *et al.*, 1987)

Nickel

An excess risk of lung and sinonasal cancers following exposure to nickel compounds in refining processes has been reported from Wales, Canada, Norway and the Soviet Union (IARC, 1976, 1984, 1987; Pedersen *et al.*, 1982). The IARC (1987) monograph has concluded that 'the risk is particularly high in those exposed to certain processes, mainly those entailing exposure to nickel (sub)-sulphites and oxides', but that 'it is still not possible to state with certainty which specific nickel compounds are human carcinogens and which are not'. Soluble nickel has also been implicated. These tumors are predominantly squamous carcinomas.

Wood-dust

This is one of the few cancers where a record linkage system has successfully related a tumor to an occupational hazard. A raised risk of sinonasal cancer has been established among furniture-makers (Acheson *et al.*, 1984), the tumors being predominantly adenocarcinomas of the ethmoid and middle turbinate. An association has also been found with wood working, especially among furniture manufacturers (IARC, 1981, 1987) and in the lumber and saw-mill industry, including logging in Scandinavia and Canada. While beech, oak and possibly other hard woods are implicated, the nature of the carcinogenic agent has not been determined.

Boot and shoe manufacture

Nasal carcinoma has been observed among employees in boot and shoe manufacturing work-shops, both in England and in Italy (IARC, 1981, 1987; Decoufle & Walrath, 1983), the risk being highest in the dustiest operations. Exposure to solvents or tobacco did not account for the increased risk. The increased risk seen in the UK shoe manufacturing industry is not observed in the US, possibly since mineral oil is not used in the latter.

Leather goods manufacture

A few studies deal specifically with workers in leather manufacture, leather tanning or processing. The risk may be related to leather dust (IARC, 1981, 1987).

Chromium

While clearly involved in lung cancer, a role for nasal cancer is less certain (IARC, 1987).

Formaldehyde

A proven nasal carcinogen in rodents, formaldehyde is of specific interest in view of widespread human exposure. A review (UAREP, 1987), concluded that there was no convincing evidence for an effect in humans and that if such an effect did exist, it was, in absolute terms, exceedingly small. No increased risk was found in the analysis of a large multifactorial work force analysis from Canada (Gérin *et al.*, 1989).

Other causes

Occasional cancers have been ascribed to mustard gas, radioisotopes, the manufacture of hydrocarbon gas, cutting oils (Redmond *et al.*, 1982) and chlorophenol (Hardell *et al.*, 1982). Reports of increased rates due to coal or coke exposures may be spurious (Acheson *et al.*, 1984). Roush *et al.* (1987) found a suggestive association for SNC and NPC in the printing industry. Most of these studies involve numbers too low to achieve adequate statistical power. Some other suspected factors are given in Table 32.1.

Non-occupational exposures
Snuff

The high frequencies of antral cancer reported from southern Africa have been associated with the use of aloe-containing snuffs with a high nickel and chrome content. Increases are anticipated with the use of snuffs in North America (Hayes *et al.*, 1987); others disagree (Olson, 1987).

Table 32.1 *Sinonasal cancer: summary of risk factors.*

Known	Suspected	Equivocal
Nickel processing	Boot/shoe manufacture	Chromium
Wood dust – beechwood dust;	Leather dust	Formaldehyde
oak wood dust	Radioisotopes	Coal or coke
Snuff/smokeless tobacco	Mustard gas	Cigarette smoking
Zinc chromate	Manufacture of	
bis-Chloromethylether	hydrocarbon gas	
2, 2¹-dichlorethyl sulphide	Cutting oils	
Monochlorodimethylether		
Respirable dusts		

Cigarette smoking

While smoking was not originally implicated as a causative factor, some reports have suggested an effect (Hirayama, 1984; Brinton *et al.*, 1984; Hayes *et al.*, 1987).

Miscellaneous

Case-control studies in Japan have consistently noted a high frequency of antecedent chronic sinusitis, but it is difficult to know whether this is cause or effect.

32.6   Attributable risks

The etiology of these cancers in the general public is unknown but in certain groups, work-place exposures may be responsible for almost all cases.

32.7   Relevant laboratory studies

Nasal cancer can be produced in rodents by direct contact with a carcinogen or by systemic carcinogens, notably tobacco specific nitrosamines. The nasal mucosa has a high capacity for metabolic activation of these latter compounds. There is evidence that epithelial damage, which correlates with DNA protein cross link formation, is a necessary precursor in formaldehyde-induced cancers in rodents. Studies in rats and mice have demonstrated species differences in nasal air flow which correlates with nasal tumor induction.

Certain fractions of beech wood show mutagenic activity which may be relevant to nasal cancer in hardwood workers.

32.8   Conclusions

At present, prevention is confined to controlling known workplace agents.

32.9 References

Acheson, E.D., Cowdell, R.H. & Rang, E.H. (1984). Nasal cancer in England and Wales: An occupational survey. *Br. J. Ind. Med.*, **38**, 218–24.

Boysen, M., Voss, R. & Solberg, L.A. (1986). The nasal mucosa in softwood exposed furniture workers. *Acta Otolaryngol.* (Stockh.), **101**, 501–8.

Brinton, L.A., Blot, W.J., Becker, J.A., Winn, D.M., Browder, J.P., Farmer, J.C., Jr. & Fraumeni, J.F., Jr. (1984). A case-control study of cancers of the nasal cavity and paranasal sinuses. *Am. J. Epidemiol.*, **119**, 896–906.

Decoufle, P. & Walrath, J. (1983). Proportionate mortality among US shoeworkers. *Am. J. Ind. Med.*, **4**, 523–32.

Gérin, M., Siemiatycki, J., Nadon, L., Dewar, R. & Krewski, D. (1989). Cancer risks due to occupational exposure to formaldehyde: Results of a multi-site case-control study in Montreal. *Int. J. Cancer*, **44**, 53–8.

Hardell, L., Johansson, B. & Axelson, O. (1982). Epidemiological study of nasal and nasopharyngeal cancer and their relation to phenoxy acid or chlorophenol exposure. (1982). *Am. J. Ind. Med.*, **3**, 247–57.

Hayes, R.B., Kardaun, J.W. & de Bruyn, A. (1987). Tobacco use and sinonasal cancer: a case-control study. *Br. J. Cancer*, **56**, 843–6.

Hirayama, T. (1984). Cancer mortality in nonsmoking women with smoking husbands based on a large-scale cohort study in Japan. *Prev. Med.*, **6**, 680–90.

IARC (1976). *IARC Monographs on the Evaluation of Carcinogenic Risk of Chemicals to Man*. Cadmium, nickel, some epoxides, miscellaneous industrial chemicals and general considerations on volatile anaesthetics. vol. 11, pp. 75–112. Lyon: International Agency for Research on Cancer.

IARC (1981). *IARC Monographs on the Evaluation of the Carcinogenic Risk of Chemicals to Humans*. Wood, leather and some associated industries. vol. 25. Lyon: International Agency for Research on Cancer.

IARC (1984). *Nickel in the Human Environment*. IARC Scientific Publications No. 53, ed. F.W. Sunderman, Jr., pp. 1–530. Lyon: International Agency for Research on Cancer.

IARC (1987). *IARC Monographs on the Evaluation of Carcinogenic Risks to Humans*. Overall evaluations of carcinogenicity: an updating of IARC Monographs Volumes 1 to 42. Supplement 7, pp. 264–9. Lyon: International Agency for Research on Cancer.

Olson, J.H. (1987). Epidemiology of sinonasal cancer in Denmark, 1943–1982. *Acta Path. Microbiolol. Immunol. Scand. Sect.* A, **95**, 171–5.

Pedersen, E., Andersen, A. & Hgetveit, A. (1982). Second study of the incidence and mortality of cancer of respiratory organs among workers at a nickel refinery (Abstract). *Ann. Clin. Lab. Sci.*, **8**, 503–4.

Redmond, C.K., Sass, R.E. & Roush, G.C. (1982). Nasal cavity and paranasal sinuses. In *Cancer Epidemiology and Prevention*, ed. D. Schottenfeld & J.F. Fraumeni, Jr., pp. 519–35. Philadelphia: W.B. Saunders.

Roush, G.C., Walrath, J., Stayner, L.T., Kaplan, S.A., Flannery, J.T. & Blair, A. (1987). Nasopharyngeal cancer, sinonasal cancer, and occupations related to formaldehyde: A case-control study. *J. Natl. Cancer Inst.*, **79**, 1221–4.

UAREP (1987). *Epidemiology of Chronic Occupational Exposure to Formaldehyde*, Report of the Ad Hoc Panel on Health Aspects of Formaldehyde. Washington: *Toxicol. Ind. Health*, **4**, 77–90.

33

Larynx

ICD-9 161

33.1 Introduction

Tumors of the larynx are the dominant cancer of the upper respiratory tract, sharing causal factors with the contiguous oropharynx and hypopharynx.

33.2 Histology, classification and diagnosis

Cancers are nearly all squamous carcinomas. The ICD separates the larynx into supraglottis (laryngeal aspect of the epiglottis, false cord, etc.); glottis (true vocal cord), and the subglottis (endolarynx) a separation which has etiological and therapeutic validity. It may be difficult to distinguish between advanced hypopharyngeal and supraglottic cancers. Preneoplastic lesions can be identified in the larynx of a high percentage of cigarette smokers as well as of tobacco chewers. Benign papillomas, which often regress, occur in children.

33.3 Descriptive epidemiology

Incidence (Fig. 33.1)

The highest male incidence rates, in the range of 12 to 17, are reported from Brazil, Italy, France and Spain which, with Luxembourg and Uruguay, also show the highest mortality rates. Rates are low in the UK, between 3 and 5, in contrast to the very high lung cancer rates.

Interesting variations in the distribution of tumors within the larynx are observed. Tumors of the glottis are predominant in Anglo-Saxon populations, whereas in France, in India and in the black populations of

Fig. 33.1 Incidence rates around 1980: Larynx (ICD-9 161).

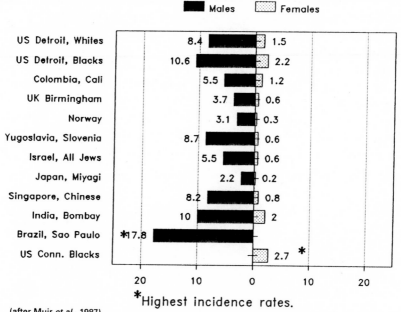

(after Muir *et al.*, 1987)

the United States the numbers of glottic and supraglottic tumors are approximately equal. High relative frequencies have been reported for several populations such as in Rangoon, Burma: (M6.4%, F2.1%) Turkey: (M12.8%, F1.1%) Cairo, Egypt: (M8.1%, F1.5%) and Chiangmai, Thailand: (M18.4%, F3.4%), many tumors being supraglottic.

Time trends

In males, both incidence and mortality rates are increasing in many countries in southern and eastern Europe, also in Scandinavia and Australia. Significant rises have been noted in mortality for US black and white females as predicted by Wynder *et al.* (1976), due to increased tobacco use.

Sex distribution

Larynx cancer is very rare in females, the highest sex ratios in the order of 25 being observed in the Latin countries of Europe.

Age distribution

Even in the high risk populations, this is an unusual tumor before the age of 40.

33.4   Etiological inferences

The distribution of laryngeal cancer is not completely consistent with that of lung cancer (see below) suggesting that the relationship with smoking is either qualitatively different or that other factors are important, as in parts of Asia. The discrepancy is consistent with the view that different types of tobacco vary in their carcinogenic potential (Chapter 9).

Tuyns and Audigier (1976) found that incidence of cancers of the lung, larynx and esophagus were all elevated in France among young adult males prior to World War II. A fall was observed in both laryngeal and esophageal tumors in those cohorts who were young adults during World War II followed by a rise after the end of the war. These trends correlated with tobacco consumption.

33.5   Known or suspected causes

The causes of this cancer have been reviewed (Adelstein, 1972; Austin, 1982; Brown *et al.*, 1988; De Stefani *et al.*, 1987).

Tobacco and alcohol

The principal cause of laryngeal cancer is tobacco and the effects of smoking have been known for many years. This has been confirmed by many studies (Austin, 1982; Schottenfeld *et al.*, 1974; Jussawalla & Deshpande, 1971). However, there are some inconsistencies in the relationship between larynx, other tobacco-related cancers and tobacco consumption (Blot *et al.*, 1978). Thus, while lung cancer has increased markedly in some countries, there has been no significant change in laryngeal cancer. There is evidence (Wynder *et al.*, 1976; Jensen, 1979; Tuyns *et al.*, 1988) that consumption of alcoholic beverages exacerbates the effect of cigarette smoking (Fig. 33.2). The decreases in France reported by Tuyns *et al.*, (1988) and Tuyns and Audigier (1976), were probably due to the fact that during World War II alcohol was not readily available. There is some evidence that the interaction of the two factors is greatest in supraglottic tumors which may explain some of the geographic discrepancies (Tuyns & Audigier, 1976). There is also evidence that light and dark tobacco vary in their effect, the latter carrying a higher risk (Tuyns *et al.*, 1988).

Occupational factors

These have been reviewed by Austin (1982) and Brown *et al.* (1988). There is some evidence that asbestos exposure is a risk factor. Laryngeal cancer has also been associated with various aspects of nickel refining, notably electrolysis (IARC, 1987), and the strong acid process of

Fig. 33.2 Combined effect of alcohol and tobacco.

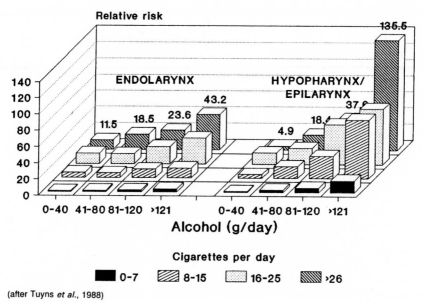

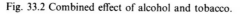

(after Tuyns *et al.*, 1988)

ethanol production and mustard gas manufacture. Although the relative risk in the nickel industry is high, the absolute number of cancers was small. Increased risks of borderline significance have been reported in a number of industries (Brown *et al.*, 1988), but the confounding role of personal habits cannot be excluded.

In the UK laryngeal cancer is common among occupations such as barmen where excessive smoking and drinking are frequent (Adelstein, 1972).

Miscellaneous

The possible role of a virus (HPV I and II) has never been confirmed, although believed to be involved in benign laryngeal papillomas in which malignant change has occurred (Shapiro *et al.*, 1976). The role of genetic susceptibility is still unestablished.

33.6 Relevant laboratory studies

The experimental data are uninformative apart from general studies on tobacco.

33.7 Attributable risks

Smoking and alcohol account for 80–90% of laryngeal cancer.

33.8   Conclusions

Abstinence from smoking and moderation in alcohol drinking habits would result in significant reduction in this cancer.

33.9   References

Adelstein (1972). Occupational mortality: Cancer. *Ann. Occup. Hyg.*, **15**, 53–7.

Austin, D.F. (1982). Larynx. In *Cancer Epidemiology and Prevention*, ed. D. Schottenfeld & J.F. Fraumeni, Jr., pp. 554–63. Philadelphia: W.B. Saunders.

Blot, W.I., Fraumeni, J.F., Jr. & Morris, L.E. (1978). Patterns of laryngeal cancer in the United States. *Lancet*, **ii**, 674–5.

Brown, L.M., Mason, T.J., Pickle, L.W., Stewart, P.A., Buffler, P.A., Burau, K., Ziegler, R.G. & Fraumeni, J.F., Jr. (1988). Occupational risk factors for laryngeal cancer on the Texas Gulf Coast. *Cancer Res.*, **48**, 1960–4.

De Stefani, E., Correa, P., Oreggia, F., Leiva, J., Rivero, S., Fernandez, G., Deneo-Pellegrini, H., Zavala, D. & Fontham, E. (1987). Risk factors for laryngeal cancer. *Cancer*, **60**, 3087–91.

IARC (1987). *IARC Monographs on the Evaluation of Carcinogenic Risks to Humans*, Overall evaluations of carcinogenicity: an updating of IARC Monographs volumes 1 to 42, Supplement 7. Lyon: International Agency for Research on Cancer.

Jensen, O.M. (1979). Cancer morbidity and causes of death among Danish brewery workers. *Int. J. Cancer*, **23**, 251–5.

Jussawalla, D.J. & Deshpande, V.A. (1971). Evaluation of cancer risk in tobacco chewers and smokers: an epidemiologic assessment. *Cancer*, **28**, 244–52.

Muir, C., Waterhouse, J., Mack, T., Powell, J. & Whelan, S. (eds.) (1987). *Cancer Incidence in Five Continents*, volume V, IARC Scientific Publication No. 88. Lyon: International Agency for Research on Cancer.

Schottenfeld, D., Gantt, R.C. & Wynder, E.L. (1974). The role of alcohol and tobacco in multiple primary cancers of the upper digestive system, larynx and lung: A prospective study. *Prev. Med.*, **3**, 277–93.

Shapiro, R.S., Marlowe, F.I. & Butcher, J. (1976). Malignant degeneration of non-irradiated juvenile laryngeal papillomatosis. *Ann. Otol.*, **85**, 101–4.

Tuyns, A.J. & Audigier, J.C. (1976). Double wave cohort increase for esophageal and laryngeal cancer in France in relation to reduced alcohol consumption during the second world war. *Digestion*, **14**, 197–208.

Tuyns, A.J., Estve, J., Raymond, L., Berrino, F., Benhamou, E., Blanchet, F., Boffetta, P., Crosignani, P., del Moral, A., Lehmann, W., Merletti, F., Péquignot, R., Riboli, E., Sancho-Garnier, H., Terracini, B., Zubiri, A. & Zubiri, L. (1988). Cancer of the larynx/hypopharynx, tobacco and alcohol: IARC international case-control study in Turin and Varese (Italy), Zaragoza and Navarra (Spain), Geneva (Switzerland) and Calvados (France). *Int. J. Cancer*, **41**, 483–91.

Wynder, E.L., Covey, L.S., Mabuchi, K. & Mushinski, M. (1976). Environmental factors in cancer of the larynx. A second look. *Cancer*, **38**, 1591–601.

34

Bronchus and lung

ICD-9 162

34.1   Introduction

Beginning in mid-century, a pandemic of lung cancer affected the industrial countries of Europe and North America, later spreading to nearly all other nations. This was due to the increasing widespread use of tobacco.

34.2   Histology, classification and diagnosis

Lung cancer can be classified into four major histological types, which have been shown to have etiological significance (IARC, 1988). As interpretation of epidemiological findings has been hampered by variations in nomenclature and criteria, the WHO Classification should be followed (Table 34.1).

The association with cigarette smoking is strongest for squamous cell carcinoma (and its variants), and least for adenocarcinoma. The proportion of the histological types changes according to sex and age group. It is also influenced by the source of biopsy, since peripheral tumors are more likely to be adenocarcinomas. There is evidence that the small (oat) cell type of carcinoma is a biological entity associated with the *ras* oncogene, and possibly a human papilloma virus (HPV).

34.3   Descriptive epidemiology
Incidence

Large international variations are seen (Fig. 34.1 and Appendix 1). In 1980, lung cancer was globally estimated to comprise one in ten of all newly diagnosed cancers for both sexes combined and was the most common tumor in males. The highest rates (100 to 110) are observed in the US black population, in New Zealand Maoris and in Scotland. Somewhat lower rates in range of 50 to 75 are seen in many European countries and

Table 34.1 *World Health Organization classification of lung cancer.*

1. Squamous cell carcinoma (epidermoid carcinoma)
    Variant:
    a. Spindle cell (squamous carcinoma)

2. Small cell carcinoma
    a. Oat cell carcinoma
    b. Intermediate cell type
    c. Combined oat cell carcinoma

3. Adenocarcinoma
    a. Acinar adenocarcinoma
    b. Papillary adenocarcinoma
    c. Bronchiolo-alveolar carcinoma
    d. Solid carcinoma with mucus formation

4. Large cell carcinoma
    Variants:
    a. Giant cell carcinoma
    b. Clear cell carcinoma

5. Adenosquamous carcinoma

6. Carcinoid tumor

7. Bronchial gland carcinomas
    a. Adenoid cystic carcinoma
    b. Mucoepidermoid carcinoma
    c. Others

8. Others

in the white populations of North America. Rates in Israel and Japan are around 30. Much higher levels, however, are recorded in the male Chinese of Singapore (73), Hong Kong (59) and Shanghai (55), which correspond to those found in Chinese living in the San Francisco Bay Area and Los Angeles in California.

Rates are usually lower in women, rates, in the order of 20 to 35, being observed in white Californian populations, in black females in New Orleans and Detroit, in Chinese in Tianjin, Hong Kong and Singapore. However, higher rates (based on small numbers) occur in Maori women (68), in female Hawaiians (40) and in women in the North West Territories and Yukon of Canada (54) which are believed due to local smoking habits (Fig. 34.2).

Time changes

This cancer continues to increase at about 0.5% per annum in Europe and North America. However, overall rates do not reflect the changes occurring in different age cohorts and segments of the community.

Fig. 34.1 Incidence rates around 1980: Bronchus, lung (ICD-9 162).

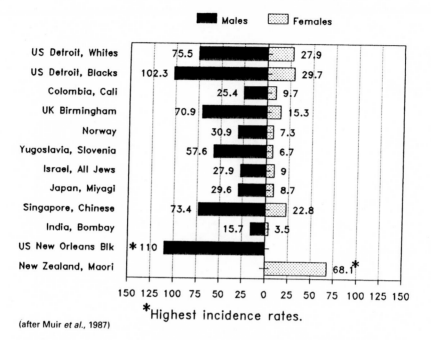

(after Muir *et al.*, 1987)

Fig. 34.2 Highest incidence rates: Bronchus, lung (ICD-9 162) New Orleans black males and New Zealand Maori females.

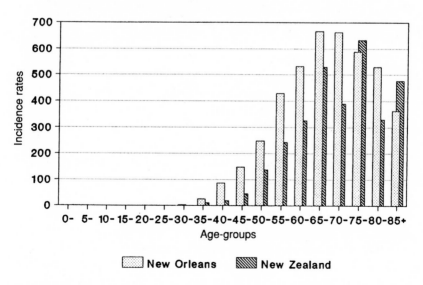

(after Muir *et al.*, 1987)

Fig. 34.3 Age-specific incidence rates per 100,000 per annum. Bronchus, lung (ICD-9 162), Detroit, Michigan, whites.

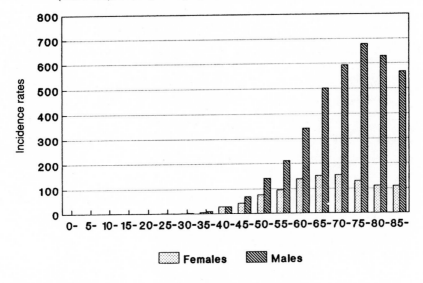

(after Muir *et al.*, 1987)

Thus, the lower age-groups and more educated males show a decrease. This is not true for females. Figure 2.7 depicts a typical birth cohort analysis for lung cancer. On reaching a specified age, successive birth cohorts of white females in Detroit had a higher age-specific incidence rate.

Sex distribution

Sex ratios are fairly high, values around 3 to 5 being common, but are falling as smoking becomes commoner in women (Fig. 34.3).

The relative frequency of adenocarcinoma of the lung is high in southern Chinese and Japanese females, which probably reflects a true increase in the former (Hanai *et al.*, 1987). In Japan, rather, it is due to a lower incidence of the squamous and other histological types.

Age distribution

Cross-sectional incidence and mortality tend to rise smoothly with age, from approximately 40 onwards. In many populations, the rise in incidence becomes less steep and age-specific rates may fall in older age-groups. While this has been interpreted as due to under-reporting in older age-groups, it largely reflects the fact that earlier birth cohorts did not smoke as much as those born later.

34.4 Etiological inferences

The descriptive epidemiological data for lung cancer, notably birth cohort analysis (Fig. 2.7), are consistent with the existence of a powerful carcinogenic factor with an approximately 20–30 year latent period which entered the environment during this century. Incidence closely correlates with tobacco usage, if this induction period be taken into account. Where current tobacco usage trends are known, fairly accurate calculations of the numbers of lung cancer cases that are likely to occur during the next three decades are possible. Over a million cases a year are forecast in China in the twenty-first century (Peto, 1986).

34.5 Known or suspected causes

The impact of tobacco is so large in relation to lung cancer causation that there is a tendency to forget that a number of other factors are important.

Tobacco

The role of the tobacco habit in lung cancer is the subject of an immense literature which is adequately covered by two recent reviews (IARC, 1986*a,b*). The following section briefly summarizes the evidence relating lung cancer to smoking and other factors modifying the association. Certain general issues associated with tobacco are further discussed in Chapter 9.

Evidence that lung cancer was related to tobacco use, notably cigarettes, was first provided in a case-control study by Muller (1939) whose work was largely ignored. Only after the reports of Wynder and Graham (1950) in the USA and Doll and Hill (1950) in the UK was the seriousness of the situation fully realized. The early studies were generally case control in nature showing very high and consistent relative risks and clear dose–responses. Later, large-scale cohort studies in the USA and the UK, helped to establish the relationship without doubt, as did recognition of the long latent period. Since then, the causal association has been consistently confirmed in different environments and countries (IARC, 1986*a*). A few of the major cohort studies that have provided the strongest evidence are summarized in Tables 34.2 and 34.3. The risk increases with the duration of smoking, tar yield and degree of inhalation (Tables 34.4 and 34.5).

Although the causal relationship is well known, epidemiological studies of tobacco continue to form a high proportion of all epidemiological studies on cancer causation.

Table 34.2 *Dose–response relationship between amount smoked and risk of lung cancer in men in selected cohort studies.*

Study	Cigarettes per day	Relative risk	Death rate per 100,000
American cancer	0	1.0	12
society 25-state	1–9	4.6	56
study	10–19	7.5	90
(Hammond, 1966)	20–39	13.1	159
	40 +	16.6	201
Japanese study	0	1.0	23
16-year follow-up	1–9	2.3	49
(Hirayama, 1985)	10–19	4.0	93
	20–29	5.9	137
	30–39	6.1	141
	40–49	7.2	170
	50 +	15.2	352
British doctors study	0	1.0	10
(Doll & Peto	1–14	7.8	78
1976)	15–24	12.7	127
	25 +	25.1	251
Norwegian study	0	1.0	
(Lund & Zeiner-	1–9	6.0	
Hennksen, 1981)	10–19	9.9	
	20 +	18.2	

(After IARC, 1986*a*.)

Types of smoking
Cigarettes, cigars, pipes and tobacco

As shown in Table 34.3, the association of lung cancer is greatest with cigarettes, and less strong for pipes and cigars. However, inhalers of cigar smoke, especially those who have switched from cigarettes to cigars (Fraumeni & Blot, 1982) have shown to have greater risks than described earlier. An association between lung cancer and the smoking of bidis (p. 111) has been established.

Duration of smoking
Peto (1986) has pointed out that the relationship of lung cancer to smoking is more dependent on the duration of smoking than the number of cigarettes smoked. This is consistent with the view that cigarette smoke contains strong promoting factors as well as initiators. Thus the risk is much greater for smoking the same number of cigarettes spread over 40 years than over 20 years (Table 34.4). Such considerations explain some of the inconsistencies that arise when attempting to correlate direct

Table 34.3 *Relative risk of lung cancer in some large cohort studies among men smoking cigarettes and other types of tobacco.*

Study	Smoking category	Relative risk	Death rate per 100,000
American cancer society 25-state study	Never smoked	1.0	12
	Cigarettes only	9.2	111
	Cigars only	1.9	22
	Pipes only	2.2	27
	Cigarettes + other	8.2	89
Swedish study	Non-smokers	1.0	
	Cigarettes only	7.0	
	Cigarettes & pipe	10.9	
	Pipe only	7.1	
	Cigars only	9.2	
	Ex-smokers	6.1	
British doctors study	Non-smokers	1.0	10
	Current smokers	10.4	104
	Cigarettes only	14.0	140
	Pipes and/or cigars	5.8	58
	Cigarettes + other	8.2	82
	Ex-smokers	4.3	43
Norwegian study	Non-smokers	1.0	
	Cigarettes	9.7	
	Cigarettes only	9.5	
	Pipes or cigars only	2.6	
	Ex-smokers	2.8	

(After IARC, 1986*a*.)

Table 34.4 *Approximate effects of various durations of cigarette smoking on annual incidence of lung cancer.*

Years of cigarette smoking	Annual excess incidence	
	Moderate smokers	Heavy smokers
15	0.005%	0.01%
30	0.1%	0.2%
45	0.5%	1.0%
(60)	(1.5%?)	(3.0%?)

(After Peto, 1986.)

consumption per capita with incidence and also explain why the risk increases with an early age of starting to smoke. Sufficient evidence exists to show that, following cessation of smoking, 80% of the risk that would have accrued with continuation of smoking is avoided.

Table 34.5 *Ten-year lung cancer mortality rates (and number of deaths)*[a] *among 17,475 male British civil servants in the Whitehall study, according to quantity smoked, tar yield, and inhalation.*

Number of cigarettes smoked per day	Tar yield (mg)		
	18–23	24–32	33+
Inhalers			
1–9	0.39 (2)	0.53 (1)	1.62 (7)
10–19	1.46 (19)	1.55 (8)	2.61 (20)
20+	2.23 (35)	2.00 (13)	1.79 (3)
Non-inhalers			
1–9	1.08 (4)	0.00 (0)	0.93 (1)
10–19	1.25 (5)	1.28 (2)	4.18 (5)
20+	1.71 (7)	5.81 (9)	5.85 (2)

[a] in parentheses.
(After Stellman, 1986.)

Low tar cigarettes

There is evidence that the introduction of low tar and filter cigarettes has reduced lung cancer risk (IARC 1986*b*) (pp. 120–1). There are difficulties in analyzing cohort effects, and reference should be made to IARC (1986*a*) for discussion on this point.

Passive smoking

In recent years, there has been growing interest regarding the relationship between cancer of the lung and passive smoking – that is the exposure of non-smokers to the cigarette smoke of nearby smokers. The various forms of exposure include main-stream smoke, side-stream smoke and smoke inhaled/exhaled: in all, carcinogenic and mutagenic substances are present, although the amount absorbed by passive smokers is small. Early studies by Hirayama (1981) in Japan showed that the mortality rate of lung cancer in non-smoking women rose according to whether they lived with non-smokers, ex-smokers, or smokers of 1–14, 15–19 and more than 20 cigarettes a day. A dose–response relationship was also observed in sub-categories defined by age and occupation. No other causal explanation appeared feasible. In contrast, no significant increase in non-smoking women, according to their husbands habits, was reported by Garfinkle in the USA (1981). Some 20 studies have now been carried out in Greece, United States, Hong Kong, etc., showing varying degrees of increase (Chapter 4). The IARC (1986*a*) concluded, taking into consideration the impact of active smoking and the quantitative relationship between dose and effect, that passive smoking probably does give rise to some risk of cancer. In evaluating the risk associated with passive smoking, accurate assessment of exposure is needed. Urinary cotinine excretion has now been shown to reflect exposure to environmental tobacco smoke reliably, and this should allow for better studies (Chapter 5).

Occupation
Asbestos

Substantial increases in the incidence of lung cancer have been found among workers exposed to asbestos dust, including miners, millers, textile and insulation workers, shipyard and cement workers, etc. (Chapter 13). Indeed, lung cancer has caused approximately 20% of all deaths in some exposed cohorts (Bogovski *et al.*, 1973). Combined exposure to asbestos and cigarette smoking appears to have a multiplicative effect so that the risk among smoking asbestos workers is very high (IARC, 1973) (Table 34.6).

There is less evidence that differences in the type of asbestos are as important for lung cancer as for mesothelioma; however, chrysotile appears less potent than the amphiboles possibly due to containing less long fibers and being more rapidly cleared from the lungs. It is stated that asbestos-related tumors occur more commonly in the lower lobe. The lungs of most persons with asbestos-related cancers show some asbestosis. Where asbestos exposure has been controlled, the risk in non-smokers or ex-smokers is markedly reduced (Elmes, 1981).

Other fibers

Since other fibers, e.g. glass, mineral wool, etc., produce mesothelioma when instilled in the pleural cavity of animals, their impact on human lung cancer has been studied. A slight increase in lung cancer mortality has been reported among workers in the early technology phase of rock-wool/slag wool production, but no such increase has been observed in recent years (Simonato *et al.*, 1987).

Arsenic and other chemicals

Lung cancer rates are raised in workers involved in the manufacture of sheep dip and vineyard workers who were heavily exposed to arsenical insecticides, and in workers in gold mines in Zimbabwe and in smelters exposed to ores where arsenic was present (IARC, 1987).

Increased lung cancer mortality has been observed in workers manufacturing mustard gas (chloromethyl (pyriline) ethers) (IARC, 1976,

Table 34.6 *Age-standardized death rates from lung cancer in cigarette smokers and non-smokers with or without occupational exposure to asbestos dust.*

Smoking status	Asbestos exposure	Death rate	Mortality ratio
Non-smoker	No	11.3	1.00
	Yes	58.4	5.17
Smoker	No	122.6	10.85
	Yes	601.6	53.24

(After IARC, 1986*a*.)

1987), and those exposed heavily to polycyclic aromatic hydrocarbons in gas generating plants, steel works, etc. Several studies have reported an increased incidence in workers handling chromates and chromium products. The nature of the carcinogenic compound is unclear, but the evidence points to the hexavalent forms. Nickel workers, especially those involved in heavy exposure to dust from relatively crude ore, also show an increase.

Air pollution

In view of its impact in the occupational setting, ambient urban air pollution has long been suspected in the etiology of lung cancer and has been extensively studied, especially in the United States. However, it is now recognized that much of the difference between urban and rural areas depends on differences in tobacco habits. To date, its role and significance in non-smokers has not been established with certainty, but a small additional increase in risk in smokers may be present (Cederlöf *et al.*, 1978, Vena, 1982).

Ionizing radiation

The famous Schneeberg cancer among uranium miners in Czechoslovakia represents one of the earliest demonstrations of this association. An increased risk of lung cancer among uranium miners, believed to be due to the inhalation of radon gas products, has been established. The risk appears higher among smokers (IARC, 1988) (Chapter 16).

Domestic radon exposures (Chapter 16) may be considerable in certain countries where domestic insulation against heat, or more usually cold, has been made highly effective. The radon arises from natural sources in the soil and building materials and varies according to local geological conditions (IARC, 1988). In the United States, 5000 to 25,000 excess lung cancer cases have been ascribed to domestic sources (National Research Council, 1988). It has been noted that one in 1000 British homes will give rise to a dose of about 1 msv. y^{-1}, an amount estimated to cause a lifetime risk of fatal cancer of 10%. Further epidemiological studies are needed, since the investigation of the impact of domestic radon is highly complex.

Miscellaneous
Nutritional status
Following the observation that lung cancer was more common in individuals with low serum levels of Vitamin A, there have been several follow-up studies. However, there are a number of biological inconsistencies and the relative role of Vitamin A, beta carotenes and other retinoids is still not understood (Friedman *et al.*, 1986) (Chapter 12).

Host factors
It is believed that genetic factors may be important in lung cancer and a number of markers of susceptibility have been studied, notably inducible aryl hydroxylase activity and debrisoquine metabolism (Chapter 18). An ethnic factor was considered to be a possible explanation for the high rate of lung adenocarcinoma among Chinese females. Gao *et al.* (1988) showed that in Shanghai, smoking accounted for only about one-quarter of female lung cancers and less than 10% of lung adenocarcinomas. In this population, the increased risk has been attributed to the oils used in cooking. There may be an increased incidence of lung cancer among recipients of immunosuppressant drugs.

34.6   Relevant laboratory studies
Tobacco smoke contains many carcinogens and promoters (Hoffman & Wynder, 1986) (Table 9). Laboratory studies on lung cancer, which require quite complex methodology, mostly relate to the production of experimental tumors in rodents. Pertinent reviews of major studies on tobacco components are covered in the IARC Monograph (1986*a*) and on fibers in Chapter 13. Methods to evaluate individual susceptibility are described in Chapter 18.

34.7   Attributable risks
In most investigations, the attributable risk from tobacco smoking is around 80–85% (Doll & Peto, 1981). In those highly exposed to asbestos the attributable risk is about the same for both tobacco and asbestos since the two risks are multiplicative.

34.8   Conclusions

The overwhelming role of tobacco smoking in the causation of lung cancer and the widespread nature of the exposure mean that this is now the commonest fatal form of cancer. Although consumption is decreasing at about 1% per annum in the developed world, it is rising by 1–2% in developing countries where two-thirds of the globe's population lives. The fall in incidence observed in males in England and Wales and in Finland as well as in groups such as British physicians who have reduced tobacco consumption clearly demonstrates that prevention works. Several occupational sources of increased risk have been identified and these are controllable by appropriate industrial hygiene.

The unresolved questions relate to the degree of influence of atmospheric pollution and domestic radon exposure. High radon levels can be reduced by modifying the floor of buildings or installation of exhaust fans. This requires large-scale surveys to identify homes with potentially high levels.

34.9   References

Bogovski, P., Gilson, J.C., Timbrell, V. & Wagner, J.C. (eds.) (1973). *Biological Effects of Asbestos*, IARC Scientific Publications No. 8. Lyon: International Agency for Research on Cancer.

Cederlöf, R., Doll, R., Fowler, B., Friberg, L., Nelson, N. & Vouk, V. (1978). Air pollution and cancer: risk assessment methodology and epidemiological evidence. (Report of a task group). *Environ. Health Perspect.*, **22**, 1–12.

Doll, R. & Hill, A.B. (1950). Smoking and carcinoma of the lung. Preliminary report. *Br. Med. J.*, **ii**, 739–48.

Doll, R. & Peto, R. (1981). The causes of cancer: quantitative estimates of avoidable risks of cancer in the United States today. *J. Natl. Cancer Inst.*, **66**, 1191–308.

Elmes, P.C. (1981). Relative importance of cigarette smoking in occupational lung disease. *Br. J. Ind. Med.*, **38**, 1–13.

Fraumeni, J.F., Jr. & Blot, W.J. (1982). Lung and pleura. In *Cancer Epidemiology and Prevention*, ed. D. Schottenfeld & J.F. Fraumeni, Jr., pp. 564–82. Philadelphia: W.B. Saunders.

Friedman, G.D., Blaner, W.S., Goodman, D.S., Vogelman, J.H., Brind, J.L., Hoover, R., Fireman, B.H. & Orentreich, N. (1986). Serum retinol and retinol-binding protein levels do not predict subsequent lung cancer. *Am. J. Epidemiol.*, **123**, 781–899.

Garfinkle, L. (1981). Time trends in lung cancer mortality among nonsmokers and a note on passive smoking. *J. Natl. Cancer Inst.*, **66**, 1061–6.

Gao, Y.-T., Blot, W.J. & Zheng, W. (1988). Lung cancer among Chinese women. *Int. J. Cancer*, **40**, 604–9.

Hanai, A., Whittaker, J.S., Tateishi, R., et al. (1987). Concordance of histological classification of lung cancer with special reference to adenocarcinoma in Osaka, Japan and the north-west region of England. *Int. J. Cancer*, **39**, 6–9.

Hirayama, T. (1981). Non-smoking wives of heavy smokers have a higher risk of lung cancer; a study from Japan. *Br. Med. J.*, **282**, 183–5.

Hoffman, D. & Wynder, E.L. (1986). Chemical constituents and bioactivity of tobacco smoke. In *Tobacco: A Major International Health Hazard*, ed. D. Zaridze & R. Peto, pp. 145–65. Lyon: International Agency for Research on Cancer.

IARC (1973). *Biological Effects of Asbestos*, IARC Scientific Publications No. 8, ed. P. Bogovski, J.C. Gilson, V. Timbrell & J.C. Wagner. Lyon: International Agency for Research on Cancer.

IARC (1976). *IARC Monographs on the Evaluation of Carcinogenic Risk of Chemicals to Man*, Cadmium, nickel, some epoxides, miscellaneous industrial chemicals and general considerations on volatile anaesthetics, volume 10, pp. 113–9. Lyon: International Agency for Research on Cancer.

IARC (1986a). *IARC Monographs on the Evaluation of the Carcinogenic Risk of Chemicals to Humans*, Tobacco Smoking, volume 38. Lyon: International Agency for Research on Cancer.

IARC (1986b). *Tobacco: A Major International Health Hazard*, IARC Scientific Publications No. 74, ed. D.G. Zaridze & R. Peto, pp. 1–324. Lyon: International Agency for Research on Cancer.

IARC (1987). *IARC Monographs on the Evaluation of Carcinogenic Risks to Humans*, Overall evaluations of carcinogenicity: an updating of IARC Monographs volumes 1 to 42, Supplement 7. Lyon: International Agency for Research on Cancer.

IARC (1988). *IARC Monographs on the Evaluation of Carcinogenic Risks to Humans*, Man-made mineral fibres and radon, volume 43. Lyon: International Agency for Research on Cancer.

Muller, F.H. (1939). Tobacco abuse and lung carcinoma. *Z. Krebsforsch.*, **49**, 57–85.

National Research Council Committee on the biological effects of ionizing radiations (1988). *Health Risks of Radon and Other Internally Deposited Alpha-Emitters*. Washington: National Academy Press.

Peto, R. (1986). Influence of dose and duration of smoking on lung cancer rates. In *Tobacco, A Major International Health Hazard*, IARC Scientific Publications No. 74, ed. D. Zaridze & R. Peto, pp. 23–33.

Simonato, L., Fletcher, A.C., Cherrie, J.W., Andersen, A., Bertazzi, P., Charnay, N., Claude, J., Dodgson, J., Esteve, J., Frentzel-Beyme, R., Gardner, M.J., Jensen, O., Olsen, J., Teppo, L., Winkelmann, R., Westerholm, P., Winter, P.D., Zocchetti, C. & Saracci, R. (1987). The International Agency for Research on Cancer historical cohort study of MMMF production workers in seven European countries: Extension of the follow-up. *Ann. Occup. Hyg.*, **31**, 603–23.

Stellman, S.D. (1986). Cigarette yield and cancer risk: Evidence from case-control and prospective studies. In *Tobacco: A Major International Health Hazard*, IARC Scientific Publications No. 74, ed. D.G. Zaridze & R. Peto, pp. 197–210. Lyon: International Agency for Research on Cancer.

Vena, J.E. (1982). Air pollution as a risk factor in lung cancer. *Am. J. Epidemiol.*, **116**, 42–56.

Wynder, E.L. & Graham, E.A. (1950). Tobacco smoking as a possible etiologic factor in bronchiogenic carcinoma. *JAMA*, **143**, 329–36.

35

Pleura/mesothelioma

ICD-9 163

35.1 Introduction

Mesothelioma is a rare tumor, which may arise from pleura, peritoneum or pericardium. Its existence as an entity was formerly doubted. In industrial countries the majority of cases (about 80%), are believed to be due to occupation-related exposures to asbestos.

35.2 Histology, classification and diagnosis

The histological diagnosis of mesothelioma is not easy and the appearance can be mimicked by secondary tumors, thus leading to overestimation of frequency. The former absence of clearly defined criteria for diagnosis and its rarity make earlier studies of incidence unreliable. The practice today is to submit equivocal cases to a consultant pathology panel for diagnosis.

The coding of mesothelioma may result in an under-estimation of incidence. In the eighth revision of the ICD, mesothelioma NOS was indexed to benign neoplasms, whereas in the ninth revision, if not specifically stated to be benign (which are very rare tumors) the coder was instructed to use a malignant code number. However, due to the interest in this tumor, and better histological diagnosis, rates in registers such as in Denmark, or in the SEER program, are probably quite accurate.

35.3 Descriptive epidemiology

Incidence (Figure 35.1)

Rates over 1 are rare, being recorded in Recife, Brazil, the white population of the San Francisco Bay Area and New Orleans, Seattle, Hamburg, the department of Calvados in France, the German Democratic Republic, Sweden (2.3), Basel and Zurich in Switzerland, New South Wales and West Australia (2.8) and in the white population of Hawaii

Fig. 35.1 Incidence rates around 1980: Pleura (ICD-9 163).

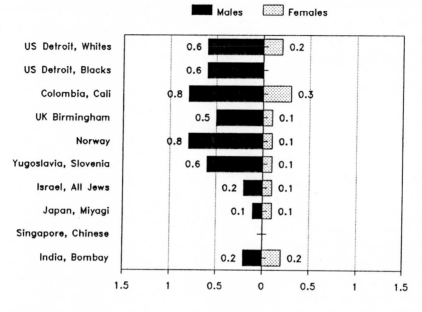

(after Muir *et al.*, 1987)

(2.0). Rates in females are usually around 0.3. The sex ratio thus tends to be fairly high. In the USA, the SEER program, covering slightly more than 10% of the total population, reported 1648 cases from 1978–1984.

These overall rates contrast with the very high levels reported in certain industries, for example, PMRs of nearly 2000% may be found in some works processing crocidolite. In Turkey rates of 1000 have been recorded following exposures to high levels of erionite in the ambient environment. Thus, the overall rate in a country is largely dependent on the number of mesotheliomas occurring in specific subgroups of the population, usually occupational, as distinct from the background rate.

Time trends

In males, rates in the USA have been steadily increasing but in females rates have held steady about 0.2 to 0.4 (Mossman & Gee, 1989; Mossman *et al.*, 1990).

35.4 Etiological inferences

The geographical distribution of mesothelioma such as proximity to shipyards and manufacturing plants, or in rare Turkish villages, has provided a classic example of linking a 'sentinel' cancer with its suspected cause (Langer *et al.*, 1987). The increasing trends in males in the USA have been attributed to previous occupational exposures to asbestos. In contrast, the stability of rates in women suggests that these may represent a background rate and that the ambient causal factors concerned have not significantly changed.

35.5   Known and suspected causes
Asbestos

This is by far the most important cause and is discussed in more detail in Chapter 13.

Occupational exposures

Although mesothelioma was originally considered to be a very rare tumor, the report by Wagner and co-workers in 1960 of nearly 30 cases in Southern Africa changed the situation dramatically. Later, in 1964, Selikoff *et al.* (1965) reported numerous cases in insulation workers and these observations were soon supplemented by numerous reports in other workplaces where asbestos usage was common. Today, occupational exposure to asbestos is responsible in industrial states for approximately 80% of all mesotheliomas. The latent period may be as long as 40 years. The majority of these tumors are due to exposure to amphiboles, notably amosite and crocidolite, rather than chrysolite (white asbestos) which seems less hazardous (Mossman *et al.*, 1990). Early evidence regarding chrysotile however, is often confounded by exposures to crocidolite and tremolite. In a recent study, the number of amphiboles fibers in the lung was significantly higher in mesothelioma cases than in controls, but the numbers of chrysolite and non-asbestos fibers were similar (Bignon *et al.*, 1989). The physical characteristics of fibers most likely to cause mesotheliomas in humans are discussed further in Chapter 13.

Non-occupational exposure

This subject has been discussed in Chapter 13.

Non-asbestos related mesotheliomas

Whereas the role of asbestos is well accepted, there still remain a number of cases of mesothelioma in the general population (around 20%), for which no unusual exposures to asbestos can be identified and a variety of hypotheses, including radiation, have been put forward. Unlike lung cancer, there is no relationship to tobacco. No convincing association with man-made mineral fibers (MMMF) has been demonstrated (Simonato *et al.*, 1987).

35.6   Relevant laboratory studies

In rodents, following intra-pleural and intra-peritoneal injection, mesothelioma has been produced by a range of fibers, not only asbestos, but also by granular non-fibrous materials such as barium sulphate. The relevance of the latter observation to humans is doubtful as, in general, such material does not reach the serosal surface of the lung on inhalation. In contrast to humans, there is comparatively little variation in potency between the various types of fibers administered by the pleural route. Most asbestos inhalation studies result in few mesotheliomas with the exception of erionite.

35.7   Attributable risks

It is believed that nearly all cases of mesothelioma in industries with significant exposure to asbestos, especially amphiboles, are due to these fibres. On the other hand, taking the general population as a whole, there remains a residue of some 20% of mesotheliomas for which no evidence of unusual asbestos exposure can be found. A number of calculations have been made regarding the incidence of mesothelioma due to asbestos compared to other agents (Peto 1989; Hughes & Weill, 1989; McDonald *et al.*, 1989).

35.8   Conclusions

A textbook example of the relationship between a specific tumor and a defined exposure, mesothelioma of occupational origin is now controllable. However, cases resulting from past exposure will continue to occur.

35.9   References

Bignon, J., Peto, J. & Saracci, R. (eds.) (1989). *Non-Occupational Exposure to Mineral Fibres*, IARC Scientific Publications No. 90. Lyon: International Agency for Research on Cancer.

Hughes, J.M. & Weill, H. (1989). Development and use of asbestos risk estimates. In *Non-occupational Exposure to Mineral Fibres*, IARC Scientific Publications No. 90, ed. J. Bignon, J. Peto & R. Saracci, pp. 471–5. Lyon: International Agency for Research on Cancer.

Langer, A.M., Nolan, R.P., Constantopoulos, S.H. & Moutsopoulos, H.M. (1987). Association of metsovo lung and pleural mesothelioma with exposure to tremolite-containing whitewash. *Lancet*, i, 965–7.

McDonald, J.C., Sébastien, P., McDonald, A.D. & Case, B. (1989). Epidemiological observations on mesothelioma and their implications for non-occupational exposure. In *Non-occupational Exposure to Mineral Fibres*, IARC Scientific Publications No. 90, ed. J. Bignon, J. Peto & R. Saracci, pp. 420–7. Lyon: International Agency for Research on Cancer.

Mossman, B.T. & Gee, J.B.L. (1989). Asbestos-related disease. *N. Engl. J. Med.*, **320**, 1721–30.

Mossman, B.T., Bignon, J., Corn, M., Seaton, A. & Gee, J.B.L. (1990). Asbestos: Scientific developments and implications for public policy. *Science*, **247**, 294–301.

Peto, J. (1989). Fibre carcinogenesis and environmental hazards. In *Non-occupational Exposure to Mineral Fibres*, IARC Scientific Publications No. 90, ed. J. Bignon, J. Peto & R. Saracci, pp. 457–70. Lyon: International Agency for Research on Cancer.

Selikoff, I.J., Churg, J. & Hammond, E.C. (1965). The occurrence of asbestosis among insulation workers in the United States. *Ann. NY Acad. Sci.*, **132**, 139–55.

Simonato, L., Fletcher, A.C., Cherrie, J.W., Andersen, A., Bertazzi, P., Charnay, N., Claude, J., Dodgson, J., Esteve, J., Frentzel-Beyme, R., Gardner, M.J., Jensen, O., Olsen, J., Teppo, L., Winkelmann, R., Westerholm, P., Winter, P.D., Zocchetti, C. & Saracci, R. (1987). The International Agency for Research on Cancer historical cohort study of MMMF production workers in seven European countries: Extension of the follow-up. *Ann. Occup. Hyg.*, **31**, 603–23.

Wagner, J.C., Steggs, C.A. & Marchand, P. (1960). Diffuse pleural mesothelioma and asbestos exposure in the north western Cape Province. *Br. J. Ind. Med.*, **17**, 260–71.

Part VIII

Bone and soft tissue

36

Bone

ICD-9 170

36.1 Introduction

Tumors arising in the bone and cartilage are rare, accounting for about 0.5% of all malignant neoplasms. Mortality data tend to be imprecise as metastatic tumors are frequently miscoded as primary (Percy *et al.*, 1981; Percy & Muir, 1989). Radiation apart, little is known of their etiology.

36.2 Histology, classification and diagnosis

Osteogenic sarcoma (osteosarcoma), chondrosarcoma and Ewing's tumor are the three main clinicopathological entities grouped under this single ICD rubric.

36.3 Descriptive epidemiology

Incidence and time trends (Fig. 36.1)

The highest reported rates for bone cancers, between 2.6 and 4.3, are encountered in males from South America. Rates around 2 to 3 are seen in several parts of Europe, whereas, in most countries, rates are close to or below unity. High relative frequencies, around 5% in both sexes, have been reported from the North West Frontier Province of Pakistan, as compared to other parts of the country (Parkin, 1986), but the histological nature of these tumors is not known. The raised frequency may reflect the higher proportion of younger persons in the population.

Age and sex distribution

Male rates tend to be slightly higher than those in females. There are variations in the peak incidence with age (Table 36.1.). Osteosarcoma

Fig. 36.1 Incidence rates around 1980: Bone (ICD-9 170).

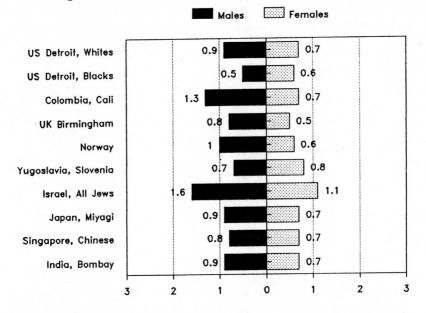

(after Muir *et al.*, 1987)

is characterized by incidence peaks around 15–19 and thereafter in old age, whereas chondrosarcoma shows a gradual increase with age. Ewing's sarcoma is almost entirely confined to childhood and early adult life, being rare in black and Asian populations. Osteosarcomas, on the contrary, are somewhat more frequent in black than in white children. Parkin *et al.* (1988) give incidence rates for these cancers in many parts of the world in the age-group 0–14.

36.4   Etiological inferences

The relative lack of geographical variation in incidence suggests a minimal environmental component. The age, sex and site distribution of the main types, notably osteosarcoma, chondrosarcoma and Ewing's sarcoma, argues against a common etiology.

36.5   Known and suspected causes

While a variety of agents, chemical, physical and viral, have been reported to cause bone tumors in animals, human data are limited (Fraumeni & Boice, 1982).

Familial and heredity factors

There is some evidence of a familial tendency, especially for osteogenic sarcoma, in some families with multiple tumors. Survivors of

Table 36.1. *Primary bone cancer by histological type with site, sex and age distribution.*

Histology	Major sites	% Male	Age distribution Middle 80% of cases (years)	Peak incidence (years)
Osteosarcoma	Femur, tibia, humerus, innominate bones	60	10–55	10–20
Chondrosarcoma	Femur, innominate bones, ribs, tibia, shoulder girdle	65	25–65	50–60
Ewing's sarcoma	Femur, innominate bones, ribs, tibia, humerus	60	10–30	10–20
Reticulum cell sarcoma	Innominate bones, ribs, femur, humerus, vertebrae	60	15–70	50–60
Fibrosarcoma	Femur, tibia, humerus, innominate bones, mandible	45	25–60	30–40
Giant cell tumor	Femur, humerus, tibia	60	40–60	40–55
Chordoma	Sacrum, skull, vertebrae	65	40–70	55–65
Periosteal osteosarcoma	Femur, tibia, humerus	35	20–45	30–40

(After Fraumeni & Boice, 1982.)

bilateral retinoblastoma have an increased risk of osteosarcoma. Certain syndromes, skeletal malformations, and various other hereditary dysplasias are prone to bone tumors including osteochondromas and chondrosarcoma (Unni & Dahlin, 1979; Fraumeni & Boice, 1982). Paget's disease is the most important and predisposes mainly to osteogenic sarcoma and to other sarcomas (Seret *et al.*, 1987), especially in older adults. Although environmental influences have been suggested, their nature is unknown.

Trauma

Trauma has been frequently ascribed as a cause of bone cancer, but convincing evidence is lacking. The association probably represents observer recall bias following the discovery of a tumor after a local injury.

Radiation

Martland (1929) described occupational radium poisoning in the manufacture of luminous watch dials as a cause of bone cancer. Ionizing radiation, including radioisotopes, have been conclusively linked to bone cancer, especially to osteosarcoma, but the role of external beam radiation (X- and gamma rays) is less well documented (Tucker *et al.*, 1987).

Carcinogenic chemicals

While certain chemicals may induce bone tumor in animals, there is no convincing evidence that these have done so in humans (Fraumeni & Boice, 1982). An increase in bone cancer has been reported, however, following alkylating drugs in childhood (Tucker *et al.*, 1987).

Viruses

Viruses can cause osteosarcoma in experimental animals but have yet to be implicated in humans. While there is some support for the view that a slow viral infection may be involved in Paget's disease (Mirra, 1987), the evidence remains circumstantial.

36.6   Relevant laboratory studies

These so far have been uninformative: those related to genetic disposition are described in Chapter 18.

36.7   Attributable risks

About one-quarter of those with Paget's disease eventually develop an adult osteosarcoma. The attributable risk due to radiation is probably less than 10%, although high radiation risks are reported in individual studies.

36.8   Conclusions

The relative rarity of histological types makes study difficult and traditional analytical studies are unlikely to indicate new causal agents unless some specific biomarkers can be identified.

36.9   References

Fraumeni, J.F., Jr. & Boice, J.D., Jr. (1982). Bone. In *Cancer Epidemiology and Prevention*, ed. D. Schottenfeld & J.F. Fraumeni, Jr., pp. 814–26. Philadelphia: W.B. Saunders.

Martland, H.S. (1929). Occupational poisoning in manufacture of luminous watch dials. *JAMA*, **92**, 466–73.

Mirra, J.M. (1987). Pathogenesis of Paget's disease based on viral etiology. *Clin. Orthop.*, **217**, 162–70.

Muir, C., Waterhouse, J., Mack, T., Powell, J. & Whelan, S. (eds.) (1987). *Cancer Incidence in Five Continents*, Volume V, IARC Scientific Publications No. 88. Lyon: International Agency for Research on Cancer.

Parkin, D.M. (ed.) (1986). *Cancer Occurrence in Developing Countries*, IARC Scientific Publications No. 75. Lyon: International Agency for Research on Cancer.

Parkin, D.M., Stiller, C.A., Draper, G.J., Bieber, C.A., Terracini, B. & Young, J.L. (eds.) (1988). *International Incidence of Childhood Cancer*, IARC Scientific Publications No. 87. Lyon: International Agency for Research on Cancer.

Percy, C. & Muir, C. (1989). The international comparability of cancer mortality data. Results of an international death certificate study. *Am. J. Epidemiol.*, **129**, 934–46.

Percy, C., Stanek, E., III & Gloeckler, L. (1981). Accuracy of cancer death certificates and its effect on cancer mortality statistics. *Am. J. Public Health*, **71**, 242–50.

Seret, P., Basle, M.F., Rebel, A., Renier, J.C., Saint-Andre, J.P., Bertrans, G. & Audran, M. (1987). Sarcomatous degeneration in Paget's bone disease. *J. Cancer Res. Clin. Oncol.*, **113**, 392–9.

Tucker, M.A., D'Angio, G.J., Boice, J.D., Jr., Strong, L.C., Li, F.P., Stovall, M., Stone, B.J., Green, D.M., Lombardi, F., Newton, W., Hoover, R.N., & Fraumeni, J.F., Jr. (1987). Bone sarcoma linked to radiotherapy and chemotherapy in children. *N. Eng. J. Med.*, **317**, 588–93.

Unni, K.K. & Dahlin, D.C. (1979). Premalignant tumors and conditions of bone. *Am. J. Surg. Pathol.*, **3**, 47–60.

37

Soft tissue sarcoma (STS)

ICD-9 171

37.1   Introduction

Tumors of soft tissues (STS) represent sarcomas covering a range of histological types which are classified according to tissue of origin. They occur relatively rarely, and incidence rates between countries do not differ significantly.

37.2   Histology, classification and diagnosis

Soft tissue sarcomas are derived from mesenchymal tissues such as muscle, fat, blood vessels and other connective tissues, a heterogeneity of cell type concealed by site-oriented classifications such as the ICD. There is no evidence that these diverse neoplasms have a common etiology.

The Third National Cancer Survey and the SEER Programme (Surveillance, Epidemiology and End Results) in the USA have provided tabulations for these cancers both by site and cell type for 1969–1971 and 1972–77 (Young *et al.*, 1981). Leiomyosarcoma (30%) appears to be the most common form affecting mainly the uterus in females and the gastro-intestinal tract in males. Liposarcomas (17%), fibrosarcomas (14%) and rhabdomyosarcomas (11%) are predominant in males. An increasing number of cancer registries are providing this type of information, although numbers are much smaller. However, the indexing of these cancers is such that some connective tissue malignancies are currently coded to specified organs such as uterus, stomach, rather than ICD-9 171. Kaposi's sarcoma (see below) is coded to malignant neoplasm of skin ICD-9 173. Unless diagnoses are coded by ICD-O (WHO, 1976, 1990), such neoplasms can be 'lost'.

37.3   Descriptive epidemiology
Incidence

In much of the world the incidence of these tumors is around 2 in males. The incidence in Brazilian males is somewhat higher, around 3. Due to their rarity, estimation of the incidence rates for each histological type is very uncertain, unless a registry covers a very large population.

Age, sex and time distribution

A slight male excess is usually observed. Unlike most epithelial cancers, the increase with age is very slight. Most STS occur at relatively young ages.

Angiosarcoma

In children age 0–14, from 1973–1986, the US SEER Program registered a total of six angiosarcomas of which none was in the liver. The rate for all ages, both sexes combined, averaged 0.23 prior to the AIDS epidemic. Slight increases since then may include a few cases of Kaposi's sarcoma.

Kaposi's sarcoma

Although Kaposi's sarcoma has hitherto been rare in western countries and uncommon in American blacks, these neoplasms represent 5–12% of all cancers in some African countries, arising mainly in older males and affecting principally the legs. Between 1982 and 1983, in parallel with the AIDS epidemic, the incidence of Kaposi's sarcoma in the SEER areas doubled among men age 20–54, increasing by another 85% in the next biennium. In San Francisco city and county, incidence rates increased from 2.0 in 1980 to 56.7 in 1983 and 112.7 in 1985. The classical African Kaposi's sarcoma runs an indolent course unlike the AIDS-associated form.

37.4   Etiological inferences

Relatively minor geographical variations suggest that most of these tumors are not significantly affected by general environmental factors. The occurrence of Kaposi's sarcoma in Africa and also in AIDS patients indicates the possibility of some common biological agent.

37.5   Known and suspected causes

Rarely is there a history of an unusual local stimulus such as radiation or the injection of a potential carcinogen. When present, such isolated cases are usually insufficient to affect overall cancer rates.

Hereditary factors

A small proportion of patients with soft-tissue tumors appear to have a dominant inherited single gene such as in neurofibromatosis, in which some neurofibromas progress to sarcomas. Occasionally there has been a degree of clustering in siblings associated with tumors of other sites within the same family (Tucker & Fraumeni, 1982).

Radiation

Nearly all types of soft-tissue tumors have been found following radiation. Angiosarcomas have followed thorotrast injection for radiography of blood vessels. Other types have occurred at the edge of such deposits. Lymphosarcomas also arise in areas of lymphedema following radical mastectomy.

Chemicals

Falk (1988) concluded that of 168 hepatic hemangiosarcomas (HAS) in the USA between 1964 and 1976, 7% were related to vinyl chloride monomer (VCM), 12% to thorotrast, 4% to arsenic and 2% were associated with androgenic anabolic steroids. With modern industrial hygienic and radiological practices, VCM and thorotrast related tumors will probably disappear (pp. 306–7).

Pesticides and herbicides

Agricultural chemical exposures have caused concern (Hardell & Sandström, 1979), especially phenoxy-acetic acids and chlorophenols. However, a number of these studies have technical deficiencies and the available evidence is not convincing (Lynge *et al.*, 1987; IARC, 1987). Other studies on veterans in Vietnam and elsewhere have not confirmed earlier reports (Balarajan & Acheson, 1984; Hogstedt & Westerlund, 1980; Riihimaki, 1982; Royal Commission, 1985; Smith *et al.*, 1984; Johnson, 1990). There is no evidence of an effect in animals.

Apart from HAS, evidence of a major role of chemicals remains unconvincing.

Viruses

Although an association between viruses and human sarcoma has long been postulated,it remains to be confirmed. However, in recent years, certain types of Kaposi's sarcoma have been found to be related to human immunodeficiency disease (AIDS) and its related virus (HIV). Kaposi's hemangiosarcoma has been long recognized in Africa but it is now suggested that there are two types, one of which is related to the HIV virus infection (Weiss, 1989). Evidence is accumulating that a virus other than HIV may be involved, but no agent has, as yet, been definitively implicated. Mueller and Hatzakis (1988) describe this tumor, in relation to AIDS, as an opportunistic malignancy.

Miscellaneous

There is some evidence that immunosuppressive states may be related to STS possibly by increasing susceptibility to a virus.

No convincing evidence has been found that soft-tissue tumors can be ascribed to the injection of Penicillin-G, saccharated iron oxide, and other chemicals which cause sarcomas in rodents (Weinbren *et al.*, 1978). Occasional cases related to implants in humans (Ryu *et al.*, 1987) and war wound foreign bodies are reported (Chapter 14).

37.6   Relevant laboratory studies

Although STS, subsequent to implanted membranes, are well recognized in rodents (i.e. Oppenheimer effect), this effect is very rarely observed in humans. There is now evidence that the relevant gene in neurofibromatosis (NF Type I) has been isolated. HIV related Kaposi's sarcoma is now the subject of extensive studies.

37.7   Attributable risks

No meaningful data, apart from the studies of Falk (1988) on HAS, has been reported.

37.8   Conclusions

In general, the majority of soft tissue sarcomas cannot be attributed to any definite factor, and the number with defined causes is probably less than 5%. However, the proportion may rise as more HIV-related cases are identified in Western countries.

37.9   References

Balarajan, R. & Acheson, E.D. (1984). Soft tissue sarcomas in agriculture and forestry workers. *J. Epidemiol. Community Health*, **38**, 113–16.

Falk, H. (1988). Vinyl chloride-induced hepatic angiosarcoma. In *Unusual Occurrences as Clues to Cancer Etiology*, Proceedings of the 18th International Symposium of The Princess Takamatsu Cancer Research Fund, Tokyo, 1987, ed. R.W Miller, S. Watanabe, J.F. Fraumeni, Jr., T. Sugimura, S. Takayama & H. Sugano. Tokyo: Japan Scientific Societies Press.

Hardell, L. & Sandström, A. (1979). A case-control study: Soft-tissue sarcomas and exposure to phenoxyacetic acids or chlorophenols. *Br. J. Cancer*, **39**, 711–17.

Hogstedt, C. & Westerlund, B. (1980). Cohort studies of cause of death of forest workers with and without exposure to phenoxyacid preparations. *Lakartidningen*, **77**, 1828–31.

IARC (1987). *IARC Monographs on the Evaluation of Carcinogenic Risks to Humans*, Overall evaluations of carcinogenicity: an updating of IARC Monographs volume 1 to 42, Supplement 7, pp. 156–60. Lyon: International Agency for Research on Cancer.

Johnson, E.S. (1990). Association between soft tissue sarcomas, malignant lymphomas, and phenoxy herbicides/chlorophenols: Evidence from occupational cohort studies. *Fundam. Appl. Toxicol.*, **14**, 219–34.

Lynge, E., Storm, H.H. & Jensen, O.M. (1987). The evaluation of trends in soft tissue sarcoma according to diagnostic criteria and consumption of phenoxy herbicides. *Cancer*, **60**, 1896–901.

Mueller, N. & Hatzakis, A. (1988). Opportunistic malignancies and the acquired immunodeficiency syndrome. In *Unusual Occurrences as Clues to Cancer Etiology*, Proceedings of the 18th International Symposium of The Princess Takamatsu Cancer Research Fund, Tokyo, 1987, ed. R.W. Miller, S. Watanabe, J.F. Fraumeni, Jr., T. Sugimura, S. Takayama & H. Sugano, pp. 159–71. Tokyo: Japan Scientific Societies Press.

Riihimaki, V. (1982). *Mortality of Chlorinated Phenoxyacid Herbicide 2,4-D and 2,4,5-T Applicators in Finland*. First Report of an Ongoing Prospective Follow-Up Study, 20 pp., Helsinki: Institute of Occupational Health.

Royal Commission on the Use and Effects of Chemical Agents on Australian Personnel in Vietnam. (1985). *Final Report*, Volume 4, pp. 71–4. Canberra: Australian Government Publishing Service.

Ryu, R.K., Bovill, E.G. Jr, Skinner, H.,B. & Murray, W.R. (1987). Soft tissue sarcoma associated with aluminum oxide ceramic total hip arthroplasty. A case report. *Clin. Orthop.*, **216**, 207–12.

Smith, A.H., Pearce, N.E., Fisher, D.O., Giles, H.J. & Teague, C.A. (1984). Soft tissue sarcoma and exposure to phenoxyherbicides and chlorophenols in New Zealand. *J. Natl. Cancer Inst.*, **73**, 1111–17.

Tucker, M.A. & Fraumeni, J.F., Jr. (1982). Soft tissue. In *Cancer Epidemiology and Prevention*, ed. D. Schottenfeld & J.F. Fraumeni, Jr., pp. 827–36. Philadelphia: W.B. Saunders.

Weinbren, K., Salm, R. & Greenberg, G. (1978). Intramuscular injections of iron compounds and oncogenesis in man. *Br. Med. J.*, **1**, 683–5.

Weiss, R.A. (1989). HIV and Kaposi's Sarcoma in Mice. *Nature*, **337**, 112–13.

WHO (1976). *ICD-O International Classification of Diseases for Oncology*. Geneva: World Health Organization.

WHO (1990). *ICD-O International Classification of Diseases for Oncology*, 2nd Edition, ed. C. Percy, V. Van Holten, & C. Muir. Geneva: World Health Organization.

Young, J.L., Percy, C.L. & Asire, A.J. (1981). *Surveillance, epidemiology and end results: Incidence and mortality data 1973–77*, National Cancer Institute Monograph No. 57. Bethesda, MD: US Department of Health and Human Services.

Part IX

Skin

38

Malignant Melanoma

ICD-9 172

38.1 Introduction

In 1950, the sixth revision of the ICD separated malignant melanoma (MM) of the skin from other forms of cutaneous cancer for the first time. Its clinical behavior is considerably more aggressive than the latter. The five-year survival rate is at best around 80% compared to virtually 100% for basal cell carcinoma.

38.2 Histology, classification and diagnosis

Malignant melanoma arises from the pigment-producing cells of the skin. Clinical diagnosis, which may not always be easy, is confirmed by histology. Approximately 70% of tumors probably arise in an existing pigmented nevus. The *superficial spreading* form constitutes around 60% of all malignant melanomas and is frequently indolent. *Nodular melanoma* (15%) grows rapidly being invasive *ab initio*. *Lentigo malignant melanoma* is very slow growing and occurs usually on the face of older persons and represents the most frequent of other forms. Prognosis is deduced from histological examination (Clark, 1969). Tumors less than 0.85 mm thick have a 90% five-year survival; over 4.65 mm a 40% five-year survival (Breslow, 1980).

The topographical distribution of malignant melanoma varies by sex, being commoner on the trunk in males and on the extremities in females.

38.3 Descriptive epidemiology
Incidence

The incidence of malignant melanoma of the skin varies by about 100 fold. Incidence is greatest in fair-skinned populations living in sunny climates, e.g. Hawaii, New Zealand. Rates in whites in Los Angeles and

New Mexico are double those in New York State. The highest rates are in Australasia. There is a substantial north-to-south gradient within Australia. The highest rates 30.9 (M) and 28.5 (F) occur in Queensland, the lowest in Tasmania 11.0 (M) and 13.7 (F). A gradient is also found in Scandinavia, the highest rates being seen along the coast of southern Norway, south-western Sweden, extending into Denmark (Osterlind *et al.*, 1988*b*). The cancer is commoner in the Israeli-born population than in migrants born in Europe or North America or Africa/Asia, the respective rates being 9.0 (M) and 14.5 (F); 7.3 (M) and 9.3 (F); as compared to 1.3 (M) and 1.6 (F).

Time trends
Rates in deeply pigmented populations are increasing by some 0.5% per annum, but, in contrast, annual increases have been in the order of 5–7% in white North American populations and in Nordic countries, and about 10% in Israel. These increases, even in low-risk populations such as in Japan, are most marked in recent birth-cohorts.

Sex distribution
The sex ratio is, in general, about unity, but some populations show a male predominance, e.g. white males in Atlanta. In contrast, a substantial excess in white females is observed in New Zealand.

Age distribution
Incidence increases with age, but there is a marked cohort effect in some countries, e.g. Denmark, where adults show a substantial increase in risk as compared to 30 years ago.

38.4   Etiological inferences
The dependency on latitude, the predilection for fair-skinned persons, the increased risk after migration to regions nearer to the Equator and the differing body distribution patterns of increase in each sex, support a role for solar radiation. The evidence from birth-cohorts in Europe and North America suggests a change of lifestyle after 1880 leading to increased solar exposure.

38.5   Known and suspected causes
Predisposing factors
Many malignant melanomas are related to a pre-existing benign nevus, the number of palpable nevi being a strong marker of risk (Osterlind *et al.*, 1988*a*). These nevi are probably sun induced rather than

Fig. 38.1 Incidence rates around 1980: Melanoma (ICD-9 172).

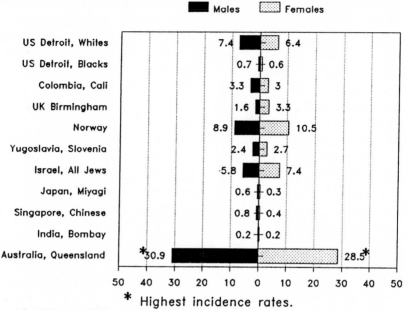

(after Muir *et al.*, 1987)

of genetic origin. In Africans, melanomas develop from pigmented nevi on the soles of the feet. High frequencies of plantar melanoma have been found in India and in non-caucasians in Hawaii, which possibly reflect a relative absence of melanoma on other parts of the body.

The *dysplastic nevus syndrome* is characterized by numerous large nevi on the body which are irregular in shape and color. Mendelian inheritance for the syndrome has not been demonstrated and autosomal transmission of malignant melanoma in these persons, possibly linked to the HLA gene, has been suggested.

Ultra-violet light

While a direct etiological association with UV B light (280–350 nm) is readily demonstrated for squamous cell and basal cell carcinomas, a simple direct association is less evident for malignant melanoma (Chapter 15). There is, however, strong presumptive evidence that exposure to solar radiation, especially when sporadic, increases risk.

A population-based case-control study in eastern Denmark covering 45% of the total Danish population (Osterlind *et al.*, 1988*a*, *b*) examined several hypotheses, including genetically determined pigmentation as reflected by color of skin, hair and eyes; freckling, skin reactions to solar exposure; and the presence of palpable nevi (which were considered to reflect either genetic predisposition or an environmental factor). Light-skinned and red-haired individuals were at increased risk, which, however, reflected their susceptibility to freckling. The increased risk in persons with a tendency to burn easily was also linked to freckling. The strongest determinant of risk was the number of palpable benign pigmented nevi, the risk being related to number not size. Persons with nevi and a tendency to develop many freckles, had a 14 times higher risk than those with no nevi and freckles. This observation suggests a synergistic effect. These results are consistent with studies from Australia and Western Canada (Elwood *et al.*, 1987). There is evidence that exposure to the sun in childhood is of major importance. Thus, in Western Australia, it has been shown that, for superficial spreading melanoma, individuals migrating to Australia before the age of 10 years have the same risk as the Australian born; those migrating at a later age have a risk similar to those in the country of origin. Walter *et al.* (1990) found a modest dose-dependent increase of risk (around 1.5) following use of a sunbed or a sunlamp, particularly at home.

There is controversy over the possible role of the ultraviolet radiation emanating from fluorescent lamps (Beral *et al.*, 1982), as confounding cannot be excluded.

Other risk factors

Therapeutic immunosuppression (Hoover, 1977; Kinlen *et al.*, 1979) may result in an increased risk. Pregnancy, subsequent to the occurrence of melanoma, may worsen the prognosis especially where secondary spread has occurred. An increase with use of oral contraceptives has also been reported, but others disagree (Green & Bain, 1985). There is no evidence of an incidence difference between married and single women.

Psoralen, a photosensitizing agent incorporated in some sun protection creams (Gupta & Anderson, 1987), in combination with ultraviolet A light can induce non-melanoma skin tumors in experimental animals but, to date, has not been implicated in humans.

38.6   Relevant laboratory studies

Minipigs are reported to have a high incidence of spontaneous malignant melanoma. Melanoma can be produced by estrogens in hamsters which may be pertinent to the effect of pregnancy in humans. Melanomas are also highly antigenic and the role of immunosuppression in their origin is under study. The site of the primary tumor is strongly associated with the presence of the *ras* oncogene mutation.

38.7 Attributable risks

The majority of MM are believed due to sunlight and hereditary susceptibility.

38.8 Conclusions

Although dose–effect relationships have not been established there is little doubt that cutaneous malignant melanoma is linked to solar exposure, possibly involving sunburn, in fair-skinned persons prone to freckling. The rapid rate of increase in incidence in many populations has evoked, notably in Australia, public information campaigns on 'wise use of the sun', suggesting measures to reduce solar exposure. While the mean thickness of lesions at diagnosis has fallen substantially (i.e. earlier diagnosis), no comparable decrease in incidence has yet been recorded.

38.9 References

Beral, V., Evans, H., Shaw, H. & Milton, G. (1982). Malignant melanoma and exposure to fluorescent lighting at work, *Lancet*, **ii**, 290–3.

Breslow, A. (1980). Prognosis in cutaneous melanoma: Tumor thickness as a guide to treatment. In *Pathology Annual*, Part I, vol. 15, ed. S.C. Sommers & O.O. Rosen, pp. 1–22. New York: Appleton-Century Crofts.

Clark, W.H., Jr. (1969). The histogenesis and biological behavior of primary human malignant melanoma of the skin. *Cancer Res*,. **29**, 705–26.

Elwood, J.M., Gallagher, R.P., Worth, A.J., Wood, W.S. & Pearson, J.C. (1987). Etiological differences between subtypes of cutaneous malignant melanoma: Western Canada melanoma study. *J. Natl. Cancer Inst.*, **78**, 37–44.

Green, A. & Bain, C. (1985). Hormonal factors and melanoma in women. *Med. J. Aust.*, **142**, 446–734.

Gupta, A.K. & Anderson, T.F. (1987). Psoralen Photochemotherapy. *J. Am. Acad. Dermatol.*, 703–34.

Hoover, R. (1977). Effects of drugs – immunosuppression. In *Origins of Human Cancer*, Cold Spring Harbor Conference on Cell proliferation, ed. H. Hiatt, J.D. Watson & J.A. Winston, pp. 296–301. New York: Cold Spring Harbor Laboratory.

Kinlen, L.J., Sheil, A.G.R., Peto, J. & Doll, R. (1979). Collaborative United Kingdom Australasian study of cancer in patients treated with immunosuppressive drugs. *Br. Med. J.*, **2**, 1461–6.

Osterlind, A., Tucker, M.A., Hou-Jensen, K., Stone, B.J., Englom, G. & Jensen, O.M. (1988a). The Danish case-control study of cutaneous malignant melanoma. I. Importance of host factors. *Int. J. Cancer*, **42**, 200–6.

Osterlind, A., Tucker, M.A., Stone, B.J. & Jensen, O.M. (1988b). The Danish case-control study of cutaneous malignant melanoma. II. Importance of UV light exposure. *Int. J. Cancer*, **42**, 319–24.

Walter, S.D., Marrett, D., From, L., Hertzman, C., Shannon, H.S. & Roy, P. (1990). The association of cutaneous malignant melanoma with the use of sunbeds and sunlamps. *Am. J. Epidemiol.*, **131**, 232–430.

Skin cancers other than malignant melanoma

ICD-9 173

39.1 Introduction

The non-melanoma skin (NMS) cancers, principally basal cell and squamous cell carcinomas, are very common but rarely fatal.

39.2 Histology, classification and diagnosis

Basal cell carcinomas are usually found on the face above a line drawn from the angle of the mouth to the ear lobe. Although slow growing, and almost never mestastasizing, these cancers, if neglected, can result in large ulcers hence the term 'rodent ulcer'. Squamous cell carcinomas can occur on any part of the body, especially in the dorsum of the hand, or on the legs (notably in Africa). Other skin cancers, mainly arising from sweat glands, are very rare.

39.3 Descriptive epidemiology

Incidence

The incidence of NMS tumors shows wide variation. The true incidence is difficult to determine in view of their high frequency, low lethality and the fact that an individual may have several over a lifetime. Many cancer registries do not record basal cell carcinomas, which are also often under reported.

The highest rates of NMS cancer recently reported are from Tasmania in Australia (167.2 in males and 89.3 in females) and from British Columbia in Canada (109.1 in males and 75.5 in females). In El Paso in Texas, after a special effort to assess the true incidence, rates were as high as 144.9 in 'Anglo' males and 73.3 in 'Anglo' females (Waterhouse *et al.*, 1976). Rates in the 50 to 60 range are observed in males in Brazil, Colombia and Switzerland. NMS cancers are much more common in

Fig. 39.1 Incidence rates around 1980: Skin (ICD-9 172).

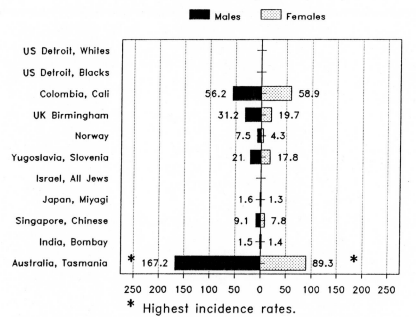

(after Muir *et al.*, 1987)

whites than in dark-skinned populations. Rates in the range of 1 to 5 are reported from Africa and Asia.

In whites, NMS cancers are most common in areas of strong sunlight, and arise mainly in the most exposed areas of the face head and neck, in contrast to the somewhat more even distribution of malignant melanoma (Pearl & Scott, 1986).

The incidence of NMS carcinomas, especially basal cell, seems to have increased in the United States in both sexes (Fears & Scotto, 1982).

Sex distribution

Rates in males tend to be about double those in females, with rare exceptions, such as the higher frequency noted in women working in the rice fields of north Thailand (Menakanit *et al.*, 1971). A male excess is seen for most sites except the legs, where female rates are higher.

Age distribution

These cancers increase with age.

39.4   Etiological inferences

Squamous cell cancers frequently arise from so-called solar keratosis, which can be considered as precancerous. Light-skinned populations, especially of Celtic origin, have much higher frequencies of NMS cancer than the darker pigmented ethnic groups. Such variations explain the fact that the correlation between sunlight exposure and the development of skin cancer is not always clear-cut. Naturally pigmented skins are at much lower risk. Thus, in Australia, individuals of Italian origin have a much lower incidence of skin cancer than Anglo-Saxons and Celts.

The influence of latitude and skin type speak strongly for a role for solar radiation, a relationship which, unlike that observed for malignant melanoma, is dose-dependent, thus giving higher rates in outdoor workers.

39.5   Known and suspected causes
Hereditary factors
In addition to level of skin pigmentation, individuals with the complex hereditary condition xeroderma pigmentosum (XP) are at very high risk due to lack of the enzymes needed to repair the DNA damaged by ultraviolet light (Chapter 18).

Sunlight
The major cause for NMS cancer is prolonged solar exposure, the role of which is discussed further in Chapter 15.

Occupation and chemicals
Following the original observation by Percival Pott of an excess of scrotal cancer among chimney sweeps, the role of various polycyclic aromatic hydrocarbons (PAH) has become better understood. Thus, NMS cancers are found among shale oil workers, jute processors, tool setters, mulespinners, etc. The majority are squamous cell carcinomas occurring at a site that is exposed to long contact with the carcinogen, such as the scrotum in the case of mineral cutting oils. Inorganic arsenic can cause cancer of the skin (IARC, 1980, 1987). In addition to such occupational exposures as sheep-dip workers, vineyard workers, etc., most such cancers arise as a result of arsenic in drinking water or, occasionally, as in the past, from the use of medicinal agents. Apart from certain specific exposures, e.g. shale oil workers, benign papillomas seldom precede squamous cell carcinoma in humans, in contrast to experimental animals.

Ionizing radiation
Skin cancers were observed early among radiation workers, notably radiologists, and this has been confirmed many times over. Heavy exposures associated with radio-dermatitis are most likely to result in

squamous cell carcinomas, but basal cell carcinomas can also occur, possibly due to a potentiating factor of UV light (Chapter 16).

Immunosuppression

An increased incidence of squamous cell carcinoma of the skin has been reported among kidney transplant recipients receiving immunosuppressive therapy. It is believed that the excess risk occurs predominantly at sun-exposed areas. The rapid increase in risk suggests a promotional effect.

Trauma and chronic ulcers

Squamous cell carcinomas in blacks in Africa have been observed in relation to burns, infections, tropical and other chronic ulcers, especially on the lower limbs, although their frequency has declined in recent years (Samitz, 1980). The lesions are often accompanied by areas of depigmented skin.

39.6   Relevant laboratory studies

Skin cancers can be readily produced in experimental animals by artificial UV exposure or by painting with polycyclic aromatic hydrocarbons.

39.7   Attributable risks

In non-pigmented races, about 90–95% of tumors can be attributed to sunlight, whereas, in blacks, most tumors are related to chronic skin trauma.

39.8   Conclusions

Eminently preventable and treatable, NMS cancers none the less consume medical care resources. Public education to avoid or protect against sunlight by barrier creams should reduce incidence and increase early detection.

39.9   References

Fears, T.R. & Scotto, J. (1982). Changes in skin cancer morbidity between 1971–72 and 1977–78. *J. Natl. Cancer Inst.*, **69**, 365–70.

IARC (1980). *IARC Monographs on the Evaluation of the Carcinogenic Risk of Chemicals to Humans*, Some metals and metallic compounds, vol. 23. Lyon: International Agency for Research on Cancer.

IARC (1987). *IARC Monographs on the Evaluation of Carcinogenic Risks to Humans, Overall Evaluations of Carcinogenicity: An Updating of IARC Monographs*, volumes 1 to 42, Supplement 7. Lyon: International Agency for Research on Cancer.

Kinlen, L.J., Sheil, A.G.R., Peto, J. & Doll, R. (1979). Collaborative United Kingdom–Australian study of cancer in patients treated with immunosuppressive drugs. *Br. Med. J.*, **2**, 1461–6.

Menakanit, W., Muir, C.S. & Jain, D.K. (1971). Cancer in Chiang Mai, North Thailand. A relative frequency study. *Br. J. Cancer*, **25**, 225–36.

Muir, C., Waterhouse, J., Mack, T., Powell, J. & Whelan, S. (eds.) (1987). *Cancer Incidence in Five Continents*, volume V, IARC Scientific Publication No. 88. Lyon: International Agency for Research on Cancer.

Pearl, D.K. & Scott, E.L. (1986). The anatomical distribution of skin cancers. *Int. J. Epid.*, **15**, 502–6.

Samitz, M.H. (1980). Dermatology in Tanzania – problems and solutions. *Int J. Dermat.*, **19**, 102–6.

Waterhouse, J., Muir, C., Correa, P. & Powell, J. (1976). *Cancer Incidence in Five Continents*, volume III, IARC Scientific Publications No. 15. Lyon: International Agency for Research on Cancer.

Part X

Breast and genitourinary system

40

Breast

ICD-9 174–175

40.1　Introduction

Globally, breast cancer is the most frequent malignancy among women with an estimated 572,000 new cases in 1980 or 18.4% of all cancers. The disease is extremely rare in males: in females it shows marked geographical variation.

40.2　Histology, classification and diagnosis

Most breast tumors arise from the ductal or lobular epithelial cells. A number of histological subgroups are described which, in general, do not appear to have etiological relevance although differences in biological behavior between Japanese and North American women have been reported. Breast biopsies have increased with growth of mammography with a resultant rise in the diagnosis of borderline *in situ* lesions which complicates interpretation of incidence and mortality trends. Mortality is also influenced by newer therapeutic techniques. The risk of cancer developing in patients with benign breast disease is directly related to the degree of epithelial atypia. While hormonal receptors appear significant for prognosis, they appear to be unrelated to specific risk factors.

40.3　Descriptive epidemiology
Incidence and mortality

The highest rates occur in North America, Israel and temperate South America (over 60). High rates (40–60) are also seen in north western Europe and in Australia. Intermediate rates (20–40) are found in parts of Eastern Europe, tropical South America, Philippines and Singapore. Low rates (less than 20) are seen in China, parts of Japan and India and in Kuwaitis. In the USA rates are higher in whites than in blacks.

In contrast to incidence, the highest mortality rates are reported from north-western Europe followed by North America. This discrepancy may be due, in part, to later diagnosis and evaluation of borderline lesions.

An urban–rural gradient has been observed in several populations, the rates being higher in urban areas. Several investigations have shown higher rates in upper socio-economic levels. Rates are somewhat lower among Mormons and Seventh Day Adventists than in the general population.

Several investigations on migrants from high- and low-risk countries to the USA and Australia have shown that they slowly acquire breast cancer rates that approach those of the host countries. European migrants to the USA experience a faster change towards the rates of the USA population than migrants from Japan and China, in whom the increase does not become apparent until the second and third generations.

Age distribution

The rates increase progressively with age from the third decade. A plateau or inflexion (Clemmesen's hook) is present in the age-specific incidence curve around ages 45–55 and marks the division into pre- and post-menopausal types of cancer.

Sex distribution

Female-to-male ratios range from 70 to 130. In males, incidence rates are below 1.0 in most countries, and are based on very few cases, so differences are unlikely to be significant.

Time trends

In most populations, increasing incidence trends of breast cancer have been observed, notably in post-menopausal women. There are data indicating, however, that the rate of increase in younger cohorts is levelling off or even falling in some areas. Singapore is an exception and the increase is most noticeable in those under 50 years of age. In contrast, mortality rates in most populations have been stable or shown only very small increases, except in southern and eastern Europe and in some Latin American countries.

40.4   Etiological inferences

An important role of environmental factors can be deduced from the considerable geographical variation reported and the changes in rates among migrants toward those of the host country. Since the change in risk occurs slowly, and over several generations, as illustrated by migrants

Fig. 40.1 Incidence rates around 1980: Breast (ICD-9 173–174).

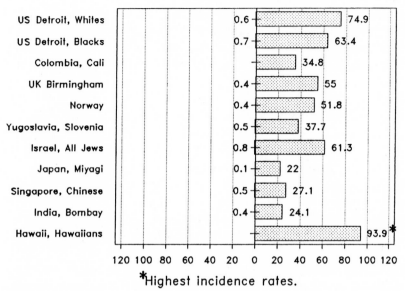

░░ Females

US Detroit, Whites — 0.6 — 74.9
US Detroit, Blacks — 0.7 — 63.4
Colombia, Cali — 34.8
UK Birmingham — 0.4 — 55
Norway — 0.4 — 51.8
Yugoslavia, Slovenia — 0.5 — 37.7
Israel, All Jews — 0.8 — 61.3
Japan, Miyagi — 0.1 — 22
Singapore, Chinese — 0.5 — 27.1
India, Bombay — 0.4 — 24.1
Hawaii, Hawaiians — 93.9 *

120 100 80 60 40 20 0 20 40 60 80 100 120

*Highest incidence rates.

(after Muir *et al.*, 1987)

from Japan and China to the USA, some of the determinants of the risk must act early in life. The shape of age–incidence curves and temporal changes also suggest differences in etiology between pre- and post-menopausal tumors. The higher frequency of breast cancer in upper income groups and the lower risk in certain religious groups may reflect the influence of reproductive and dietary factors.

40.5   Known and suspected causes
Hereditary factors

A history of breast cancer in a mother or in a sister increases a woman's chance of developing the disease. The magnitude of the increased risk depends on the age at diagnosis, tumor laterality, and number of first-degree relatives affected (Anderson, 1977). Particularly dramatic increases in risk are associated with a family history of breast cancer in a young sister or mother or of bilateral disease. Among such women, empirical risks of breast cancer by age 65 approach 50%, a risk similar to that expected for a fully penetrant dominant condition (Schwartz *et al.*, 1985). However, multiple cases of post-menopausal breast cancer can occur in families due to chance. Clustering of breast cancer in high-risk families may be explained by the influence of major genes, polygenic effects, culturally transmitted risk factors, a shared environment or a combination of these (King *et al.*, 1984). The relative contribution of these various factors remains to be assessed. Recent complex segregation analysis of breast cancer in families is compatible with an autosomal dominant transmission, although genetic susceptibility was identified in only 4% of the families studied (Newman *et al.*, 1988; Bishop *et al.*, 1988).

Reproductive habits (see also Chapter 11)
Marital status
The protective role of marriage in breast cancer and the high incidence in single females was recognized by Ramazzini in the eighteenth century. Current breast cancer patterns still show a higher absolute risk for single women. This difference is generally confined to the post-menopausal period (Lilienfeld, 1956).

Lactation
The historical view of the protective effect of breast-feeding was challenged by MacMahon *et al.* (1970*a,b*) who, finding no relationship with lactation in an international study, concluded that the most important factor was age at first pregnancy. However, a beneficial effect of lactation after controlling for the effects of age, parity and age at first pregnancy has been detected in subsequent studies carried out in high-risk populations in the USA (Byers *et al.*, 1985; McTiernan & Thomas, 1986) as well as in low-risk Chinese women (Yuan *et al.*, 1988; Tao *et al.*, 1988).

Menstruation and menopause
Menstrual and reproductive events are among the most important breast cancer risk factors and are probably related to estrogen exposure (Henderson *et al.*, 1988). Most case-control studies and all prospective studies have shown a moderately increased risk of breast cancer associated with an early age at menarche (Staszewski, 1971; Byers *et al.*, 1985) and late age at menopause. A protective effect of early age at menopause (natural or artificial) has also been demonstrated (Lilienfeld, 1956; Trichopoulos *et al.*, 1972). Epidemiological and experimental evidence suggests that the cumulative number of ovulatory cycles is directly related to breast cancer risk. Women with early menarche (age 12 or younger) and rapid establishment of regular cycles have an almost four-fold increased risk compared to women with late menarche (age 13 or older) and long duration of irregular cycles (MacMahon *et al.*, 1982; Henderson *et al.*,

1985). Further, women with early menarche have higher serum estradiol concentrations and lower levels of sex-hormone-binding globulin during the follicular phase of the menstrual cycle than women with later menarches, suggesting that such women are subject to greater estrogen stimulation (Apter *et al.*, 1989).

There is conflicting evidence regarding an association between breast cancer risk and menstrual irregularity, length of menstrual cycles, amount of menstrual flow and menstrual cramps.

Age at first birth and parity

MacMahon *et* al. (1970*a*) found that women with a first birth before age 20 had half the cancer risk of nulliparous women or of women delaying the first birth until age 30. In a reanalysis, it was found that the critical age was 35. Thus, before this age each full-term pregnancy conferred some protection, whereas, afterwards, any full term pregnancy was associated with an increased risk (Trichopoulos *et al.*, 1983). These authors also concluded that the apparent protective effect of increased parity was actually due to early age at first full-term pregnancy. However, other studies have shown a residual protective effect of an increasing number of births after controlling for the effects of age at first pregnancy (Thein-Hlaing & Thein-Maung-Myint, 1978; Tulinius *et al.*, 1978; Yuan *et al.*, 1988; Leon, 1989).

Endogenous and exogenous hormones

There is considerable indirect evidence suggesting a role for endogenous estrogens in the etiology of human breast cancer. Studies in experimental animals have shown that hormones can modulate mammary carcinogenesis (Bittner, 1936). In humans, inferences on their role can be deduced indirectly from epidemiological studies linking biological indicators of endogenous estrogenic stimulus (e.g. age at menarche, menopause, cumulative number of ovulatory cycles) to breast cancer risk, as well as from studies correlating sex hormone levels in blood or urine to breast cancer risk. Such studies have been difficult to interpret because it is not clear whether the altered hormone levels in breast cancer patients are the result of or precede the disease. Henderson *et al.* (1982, 1988) have concluded that the data overall support the hypothesis that breast cancer risk is determined primarily by the total cumulative exposure of breast tissue to bioavailable estrogens and the associated cumulative mitotic activity. The sources of endogenous estrogens are the ovary, during menstrual life, and the peripheral conversion of adrenal-derived androgens to estrogen in fat cells. In this context, there is a strong relationship between weight and post-menopausal breast cancer risk (de Waard *et al.*, 1977) and Begg *et al.* (1987) have described a relationship between obesity and increased endogenous estrogen levels in siblings of women with post-menopausal breast cancer.

Oral contraceptives

The use of oral contraceptives and estrogen replacement therapy (ERT) has been suspected to be associated with breast cancer. Oral contraceptives (OC) have been widely used since the early 1960s, and a considerable number of case-control and cohort studies investigating this relationship have been published. The present consensus is that the use of OCs during most of a woman's reproductive life (e.g. 25–40 years) has no adverse effect on breast cancer risk (Vessey, 1987; Prentice & Thomas, 1987). No evidence of increasing trends in breast cancer rates with increasing duration of use of OCs has been produced.

There is, however, considerable concern about the effects of OC use at an early age and specially in the late adolescent period. The studies on OC use in young breast cancer cases and controls have produced conflicting results. However, in most studies, a clear but low increase in risk in young women who have used OCs has been demonstrated (Henderson *et al.*, 1988, UK National Case-control Study Group, 1989). In the largest of the so-called 'negative' studies, an increase in risk was also detected after reanalysis of the data (Peto, 1989).

Estrogen-replacement therapy after menopause has not been associated with an increased risk in most studies; however, recent case-control studies which have used healthy population comparison groups show a moderately increased risk of breast cancer for long-term users (Henderson *et al.*, 1988).

Diet

High-fat intake, and animal fat in particular, has been proposed as a major risk determinant for breast cancer during the last decade. This hypothesis is based essentially on animal experiments showing that diets high in fat increase mammary tumor induction and on ecological studies showing striking correlations between per capita consumption of fat and breast cancer rates (Armstrong & Doll, 1975). Experimental studies are usually performed with severe dietary manipulations not extrapolable to human situations. Further, the correlation studies provide only weak evidence of a causal association since other confounding factors related to economic development are uncontrolled. Subsequent evidence from case-control and cohort studies, however, has not, overall, supported the hypothesis (Willett, 1989). In a large cohort study of over 89,000 nurses in the USA, weak inverse associations with breast cancer risk were seen for total, saturated and polyunsaturated fat (Willett *et al.*, 1987*a*). It has been postulated that diet and in particular fat intake during adolescence may be a more important determinant; however, no association with adolescent diet was detected in a recent case-control study (Pryor *et al.*, 1989). The plausibility of the hypothesis on the role of fat would be enhanced if fat could be shown to be a mediator of breast cancer risk by influencing hormonal levels. However, the relationship remains unclear at present.

A relationship between excess caloric intake, irrespective of food source and increased breast cancer risk has been proposed (Carroll, 1984). This association is supported by animal experiments showing that restriction of energy intake reduces the occurrence of mammary tumors. It is possible that reduced energy intake, particularly in early life, such as found in protein-calorie deficiency (kwashiorkor) in Africa, may reduce the incidence of breast cancer. A high correlation between the average height of adult women (determined in great part by energy intake before 20 years) and breast cancer rates in various countries has been observed. Moreover, a positive association has been found between height and risk of breast cancer in several countries that experienced famine (Willett, 1989). The above data may indicate that any dietary contribution to the breast cancer risk is due to the amount of calories consumed and utilized, specially during critical periods such as adolescence, and not to the intake of specific nutrients. De Waard and Trichopoulos (1988) have concluded that an energy-rich diet in later life contributes to the occurrence of obesity which, after menopause, enhances the development of breast cancer (see also Chapter 12).

Miscellaneous
Tobacco

An association with cigarette smoking has also been suspected but the evidence is weak and inconsistent. In some studies, a slight increase in risk has been detected in smokers while, in others, a protective effect has been suggested (IARC, 1986).

Alcohol

Intake of alcoholic beverages has also been associated with an increased risk for breast cancer (Willett *et al.*, 1987*b*). However, the possibility that some other characteristic of women who drink alcohol might explain this association cannot currently be entirely excluded.

Ionizing radiation

Exposure to high doses of ionizing radiation, specially during adolescence, has been associated with an increased risk of breast cancer (Boice & Monson, 1977), and there may be an increased risk associated also with exposure to low doses (Modan *et al.*, 1989).

Viruses

Despite the discovery of a B-type RNA tumor virus in mice over 50 years ago (Bittner, 1936), no convincing evidence of a viral agent linked to human breast cancer has been detected in epidemiological and associated laboratory studies.

Male breast cancer

The etiology of this cancer is unknown. The linkage of such cancers to gynecomastia, a common condition in early life, has been an attractive hypothesis, although no clear or consistent association has been proved. A small number of cases have been reported following hormonal therapy in prostatic cancer, but metastases cannot always be excluded. Despite the reported relationship of gynecomastia to malnutrition or obesity, there is no convincing evidence for an etiological association (Casagrande *et al.*, 1988). Because of the rarity of the disease only a few case-control studies have been reported. Some indicate that hormonal factors may be important (Casagrande *et al.*, 1988, Lenfant-Pejovic *et al.*, 1990).

40.6   Relevant laboratory studies

The relevance to man of early studies on viral transmission in mice has never been established. Many dietary studies on naturally occurring and chemically induced tumors in rodents support the concept of a multifactorial process with major impact on the later stages of carcinogenesis. Recent studies have identified biological features which may be of value in predicting prognosis but their etiological implications are unknown. They include hormone receptors, epidermal growth factor-receptor (EGFR), gene expression and oncogene abnormalities.

Estrogen receptors have been detected in over 50% of breast cancer patients, and most patients with these receptors respond well to endocrine therapy. However, it is not yet established whether the presence or absence of these receptors reflect different stages of the same disease or two different diseases. A few case-control studies show that there is an overlap in the risk factors suggesting that there is a progression from one type to the other (Cooper *et al.*, 1989). Among oncogene abnormalities, amplifications of the proto-oncogenes c-*myc* and HER2/*neu* have been shown to be associated with a poor prognosis (Slamon *et al.*, 1987; Seshadri *et al.*, 1989).

The significance of mutagens formed from cholesterol in breast secretions remains to be evaluated.

40.7   Attributable risks

Although an energy-rich diet and hormonal factors which reflect reproductive habits are probably major determinants of breast cancer risk, the proportion of breast cancer cases that can be attributed to these individually is, at present, difficult to estimate.

Genetic susceptibility alone probably accounts for a small proportion of breast cancer, at most 4%.

40.8   Conclusions

The overall epidemiological data suggest that the major determinant of breast cancer risk is the total cumulative exposure of breast tissue to bioavailable estrogens and that this exposure is influenced by nutritional factors and reproductive history. Energy-rich diet during adolescence may enhance the occurrence of precancerous lesions. This process is counteracted by full-term pregnancies, earlier pregnancies having the strongest protective effect.

40.9   References

Anderson, D.E. (1977). Breast cancer in families. *Cancer*, **40**, 1855–60.

Apter, D., Reinilä, M. & Vihko, R. (1989). Some endocrine characteristics of early menarche, a risk factor for breast cancer, are preserved into adulthood. *Int. J. Cancer*, **44**, 783–7.

Armstrong, B. & Doll, R. (1975). Environmental factors and cancer incidence and mortality in different countries, with special reference to dietary practices. *Int. J. Cancer*, **15**, 617–31.

Begg, L., Kuller, L.H., Gutai, J.P., Caggiula, A.G., Wolmark, N. & Watson, C.G. (1987). Endogenous sex hormone levels and breast cancer risk. *Genet. Epidemiol.*, **4**, 233–47.

Bishop, D.T., Cannon-Albright, L., Mclellan, T., Gardner, E.J., Skolnick, M.H. (1988). Segregation and linkage analysis of nine Utah breast cancer pedigrees. *Genet. Epidemiol.*, **5**, 151–69.

Bittner, J.J. (1936). Some possible effects of nursing on the mammary gland tumor incidence in mice. *Science*, **84**, 162.

Boice, J.D. & Monson, R.R. (1987). Declining breast cancer mortality among young American women. *J. Natl. Cancer Inst.*, **78**, 451–4.

Byers, T., Graham, S., Rzepka, T. & Marshall, J. (1985). Lactation and breast cancer: Evidence for a negative association in premenopausal women. *Am. J. Epidemiol.*, **121**, 664–74.

Carroll, K.K. (1984). Influence of diet on mammary cancer. *Nutr. Cancer*, **2**, 232–6.

Casagrande, J.T., Hanisch, R., Pike, M.C., Ross, R.K., Brown, J.B. & Henderson, B.E. (1988). A case-control study of male breast cancer. *Cancer Res.*, **48**, 1326–30.

Cooper, J.A., Rohan, T.E., McK. Cant, E.L., Horsfall, D.J. & Tilley, W.D. (1989). Risk factors for breast cancer by oestrogen receptor status: a population-based case-control study. *Br. J. Cancer*, **59**, 119–25.

de Waard, F. & Trichopoulos, D. (1988). A unifying concept of the aetiology of breast cancer. *Int. J. Cancer*, **41**, 666–9.

de Waard, F., Cornelis, J.P., Aoki, K. & Yoshida, M. (1977). Breast cancer incidence according to weight and height in two cities of the Netherlands and in Aichi Prefecture, Japan. *Cancer*, **40**, 1269–75.

Henderson, B.E., Ross, R.K., Pike, M.C. & Casagrande, J.T. (1982). Endogenous hormones as a major factor in human cancer. *Cancer Res.*, **43**, 3232–9.

Henderson, B.E., Ross, R.K., Judd, H.L., Krailo, M.D. & Pike, M.C. (1985). Do regular ovulatory cycles increase breast cancer risk? *Cancer*, **56**, 1206–8.

Henderson, B.E., Ross, R. & Bernstein, L. (1988). Estrogens as a cause of human cancer; The Richard and Hinda Rosenthal Foundation Award Lecture. *Cancer Res.*, **48**, 246–53.

IARC (1986). *Monographs on the Evaluation of the Carcinogenic Risk of Chemicals to Humans*, Tobacco smoking, volume 38. Lyon: International Agency for Research on Cancer.

King, M.-C., Lee, G.T., Spiner, N.R., Thompson, G. & Wrensch, M.R. (1984). Genetic epidemiology. *Annu. Rev. Public Health*, **5**, 1–52.

Lenfant-Pejovic, M.-H., Mlika-Cabanne, N., Bouchardy, C., & Auquier, A. (1990). Risk factors for male breast cancer: a Franco-Swiss case-control study. *Int. J. Cancer*, **45**, 661–5.

Leon, D.A. (1989). A prospective study of the independent effects of parity and age at first birth on breast cancer incidence in England and Wales. *Int. J. Cancer*, **43**, 986–91.

Lilienfeld, A. (1956). The relationship of cancer of the female breast to artificial menopause and marital status. *Cancer*, **9**, 927–34.

MacMahon, B., Cole, P., Lin, T.M., Lowe, C.R., Mirra, A.P., Ravnihar, B., Salber, E.J., Valaoras, V.G. & Yuasa, S. (1970a). Age at first birth and breast cancer risk. *Bull. WHO*, **43**, 209–21.

MacMahon, B., Lin, T.M., Lowe, C.R., Mirra, A.P., Ravnihar, B., Salber, E.J., Trichopoulos, D., Valaoras, V.G. & Yuasa, S. (1970b). Lactation and cancer of the breast. A summary of an international study. *Bull. WHO*, **42**, 186–94.

MacMahon, B., Trichopoulos, D., Brown, J., Andersen, A.P., Aoki, K., Cole, P., de Waard, F., Kaurantemi, T., Morgan, R.W., Purde, M., Ravnihar, B., Stormby, N., Westlund, K. & Woo, N.-C. (1982). Age at menarche, probability of ovulation and breast cancer risk. *Int. J. Cancer*, **29**, 13–16.

McTiernan, A. & Thomas, D.B. (1986). Evidence for a protective effect of lactation on risk of breast cancer in young women: results from a case-control study. *Am. J. Epidemiol.*, **124**, 353–8.

Modan, B., Alfandary, E., Chetrit A. & Katz, L. (1989). Increased risk of breast cancer after low-dose irradiation. *Lancet*, **i**, 629–31.

Newman, B., Austin, M.A., Lee, M. & King, M.C. (1988). Inheritance of human breast cancer: evidence for autosomal dominant transmission in high-risk families. *Proc. Natl. Acad. Sci. USA*, **85** 3044–8.

Peto, J. (1989). Oral contraceptives and breast cancer: is the CASH study really negative? *Lancet*, **i**, 522.

Prentice, R.L. & Thomas, D.B. (1987). On the epidemiology of oral contraceptives and disease. In *Advances in Cancer Research*, Vol. 49, ed. G. Klein & S. Weinhouse, pp. 285–401. San Diego: Academic Press.

Pryor, M., Slattery, M.L., Robison, L.M. & Egger, M. (1989). Adolescent diet and breast cancer in Utah. *Cancer Res.*, **49**, 2161–7.

Schwartz, A.G, King, M.D., Belle, S.H. & Satariano, V.A. (1985). Risk of breast cancer to relatives of young breast cancer patients. *J. Natl. Cancer Inst.*, **75**, 665–8.

Seshadri, R., Matthews, C., Dobrovic, A. & Horsfall, D.J. (1989). The significance of oncogene amplification in primary breast cancer. *Int. J. Cancer*, **43**, 270–2.

Slamon, D.J., Clark, G.M., Wong, S.G., Levin, W.J., Ullrich, A. & McGuire, W.L. (1987). Human breast cancer: correlation of relapse and survival with amplification of the HER-2/neu oncogene. *Science*, **235**, 177–82.

Staszewski, J. (1971). Age at menarche and breast cancer. *J. Natl. Cancer Inst.*, **47**, 935–40.

Tao, S.-C., Yu, M.C., Ross, R.K. & Xiu, K.-W. (1988). Risk factors for breast cancer in Chinese women of Beijing. *Int. J. Cancer*, **42**, 495–8.

Thein-Hlaing & Thein-Maung-Myint (1978). Risk factors of breast cancer in Burma. *Int. J. Cancer*, **21**, 432–7.

Trichopoulos, D., MacMahon, B. & Cole, P. (1972). Menopause and breast cancer risk. *J. Natl. Cancer Inst.*, **48**, 605–13.

Trichopoulos, D., Hsieh, C.C., MacMahon, B., Lin, T.M., Lowe, C.R., Mirra, A.P., Ravnihar, B., Salber, E.J., Valaoras, V.G. & Yuasa, S. (1983). Age at any birth and breast cancer risk. *Int. J. Cancer*, **31**, 701–4.

Tulinius, H., Day, N.E., Johannesson, B., Bjarnason, O. & Gonzales, M. (1978). Reproductive factors and risk for breast cancer in Iceland. *Int. J. Cancer*, **21**, 724–30.

U.K. National Case-Control Study Group (1989). Oral contraceptive use and breast cancer risk in young women. *Lancet*, **i**, 973–82

Vessey, M.P. (1987). Oral contraceptives and breast cancer. *IPPF Med. Bull.*, **21**, 1.

Willett, W.C., Stampfer, M.J., Colditz, G.A., Rosner, B.A., Hennekens, C.H. & Speizer, F.E. (1987a). Dietary fat and the risk of breast cancer. *N. Engl. J. Med.*, **316**, 22–8.

Willett, W.C., Stampfer, M.J., Colditz, G.A., Rosner, B.A., Hennekens, C.H. & Speizer, F.E. (1987b). Moderate alcohol consumption and the risk of breast cancer. *N. Engl. J. Med.*, **316**, 1174–80.

Willett, W.J. (1989). The search for the causes of breast and colon cancer. *Nature*, **338**, 389–93.

Yuan, J.-M., Yu, M.C., Ross, R.K., Gao, Y.-T. & Henderson, B.E. (1988). Risk factors for breast cancer in Chinese women in Shanghai. *Cancer Res.*, **48**, 1949–53.

41

Uterine cervix

ICD-9 180

41.1　Introduction

Cervical cancer is the second most frequent cancer in women on a worldwide basis, but it is the most frequent cancer in developing countries even when both sexes are considered (Parkin *et al.*, 1988). It shows large geographical variations and temporal changes.

41.2　Histology, classification and diagnosis

About 95% of these cancers are squamous cell carcinomas, the others adenocarcinomas. It is now accepted that invasive squamous cell carcinoma arises from precursor lesions of the cervix such as dysplasia and carcinoma *in situ*. There is a recent trend to use the term *cervical intra epithelial neoplasia* (CIN) to cover the postulated sequence of cellular changes from mild dysplasia to *in situ* carcinoma. Information on the lesions preceding dysplasia is limited.

While the pathological diagnosis of invasive carcinoma is straight-forward, the cytological and histological diagnosis of CIN can be difficult, as illustrated in distinguishing CIN from sub-clinical human papilloma virus (HPV) infection by morphology only. The use of nomenclature based on the three degrees of CIN instead of three degrees of dysplasia plus carcinoma *in situ* may be ambiguous in regard to the clinical implications and complicate the interpretation of reports on prevalence. Accordingly, a new classification for cytology (The Bethesda System) has been proposed grouping squamous intraepithelial lesions (SIL) in two categories: low-grade SIL (previously mild dysplasia or CIN-I) and high-grade SIL (previously moderate and severe dysplasia, carcinoma *in situ* or CIN-II and CIN-III).

Fig. 41.1 Incidence rates around 1980: Cervix uteri (ICD-9 180).

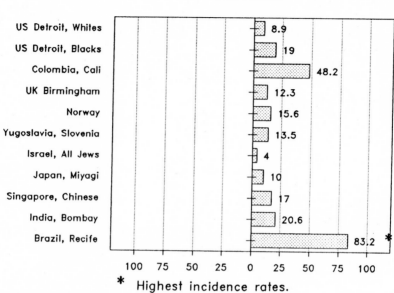

Females

US Detroit, Whites	8.9
US Detroit, Blacks	19
Colombia, Cali	48.2
UK Birmingham	12.3
Norway	15.6
Yugoslavia, Slovenia	13.5
Israel, All Jews	4
Japan, Miyagi	10
Singapore, Chinese	17
India, Bombay	20.6
Brazil, Recife	83.2 *

100 75 50 25 0 25 50 75 100

* Highest incidence rates.

(after Muir *et al.*, 1987)

41.3   Descriptive epidemiology
Incidence

Very high incidence rates (over 30) are observed in most Latin American countries, some Polynesian Islands, many Indian communities and parts of Sub-Saharan Africa. Relatively high rates (15–30) are found in areas of eastern, western and northern Europe, and in black and Hispanic groups in the USA. Low rates (below 15) are observed in caucasian populations in North America, Southern Europe, Middle East and Australia, with the lowest rates (below 7) being found in Finland, Israel, Kuwait, Ireland and Spain (Fig. 41.1).

Time trends

Incidence and mortality rates steadily declined in most populations during the last half century partly due to increased use of cervical cytology screening. In contrast, a poorly understood increase in incidence and mortality has been observed among young women in the UK, Canada, Australia, New Zealand, Norway and the German Democratic Republic (Muñoz & Bosch, 1989).

Fig. 41.2 Cervical cancer incidence by age-group for selected registries.

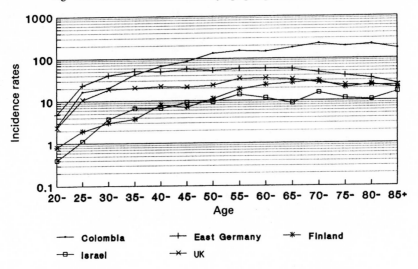

(after Muir *et al.*, 1987)

Age distribution

In most populations, invasive cancer is very rare before 20 years of age. Rates increase progressively with age until the fifth decade when the rates either decrease or level off. Examples of this pattern, and exceptions to it, are shown in Figure 41.2. In Cali, Colombia, the incidence continues to increase with age up to 60 years and even older. In Finland, the incidence is as low as in Israel until about 50 years of age and then increases to about double the Israeli rate. The incidence in East Germany is higher than it is in Colombia before 40 years of age but lower thereafter.

41.4   Etiological inferences

The large geographical variations in incidence and very high rates in developing countries suggest a role of cultural and exogenous factors. These include sexually transmitted infections, high parity, and inadequate medical services which are prevalent among low socio-economic groups. The recent increase in young women in some developed countries suggest the introduction of possibly new risk factor(s), mostly affecting the younger generations. The very low rates in North America and in European Jewish women, and the lower rates in Moslem as compared to Hindu women is consistent with circumcision practices (see below). The extremely low rates in Finland are probably the result of a population-wide screening program in that country over the last 30 years. In contrast, rates in Israel, Kuwait, Ireland and Spain are believed consistent with low exposures to a putative sexually transmitted agent, due to conservative sexual behavioral habits. Increasing sexual freedom has been postulated as a cause of the increase in young women and is supported by the parallel trends between rates of sexually transmitted disease and mortality from cancer of the cervix. Since the rise has occurred in those 25–29 years of age, the latent period for the effect of the putative agent has been estimated as 10–15 years.

41.5   Known and suspected causes
Sexual behavior

The role of sexual behavior is discussed in Chapter 11. The associations demonstrated with certain sexual behavioral patterns in both females and males are consistent with a role of a sexually transmitted infectious agent (Chapter 17).

Reproductive factors

These are discussed in Chapter 11. The association with age at first pregnancy and number of pregnancies has been interpreted as indirect, reflecting mainly early age at first sexual intercourse.

Sexually transmitted infectious agents

Various sexually transmitted infections have long been described as associated with cervical cancer, including *syphilis, Trichomonas vaginalis, Candida albicans, Chlamydia trachomatis, herpes simplex virus* Type 2 (HSV-2), *cytomegalovirus* (CMV), and *human papillomavirus* (HPV) as described in Chapter 17. HSV-2 has been the most extensively studied but the evidence remains inconclusive.

The current hypotheses favor a key etiological role for certain types of HPV. Although certain types of HPV (16, 18, 31, 33, 35, 39, 41–45, 51–56), and, in particular, HPV 16 and 18 are associated with an increased risk of cervical cancer, most studies do not completely satisfy basic epidemiological criteria for causality, and are, hence, difficult to interpret. Moreover, the findings of several well-designed studies have been inconsistent. Thus, while the experimental data suggest an oncogenic potential for HPV, the human data remain limited (Muñoz *et al.*, 1988).

Oral contraceptives

The relationship between oral contraceptives (OC) and cervical neoplasia has been extensively studied with conflicting results. This may be partly due to the fact that OC use is highly correlated with other key risk factors, such as number of sexual partners, age at first intercourse, screening history, etc. Some case-control studies show a moderate increase in risk for both squamous cell and adenocarcinoma of the cervix (Brinton *et al.*, 1987) but others do not (Peters *et al.*, 1986; Parazzini *et al.*, 1988). Further, the degree of adjustment for confounders varies among studies. Thus, a cohort study which showed an increased risk among ever-users, despite correction for social class, parity, screening history, history of STD and smoking did not adjust for sexual behavioral variables (Beral *et al.*, 1988).

Barrier contraceptives

A protective effect of barrier contraceptives has been noted in some studies (Peters *et al.*, 1986) which is consistent with the hypothesis of a sexually transmitted agent.

Genital hygiene

Poor genital hygiene has been associated with an increased risk of cervical cancer in Indian women (Jayant *et al.*, 1987). No consistent causal relationship has been found in the USA, nor with vaginal douching (Brinton, 1987; Peters *et al.*, 1986).

Male circumcision

Low rates in Jewish women have been ascribed to early circumcision in males. In populations where males are circumcised around puberty, e.g. Muslim and African, cervical cancer rates in females tend to be somewhat lower than in other groups of similar reproductive habits where males are not circumcised. Evaluation of this association may be complicated by difficulties in defining circumcision status. Thus, in a recent study in Latin America, circumcision as assessed by physical examination did not affect the risk of cervical cancer in monogamous women, but poor penile hygiene did increase the risk (Brinton *et al.*, 1989).

Tobacco smoking

Since tobacco smoking correlates with the key sexual variables, epidemiological studies investigating its role in cervical carcinogenesis have yielded conflicting results (Brinton *et al.*, 1986; Peters *et al.*, 1986; IARC, 1986). Adjustment for potential confounders can be only partial since adjustment for other as yet unknown agents is not possible (Muñoz & Bosch, 1989).

Other factors

An increased risk associated with primary and acquired immunodeficiencies has been suggested, as has a protective effect of beta-carotene or other unidentified components of a diet rich in vegetables, but the evidence is not conclusive.

41.6   Relevant laboratory studies

These have largely related to the identification of biological agents (Chapter 17). The significance of early hormonal studies in mice is unclear.

41.7   Attributable risks

Since the AR for the suspected infectious causal agents cannot be determined, evaluation of the significance of other suspected risk factors is not yet possible.

41.8   Conclusions

The data suggest that a sexually transmitted agent, notably HPV, may be the major cause of cervical cancer, although the evidence is not yet conclusive. Thus, while the future development of a viral vaccine is attractive, its effectiveness remains speculative. If a viral etiology is confirmed, the perspectives for primary prevention through vaccination would change. In the meantime, prevention can be implemented by well-conducted screening programs and by modification of sexual behavior that facilitates the transmission of putative infectious agent(s), such as use of condoms.

41.9   Vaginal adenocarcinoma

Tumors of the vagina are exceedingly rare. In the 1970s, a small epidemic of clear cell adenocarcinomas was reported in young females reaching a peak between 17 and 19 years of age. These arose in the offspring of women treated during pregnancy with large doses of diethylstilbestrol (DES) to prevent spontaneous abortion (Herbst *et al.*, 1975*a, b*). As the treatment proved to be ineffective, it was discontinued and these tumors have essentially disappeared. The possibility of further occurrence in adults, who were previously exposed, although improbable, cannot as yet be completely excluded. The association between reproductive factors and adenocarcinoma of the cervix is not clear, being reported in some studies (Parazzini *et al.*, 1988) but not in others (Brinton *et al.*, 1987) (Chapter 11). Minor developmental abnormalities of the

vagina possibly relevant to pathogenesis have also been found in offspring
without cancer (IARC, 1979).

41.10   References

Beral, V., Hannaford, P. & Kay, C. (1988). Oral contraceptive use and malignancies of the
genital tract. Results from the Royal College of General Practitioners Oral Contraceptive
Study. *Lancet*, **ii**, 1331–5.

Brinton, L.A., Schairer, C., Haenszel, W., Stolley, P., Lehman, H.F., Levine, R. & Savitz,
D.A. (1986). Cigarette smoking and invasive cervical cancer. *JAMA*, **255**, 3265–9.

Brinton, L.A., Tashima, K.T., Lehman, H.F., Levine, R.S., Mallin, K., Savitz, D.A., Stolley,
P.D. & Fraumeni, J.F., Jr. (1987). Epidemiology of cervical cancer by cell type. *Cancer
Res.*, **47**, 1706–11.

Brinton, L.A., Reeves, W.C., Brenes, M.M., Herrero, R., Gaitan, E., Tenorio, F., Garcia,
M.R., Rawls, W.E. (1989). The male factor in the etiology of cervical cancer among
sexually monogamous women. *Int. J. Cancer*, **44**, 199–203.

Herbst, A.L., Poskanzer, D.C., Robboy, S.J., Friedlander, L. & Scully, R.E. (1975a).
Prenatal exposure to stilbestrol. A prospective comparison of exposed female offspring
with unexposed controls. *New Engl. J. Med.*, **292**, 334–9.

Herbst, A.L., Scully, R.E. & Robboy, S.J. (1975b). Vaginal adenosis and other
diethylstilbestrol related abnormalities. *Clin. Obstet. Gynecol.*, **18**, 185–94.

IARC (1979). *IARC Monographs on the Evaluation of the Carcinogenic Risk of Chemicals to
Humans*, Sex Hormones (II), volume 21. Lyon: International Agency for Research on
Cancer.

IARC (1986). *IARC Monographs on the Evaluation of the Carcinogenic Risk of Chemicals to
Humans*, Tobacco smoking, volume 38. Lyon: International Agency for Research on
Cancer.

Jayant, K., Notani, P.N., Gadre, V.V., Gulati, S.S. & Shah, P.R. (1987). Personal hygiene
in groups with varied cervical cancer rates: a study in Bombay. *Ind. J. Cancer*, **24**, 47–52.

Muir, C., Waterhouse, J., Mack, T., Powell, J. & Whelan, Sh. (eds.) (1987). *Cancer Incidence
in Five Continents*, volume V, IARC Scientific Publication No. 88. Lyon: International
Agency for Research on Cancer.

Muñoz, N., Bosch, X. & Kaldor, J.M. (1988). Does human papillomavirus cause cervical
cancer? The state of the epidemiological evidence. *Br. J. Cancer*, **57**, 1–5.

Muñoz, N. & Bosch, F.X. (1989). Epidemiology of cervical cancer. In *Human Papillomavirus
and Cervical Cancer*, IARC Scientific Publications No. 94, ed. N. Muñoz, F.X. Bosch &
O.M. Jensen, pp. 9–39. Lyon: International Agency for Research on Cancer.

Parazzini, I., La Vecchia, C., Negri, E., Fasoli, M. & Ceccheti, G. (1988). Risk Factors for
adenocarcinoma of the cervix: a case-control study. *Br. J. Cancer*, **57**, 201–4.

Parkin, D.M., Läärä, E. & Muir, C.S. (1988). Estimates of the worldwide frequency of
sixteen major cancers in 1980. *Int. J. Cancer*, **41**, 184–97.

Peters, R.K., Thomas, D., Hagan, D.G., Mack, T.M. & Henderson, B.E. (1986). Risk
factors for invasive cervical cancer among Latins and non-Latins in Los Angeles County.
J. Nat. Cancer Inst., **77**, 1063–77.

42

Choriocarcinoma

ICD-9 181

42.1 Introduction

These rare tumors, although formerly fairly common in South East Asia, now appear to be declining in incidence.

42.2 Histology, classification and diagnosis

Choriocarcinoma arises from the trophoblastic epithelium of the placenta. It frequently, but not invariably, follows a hydatidiform mole, and invades maternal tissues. Very rarely, these cancers may arise in the mediastinum, the ovary, and the testis.

The International Classification of Diseases (ICD) regards only tumors denoted as choriocarcinomas as being classifiable to this rubric. The invasive or so-called malignant hydatidiform mole (chorioadenoma destruens) is assigned to tumors of uncertain behavior. The diagnostic criterion which distinguishes these two entities is the presence of chorionic villi in the latter. Diagnosis is made either through examination of endometrial scrapings or metastatic deposits, or through demonstration of increased chorionic gonadotrophin in urine.

42.3 Descriptive epidemiology
Incidence and time trends

The incidence rates for this tumor are usually very low, around 0.1 or less. They tend to be somewhat higher in South East Asia, for example, in Rizal province, of the Philippines (0.7) and in Chinese in Singapore and Shanghai (0.5).

Some registries, however, include malignant mole with chorio-carcinoma. Shanmugaratnam *et al.* (1971) calculated age-standardized rates for histologically diagnosed choriocarcinoma for Chinese and Malays in Singapore as 1.0 and 1.2 respectively. The rates for histologically diagnosed malignant trophoblastic disease (both choriocarcinoma and invasive mole) were 18 per 100,000 live births and still-births. Comparable figures for Connecticut, Norway and Sweden were 2, 6 and 4.

Data on hydatidiform mole – the common precursor – are not collected by most cancer registries – Sweden is a notable exception.

The incidence of choriocarcinoma seems to be falling in Asia, and modern chemotherapy has substantially reduced mortality.

Age and sex distribution
Most of these pregnancy-related tumors occur in women of child-bearing age.

42.4   Etiological inferences
High Asian rates suggest the possibility of factors relating to prenatal events.

42.5   Known and suspected causes
The causes are essentially unknown (Bagshawe & Lawler, 1982; Bracken, 1987; Buckley *et al.*, 1988; Messerli *et al.*, 1985). Pregnancies with a hydatidiform mole are about 1000 times more likely to progress to choriocarcinoma than non-molar pregnancies. An increased frequency is observed following pregnancies in mothers over 40 (La Vecchia *et al.*, 1984). The higher rates observed in South East Asia may be linked to the human leukocyte antigen (HLA) profile but data are inconsistent.

Chromosomal changes
About 25% of hydatidiform moles are described as *partial*, i.e. they are triploid, the extra chromosomes being usually paternally derived. These have not so far been demonstrated to be associated with subsequent choriocarcinoma. The *complete* hydatidiform mole is diploid but all chromosomes are of paternal origin, the cytoplasm being maternally derived as in normal conception. It has been suggested that the rare heterozygous complete moles arising by dispermy, i.e. the fertilization of an anucleated ovum by two sperm are more likely to give rise to choriocarcinoma (Fisher *et al.*, 1988).

42.6   Relevant laboratory studies
Laboratory studies have not been of value in determining etiology.

42.7 Attributable risks

The attributable risk for choriocarcinoma is unknown at this time.

42.8 Conclusions

Recent decreases in Asia have been ascribed to improved diet or to better antenatal care, but there are no studies to substantiate these possibilities.

42.9 References

Bagshawe, K.D. & Lawler, S.D. (1982). Choriocarcinoma. In *Cancer Epidemiology and Prevention*, ed. D. Schottenfeld & J.F. Fraumeni, Jr., pp. 909–24. Philadelphia: W.B. Saunders.

Bracken, M.B. (1987). Incidence and aetiology of hydatidiform mole: An epidemiological review. *Br. J. Obstet. Gynaecol.*, **94**, 1123–35.

Buckley, J.D., Henderson, B.E., Morrow, C.P., Hammond, C.B., Kohorn, E.I. & Austin, D.F. (1988). Case-control study of gestational choriocarcinoma. *Cancer Res.*, **48**, 1004–10.

Fisher, R.A., Lawler, S.D., Povey S. & Bagshawe, K.D. (1988). Genetically homozygous choriocarcinoma following pregnancy with hydatidiform mole. *Br. J. Cancer*, **58**, 788–92.

La Vecchia, C., Parazzsini, F., Decarli, A., Francheschi, S., Fasoli, M., Favalli, G., Negri, E. & Pampallona, S. (1984). Age of parents and risk of gestational trophoblastic disease. *J. Natl. Cancer Inst.*, **73**, 639–42.

Messerli, M.L., Lilienfeld, A.M., Parmley, T., Woodruff, J.D. & Rosenshein, N.B. (1985). Risk factors for gestational trophoblastic neoplasia. *Am. J. Obstet. Gynecol.*, **153**, 294-300.

Muir, C., Waterhouse, J., Mack, T., Powell, J. & Whelan, S. (eds.) (1987). *Cancer Incidence in Five Continents*, volume V, IARC Scientific Publication No. 88. Lyon: International Agency for Research on Cancer.

Shanmugaratnam, K., Muir, C.S., Tow, S.H., *et al.* (1971). Rates per 100,000 births and incidence of choriocarcinoma and malignant mole in Singapore Chinese and Malays. Comparison with Connecticut, Norway and Sweden. *Int. J. Cancer*, **8**, 165–75.

43

Endometrium (corpus uteri)

ICD-9 182

43.1   Introduction
Cancer of the corpus uteri is twice as common in the developed as in the developing world and is apparently very rare in Africa. Globally it is one-third as frequent as cervical cancer.

43.2   Histology, classification and diagnosis
These tumors are predominantly adenocarcinomas. The marked rise in endometrial cancer that occurred following estrogen replacement therapy was not accompanied by an equivalent increase in mortality. This suggests that certain types of endometrial hyperplasia may mimic malignancy or represent carcinoma *in situ*. Despite the frequency of benign fibromas, fibrosarcomas of the corpus uteri are rare.

43.3   Descriptive epidemiology
Incidence
The highest reported incidence is from La Plata in Argentina. Rates in the range of 15 to 25 are found in US whites, in Hawaii and in much of Canada (Fig. 43.1). Within the USA, rates in blacks tend to be half those of whites. In Europe, rates are between 10 to 15, being somewhat lower in southern Ireland and the UK. The lowest rates, in the 3 to 5 range or even lower, are found in Asian and in African populations. In Israel, the incidence in Jews born in Europe or America (12.5) is higher than in those born in Africa or Asia (6.1) and in Israel (8.9) The Chinese and Japanese in the USA experience rates which are more than four times those in China and Japan.

Whereas mortality rates from cancer of the corpus uteri have shown large declines, incidence trends are more variable. In the United States, a

Fig. 43.1 Incidence rates around 1980: Corpus uteri (ICD-9 182).

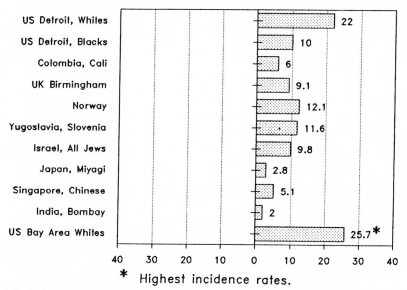

(after Muir *et al.*, 1987)

substantial increase in incidence, but not mortality, notably in ages 55–64, occurred in the 1970s due to the use of post-menopausal estrogens (ERT). Incidence rates declined to, or below, previous levels after use of these drugs ceased (Henderson *et al.*, 1988).

Age distribution

Although, in most populations, the incidence of endometrial cancer rises rapidly until age 50 and thereafter increases at a much reduced rate, most tumors appear after the menopause.

43.4   Etiological inferences

The wide range in incidence observed between countries suggests the influence of exogenous factors, which probably operate indirectly through endogenous hormonal factors. These effects appear different in pre- and post-menopausal women. Current hypotheses do not, however, explain fully the much lower incidence found in Africa as compared to North America and Europe. The association with estrogen replacement therapy (ERT) is consistent with a promoting effect (Hulka *et al.*, 1980).

43.5   Known and suspected causes
There are a number of excellent reviews (Wynder *et al.*, 1966, La Vecchia *et al.*, 1984, De Waard, 1982). Henderson *et al.* (1988) have discussed the role of hormones in depth. It is usual to distinguish between pre- and post-menopausal tumors.

Endogenous factors
The cancer is more common in unmarried and nulliparous women. The most important associated host factor is obesity, the tall obese woman being at even greater risk. This is believed due to the increased endogenous production of estradiol in such women (Enriori & Reforzo-Membrives, 1984). Amenorrhea, low progesterone, and irregular menses are all associated with obesity. According to Henderson *et al.*, (1988), in pre-menopausal women, the increased risk is due to induction of anovulation with resulting progesterone deficiency. Other factors include later menopause, heavy menstrual bleeding and pre-menstrual breast swelling, again suggesting that the etiological base may be an increase in certain endogenous hormones also partly dependent on obesity. Pike (1987) considers the menopause to have a major protective effect reducing the hypothetical rate by four- to eight-fold at 70 years. Studies have also reported an association between diabetes and endometrial cancer, possibly due to the relationship with obesity. Several authors have suggested an association between carcinomas of the breast and corpus uteri. MacMahon *et al.* (1973) concluded that there may be no single causal association between these diseases, but that there is possibly a sub-group of women with endocrine characteristics predisposing to both conditions.

Exogenous factors
The important role of exogenous estrogens was shown with the demonstration that oral conjugated equine estrogens, widely administered for replacement therapy (ERT), caused a marked rise in endometrial cancer (Shapiro *et al.*, 1985; Hunt *et al.*, 1987). Increases were also demonstrated following use of sequential oral contraceptives (OC), which deliver an unopposed estrogen during most of the monthly cycle. This increase was not found with combination OCs. When it was demonstrated that incorporation of progesterone prevented the effect of estrogens, this led to increased research on hormone inhibiting effects (Henderson *et al.*, 1982; Kreiger *et al.*, 1986, IARC, 1979). These small cancer 'epidemics' disappeared following changes in the drugs used for ERT and oral contraception.

Miscellaneous

Women with Stein–Leventhal syndrome, i.e. infertility, ano-vulation, obesity and/or hirsutism, are at a high risk.

A small number of tumors are associated with ovarian dysgenesis in young females and granulosa-cell tumors of the ovary. The latter produce estrogenic hormones.

It has been suggested that smoking is associated with a reduced risk due to its inhibiting effects on estrogen metabolism (Franks *et al.*, 1987).

Apart from its role in obesity, the influence of diet remains uncertain (La Vecchia *et al.*, 1986).

43.6 Relevant laboratory studies

These are largely directed to studying the role of endocrine metabolism in endometrial hyperplasia and neoplasia.

43.7 Attributable risks (AR)

While there is general agreement on risk factors (Ewertz *et al.*, 1988), no meaningful ARs are possible. The number due to ovarian dysgenesis is very small, and ERT related tumors are now rare.

43.8 Conclusion

Body mass and exogenous estrogen use are the main determinants of endometrial cancer risk, but they are insufficient to explain the marked geographical variations that occur between Africa and more industrialized states.

43.9 References

De Waard, F. (1982). Uterine corpus. In *Cancer Epidemiology and Prevention*, ed. D. Schottenfeld & J.F. Fraumeni, Jr., pp. 901–8. Philadelphia: W.B. Saunders.

Enriori, C.L. & Reforzo-Membrives, J. (1984). Peripheral aromatization as a risk factor for breast and endometrial cancer in postmenopausal women: A review. *Gynecol. Oncol.*, **17**, 1–21.

Ewertz, M., Schou, G. & Boice, J.D., Jr. (1988). The joint effect of risk factors on endometrial cancer. *Eur. J. Cancer Clin. Oncol.*, **24**, 189–94.

Franks, A.L., Kendrick, J.S. & Tyler, C.W., Jr. (1987). Postmenopausal smoking, estrogen replacement therapy, and the risk of endometrial cancer. *Am. J. Obstet. Gynecol.*, **156**, 20–3.

Henderson, B.E., Ross, R., & Bernstein, L. (1988). Estrogens as a cause of human cancer: the Richard and Hinda Rosenthal Foundation Award Lecture. *Cancer Res.*, **48**, 246–53.

Hulka, B.S., Fowler, W.C. & Kaufman, D.G., Grimson, R.C., Greenberg, B.G., Hogue, C.J.R., Berger, G.S. & Pulliam, C.C. (1980). Estrogen and endometrial cancer: cases and two control groups from North Carolina. *Am. J. Obstet. Gynecol.*, **137**, 92–101.

Hunt, K., Vessey, M., McPherson, K. & Coleman, M. (1987). Long-term surveillance of mortality and cancer incidence in women receiving hormone replacement therapy. *Br. J. Obstet. Gynaecol.*, **94**, 620–35.

IARC (1979). *IARC Monographs on the Evaluation of the Carcinogenic Risk of Chemicals to Humans*, Sex hormones (II), volume 21. Lyon: International Agency for Research on Cancer.

Kreiger, N., Marrett, L.D., Clarke, E.A., Hilditch, S. & Woolever, C.A. (1986). Risk factors for adenomatous endometrial hyperplasia: A case-control study. *Am. J. Epidemiol.*, **123**, 291–301.

La Vecchia, C., Decarli, A., Fasoli, M. & Gentile, A. (1986). Nutrition and diet in the etiology of endometrial cancer. *Cancer*, **57**. 1248–53.

La Vecchia, C., Franceschi, S., Decarli, A., Gallus, G. & Tognoni, G. (1984). Risk factors for endometrial cancer at different ages. *J. Natl. Cancer Inst.*, **73**, 667–71.

MacMahon, B., Cole, P. & Brown, J. (1973). Etiology of human breast cancer: A review. *J. Natl. Cancer Inst.*, **50**, 21–42.

Muir, C., Waterhouse, J., Mack, T., Powell, J. & Whelan, S. (eds.) (1987). *Cancer Incidence in Five Continents*, volume V, IARC Scientific Publication No. 88. Lyon: International Agency for Research on Cancer.

Pike, M.C. (1987). Age-related factors in cancers of the breast, ovary, and endometrium. *J. Chronic Dis.*, **40** (Suppl), 59s-69s.

Shapiro, S., Kelly, J.P., Rosenberg, L., Kaufman, D.W., Helmrich, S.P., Rosenshein, N.B.. Lewis, J.L., Jr., Knapp, R.C., Stolley, P.D. & Schottenfeld, D. (1985). Risk of localized and widespread endometrial cancer in relation to recent and discontinued use of conjugated estrogens. *N. Engl. J. Med.*, **313**, 969–72.

Wynder, E.L., Escher, G.C. & Mantel, N. (1966). An epidemiological investigation of cancer of the endometrium. *Cancer*, **19**, 489–520.

44

Ovary

ICD-9 183

44.1 Introduction

Although ovarian cancer is only moderately frequent, it is the most common cause of death from gynecological neoplasms in western countries. The range of geographical variation is modest.

44.2 Histology, classification and diagnosis

The majority of tumors are serous or pseudomucinous cystadenocarcinomas which arise from celomic epithelium. Malignant germ cell tumors, such as granulosa-cell carcinoma, are comparatively rare, and occur at younger ages. As many cancers remain clinically silent for a considerable period, prognosis tends to be poor.

44.3 Descriptive epidemiology
Incidence

Highest rates are observed in Hawaiian and Pacific Island Polynesians (25.8). In contrast, rates in New Zealand Maoris (10.9) are much lower, the incidence being the same as in non-Maoris. The highest rates reported from Europe are 17.3 in the Ardeche in France and just over 15 for Norway, Sweden and migrants to Israel born in Europe or North America. Most rates in Europe and North America range between 8 and 12. Rates for US blacks are about two-thirds of those for whites (Fig. 44.1). While women in Asia have a relatively low incidence, in the 5 to 7 range, Chinese and Japanese who reside in the USA tend to show slightly higher rates.

In most registries, few changes over time have been observed but slight rises have been reported in both Japanese and Singapore Chinese.

Fig. 44.1 Incidence rates around 1980: Ovary, etc. (ICD-9 183).

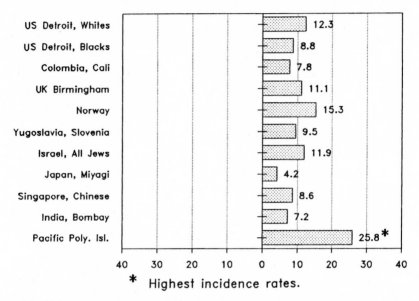

(after Muir *et al.*, 1987)

Age distribution
Incidence rates rise smoothly with age.

44.4   Etiological inferences
The moderate differences in geographical variations and the higher frequency in infertile women suggest that endogenous host factors related to reproduction, including hormonal status, are more important than environmental factors related to diet or chemical exposures. Some of the geographical variation is probably dependent on the proportion of nulliparous women or those with few pregnancies in a population (Ewertz & Kjaer, 1988; Voigt *et al.*, 1986).

44.5   Known and suspected causes
The causes of ovarian cancer remain essentially unknown. Suspected factors have been extensively reviewed (Armstrong, 1982; Cramer *et al.*, 1983; Heintz *et al.*, 1985; Henderson *et al.*, 1988; Weiss, 1982). Pike (1987) has compared age related factors in ovary, breast and endometrium.

Reproductive and host factors

These cancers are more frequent in women who find it difficult to conceive (Whittemore *et al.*, 1989) and the risk increases with years of unprotected intercourse. Phenotypic females with Y chromosomes in their genomes show increased gonadal malignancy. A small familial association has been observed (Schildkraut & Thompson, 1988).

It has long been suspected that excessive gonadotropin stimulation is involved. Multiple pregnancies, independent of age at first pregnancy, appear to be protective. Further, oral contraceptives (OC), which reduce gonadotropin production also effectively reduce the incidence (CDC, 1987). Artificial menopause is associated with a reduced risk (Hartge *et al.*, 1988). Mumps and resultant oophoritis are also held to have a protective effect. These findings have given rise to the hypothesis of 'incessant ovulation', especially in nulliparous women (Casagrande *et al.*, 1979).

The presence of dysgenetic gonads predispose to germ cell tumors which form, however, a very small proportion of ovarian cancers.

Miscellaneous

No convincing evidence for a role for diet or alcohol has been observed (Byers *et al.*, 1983; La Vecchia *et al.*, 1987). Recently, however, Cramer *et al.* (1989) have reviewed the hyper-gonadotropic hypothesis due to lack of pituitary feedback or ovarian failure. Galactose consumption and a key enzyme involved in its metabolism, galactose-1-phosphate uridyl transferase, have been linked with hypergonadotropic gonadotropism. They found a significant trend for increasing lactose/transferase ratio in the blood and suggested that lactose may be a dietary risk factor and transferase a genetic risk factor. An etiological role for asbestos has not been confirmed.

44.6   Relevant laboratory studies

Ovarian tumors can be produced by radiation and by certain chemicals, but as the majority are of germ cell origin, their relevance to humans is uncertain. Gonadotropin stimulation has been shown to play a role in both radiation and chemically induced tumors in animals. Follicular fluid has been shown to have a strong mitogenic effect on ovarian epithelium.

44.7   Attributable risks

Early and frequent parity may be associated with a reduction in risk over 50%.

44.8   Conclusions

Endometrial and ovarian cancers seem to be influenced by endogenous and exogenous steroid hormones. Reproduction-associated factors, including parity, have a role but it has not yet been possible to combine the available data into a unified hypothesis.

44.9   References

Armstrong, B. (1982). Endocrine factors in human carcinogenesis. In *Host Factors in Human Carcinogenesis*, IARC Scientific Publications, Vol. 39, ed. H. Bartsch, B. Armstrong, & W. Davis, pp. 193–221. Lyon: International Agency for Research on Cancer.

Byers, T., Marshall, J., Graham, S., Mettlin, C. & Swanson, M. (1983). A case-control study of dietary and nondietary factors in ovarian cancer. *J. Nat!. Cancer Inst.* **71**, 681–6.

CDC (Cancer and Steroid Hormone Study of the Centers for Disease Control and National Institute of Child Health and Human Development.) (1987). The reduction in risk of ovarian cancer associated with oral-contraceptives. *N. Engl. J. Med.*, **316**, 650–5.

Casagrande, J.T., Pike, M.C., Ross, R.K., Louie, E.W., Roy, S. & Henderson, B.E. (1979). 'Incessant ovulation' and ovarian cancer. *Lancet*, **ii**, 170–2.

Cramer, D.W., Hutchinson, G.B., Welch, W.R., Scully, R.E. & Ryan, K.J. (1983). Determinants of ovarian cancer risk. I. Reproductive experiences and family history. *J. Natl. Cancer Inst.*, **71**, 711–16.

Cramer, D.W., Harlow, B.L., Willett, W.C., Welch, W.R., Bell, D.A., Scully, R.E., Ng, W.G., Knapp, R.C. (1989). Galactose consumption and metabolism in relation to the risk of ovarian cancer. *Lancet*, **ii**, 66–71.

Ewertz, M. & Kjaer, S.K. (1988). Ovarian cancer incidence and mortality in Denmark, 1943–1982. *Int. J. Cancer*, **42**, 690–6.

Hartge, P., Hoover, R., McGowan, L., Lesher, L. & Norris, H.J. (1988). Menopause and ovarian cancer. *Am. J. Epidemiol.*, **127**, 990–8.

Heintz, A.P.M., Hacker, N.F. & Lagasse, L.D. (1985). Epidemiology and etiology of ovarian cancer: a review. *Obstet. Gynecol.*, **66**, 127–35.

Henderson, B.E., Ross, R. & Bernstein, L. (1988). Estrogens as a cause of human cancer: the Richard and Hinda Rosenthal Foundation Award Lecture. *Cancer Res.*, **48**, 246–53.

La Vecchia, C., Decarli, A., Negri, E., Parazzini, F., Gentile, A., Cecchetti, G., Fasoli, M. & Franceschi, S. (1987). Dietary factors and the risk of epithelial ovarian cancer. *J. Natl. Cancer Inst.*, **79**, 663–9.

Muir, C., Waterhouse, J., Mack, T., Powell, J. & Whelan, S. (eds.) (1987). *Cancer Incidence in Five Continents*, volume V, IARC Scientific Publication No. 88. Lyon: International Agency for Research on Cancer.

Pike, M.C. (1987). Age-related factors in cancers of the breast, ovary, and endometrium. *J. Chron. Dis.*, **40**, 59s–69s.

Schildkraut, J.M. & Thompson, W.D. (1988). Familial ovarian cancer: A population-based case-control study. *Am. J. Epidemiol.*, **128**, 456–66.

Voigt, L.F., Harlow, B.L. & Weiss, N.S. (1986). The influence of age at first birth and parity on ovarian cancer risk. *Am. J. Epidemiol.*, **124**, 490–1.

Weiss, N.S. (1982). Ovary. In *Cancer Epidemiology and Prevention*, ed. D. Schottenfeld & J.F. Fraumeni, Jr., pp. 871–80. Philadelphia: W.B. Saunders.

Whittemore, A.S., Wu, M.L., Paffenbarger, R.S., Jr., Sarles, D.L., Kampert, J.B., Grosser, S., Jung, D.L., Ballon, S., Hendrickson, M. & Mohle-Boetani, J. (1989). Epithelial ovarian cancer and the ability to conceive. *Cancer Res.*, **49**, 4047–52.

45

Prostate

ICD-9 185

45.1 Introduction

Prostatic cancer is the most common neoplasm in elderly males in many countries. There are large ethnic and international differences, the disease being particularly common in American blacks. The cause is essentially unknown.

45.2 Histology, classification and diagnosis

Routine histopathological examination of the prostate at autopsy or after resection reveals an age-dependent high frequency of small *latent carcinomas*, which are not clinically manifest. These represent a step in the progression of the disease. Association of prostatic cancer with benign adenomatous hyperplasia has not been established with certainty (Armenian *et al.*, 1974).

45.3 Descriptive epidemiology

The interpretation of time trends and incidence levels is complicated by local practices concerning registration of *latent* cancers, discovered incidentally at resection or autopsy. In Malmo, Sweden the incidence rate of prostate cancer was 50% higher than the national level. In the latter, only 7.6% of 298 cases were discovered at autopsy compared to 36.4% of 177 in Malmo (National Board of Health and Welfare, 1984).

Incidence

The highest rates of clinical prostatic cancer have been recorded in the black population of the USA. Rates as high as 87.8 in Alameda County, California, and over 70 elsewhere, are often double those among whites in the same locality. Intermediate rates in the 30 to 50 range are found in Connecticut whites, Canada, South America, Scandinavia,

Fig. 45.1 Incidence rates around 1980: Prostate (ICD-9 185).

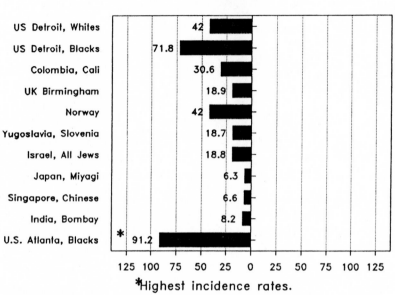

■ Males

US Detroit, Whites	42
US Detroit, Blacks	71.8
Colombia, Cali	30.6
UK Birmingham	18.9
Norway	42
Yugoslavia, Slovenia	18.7
Israel, All Jews	18.8
Japan, Miyagi	6.3
Singapore, Chinese	6.6
India, Bombay	8.2
U.S. Atlanta, Blacks	*91.2

125 100 75 50 25 0 25 50 75 100 125

*Highest incidence rates.

(after Muir *et al.*, 1987)

Switzerland and Oceania, whereas lower rates, around 20, are seen in most European countries and in the Jewish population of Israel. Rates in South African blacks are similar to Denmark. Very low rates, below 10, are present in China, Japan, India, other Asian countries, and in the Middle East (Fig. 45.1).

Japanese migrants to the USA have experienced a marked increase in prostatic cancer, although the rates of the Japanese in San Francisco Bay Area (16.5) and in Los Angeles (22.8) are still considerably lower than in whites. The contrasts between US Chinese and those elsewhere are even greater. Polish migrants to the USA also show increased mortality rates. Despite the large variations in clinical cancer incidence, the prevalence of latent cancer shows only modest geographical variation. In many countries, such cancers may be found in over 50% of males over 80 years.

Time trends

The incidence and mortality of prostatic cancer have been rising over time in many areas. While an average annual increase of 4.9% has been observed in Singapore Chinese and of 1.7% in the US black population, a decrease in mortality in American blacks is anticipated as reduced rates have recently been observed in the younger birth cohorts

(Fig. 2.6). Similar observations have been made in Australia and in England and Wales. It is not clear to what extent increased morbidity rates may be related to more frequent diagnosis of latent tumors following surgical biopsy.

Age distribution
Both clinical and latent tumors are rare before the age of 50 years but the incidence rises fairly steeply thereafter.

45.4   Etiological inferences
The prevalence of latent prostatic cancer seems to be of the same order in countries with high and low clinical cancer rates (Breslow *et al.*, 1977). Accordingly, a promoting or enhancing role for endogenous or exogenous factors in high-risk populations is considered probable. However, in view of the marked difference in incidence among blacks and whites in the USA (Fig. 45.1), the possibility of ethnic factors cannot be ignored or excluded (Blair & Fraumeni, 1978; Ross *et al.*, 1987).

45.5   Known and suspected causes
Diet
There have been attempts to associate prostatic cancer and diet (Hirayama, 1979; Schuman *et al.*, 1982; Ross *et al.*, 1987; Zaridze & Boyle, 1987). An association between total fat intake and mortality has been reported. The highest mortality in American whites is from counties with the greatest per capita intake of beef products, milk products, fats and oils. Dietary factors have been implicated as partly responsible for the significant changes that have occurred in Japanese migrants to the USA and for the relatively lower frequency in certain countries, as in parts of Africa. Retinoids and vitamin A have been suggested as enhancing the risk (Kolonel *et al.*, 1988) but others disagree (Kaul *et al.*, 1987; Ohno *et al.*, 1988). Dietary changes do not explain the existing differences between blacks and whites, nor general geographical variations in incidence in North America. The NAS report (1982) was equivocal in an evaluation of the dietary relationship, but Kolonel *et al.* (1988) suggest that, in Hawaii, several different dietary components are involved independently.

Endogenous hormones
Hormonal stimulation (estrogen and testosterone) and increased sexual activity have been associated with prostatic cancer (Hill *et al.*, 1982; Ross *et al.*, 1987). An increased incidence in cirrhotic patients, characterized by hyper-estrogenism, has been reported. While differences

in hormonal profiles have been demonstrated between North American and African men which can plausibly be related to prostate cancer incidence (Hill *et al.*, 1982), other studies are equivocal (Nomura *et al.*, 1988). Some suggest a possible relationship to circulating levels of testosterone (Chapter 18). Dietary factors however, have a significant influence on hormonal status which is thus difficult to evaluate *per se*.

Occupation and socio-economic class

There is little convincing evidence that prostatic cancer is directly related to specific work-place exposures. Earlier reports on the role of cadmium have not been confirmed (Zaridze & Boyle, 1987). There is considerable evidence that individuals in higher socio-economic groups have an increased frequency of prostatic cancer with higher rates reported in clergymen, managers, and farmers, in whom no common factor has been identified.

Viruses

A history of sexually transmitted disease is a strong predictor of risk in blacks and whites (Ross *et al.*, 1987). Virus-like particles in human prostatic cancers, and reported increases in cervical cancer in the wives of patients, led to suggestions of a viral transmission. This has never been confirmed.

Sexual habits

Evidence of the role of sexual activity is not clear-cut, but a higher risk is reported among married males a number of years after vasectomy (Honda *et al.*, 1988). These relationships have not been confirmed.

45.6   Relevant laboratory studies

Most studies largely relate to diagnosis and are not etiologically informative. While the rat prostate is susceptible to endocrine manipulation, such studies have not so far been helpful in evaluating the human disease.

45.7   Attributable risks

No meaningful comment can be made.

45.8   Conclusions

Although the role of endocrine status in prostatic cancer has some biological plausibility, the influence of environmental factors, including diet, remains unclear. In the absence of suitable hypotheses for testing, especially in relation to metabolism and promotion, their role probably cannot be elucidated by simple observational studies in humans.

45.9   References

Armenian, H.K., Lilienfeld, A.M., Diamond, E.L., & Bross, I.D.J. (1974). Relation between benign prostatic hyperplasia and cancer of the prostate – a prospective and retrospective study. *Lancet*, **ii**, 115–7.

Blair, A. & Fraumeni, J.F. (1978). Geographic patterns of prostate cancer in the United States. *J. Natl. Cancer Inst.*, **61**, 1379–84.

Breslow, N., Chan, C.W., Dhom, G., Drury, R.A.B., Franks, L.M., Gellei, B., Lee., Y.S., Lundberg, S., Sparke, B., Sternby, N.H. & Tulinius, H. (1977). Latent carcinoma of prostate at autopsy in seven areas. *Int. J. Cancer*, **20**, 680–8.

Hill, P., Wynder, E.L., Garbaczewski, L., Garnes, H. & Walker, A.R. (1982). Response to luteinizing releasing hormone, thyrotrophic releasing hormone, and human chorionic gonadotrophin administration in healthy men at different risks for prostatic cancer and in prostatic cancer patients. *Cancer Res.*, **42**, 2074–80.

Hirayama, T. (1979). Epidemiology of prostate cancer with special reference to the role of diet. *Natl. Cancer Inst. Monogr.*, **53**, 149–55.

Honda, G.D., Bernstein, L., Ross, R.K., Greenland, S., Gerkins, V. & Henderson, B.E. (1988). Vasectomy, cigarette smoking, and age at first sexual intercourse as risk factors for prostate cancer in middle-aged men. *Br. J. Cancer*, **57**, 326–31.

Kaul, L., Heshmat, M.Y., Kovi, J., Jackson, M.A., Jackson, A.G., Jones, G.W., Edson, M., Enterline, J.P., Worrell, R.G. & Perry, S.L. (1987). The role of diet in prostate cancer. *Nutr. Cancer*, **9**, 123–8.

Kolonel, L.N., Yoshizawa, C.N., & Hankin, J.H. (1988). Diet and prostatic cancer: a case-control study in Hawaii. *Am. J. Epidemiol.*, **127**, 999–1012.

Muir, C., Waterhouse, J., Mack, T., Powell, J. & Whelan, S. (eds.) (1987). *Cancer Incidence in Five Continents*, Volume V, IARC Scientific Publication No. 88. Lyon: International Agency for Research on Cancer.

NAS (National Academy of Sciences, Committee on Diet, Nutrition and Cancer) (1982). *Diet, Nutrition, and Cancer*, pp. 17–21. Washington: National Academy Press.

National Board of Health and Welfare (1984). *The Cancer Registry. Cancer incidence in Sweden*, 1981. Stockholm: Socialstuyrelsen.

Nomura, A., Heilbrun, L.K., Stemmermann, G.N. & Judd, H.L. (1988). Prediagnostic serum hormones and the risk of prostate cancer. *Cancer Res.*, **48**, 3515–17.

Ohno, Y., Yoshida, O., Oishi, K., Okada, K., Yamabe, H. & Schroeder, F.H. (1988). Dietary β-carotene and cancer of the prostate: a case-control study. *Cancer Res.*, **48**, 1331–6.

Ross, R.K., Shimizu, H., Paganini-Hill, A., Honda, G. & Henderson, B.E. (1987). Case-control studies of prostate cancer in blacks and whites in Southern California. *J. Natl. Cancer. Inst.*, **78**, 869–74.

Schuman, L.M., Mandel, J.S., Radke, A., Seal, U. & Halberg, F. (1982). Some selected features of the epidemiology of prostatic cancer: Minneapolis-St. Paul, Minnesota case-control study, 1976–1979. In *Trends in Cancer Incidence: Causes and Practical Implications*, ed. K. Magnus, pp. 345–54. New York: Hemisphere Publishing.

Zaridze, D.G. & Boyle, P. (1987). Cancer of the prostate: epidemiology and aetiology. *Br. J. Urol.*, **59**, 493–502.

46

Testis

ICD-9 186

46.1 Introduction

Testicular cancers are relatively uncommon and occur primarily in white males under the age of 50. They are very rare in Africans and Asians.

46.2 Histology, classification and diagnosis

While testicular germ cell cancers predominate, a range of histological types are described by Mostofi (1977) and Schottenfeld and Warshauer (1982). About 50% of tumors are seminomas, 40% embryonal carcinomas and 6% teratomas.

46.3 Descriptive epidemiology

Incidence

The upper range of rates, between 3 and 9, is generally seen in western European countries. Although the highest rates occur in Switzerland (8.3 in Basel; 9.9 in urban Vaud) and in Denmark (7.8), a high rate is also seen in the Maoris (7.9) of New Zealand. Blacks in the USA, with rates around unity, have a much lower incidence than whites, with rates in the range of 3 to 5. The reported incidence of testicular cancer is even lower for African blacks than for American blacks (Fig. 46.1). Despite the accessibility of this site, several reports from Africa (Parkin, 1986) do not describe any such tumors, in contrast to penile cancer. Most rates in Asia are below unity. In several European countries, notably Denmark, the cancer is increasing in incidence.

Mortality rates for the highest socio-economic classes have been shown to be twice those in the lowest (Logan, 1982).

Fig. 46.1 Incidence rates around 1980: Testis (ICD-9 186).

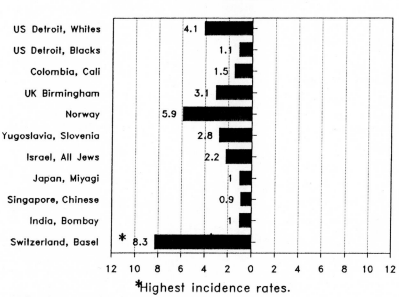

(after Muir *et al.*, 1987)

46.4   Etiological inferences

While geographical variations and higher rates in the upper social classes suggest that environmental factors may play some role, the great rarity of this cancer in both North American blacks and Africans suggest that an ethnic factor may be involved.

46.5   Known and suspected causes

The etiology of testicular cancer is basically unknown but cryptorchidism is a major factor, although the risk varies in different studies (Giwercman *et al.*, 1987). It has been suggested that cryptorchidism has increased in the USA, since the early 1940s, possibly due to the use of estrogen therapy during pregnancy. Although studies are based on small numbers, Moss *et al.*, (1986) believe that exposures to exogenous hormones explain a significant fraction. Henderson *et al.*, (1988) have suggested that the lower incidence of testicular cancer in North American blacks may be due to higher levels of circulating testosterone in black females during the early weeks of gestation. Excess maternal weight has been postulated as a risk factor since sex-hormone-binding globulin levels are decreased and free estrogen levels are increased in obese women. Other possible risk factors have been recently reviewed by Senturia (1987) and Henderson *et al.* (1988). There is evidence of a hereditary factor in some cases of testicular cancer associated with genital dysgenesis (Anderson *et al.*, 1984; Mills *et al.*, 1984; Forman *et al.*, 1990). There is little proof that trauma, or viral infections are involved (see also p. 202).

46.6   Relevant laboratory investigations
Although cadmium chloride can produce testicular tumors in rodents, the relevance of this observation to humans is unknown. There is no supportive epidemiological data.

46.7   Attributable risks
No meaningful observations.

46.8   Conclusions
A number of environmental factors, as well as cryptorchidism, gonadal dysgenesis and genetic influence, give rise to atrophy and dysfunction of the testis. These are believed to be risk factors for testicular cancer, but the biological mechanism as well as the significance of ethnic variations remain obscure.

46.9   References

Anderson, K.C., Li, F.P. & Marchetto, D.J. (1984). Dizygotic twinning, cryptorchism and seminoma in a sibship. *Cancer*, **53**, 374–6.

Forman, D.; Gallagher, R., Møller, H. & Swerdlow, T.J. (1990). Aetiology and Epidemiology of testicular cancer: Report of consensus group. In *Prostate Cancer and Testicular Cancer*, EORTC Genitourinary Group Monograph 7, pp. 245–53. New York: Wiley-Liss, Inc.

Giwercman, A., Grindsted, J., Hansen, B., Jensen, O.M. & Skakkebaek, N.E. (1987). Testicular cancer risk in boys with maldescended testis: a cohort study. *J. Urol.*, **138**, 1214–16.

Henderson, B.E., Ross, R. & Bernstein, L. (1988). Estrogens as a cause of human cancer: the Richard and Hinda Rosenthal Foundation Award Lecture. *Cancer Res.*, **48**, 246–53.

Logan, W.P.D. (1982). *Cancer Mortality of Occupation and Social Class 1851–1971.* IARC Scientific Publication No. 36. Lyon: International Agency for Research on Cancer.

Mills, P.K., Newell, G.R. & Johnson, D.E. (1984). Testicular cancer associated with employment in agriculture and oil and natural gas extraction. *Lancet*, **i**, 207–9.

Moss, A.R., Osmond, D., Bacchetti, P., Torti, F.M. & Gurgin, V. (1986). Hormonal risk factors in testicular cancer. A case-control study. *Am. J. Epidemiol.*, **124**, 39–52.

Mostofi, F. K. (1977). Epidemiology and pathology of tumors of human testis. In *Tumors of Male Genital System*, ed. E. Grundmann & W. Vahlensiek W., pp. 176–95. Berlin: Springer-Verlag.

Parkin, D.M (ed.) (1986). *Cancer Occurrence in Developing Countries*, IARC Scientific Publications No. 75, Lyon: International Agency for Research on Cancer.

Schottenfeld, D. & Warshauer, M.E. (1982). Testis. In *Cancer Epidemiology and Prevention*, ed. D. Schottenfeld & J.F. Fraumeni, Jr., pp. 947–57. Philadelphia: W.B. Saunders.

Senturia, Y.D. (1987). The epidemiology of testicular cancer. *Br. J. Urol.*, **60**, 285–91.

47

Penis and Scrotum

ICD-9 187

47.1   Introduction
Cancers of the penis and scrotum are comparatively rare in western countries but show great geographical and ethnic variation elsewhere.

47.2   Histology, classification and diagnosis
The majority of penile tumors are well-differentiated squamous carcinomas originating on the glans penis or prepuce or occasionally in giant condylomas. Precancerous lesions include Bowen's disease, Bowenoid papulosis and erythroplasia of Queyrat.

47.3   Descriptive epidemiology
Incidence and time trends
The highest incidence rates (5–8) are reported from North-east Brazil, intermediate rates (2.5–3.0) are seen in south Brazil, Colombia and India, rates ranging from 0.0–1.9 in the rest of the world (Figure 47.1). Relative frequency data indicate that cancer of the penis is particularly frequent in certain population groups in Uganda, Latin America and Asia.

Clusters of high rates of both cancer of the cervix and of the penis have been described in China (Li et al., 1982). The incidence rates appear to be decreasing in some Latin American countries but seem stable elsewhere.

Age distribution
The age-specific incidence rates increases progressively with age. This cancer is extremely rare under the age of 30.

Fig. 47.1 Incidence rates around 1980: Penis and scrotum. (ICD-9 187)

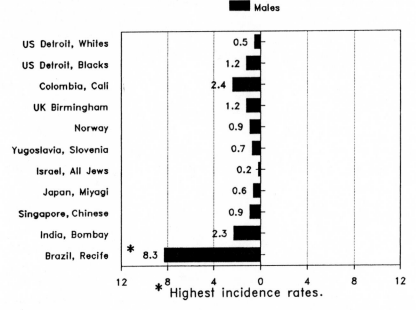

(after Muir *et al.*, 1987)

47.4   Etiological inferences

The most interesting etiological inference is the correlation of penile cancer with lack of circumcision in different religious and ethnic groups. Scrotal cancer is very rare and follows the pattern of non-UV induced skin tumors. Both penile and scrotal cancers are inversely related to socio-economic class, supporting a role for personal hygiene.

47.5   Known and suspected causes

Socio-economic factors

In all countries with a high standard of living, the rate of penile cancer is comparatively low, suggesting a protective role for personal hygiene (Raju *et al.*, 1985).

Occupational factors

As well as tumors observed in chimney sweeps (Pott, 1775), exposures to polycyclic hydrocarbons and mineral and shale oils, have been consistently associated with squamous cell tumors of the scrotum (IARC, 1987). Occupational factors do not seem to play an important role in penile cancer.

Circumcision

There is considerable evidence that where circumcision is performed in infancy, penile cancer is very rare, as among Jews. In contrast, among Muslims and many African tribes who circumcise at a later age, often at puberty, the incidence of cancer appears higher suggesting less complete protection (Hall & Schottenfeld, 1982).

Phimosis and balanitis

A relative risk of 57 (95% CI 14 to 233) was found for history of phimosis and of 2.4 (95% CI 1.0 to 5.8) for history of balanitis after adjusting for confounding variables (Hellberg *et al.*, 1987). The retention of smegma associated with phimosis may explain the increased risk.

Sexual factors

No association with the number of sexual partners was found in a large case-control study (Hellberg *et al.*, 1987). Previous studies have shown, however, that wives of men with cancer of the penis have a 3–6 greater risk of cervical cancer than control women (Graham *et al.*, 1980; Smith et al., 1980), suggesting that a sexually transmitted agent(s) could be implicated in the causation of both tumors.

Viruses

HPV has for long been suspected to be associated with penile carcinoma, based on reports of giant condylomas undergoing malignant degeneration. Recently developed hybridization techniques to detect HPV-DNA have shown that HPV 16 and 18 are found in a high proportion of tumors from Uganda (Dürst *et al.*, 1985) and Brazil (McCance *et al.*, 1986; Villa and Lopes, 1986), but no formal epidemiological studies have been carried out. A high prevalence of penile intra-epithelial neoplasia (PIN) associated with HPV 16 and 33 has also been found in male sexual partners of women with CIN lesions in France (Barrasso *et al.*, 1987). The high rates of PIN contrast with the very low rates of penile cancer in the same populations. Thus, although it is plausible that a virus could be involved in the etiology of penile cancer, convincing evidence is still lacking (Chapter 17).

47.6   Relevant laboratory investigations

Pertinent laboratory studies on HPV are discussed in Chapter 17.

47.7   Conclusions

Cancer of the penis may reflect several factors, especially lack of early circumcision and poor personal hygiene. A sexually transmitted agent is consistent with certain demographic features of this disease.

47.8   References

Barrasso, R., De Brux, J., Croissant, O. & Orth, G. (1987). High prevalence of papilloma virus-associated penile intra-epithelial neoplasia in sexual partners of women with cervical epithelial neoplasia. *N. Engl. J. Med.*, **317**, 916–23.

Dürst M., Kleinheinz, A., Hotz, M. & Gissman, L. (1985). The physical state of human papilloma virus type 16 in benign and malignant genital tumours. *J. Gen. Virol.*, **66**, 1515–22.

Graham, S., Priore, R., Graham, M., Browne, R., Burnett, W. & West D. (1980). Genital cancer in wives of penile cancer patients. *Cancer*, **44**, 1870–4.

Hall, N.E.L. & Schottenfeld, D. (1982). Penis. In *Cancer Epidemiology and Prevention*, ed. D. Schottenfeld & J.F. Fraumeni, Jr., pp. 958–67. Philadelphia: W.B. Saunders.

Hellberg, D., Valentin, J., Eklund, T. & Nilsson, S. (1987). Penile cancer: Is there an epidemiological role for smoking and sexual behavior? *Br. Med. J.*, **295**, 1306–8.

IARC (1987). *IARC Monographs on the Evaluation of Carcinogenic Risks to Humans.* Overall evaluations of carcinogenicity: an updating of IARC monographs volumes 1 to 42, Supplement 7, pp. 252–4, 339–41, 343–4. Lyon: International Agency for Research on Cancer.

Li, J.Y., Li, F.P., Blot, W.J., Miller, R.W. & Fraumeni, J.F. (1982). Correlation between cancers of the uterine cervix and penis in China. *J. Natl. Cancer Inst.* **69**, 1063–5.

McCance, D.J., Kalache, A., Ashdown, K. *et al.* (1986). Human papilloma virus types 16 and 18 in carcinomas of the penis from Brazil. *Int. J. Cancer.* **37**, 55–9.

Muir, C., Waterhouse, J., Mack, T., Powell, J. & Whelan, S. (1987). *Cancer Incidence in Five Continents*, volume V, IARC Scientific Publications No. 88. Lyon: International Agency for Research on Cancer.

Pott, P. (1775). Chirurgical observations relative to the cataract, polypus of the nose, the cancer of the scrotum, the different kinds of ruptures and the mortification of the toes and feet, pp. 63–8. London: Hawes, Clarke & Collins.

Raju, G.C., Naraynsingh, V. & Venu, P.S. (1985). Carcinoma of the penis in the West Indies: A Trinidad study. *Trop. Geogr. Med.*, **37**, 334–6.

Smith, P.G., Kinlen, L.J., White, G.C., Adelstein, A.M. & Fox, A.J. (1980). Mortality of wives of men dying with cancer of the penis. *Br. J. Cancer.*, **41**, 422–8.

Villa, L.L. & Lopes, A. (1986). Human papillomavirus DNA sequences in penile carcinomas in Brazil. *Int. J. Cancer.*, **37**, 853–5.

Urinary tract: bladder, ureter and urethra

ICD-9 188

48.1 Introduction

Cancer of the bladder is common in males in many parts of the world, exhibiting moderate variation. Geographical differences may be partly dependent on whether so-called 'benign papillomas' of the bladder are included with the overtly malignant neoplasms. Tumors of the ureter are not common, but are sometimes associated with cancer of the bladder.

48.2 Histology, classification and diagnosis

In industrial states, most bladder cancers are transitional cell or urothelial carcinomas, squamous carcinomas being usually less than 10% of all tumors. Today, the term 'benign' papillomas is rarely used for bladder tumors, and these are now regarded as malignant. A predominance of squamous cell carcinomas is observed in areas where bladder cancer is related to schistosomiasis.

48.3 Descriptive epidemiology

Incidence (Fig. 48.1)

Rates are elevated in several industrialized countries, the highest being observed in Basel, Switzerland (27.8) and in Varese, northern Italy (27.3). In most registries in Europe and North America, rates are around 20. The lowest rates occur in India, with rates between 1.7 in Nagpur and 4.3 in Bombay, being slightly higher in Japan, between 6 and 10. Rates for U.S. blacks, around 10, are uniformly lower than in white Americans by some 50%, apparently due in part to under-reporting of early stage tumors (Schairer *et al.*, 1988). Bladder cancer is also frequent in countries of the Middle East and Africa where schistosomiasis is endemic; for

Fig. 48.1 Incidence rates around 1980: Bladder (ICD-9 188).

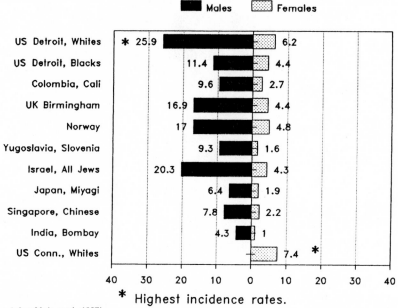

(after Muir *et al.*, 1987)

example, it accounts for some 29% of all cancer in males and 11% of those in females reported to the Cairo Metropolitan Cancer Registry. In Baghdad, bladder cancer accounts for 13% of all malignant neoplasms in males (Al-Fouadi & Parkin, 1984).

The incidence of bladder cancer is slowly increasing in many countries, with a more moderate increase in mortality.

Age distribution
Incidence increases with age.

Sex distribution
The sex ratio is about 3 to 1, and geographical variations are less prominent for females than males.

48.4   Etiological inferences
Geographical, sex and occupational variations provide convincing evidence for a role of exogenous factors. Tumors occurring as a result of chemical exposures or tobacco smoking are usually transitional cell carcinomas, whereas the distribution of *S. haematobium* correlates well with squamous cell carcinomas.

48.5   Known and suspected causes

Three major factors have been implicated in bladder carcinoma: occupation, tobacco smoking and parasitic infestation.

Occupation

Early observations in the dye industry, which had an increased incidence of bladder cancer, led to the identification of a number of aromatic amines, notably benzidine and 2-naphthylamine, which were carcinogenic in experimental animals (IARC, 1987). Similar exposures occurred in the rubber industry (Case *et al.*, 1954). Today cessation of manufacture of such aromatic amines has largely reduced or eliminated the excess of bladder cancers in these industries. Excess risks have also been reported in the leather, painting and other industries using organic chemicals, as well as among truck and locomotive drivers and miners. However, the specific agents in such occupations are unclear and confounding variables may be involved (Smith *et al.*, 1985; Claude *et al.*, 1988).

Tobacco

There are now numerous studies supporting the association between cigarette smoking and transitional cell bladder cancer (IARC, 1986). While the incidence among smokers is related to the number of cigarettes smoked, the relationship is not as striking as in lung cancer. A decrease in bladder cancer occurs in ex-smokers. This habit probably explains much of the variation between occupations, countries and sexes. Higher risks have been associated with black than with blond tobacco.

Parasitic infestation

Evidence from South Africa, Mozambique and Egypt, where *S. haematobium* is endemic, shows that a very high proportion of squamous carcinomas develops in bladders with bilharzial cystitis (Kitinya *et al.*, 1986). N-nitroso compound formation associated with a concomitant bacterial cystitis has been postulated as a mechanism (Chapter 17).

Other causes

Pelvic radiation

An increase has been reported in women receiving radiotherapy for pelvic conditions (Boice *et al.*, 1985).

Coffee drinking

Some reports have associated bladder cancer with coffee drinking but the evidence remains limited (IARC, 1990).

Artificial sweeteners

The demonstration that certain artificial sweeteners in very high doses enhanced bladder cancer in rodents led to extensive studies on humans (IARC, 1980a; 1987). A major study showed no increase in relative risk in the total study population, but some controversial increases and decreases in risk were observed in several sub-groups (Hoover & Strasser, 1980). No convincing hypotheses have been proposed to explain these inconsistencies and other studies do not indicate a risk.

Analgesic abuse

A number of studies (IARC, 1980b; 1987) have indicated that certain analgesics, notably those containing phenacetin, are associated with increased risk of tumors of the renal pelvis, ureter and bladder. The number of cases is small and the attributable risk is difficult to determine.

Other drugs

Chlornaphazine, an anti-neoplastic drug related to 2-naphthylamine, formerly used in the treatment of lymphomas, is a strong bladder carcinogen (IARC, 1987).

Water pollution

A number of ecological reports have associated bladder cancer with water pollution, notably chlorination (Cantor *et al.*, 1987). The association remains inconsistent and confounding variables, such as cigarettes are difficult to exclude.

Balkan or endemic nephropathy

An increase of bladder tumors has also been found in this disease, also tumors of the ureters (p. 428).

Individual susceptibility

There are reports indicating that individuals who are of the slow acetylator phenotype are at an increased risk (Mommsen & Aagaard, 1986). This is biologically plausible and implies past exposure to aromatic amines, either in cigarette smoke or in industry.

48.6   Relevant laboratory studies

The induction of bladder cancer in animals, especially dogs, proved of great value in identifying specific carcinogenic aromatic amines, especially those with a double ring. Tobacco smoke-derived mutagens have been found in human urine and DNA adducts in the bladder epithelium of smokers. The first mutated human *ras* oncogene was identified in a bladder carcinoma, but this observation has not proved of value in etiological studies.

48.7   Attributable risks

In western countries, approximately 40% to 50% of bladder cancers are related to smoking, and a smaller proportion (25%) to occupational factors. These percentages are probably changing as smoking consumption is reduced and industrial hygiene improves. The causes of most cases in the general population cannot be readily related to any single exposure. In contrast, schistosomal infestation is the major cause (over 50%) in parts of Africa and the Middle East.

48.8   Conclusion

Smoking still remains the most important cause in most countries except where schistosomiasis remains endemic. The number of occupational cancers will probably decrease with improved industrial hygiene. However, a rise may be anticipated in third world countries with increases in cigarette smoking and cottage industry development and uncontrolled use of outdated manufacturing processes.

48.9   References

Al-Fouadi, A. & Parkin, D.M. (1984). Cancer in Iraq: Seven years' data from the Baghdad Tumour Registry. *Int. J. Cancer*, **34**, 207–13.

Boice, J.D., Day, N.E., Andersen, A., Brinton, L.A., Brown, R., Choi, N.W., Clarke, E.A., Coleman, M.P., Curtis, R.E., Flannery, J.T., Hakama, M., Hakullinen, T., Howe, G.R., Jensen, O.M., Kleinerman, R.A., Magnin, D., Magnus, K., Makela, K., Malker, B., Miller, A.B., Nelson, N., Patterson, C.C., Pettersson, F., Pompe-Kirn, V., Primic-Zakelj, M., Prior, P., Ravnihar, B., Skeet, R.G., Skjerven, J.E., Smith, P.G., Sok, M., Spengler, R.F., Storm, H.H., Stovall, M., Tomkins, G.W.O. & Wall, C. (1985). Second cancers following radiation treatment for cervical cancer. An international collaboration among cancer registries. *J. Natl. Cancer Inst.*, **74**, 955–75.

Cantor, K.P., Hoover, R., Hartge, P., Mason, T.J., Silverman, D.T., Altman, R., Austin, D.F., Child, M.A., Key, C.R., Marrett, L.D., Myers, M.H., Narayana, A.S., Levin, L.I., Sullivan, J.W., Swanson, G.M., Thomas, D.B. & West, D.W. (1987). Bladder cancer, drinking water source, and tap water consumption: A case-control study. *J. Natl. Cancer Inst.*, **79**, 1269–79.

Case, R.A.M., Hosker, M.E., McDonald, D.B. & Pearson, J.T. (1954). Tumours of the urinary bladder in workmen engaged in the manufacture and use of certain dyestuff intermediates in the British chemical industry. *Br. J. Ind. Med.*, **11**, 75–104.

Claude, J.C., Frentzel-Beyme, R.R. & Kunze, E. (1988). Occupation and risk of cancer of the lower urinary tract among men. A case-control study. *Int. J. Cancer*, **41**, 371–9.

Hoover, R. & Strasser, P.H. (1980). Artificial sweeteners and human bladder cancer. *Lancet*, **i**, 837–40.

IARC (1980a). *IARC Monographs on the Evaluation of the Carcinogenic Risk of Chemicals to Humans*, Some non-nutritive sweetening agents, vol. 22. Lyon: International Agency for Research on Cancer.

IARC (1980*b*). *IARC Monographs on the Evaluation of the Carcinogenic Risk of Chemicals to Humans*, Some pharmaceutical drugs, Vol. 24, pp. 135–61. Lyon: International Agency for Research on Cancer.

IARC (1986). *IARC Monographs on the Evaluation of the Carcinogenic Risk of Chemicals to Humans*, Tobacco smoking, Vol. 38. Lyon: International Agency for Research on Cancer.

IARC (1987). *IARC Monographs on the Evaluation of Carcinogenic Risks to Humans*, Overall evaluations of carcinogenicity: an updating of IARC Monographs volumes 1 to 42, Supplement 7. Lyon: International Agency for Research on Cancer.

IARC (1990). *IARC Monographs on the Evaluation of Carcinogenic Risks to Humans*, Coffee, tea, maté, methylxanthines (caffeine, theophylline, thiobromine) and methylglyoxal, volume 51. Lyon: International Agency for Research on Cancer.

Kitinya, J.N., Lauren, P.A., Eshleman, L.J., Paljarvi, L & Tanaka, K. (1986). The incidence of squamous and transitional cell carcinomas of the urinary bladder in Northern Tanzania in areas of high and low levels of endemic schistosoma haematobium infection. *Trans. Roy. Soc. Trop. Med. Hyg.*, **80**, 935–9.

Mommsen, S. & Aagaard, J. (1986). Susceptibility in urinary bladder cancer: Acetyltransferase phenotypes and related risk factors. *Cancer Lett.*, **32**, 199–205.

Muir, C., Waterhouse, J., Mack, T., Powell, J. & Whelan, S. (eds.) (1987). *Cancer Incidence in Five Continents*, IARC Scientific Publication No. 88. Lyon: International Agency for Research on Cancer.

Schairer, C., Hartge, P., Hoover, R.N. & Silverman, D.T. (1988). Racial differences in bladder cancer risk: A case-control study. *Am. J. Epidemiol.*, **128**, 1027–37.

Smith, E.M., Miller, E.R., Woolson, R.F. & Brown, C.K. (1985). Bladder cancer risk among auto and truck mechanics and chemically related occupations. *Am. J. Pub. Health*, **75**, 881–3.

49

Kidney and renal pelvis

ICD 189.0 to 189.1

49.1   Introduction

Cancers of the kidney are relatively uncommon, but a steadily increasing trend in both incidence and mortality has been reported.

49.2   Histology, classification and diagnosis

Most renal parenchymal tumors are adenocarcinomas. In the past, small tumors (<3 cm) were considered benign, but today, many believe that even small nodules are potentially malignant. New methods of diagnostic imaging have also increased accuracy of diagnosis with a possible impact on incidence. Malignant tumors of the renal pelvis are usually urothelial carcinomas, as in the bladder.

Nephroblastoma (Wilms' tumor) is a rare embryonal tumor of childhood with its own distinctive histological and cytogenic patterns.

49.3   Descriptive epidemiology
Incidence

Worldwide variation in these tumors is moderate, the highest rates (> 10) being seen in North America and Europe: in the male populations of Iceland (12.2), Sweden (11.3), and the Bas-Rhin department in France (11.0). Intermediate rates are seen in most remaining areas of the western world, rates being nearly identical in blacks and whites in the USA. Rates are very low in Chinese, Japanese, and Indians. Rates in Japanese and Chinese groups in the USA are, however, frequently higher. Renal pelvic cancer incidence usually reflects that of the parenchyma. However, high rates of renal pelvis and ureter cancer occur in regions where Balkan nephropathy is endemic (Castegnaro & Chernozemsky, 1987).

Fig. 49.1 Incidence rates around 1980: Kidney, renal pelvis, ureter and urethra (ICD-9 189).

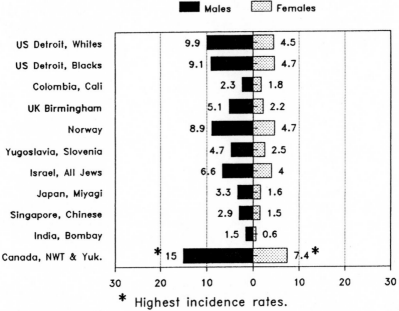

(after Muir *et al.*, 1987)

Nephroblastomas, which are relatively frequent in children between one and three years of age, are slightly commoner in blacks, especially females, than in whites (Chapter 58). The rates in the SEER registries are 7.9 and 10.0 per million white male and female children aged 0–14 and 9.9 and 12.3 in black male and female children, respectively. This excess risk has been ascribed to a hereditary predisposition. None the less, even higher rates have been recorded in Finland and in Bas-Rhin in France.

Age distribution

There are no unusual features to the age distribution of renal cell carcinoma which increases steadily with age. Nephroblastoma is characterized by peak incidence rates between ages 2 and 4 years.

Sex distribution

Renal cell carcinomas are usually twice as common in males as in females. Nephroblastoma often shows a slight female excess.

Time trends

In many countries steady increases have been reported.

49.4   Etiological inferences

Migration appears to modify renal cancer risk which supports a role for environmental factors. Socioeconomic variations are still observed in some countries, e.g. UK, but have diminished and may be related to lifestyle (Logan, 1982).

49.5   Known and suspected causes
Hereditary and familial factors

Genetic and non-genetic forms of nephroblastoma occur. The tumor is associated with a spectrum of congenital abnormalities (Breslow & Beckwith, 1982). While several factors in the preconception and gestational period have been tentatively postulated – including high blood pressure or fluid retention during pregnancy, vaginal infection, use of hair coloring products, older maternal age, and tea consumption (Bunin *et al.*, 1987) further confirmation is necessary (Chapter 58).

Tobacco smoking

Cigarette smoking and cancers of the renal pelvis are associated (Ross *et al.*, 1989). Further, several studies have shown a relationship between renal adenocarcinoma and cigarette smoking, which has been regarded by an IARC working party as probably causal (IARC, 1986). The carcinogenic effect in those who both chew and smoke tobacco is much more pronounced (Goodman *et al.*, 1986).

Chemicals and occupation

To date, no chemical has been associated unequivocally with renal cancer in humans. Most studies do not suggest a consistent relationship between renal carcinoma and any occupation (McLaughlin *et al.*, 1984). Risks tend to be higher in operatives than professionals, but tobacco confounding is always a problem (Asal et al., 1988).

Adenocarcinomas have been demonstrated in male rats following gasoline exposure (Kitchen, 1984), but there is no convincing evidence to suggest that there is any relationship between genito-urinary cancer and gasoline use in humans (Higginson *et al.*, 1984). However, workers in the petroleum-related and dry cleaning industries have shown an increased risk (Asal *et al.*, 1988). Parental occupation has been examined as a risk factor for nephroblastoma (Wilkins and Sinks, 1984) but the evidence is not persuasive.

Hormonal factors
Steroid sex hormones can produce renal tumors in hamsters, but there is no evidence that they are of significance in humans.

Diet, coffee and alcohol
There is no convincing evidence of an association of these factors with cancers of the parenchyma or pelvis.

Obesity was the most important risk factor for this cancer in both men and women in a recent case-control study (Asal *et al.*, 1988).

Miscellaneous
Analgesic nephropathy

Cancer of the renal pelvis in humans has been associated with the abuse of pain killing compounds containing phenacetin (IARC, 1980; Ross *et al.*, 1989).

Balkan nephropathy

This is a severe disease of the renal parenchyma and occurs primarily in Bulgaria, Yugoslavia and Rumania where it is localized to specific regions. It is associated with an increase in tumors of the bladder, ureter and renal pelvis but not of the parenchyma (Castegnaro & Chernozemsky, 1987). The causes are unknown but food-related mycotoxins such as ochratoxin A, are suspected.

End stage kidney and dialysis

A lesion considered to be preneoplastic lesion has been reported in dialyzed kidneys, also in chronic end-stage renal disease (Hughson *et al.*, 1986).

Kidney transplants

There is some evidence that individuals who have received kidney transplants may show an increase in renal cancer as well as tumors at other sites, possibly due to use of immunosuppressive agents (Sheil *et al.*, 1980).

49.6   Relevant laboratory studies
A wide range of natural and man-made chemicals induce renal carcinoma experimentally. These include aromatic amines, aliphatic compounds such as urethane, certain *N*-nitroso compounds, metal salts and hormones. Adenocarcinomas similar to those in man have been

reported in a number of animal species for which no causal relationship can be identified. Ochratoxin A produces mostly renal tumors in rodents.

A biochemical mechanism based on the occurrence of *alpha$_{2u}$* globulin in female rats offers a plausible biological explanation for species differences due to gasoline exposure (Charbonneau & Swenberg, 1988).

A virus associated with renal carcinoma has been identified in frogs, but there is no evidence of a comparable virus in humans.

Most renal cell carcinomas demonstrate constant loss of the 3p13-pter chromosomes segment and gain of the 5q22-qter segment (Kovacs, 1989). Papillary and non-papillary renal carcinomas appear to differ both morphologically and karyotypically.

49.7 Attributable risks

For adenocarcinoma McLaughlin *et al.* (1984) report the attributable risk (AR) for smoking as 30% in males and 24% in females. The ARs for cancer of the renal pelvis are somewhat higher (IARC, 1986).

49.8 Conclusions

A significant proportion of renal adenocarcinomas and pelvic cancers have an environmental component of which the most important identified to date is tobacco.

Nephroblastoma is further discussed in Chapters 18 and 58.

49.9 References

Asal, N.R., Lee, E.T., Geyer, J.R., Kadamani, S., Risser, D.R. & Cherng, N. (1988). Risk factors in renal cell carcinoma. II. Medical history, occupation, multivariate analysis, and conclusions. *Cancer Detect. Prev.*, **13**, 263–79.

Birkeland, S.A., Kemp, E. & Hauge, M. (1980). Renal transplantation and cancer in the Scandiatransplant material. *Scand. J. Urol. Nephrol. Suppl.*, **284**, 11–5.

Breslow, N.E. & Beckwith, J.B. (1982). Epidemiological factors of Wilms' tumor: Results of the National Wilms' Tumor Study. *J. Natl. Cancer Inst.*, **68**, 429–36.

Bunin, G.R., Kramer, S., Marrero, O. & Meadows, A.T. (1987). Gestational risk factors for Wilms' tumor: Results of a case-control study. *Cancer Res.*, 47, 2972–7.

Castegnaro, M. & Chernozemsky, I. (1987). Endemic nephropathy and urinary tract tumors in the Balkans. *Cancer Res.*, **47**, 3608–9.

Charbonneau, M. & Swenberg, J.A. (1988). Studies on the biochemical mechanism of alpha$_{2u}$-globulin nephropathy in rats. *CIIT Activities*, **8**, 1–5.

Goodman, M.T., Morgenstern, H. & Wynder, E.L. (1986). A case-control study of factors affecting the development of renal cell cancer. *Am. J. Epidemiol.*, **124**, 926–41.

Higginson, J., Muir, C. & Buffler, P. (1984). The epidemiology of renal carcinoma in humans with a note on the effect of exposure to gasoline. In *Renal Effects of Petroleum Hydrocarbons*, Advances in Modern Environmental Toxicology, Volume VII, ed. M.A. Mehlman, G.P. Hemstreet, J.J. Thorpe & N.K. Weaver, pp. 203–26. Princeton, NJ: Princeton Scientific Publishers.

Hughson, M.D., Buchwald, D. & Fox, M. (1986). Renal neoplasia and acquired cystic kidney disease in patients receiving long-term dialysis. *Arch. Pathol. Lab. Med.*, **110**, 592–601.

IARC (1980). *IARC Monographs on the Evaluation of the Carcinogenic Risk of Chemicals to Humans*, Some pharmaceutical drugs, vol. 24, pp. 135–61. Lyon: International Agency for Research on Cancer.

IARC (1986). *IARC Monographs on the Evaluation of the Carcinogenic Risk of Chemicals to Humans*, Tobacco smoking, vol. 38. Lyon: International Agency for Research on Cancer.

Kitchen, D.N. (1984). Neoplastic renal effects of unleaded gasoline in Fischer 344 rats. In *Renal Effects of Petroleum Hydrocarbons*, Advances in Modern Environmental Toxicology, Volume VII, ed. M.A. Mehlman, G.P. Hemstreet, J.J. Thorpe & N.K. Weaver, pp. 65–71. Princeton, NJ: Princeton Scientific Publishers.

Kovacs, G. (1989). Papillary renal cell carcinoma: A morphologic and cytogenetic study of 11 cases. *Am. J. Pathol.*, **134**, 27–34.

Logan, W.P.D. (1982). *Cancer Mortality by Occupation and Social Class* 1851–1971. IARC Scientific Publications No. 36. Lyon: International Agency for Research on Cancer.

McLaughlin, J.K., Mandel, J.S., Blot, W.J., Schuman, L.M., Mehl, E.S. & Fraumeni, J.F., Jr. (1984). A population-based case-control study of renal cell carcinoma. *J. Natl. Cancer Inst.*, **72**, 275–84.

Muir, C., Waterhouse, J., Mack, T., Powell, J., Whelan, S., Smans, M. & Casset, F. (1987). *Cancer Incidence in Five Continents*, volume V, IARC Scientific Publications No. 88. Lyon: International Agency for Research on Cancer.

Ross, R.K., Paganini-Hill, A., Landolph, J., Gerkins, V. & Henderson, B.E. (1989). Analgesics, cigarette smoking, and other risk factors for cancer of the renal pelvis and ureter. *Cancer Res.*, **49**, 1045–8.

Seemayer, T.A. & Cavenee, W.K. (1989). Biology of disease. Molecular mechanisms of oncogenesis. *Lab. Invest.*, **60**, 585–99.

Sheil, A.G., May, J., Mahoney, J.F., Horvath, J.S., Johnson, J.R., Tiler, D.J. & Stewart, J.H. (1980). Incidence of cancer in renal transplant recipients. *Proc. Eur. Dial. Transp. Assoc.*, **17**, 502–6.

Wilkins, J.R. & Sinks, T.H., Jr. (1984). Paternal occupation and Wilms' tumour in offspring. *J. Epidemiol. Community Health*, **38**, 7–11.

Part XI

Eye and nervous system

50

Eye

ICD-9 190

50.1　Introduction

Tumors of the eye (ICD-9 190) are infrequent (Chapters 18 and 58).

50.2　Histology, classification and diagnosis

Squamous cell carcinoma of the conjunctiva occurs with moderate frequency in parts of Africa. Intraorbital tumors are almost always retinoblastomas in children under 10 years of age, arising from the retina. In adults they are predominantly malignant melanomas arising from the choroid. Rarely, metastases from an ocular melanoma may manifest in the liver up to 20 years after diagnosis and treatment of the primary.

50.3　Descriptive epidemiology

Incidence rates for retinoblastoma are usually less than one and there is up to eight-fold geographical variation, but registration artefacts cannot be excluded. Intraocular melanomas are, however, rare in Africans and Asians. There is usually a modest male excess.

50.4　Etiological inferences

Familial studies on retinoblastoma estimate a role of inheritance by autosomal dominance in about 50% of the cases. Most of the genetic forms are bilateral. Survivors of bilateral retinoblastoma have an excess risk of osteogenic sarcoma.

50.5　Known and suspected causes

Tumors of the conjunctiva (and eyelids) are related to sunlight. The cause of ocular melanoma is unknown (Osterlind, 1987).

The pathogenesis of childhood retinoblastomas is discussed in Chapter 18. These neoplasms provide the best example of the two-hit theory of mutagenesis, although the triggering agent is unknown.

50.6   Relevant laboratory studies
See Chapter 18.

50.7   Conclusion
Control of hereditary retinoblastoma is dependent on early diagnosis.

50.8   References
Osterlind, A. (1987). Trends in incidence of ocular malignant melanoma in Denmark, 1943–1982. *Int. J. Cancer*, **40**, 161–4.

51

Brain and central nervous system

ICD-9 191–192

51.1   Introduction

Brain (ICD-9 191) and nervous system (ICD-9 192), cover a range of neoplasms arising from glial tissue and the meninges.

51.2   Histology, classification and diagnosis

Histological classification is based on the presumptive cell of origin (Rubinstein, 1972), but there are often diagnostic difficulties in determining type. Glial tumors show wide variations in aggressiveness, some being highly malignant whereas others grow relatively slowly. There are also differences in the age distribution of the various histological types, medulloblastoma being found exclusively in children (Table 51.1 and 51.2). Signs and symptoms depend on the size, rate of growth and anatomical location of the tumors. Clinically, tumors of the meninges and brain may present with similar findings, so that earlier statistics on different types may be biased. While glial tumors never metastasize, many other tumors frequently metastasize to the brain, notably bronchogenic carcinoma, and breast cancer in females. Metastases may also be present in the bones of the skull and vertebral column and thus indirectly mimic CNS lesions.

The availability of medical care clearly influences the likelihood of diagnosis, and in the past intracranial tumors were underdiagnosed. A full autopsy is often necessary for accurate diagnosis. Given the difficulty of obtaining biopsy material there may be an element of uncertainty about the diagnosis in several registries. Newer imaging procedures should increase the accuracy of registration statistics. Helseth *et al.* (1988) provide an excellent discussion of these problems.

Table 51.1. *Histologically confirmed primary intracranial neoplasms:*
frequency distribution – children.

Children (0–14 years)		
Type	Number	Percent
Medulloblastoma	74	24.2
Astrocytoma	63	20.6
Glioblastoma	62	20.3
Ependymoma	20	6.5
Craniopharyngioma	17	5.6
Meningioma	14	4.6
Hemangioma	9	2.9
Neuroblastoma	8	2.6
Teratoma	6	2.0
Pinealoma	6	2.0
Sarcoma	5	1.6
Oligodendroglioma	2	0.7
Neurilemoma	2	0.7
Others, specified	11	3.6
Others, unspecified	7	2.3
Total	306	100.2

(After Schoenberg *et al.*, 1976.)

51.3   Descriptive epidemiology

The highest rates for tumors of the central nervous system are observed in Israeli females born in Africa or Asia (15.7) and in Israel (10.8) and in the female population of Iceland (10.0), rates in males being 10.8, 8.2 and 8.5, respectively. Intermediate rates, between 6 and 9, are generally seen in most western countries. Rates in the 1 to 3 range in Asian populations are the lowest (Fig. 51.1). Rates in Chinese and Japanese living in the United States are intermediate between those of US whites and those for their country of origin. Except for Israel and Iceland, where female rates are occasionally higher than those for males, there is a tendency for males to exhibit slightly higher rates.

In children, the highest rates, around 30 per million, are observed in Nordic countries (see Chapter 58). According to Parkin *et al.* (1988), the distribution by cell type is much the same irrespective of incidence.

Time trends

Increases have been noted in many countries, notably in older age-groups, but are difficult to evaluate as they may reflect improvements in diagnosis (Davis *et al.*, 1990).

Table 51.2. *Histologically confirmed primary intracranial neoplasms:*
frequency distribution – adults.

Adults (15+ years)		
Type	Number	Percent
Glioblastoma	1105	52.1
Meningioma	389	18.4
Astrocytoma	214	10.1
Chromophobe adenoma	96	4.5
Neurilemoma	46	2.2
Hemangioma	41	1.9
Craniopharyngioma	30	1.4
Medulloblastoma	27	1.3
Ependymoma	27	1.3
Acidophilic adenoma	26	1.2
Oligodendroglioma	22	1.0
Sarcoma	19	0.9
Pinealoma	6	0.3
Others, specified	26	1.2
Others, unspecified	45	2.1
Total	2119	99.9

(After Schoenberg *et al.*, 1976.)

51.4 Etiological inferences

Differences in incidence are difficult to evaluate due to diagnostic variations.

51.5 Known and suspected causes (see Chapter 58)

The various suspected causes have been reviewed by Schoenberg (1982). These include trauma for which the evidence is largely anecdotal and probably reflects recall biases.

Hereditary and genetic factors

A number of hereditary syndromes (phakomatoses) have been described (Schoenberg *et al.*, 1976), such as tuberous sclerosis, in which an increased frequency of astrocytomas are reported. Other syndromes include Von Hippel-Lindau and Von Recklinghausen's diseases. However, such conditions are rare and can only explain a fraction of all brain tumors. Medulloblastoma and glioblastoma were over represented in a group of children whose relatives had central nervous system tumors.

Fig. 51.1 Incidence rates around 1980: Brain, nervous system (ICD-9 191–192).

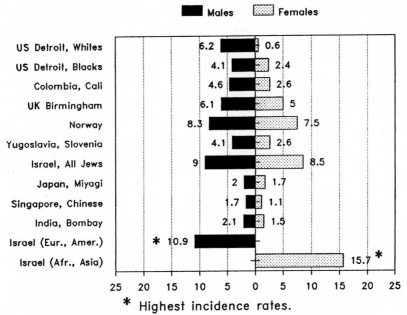

■ Males   ▦ Females

US Detroit, Whites	6.2 ▮ 0.6
US Detroit, Blacks	4.1 ▮ 2.4
Colombia, Cali	4.6 ▮ 2.6
UK Birmingham	6.1 ▮ 5
Norway	8.3 ▮ 7.5
Yugoslavia, Slovenia	4.1 ▮ 2.6
Israel, All Jews	9 ▮ 8.5
Japan, Miyagi	2 ▮ 1.7
Singapore, Chinese	1.7 ▮ 1.1
India, Bombay	2.1 ▮ 1.5
Israel (Eur., Amer.)	* 10.9
Israel (Afr., Asia)	15.7 *

25 20 15 10 5 0 5 10 15 20 25

* Highest incidence rates.

(after Muir *et al.*, 1987)

Radiation

Prenatal X-ray exposure may lead to brain tumors (MacMahon, 1962). An increased risk of brain tumors (both gliomas and meningiomas) has been found in children who received scalp radiation for tinea capitis in Israel (Modan *et al.*, 1974). Increased risks have been reported in a nuclear fuel fabrication plant, and radiation induced meningiomas have been reported (Rubinstein, 1972). Early exposure to dental X-rays increased the risk of intracranial meningiomas in women.

Occupation and chemical exposures

Many occupational exposures have been examined, and increases reported in the vinyl chloride industry and among Scandinavian rubber manufacturing plant workers. A cluster of brain tumors in a petrochemical plant could not be ascribed to any specific chemical and no coherent pattern of plausible associations has emerged (Thomas *et al.*, 1986). Another cluster was observed in laboratory workers exposed to N-methylguanine (Pleven *et al.*, 1986). An increase in brain tumors suspected as due to formaldehyde exposure in anatomists was not confirmed in other studies (UAREP, 1988).

The Cancer – Environment Registry of Sweden which linked cancer incidence (1961–1979) with census information on occupation has shown a statistically significant associations for brain tumors and meningioma in many occupations. However, it is difficult to identify any common exposure between male dentists, agricultural research workers, public prosecutors, female physicians, welders, glass, porcelain and ceramic workers, cellulose plant employees, brick and tile workers, and women employed in the wool industry. Some of the 'significant' findings probably resulted from multiple comparisons.

No reason can be given for reported increases in electrical and electronic workers (Thomas *et al.*, 1987) although electromagnetic field exposure has been suggested. An excess in farmers in Italy was attributed to use of agrochemicals.

Claims of an increased frequency of tumors in children due to exposures to insecticides, farm animals, sick pets, parental exposure to potential carcinogens (Olshan *et al.*, 1986), etc., are not convincing. In contrast an increase in gliomas is observed after chemotherapeutic cure of acute lymphoblastic leukemia (Albo *et al.*, 1985).

An excess of maternal occupations involving chemical exposures and paternal occupations involving solvents has been reported in children with brain tumors. Preston-Martin *et al.* (1982) found an increased risk associated with maternal contact with nitrosamines, such as use of nitrite-cured meats.

Viruses

An increased risk in HIV infections has been suggested (Safai & Koziner, 1985). In no case is the evidence completely convincing.

Miscellaneous factors

There is little evidence that alcohol or smoking have any impact. Although Hirayama (1984) has suggested a causative role of passive smoking, this does not seem biologically plausible.

51.6 Relevant laboratory studies

Tumors of the brain can be produced in experimental animals by viruses (Bigner, 1978). Certain chemical carcinogens, notably *N*-nitroso compounds, are capable of inducing tumors following systematic administration, especially to young rats, often following a single dose.

51.7   Attributable risks
The data available are uninformative.

51.8   Conclusions
Although many weak associations have been reported to date, epidemiology has failed to provide any satisfactory clues as to the causes of most brain tumors.

51.9   References

Albo, V., Miller, D., Leiken, S., Sather, H. & Hammond, D. (1985). Nine brain tumors (BT) as a late effect in children 'cured' of acute lymphoblastic leukemia (all) from a single protocol study. (Meeting abstract). *Proc. Ann. Meet. Am. Soc. Clin. Oncol.*, **4**, 172.

Bigner, D.D. (1978). Role of viruses in the causation of neural neoplasia. In *Biology of Brain Tumors*, ed. O.D. Laerum, D.D. Bigner & M.F. Rajewsky, pp. 85–111. Geneva: International Union Against Cancer.

Davis, D.L., Hoel, D., Fox, J. & Lopez, A. (1990). International trends in cancer mortality in France, West Germany, Italy, Japan, England and Wales, and the USA. *Lancet*, **336**, 474–81.

Helseth, A., Langmarle, F. & Mark, J.S. (1988). Neoplasms of the central nervous system: quality control of the registration at the Norwegian Cancer Registry. *APMIS*, **96**, 1002–8.

Hirayama, T. (1984). Cancer mortality in nonsmoking women with smoking husbands based on a large-scale cohort study in Japan. *Prev. Med.*, **13**, 680–90.

MacMahon, B. (1962). Prenatal x-ray exposure and childhood cancer. *J. Natl. Cancer Inst.*, **28**, 1173–91.

Modan, B., Baidatz, D., Mart, H., Steinitz, R. & Levin, S.G. (1974). Radiation-induced head and neck tumors. *Lancet*, **1**, 277–9.

Muir, C., Waterhouse, J., Mack, T., Powell, J. & Whelan, S. (eds.) (1987). *Cancer Incidence in Five Continents*, volume V, IARC Scientific Publication No. 88. Lyon: International Agency for Research on Cancer.

Olshan, A.F., Breslow, N.E., Daling, J.R., Weiss, N.S. & Leviton, A. (1986). Childhood brain tumors and paternal occupation in the aerospace industry. *J. Natl. Cancer Inst.*, **77**, 17–9.

Parkin, D.M., Stiller, C.A., Draper, G.J., Bieber, C.A., Terracini, B. & Young, J.L. (eds.) (1988). *International Incidence of Childhood Cancer*, IARC Scientific Publications No. 87. Lyon: International Agency for Research on Cancer.

Pleven, C., Falcy, M., Audran, R., Philbert, M. & Efthymion, M.L. (1984). Survenue des glioblastomes chez les personnels de laboratoires de recherche travaillent sur les produits nitrosés. *J. Toxicol. Med.*, **4**, 249–57.

Preston-Martin, S., Yu, M.C., Benton, B. & Henderson, B.G. (1982). N-nitroso compounds and childhood brain tumours: A case control study. *Cancer Res.*, **42**, 5260–5.

Rubinstein, L.J. (1972). Tumors of the central nervous system. In *Atlas of Tumor Pathology*, Second Series, Fascicle 6. Washington: Armed Forces Institute of Pathology.

Safai, B. & Koziner, B. (1985). Malignant neoplasms in AIDS. In *AIDS. Etiology, Diagnosis, Treatment, and Prevention*, ed. V.T. DeVita, S. Hellman & S.A. Rosenberg, pp. 213–22. Philadelphia: J.B. Lippincott.

Schoenberg, B.S. (1982). Nervous system. In *Cancer Epidemiology and Prevention*, ed. D. Schottenfeld & J.F. Fraumeni, Jr., pp. 968–83. Philadelphia: W.B. Saunders.

Schoenberg, B.S., Schoenberg, D.G., Christine, B.W. & Gomez, M.R. (1976). The epidemiology of primary intracranial neoplasms of childhood: a population study. *Mayo. Clinic. Proc.*, **51**, 51–6.

Thomas, T.L., Fontham, E.T., Norman, S.A., Stemhagen, A. & Hoover, R.N. (1986). Occupational risk factors for brain tumors. A case-referent death-certificate analysis. *Scand. J. Work. Environ. Health*, **12**, 121–7.

Thomas, T.L., Stolley, P.D., Stemhagen, A., Fontham, E.T., Bleecker, M.L., Stewart, P.A. & Hoover, R.N. (1987). Brain tumor mortality risk among men with electrical and electronics jobs: A case-control study. *J. Natl. Cancer Inst.*, **79**, 233–8.

UAREP, Universities Associated for Research and Education in Pathology, Inc. (1988). Epidemiology of chronic occupational exposure to formaldehyde: Report of the ad hoc panel on health aspects of formaldehyde. *Toxicol. Ind. Health*, **4**, 77–90.

Part XII

Thyroid and other endocrine glands, lymphoid and hematopoietic system

52

Thyroid and other endocrine glands

ICD-9 193–194

52.1 Introduction

Malignant tumors of the thyroid, although comparatively rare, representing 1–2% of all cancers, are the commonest cancers of the endocrine system. A number of rare tumors arise in other endocrine glands, notably the pituitary, the adrenals and pancreas.

52.2 Histology, classification and diagnosis

Thyroid tumors can be classified into several different histological types which show variations in geographical distribution (Correa *et al.*, 1969). In Colombia, papillary carcinoma predominates in areas where goiter is non-endemic, but follicular and anaplastic tumors are more common in goitrous areas, as in Israel, Norway, and Finland. Certain tumors (adenomas) of the thyroid are believed to be precursors of carcinoma and in view of their premalignant potential, benign adenomas are regarded with some suspicion. The differential diagnosis of thyroid adenoma and well-differentiated cancer is subjective and often difficult.

Pituitary tumors, although mostly histologically benign, may present as intracranial neoplasms and be fatal. Different cell types are associated with a variety of characteristic endocrine disorders.

In the adrenal gland, tumors can arise in the cortex or medulla. The latter (pheochromocytoma) may occur as part of the MEN syndrome (pp. 193, 447).

52.3 Descriptive epidemiology

Unless stated, the following comments relate to thyroid cancer since due to their rarity, little is known regarding variation in non-thyroid endocrine tumors.

Fig. 52.1 Incidence rates around 1980: Thyroid (ICD-9 193).

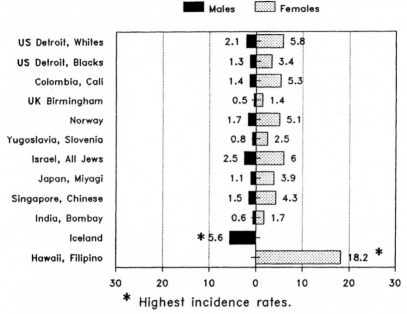

(after Muir *et al.*, 1987)

Thyroid: incidence

The highest female rates of thyroid cancer are observed in the Filipinos resident in Hawaii (18.2), the San Francisco Bay Area (12.2), Los Angeles (10.7) and in Pacific Polynesian Islanders (18.1). High rates are also seen in Iceland (13.3) and native Alaskan women (Lanier *et al.*, 1976).

Sex distribution

Incidence rates are approximately three times higher in females than in males, the female excess varying with age, being greater in the young.

Age distribution

Although relatively infrequent on a worldwide basis, thyroid cancer is one of the commonest neoplasms in adolescents and young adults. Papillary carcinoma shows a steady increase with age. Anaplastic carcinoma only becomes frequent after the sixth decade.

Time trends

A general decline in mortality rates has been observed, even in those countries such as Austria and Switzerland with traditionally high rates. Rates for both sexes, although now apparently stable, have been increasing slightly in US whites and blacks but in the Nordic countries no changes have occurred. Kerr *et al.* (1985) suggested a decline in the proportion of tumors with poor prognosis.

52.4 Etiological inferences

There appears to be a relationship of certain thyroid cancers to goiter and variations in pathogenetic pathways and time trends suggest the impact of exogenous factors.

52.5 Known and suspected causes
Hereditary and genetic factors

Significant genetic factors have not been identified (Correa *et al.*, 1969; Ron & Modan, 1982), other than for several types of the Multiple Endocrine Neoplasia (MEN) Syndrome, in which medullary cancer of the thyroid is an important feature (Sobol *et al.*, 1989) and for which the relevant gene lies on chromosome 10 (Chapter 18).

Radiation

The most significant cause identified in humans is radiation (BEIR, 1972, 1980), many studies reporting an association between radiation exposure, and subsequent development of thyroid malignancies (Chapter 16). These include children treated in the past by radiation for thymic enlargement or for enlarged tonsils. Increased risks have been described in individuals following exposure to the atomic bomb (Hoffman & Harlow, 1980). The isotope ^{131}I used for diagnostic purposes in patients with thyrotoxicosis does not appear to be a significant cause.

Chemicals

In iodine-rich areas there is some evidence of an enhanced risk of the papillary type of carcinoma, whereas the follicular type is more likely to occur in areas of endemic goiter due to iodine deficiency. So far, iodine therapy and chemotherapeutic treatment for thyrotoxicosis have not been convincingly shown to be a cause of thyroid cancer, although experimental studies suggested such a possibility.

Miscellaneous

There is some uncertainty regarding an association with thyrotoxicosis (Olen & Klinck, 1966) and thyroiditis. Although an excess of thyroid cancer has been reported in patients with breast cancer, the relationship is not clear.

52.6   Relevant laboratory studies

Experimentally, radiation, a few chemicals and increased TSH secretion have been shown to be factors in thyroid carcinogenesis, of which only TSH seems specific. This hormone is believed to act as a promoter.

52.7   Attributable risks

Iodine deficiency may be of considerable importance in areas of high risk. In certain locations the majority of carcinomas and pre-cancerous lesions are due to radiation following therapy or accidental exposure.

52.8   Conclusions

Preventive measures are largely directed to avoiding goiters and exposure to ionizing radiation.

59.9   References

BEIR (Advisory Committee on the Biological Effects of Ionizing Radiation). (1972). *The Effects on Populations of Exposure to Low Levels of Ionizing Radiation (The BEIR Report)*. Washington: National Academy of Science – National Research Council.

BEIR (Advisory Committee on the Biological Effects of Ionizing Radiation). (1980). *The Effects on Populations of Exposure to Low Levels of Ionizing Radiation (BEIR III)*. Washington: National Academy of Science – National Research Council.

Correa, P., Cuello, C. & Eisenberg., H. (1969). Epidemiology of different types of thyroid cancer. In *Thyroid Cancer* UICC Monograph Series, vol. 12, ed. C. Hedinger, pp. 81–93. New York: Springer-Verlag.

Hoffman, D.A. & Harlow, C.W. (1980). Thyroid nodularity in schoolchildren exposed to fallout radioiodine. In *Symposium on Biological Effects, Imaging Techniques, and Dosimetry of Ionizing Radiations*, FDA Publication No. 80–8126. Washington: US Government Printing Office.

Kerr, D.J., Burt, A.D., Brewin, T.B. & Boyle, P. (1985). Divergence between mortality and incidence rates of thyroid cancer in Scotland. *Lancet*, **ii**, 149.

Lanier, A.P., Bender, T.R., Blot, W.J., Fraumeni, J.F. & Hurlburt, W.B. (1976). Cancer incidence in Alaska natives. *Int. J. Cancer*, **18**, 409–12.

Muir, C., Waterhouse, J., Mack, T., Powell, J. & Whelan, S. (eds.) (1987). *Cancer Incidence in Five Continents*, volume V, IARC Scientific Publication No. 88. Lyon: International Agency for Research on Cancer.

Olen, E. & Klinck, G.H. (1966). Hyperthyroidism and thyroid cancer. *Arch. Path.*, **81**, 531–5.

Ron, E. & Modan, B. (1982). Thyroid. *In Cancer Epidemiology and Prevention, ed. D. Schottenfeld & J.F. Fraumeni, Jr.*, pp. 837–54. Philadelphia: *W.B. Saunders*.

Sobol, H., Narod, S.A., Nakamura, Y., Boneu, A., Calmettes, C., Chadenas, D., Charpentier, G., Chatal, J.F., Delepine, N., Delisle, M.J., Dupond, J.L., Gardet, P., Godefroy, H., Guillausseau, P.-J., Guillausseau-Scholer, C., Houdent, C., Lalau, J.D., Mace, G., Parmentier, C., Soubrier, F., Tourniaire, J. & Lenoir, G.M. (1989). Screening for multiple endocrine neoplasia type 2a with DNA-polymorphism analysis. *N. Engl. J. Med.*, **321**, 996–1001.

53

Burkitt's lymphoma

ICD-9 200

53.1   Introduction

Burkitt's lymphoma (BL) forms a distinct clinico-pathological entity among the non-Hodgkin's lymphomas. It is particularly frequent in children in tropical Africa and New Guinea, but outside these endemic areas the tumor is rare.

53.2   Histology, classification and diagnosis

Although BL was originally described as a clinical syndrome in African children by Burkitt (1958), the most reliable criteria for diagnosis have been its cytological and histological features. Clinically, involvement of the jaw and abdominal viscera are highly characteristic but are not specific. Histologically, it is classified as a non-Hodgkin's lymphoma of undifferentiated type. The 'starry sky' pattern given by histiocytes interspersed among malignant lymphoid cells is considered as a highly characteristic but non-specific feature. Cytologic imprints of the tumor show malignant lymphoid cells with deeply basophilic cytoplasm and lipoid vacuoles.

53.3   Descriptive epidemiology
Incidence and time trends

The highest incidence rates (5–10) are found in tropical Africa and in Papua New Guinea (see Table 58.4). Significant space-time and seasonal clustering of BL cases has been observed in some areas of Africa but not in others (Morrow, 1982). Elsewhere, the incidence is very low (0.1) (Parkin *et al.*, 1985). Tumors of the jaw are more frequently seen in African children while abdominal tumors are commoner in low-risk areas.

Age and sex distribution

The age distribution of BL in endemic areas is fairly characteristic with a peak incidence at 5–8 years of age but it is rare before age two and after adolescence. In most series, the BL rates are two-fold higher in boys than in girls.

53.4 Etiological inferences

The occurrence of BL in well-defined geographical areas of tropical Africa and Papua New Guinea characterized by low altitude, high temperatures and high rainfall, led to the suggestion that an arthropod-borne virus was etiologically involved. Subsequent observations showed a good correlation between the geographical distribution of BL and holo-endemic malaria. Significant space–time clustering in Africa and a latent period of less than a year in most cases has indicated that malaria infection was probably the trigger agent (Day *et al.*, 1985). A recent rise in malaria parasitemia in Tanzania has been followed by an increase in BL incidence (Geser *et al.*, 1989).

53.5 Known and suspected causes

Endemic and non-endemic forms of BL should be considered separately.

Endemic Burkitt's Lymphoma

Epidemiological and laboratory evidence indicate that at least two infectious agents are involved in the etiology of endemic BL, and their role is further discussed in Chapter 17.

Epstein–Barr virus (EBV)

EBV was the first virus to be associated with a human malignant tumor (Epstein & Barr, 1964). Laboratory studies have shown that EBV–DNA and membrane and nuclear antigens can be detected in at least 95% of endemic BL cases. In addition, EBV is able to transform human B lymphocytes into continuously growing cell lines carrying the viral DNA and showing most features of malignant transformation. It is oncogenic in certain South American sub-human primates.

Epidemiological evidence of a causal link has been more difficult to obtain since this virus is ubiquitous infecting 95–98% of the adult population throughout the world. The strongest evidence comes from an

IARC prospective study involving 42,000 Ugandan children. It found that those who years later developed BL had unusually high antibody titers to EBV. These high titers were interpreted as the result of an early and massive EBV infection (Geser *et al.*, 1982).

Malaria

Falciparum malaria has been causally associated with endemic BL based on a number of laboratory observations (Morrow, 1985).

Non-endemic Burkitt's Lymphoma

EBV markers are present in only 15–20% of the cells of BL in America, Europe and Asia where holoendemic malaria does not exist. However, the same chromosomal translocations observed in endemic BL are also found in non-endemic BL. The factors inducing these translocations and the subsequent malignant transformation in non-endemic areas are usually unknown. In the few BL-type cases reported in patients with AIDS or with a rare genetic syndrome, X-linked lymphoproliferative disease, the persistent stimulation of B cells by opportunistic infections may create a high risk of translocation. Subsequent EBV infection of such B cells may induce their malignant transformation.

53.6   Relevant laboratory studies

Virology, cytogenetics and molecular biological studies have been instrumental in characterizing two types of BL, endemic and sporadic, in the identification of EBV in endemic BL, and in demonstrating potential relevant mechanisms (Chapter 17). Using immunological markers, BL has now been characterized as a non-Hodgkin's lymphoma formed by B cells which synthesize heavy chain immunoglobulins (Ig) predominantly of the p subtype (Preud'homme *et al.*, 1985). In addition, cytogenetic and biochemical studies have shown that BL cells consistently show translocations of chromosome 8 with chromosomes 14, 2 and 22 (Lenoir *et al.*, 1982) which result in the activation of the cellular oncogene c-*myc* (Leder *et al.*, 1983), which is possibly responsible for the malignant transformation of the B cells.

53.7   Attributable risks

Malaria and EBV infections probably account for practically 100% of endemic BL cases. In non-endemic areas, EBV accounts for only a minority of the BL cases, and the etiological factors remain to be identified.

53.8   Conclusions

The impact of controlling malaria as a preventive strategy has been tested, but the results are not completely convincing. Continued monitoring of malaria and BL trends in endemic areas may help to understand the relationship between the two diseases.

53.9   References

Burkitt, D.P. (1958). A sarcoma involving the jaws in African children. *Br. J. Surg.*, **46**, 218–23.

Day, N.E., Smith, P.G. & Lachet, B. (1985). The latent period of Burkitt's lymphoma: the evidence from epidemiological clustering. In *Burkitt's Lymphoma: A Human Cancer Model*, IARC Scientific Publications No. 60, ed. G.M. Lenoir, G. O'Conor, & C.L.M. Olweny, pp. 187–95. Lyon: International Agency for Research on Cancer.

Epstein, M.A. & Barr, Y.M. (1964). Cultivation *in vitro* of human lymphoblasts from Burkitt's malignant lymphoma. *Lancet*, i, 252–3.

Geser, A., de-Thé, G., Lenoir, G., Day, N.E. & Williams, E.H. (1982). Final case reporting from the Ugandan prospective study of the relationship between EBV and Burkitt's lymphoma. *Int. J. Cancer*, **29**, 397–400.

Geser, A., Brubaker, G. & Draper, C.C. (1989). Effect of a malaria suppression program on the incidence of African Burkitt's lymphoma. *Am. J. Epidemiol.*, **129**, 740–52.

Leder, P., Battey, J., Lenoir, G., Moulding, C., Murphy, W., Potter, H., Stewart, T. & Taub, R. (1983). Translocation among antibody genes in human cancer. *Science*, **222**, 771–8.

Lenoir, G., Preud'homme, J.L., Bernheim, A. & Berger, R. (1982). Correlation between immunoglobulin light chain expression and variant translocation in Burkitt's lymphoma. *Nature*, **298**, 474–6.

Morrow, R.H. (1982). Burkitt's lymphoma. In *Cancer Epidemiology and Prevention*, ed. D. Schottenfeld & J.F. Fraumeni, Jr., pp. 779–94. Philadelphia: W.B. Saunders Co.

Morrow, R.H., Jr. (1985). Epidemiological evidence for the role of falciparum malaria in the pathogenesis of Burkitt's lymphoma. In *Burkitt's Lymphoma: A Human Cancer Model*, IARC Scientific Publications No 60, ed. G.M. Lenoir, G. O'Conor & C.L.M. Olweny, pp. 177–86. Lyon: International Agency for Research on Cancer.

Parkin, D.M., Sohier, R. & O'Conor, G.T. (1985). Geographic distribution of Burkitt's lymphoma. In *Burkitt's Lymphoma: A Human Cancer Model*, IARC Scientific Publications No 60, ed. G.M. Lenoir, G. O'Conor, & C.L.M. Olweny, pp. 155–64. Lyon: International Agency for Research on Cancer.

Preud'homme, J.L., Dellagi, K., Guglielmi, P., Vogler, L.B., Danon, F., Lenoir, G.M., Valensi, F. & Brouet, J.C. (1985). Immunologic markers of Burkitt's lymphoma cells. In *Burkitt's Lymphoma: A Human Cancer Model*, IARC Scientific Publications No 60, ed. G.M. Lenoir, G. O'Conor, & C.L.M. Olweny, pp. 47–64. Lyon: International Agency for Research on Cancer.

54

Hodgkin's disease (HD)

ICD-9 - 201

54.1   Introduction

In this relatively uncommon tumor, an infectious etiology has for long been suspected but never confirmed. Remarkable progress has also been made in treatment during the last 25 years which has had a significant effect on mortality rates.

54.2   Histology, classification and diagnosis

Hodgkin's disease (HD) is a malignant lymphoma characterized by the presence of multinucleated giant (Reed–Sternberg) cells. There are several histological sub-types and various classifications. The widely used Rye classification describes four sub-types that differ not only morpho-logically but in their clinical and epidemiological behavior. These four sub-types in order of best to worst prognosis are: lymphocytic pre-dominance, nodular sclerosis, mixed cellularity and lymphocytic depletion (Lukes *et al.*, 1966).

From the epidemiological point of view, three distinct forms of HD have been proposed: a childhood form (0–14 years), a young adult form (15–34 years), and an older adult form (55–74 years). Some authors regard these as separate entities (MacMahon, 1966) while others consider that they result from the interplay of environmental and host factors influencing the natural history of a single disease.

Correa and O'Conor (1971) describe three epidemiological patterns of HD:

Pattern I – is most common in developing countries and is characterized by high rates in male children, low incidence rates in the third decade and a second peak in older age groups. Most cases are classified as mixed cellularity or lymphocyte depletion with poor prognosis.

Fig. 54.1 Incidence rates around 1980: Hodgkin's disease (ICD-9 201).

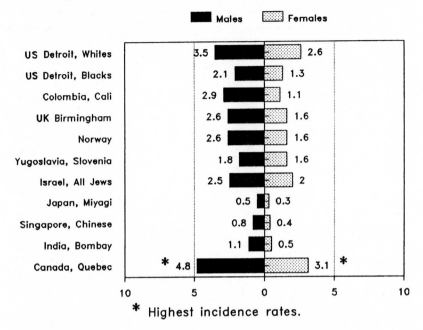

(after Muir *et al.*, 1987)

Pattern II – which is intermediate and found in rural areas of developed countries.

Pattern III – is the common type in developed countries and is characterized by very low rates in children and a pronounced initial peak in young adults (20–34 years). Most cases are of the nodular sclerosis sub-type with good prognosis.

54.3   Descriptive epidemiology
Incidence

The highest rates (ranging from 4 to 5) are reported from Italy and some registries in North America, the lowest rates (less than 1) are seen in Chinese and Japanese. Intermediate rates are observed in the rest of the world (Fig. 54.1). Most dramatic differences in incidence are seen in childhood (Chapter 58).

In the USA the incidence rates vary from 2 to 4 and are higher in whites than in blacks. The mortality rates in young adults are higher in the north than in south but have decreased in recent decades due to successful treatment and dramatic increases in survival (Rosenberg, 1989).

Time trends

Overall, the incidence rates appear to be relatively stable over time. However, different tendencies have been observed according to sex, age and histological type in the USA. Rates in children have been stable but have increased in young adults as a result of an increase in nodular sclerosis subtype. For adults over 40, rates for all sub-types have declined after 1970 (Glaser, 1986). In Japan an increase in the nodular sclerosis sub-type has also been observed. An increase in mortality rates has been observed in Japanese migrating to the USA. Time and space clustering and seasonality of cases has been described but may be possibly random (Grufferman & Delzell, 1984).

Age and sex distribution

At all ages, the rates are higher for males than for females, but the male excess is more marked in childhood.

54.4   Etiological inferences

The descriptive epidemiology and some histological characteristics of HD suggest an important role of environmental factors, possibly of an infectious nature, in the young adult form and perhaps in childhood.

54.5   Known and suspected causes
Familial aggregation

There have been many reports of the multiple occurrence of HD within the same family. An increased risk has been reported for siblings of young adults but not older adult cases. The risk is even higher for sibs of the same sex (Grufferman *et al.*, 1977). This familial aggregation may be the results of sharing a common environment in childhood or of genetic factors. An association with certain HLA types supports the latter possibility (Hors & Dausset, 1983).

Infectious origin

An infectious etiology of HD has for long been suspected, based on certain clinico-pathological characteristics resembling a chronic granulomatous infection. Further, many patients have unexplained persistent fever, frequent sweating and weight loss. Several early reports of time-space clustering and aggregation of exposure at schools, supported an infectious etiology by direct person-to-person spread. However, subsequent studies concluded that the clustering and aggregation probably resulted from bias in the ascertainment of cases (Grufferman *et al.*, 1979; Smith *et al.*, 1977).

It has also been suggested that in the young adult type of HD, i.e. nodular sclerosis, in analogy with the paralytic polio model, exposure to the infectious agent would be common in developing countries, and that infection would result either in immunity before adolescence or, in some children, development of HD. In developed countries, infection would be sporadic and delayed, leading to HD in young adults. Several epidemiological observations support this hypothesis. In developing countries the childhood type of HD is more frequent than in developed countries. Several studies in developed countries demonstrated that cases came from smaller families and a higher socio-economic class, and had fewer childhood infectious diseases than controls.

Such findings suggest that HD may be a rare manifestation of delayed infection by a common childhood virus and EBV is considered as the most likely candidate (Grufferman & Delzell, 1984; Mueller, 1987). Thus, retrospective cohort studies have shown that subjects with a previous history of serologically confirmed infectious mononucleosis have about a three-fold increased risk of HD (Muñoz *et al.*, 1978) and that EBV IgE and IgA antibody titers were higher in subjects who later developed HD than among controls (Mueller *et al.*, 1989). Recently, a high frequency of EBV genomes has been reported in HD (Herbst *et al.*, 1990). Cytomegalovirus antibody titers have also been found elevated in HD patients but not consistently. None the less, despite the long suspected relationship with an infectious agent, this has never been conclusively confirmed.

Occupation

An excess of HD reported among physicians and nurses who may have a greater contact with HD patients has not been confirmed. An increased risk reported following exposures to organic solvents, phenoxy acids and chlorophenols in Scandinavia (Hardell & Bengtsson, 1983) lacks confirmation. An association with wood-related industries is controversial.

Miscellaneous

A possible role for hormonal factors is suggested by a possible protective effect of childbearing. A weak and inconsistent association with tonsillectomy has also been described.

54.6   Relevant laboratory studies
Such studies have largely been directed to evaluating an association with suspected infectious agents, such as EBV, or genetic markers (HLA) (Herbst *et al.*, 1990).

54.7   Attributable risks
No relevant information is available.

54.8   Conclusions
Environmental factors probably play an important role in the etiology of HD as well as possible genetic susceptibility. Sex and age patterns, associated with socioeconomic development or industrialization, and aggregation within families, suggest an infectious etiology as yet unidentified, although EBV is strongly suspected.

54.9   References

Correa, P. & O'Conor, G.T. (1971). Epidemiology patterns of Hodgkins's disease. *Int. J. Cancer*, **8,**, 192–201.

Glaser, S.L. (1986). Recent incidence and secular trends in Hodgkin's disease and its histologic subtypes. *J. Chron. Dis.*, **39**, 789–98.

Grufferman, S. & Delzell, E. (1984). Epidemiology of Hodgkin's disease. *Epidemiol. Rev.*, **6**, 76–106.

Grufferman, S., Cole, P., Smith, P.G. & Lukes, R.J. (1977). Hodgkin's disease in siblings. *N. Engl. J. Med.*, **296**, 248–50.

Grufferman, S., Cole, P., & Levitan, T.R. (1979) Evidence against transmission of Hodgkin's disease in high school. *New Engl. J. Med.*, **300**, 1006–11.

Hardell, L. & Bengtsson, N.O. (1983). Epidemiological study of socioeconomic factors and clinical findings in Hodgkin's disease, and reanalysis of previous data regarding chemical exposure. *Br. J. Cancer*, **48**, 217–25.

Herbst, H., Niedobitek, G., Kneba, M., Hummel, M., Finn, T., Anagnostopoulos, I., Bergholz, M., Krieger, G. & Stein, H. (1990). High incidence of Epstein-Barr virus genomes in Hodgkin's Disease. *Am. J. Pathol.*, **137**, 13–18.

Hors, J. & Dausset, J. (1983). HLA and susceptibility to Hodgkin's disease. *Immunol. Rev.*, **70**, 167–92.

Lukes, R.J., Craver, L.F., Hall, T.C. *et al.* (1966). Report of the nomenclature committee. *Cancer Res.* **26**, 1311.

MacMahon, B. (1966). Epidemiology of Hodgkin's disease. *Cancer Res.*, **26**, 1189–200.

Mueller, N., Evans, A., Harris, N.L., Comstock, E., Jellum, E., Magnus, K., Orentreich, N., Polk, F. & Vogelman, J. (1989). Hodgkin's disease and Epstein–Barr virus. Altered antibody pattern before diagnosis. *N. Engl. J. Med.*, **32**, 689–95.

Mueller, N. (1987). Epidemiologic studies assessing the role of the Epstein–Barr virus in Hodgkin's disease. *Yale J. Biol. Med.*, **60**, 321–32.

Muir, C., Waterhouse, J., Mack, T., Powell, J. & Whelan, S. (eds.) (1987). *Cancer Incidence in Five Continents*, Volume V, IARC Scientific Publication No. 88. Lyon: International Agency for Research on Cancer.

Muñoz, N., Davidson, R.J.L., Witthoff, B. Ericsson, J.E. & de Thé, G. (1978). Infectious mononucleosis and Hodgkin's disease. *Int. J. Cancer*, **22**, 10–13.

Rosenberg, S.A. (1989). Hodgkin's disease: Challenges for the future. *Cancer Res.*, **49**, 767–9.

Smith, P.G., Kinlen, L.J., Pike, M.C., Jones, A. & Harris, R. (1977). Contacts between young patients with Hodgkin's disease: a case-control study. *Lancet*, **ii**, 59–62.

55

Non-Hodgkin's Lymphoma (NHL) and mycosis fungoides

ICD-9 200, 202

55.1 Introduction

Originally regarded as comparatively rare, this group of tumors appears to be increasing.

55.2 Histology, classification and diagnosis

Major changes in classification have occurred over the past decade. The terms 'lymphosarcoma' and 'reticulum cell sarcoma' (ICD-9 200) have gradually been abandoned by most histopathologists. This has resulted in increases in the number of neoplasms assigned to ICD-9 202 (other malignant neoplasm of lymphoid and histiocytic tissue), most being coded under rubric 202.8 (other lymphomas). Histologically such lymphomas are classified as diffuse or nodular. It has recently proved possible to classify tumors as arising from T or B lymphocytes or mononuclear phagocytes. None the less, despite attempts to formulate a uniform classification there remain areas of confusion.

Mycosis fungoides is a malignant form of non-Hodgkin's lymphoma involving the skin, arising from lymphocytes of T cell origin; *Sezary Syndrome* shares common cutaneous histopathological features.

Burkitt's lymphoma, a specific form of NHL, is described in Chapter 53.

55.3 Descriptive epidemiology
Incidence

In Canada and in the US rates vary usually between 10 and 12 in white males, but are somewhat lower, (around 7) in black populations. Rates in Australia and Israel are also around 10. In the UK and western Europe and in the Nordic countries rates average about 7. The highest rates occur in Varese in the north of Italy and in urban Vaud, Switzerland

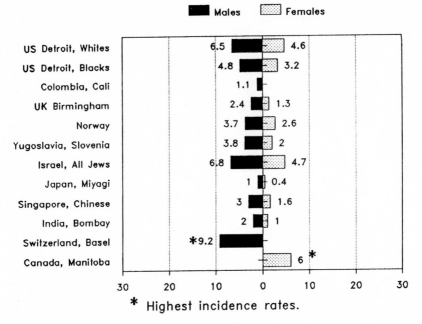

Fig. 55.1 Incidence rates around 1980: Lymphosarcoma (ICD-9 200).

* Highest incidence rates.

(after Muir *et al.*, 1987)

(12.5). In eastern Europe, as in much of Asia, rates vary between 3 and 5. (Fig. 55.1). An unusual number of cases presenting as primary intestinal lymphomas have been reported from the Mediterranean region (Chapter 27).

Time trends

In the USA, and in several other countries, there has been a slight but steady rise in incidence. It is uncertain whether this represents a reclassification and diagnostic artefact or is real, since at the same time a small fall in the incidence of Hodgkin's disease has been found. In California increases in AIDS-associated NHL have been observed.

Age distribution

These lymphomas appear at an earlier age than epithelial tumors and the risk increases relatively slowly.

Sex distribution

The sex ratio is about 4 : 3 and both sexes have the same geographic pattern.

Fig. 55.2 Incidence rates around 1980: Other reticuloses (ICD-9 202).

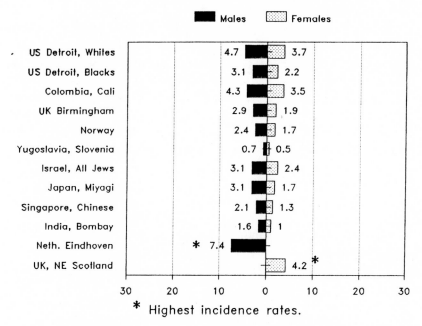

* Highest incidence rates.

(after Muir *et al.*, 1987)

Mycosis fungoides

Weinstock and Horm (1988) believe that mycosis fungoides is increasing rapidly in both incidence and mortality. In contrast to most NHL, US blacks are twice as likely to be afflicted as whites and the incidence in men is twice that in women.

55.4   Etiological inferences

Descriptive data provide evidence for only a modest effect of environmental factors. Occasional clusters have been ascribed to viral or chemical exposures without definitive confirmation.

55.5   Known and suspected causes

Comparatively little can be added to the extensive review of Greene (1982) and, at present, the cause of most cases remains unknown.

Immunodeficiency

The rare, naturally occurring immunodeficiencies carry an increased risk. A number of NHL-prone families have been reported, some of which were found to have evidence of a heritable immune dysfunction. A few cases are related to a rare X-linked lymphoproliferative syndrome in which individuals have an unregulated lymphoid response to EBV infection.

An increase has been found in renal transplant recipients especially in the first year which has suggested the possibility of viral infection (Locker & Nalesnik, 1989). Increases have also been described in patients receiving immunosuppressive therapy, and in patients with Sjogren's syndrome.

B cell lymphomas are occasionally encountered in AIDS patients (Kristal *et al.*, 1988; Hamilton-Dutoit *et al.*, 1989; Harnly *et al.*, 1988; Bernstein *et al.*, 1988). There is some evidence that very heavy exposures to radiation are associated with an increase of NHL.

Chemicals

A range of chemicals, including phenoxy acids, chlorophenols, organic solvents, pesticides and herbicides, have been suggested to be etiologically associated, combined exposures seemingly increasing risk (IARC, 1983; Hoar *et al.*, 1986; Hardell & Axelson, 1986; Woods *et al.*, 1987). Nevertheless, the evidence lacks consistency and requires confirmation.

While forestry workers in New Zealand were reported to have an increased risk of soft tissue sarcoma and non-Hodgkin's lymphoma, as well as a variety of other gastrointestinal tract tumors, such increases were not observed in sawmill workers during the same period. Following a reported outbreak of lymphoma among the employees of an underground colliery in New South Wales, Australia (standardized incidence ratio of 3.27 for non-Hodgkin's lymphoma and 7.27 for Hodgkin's disease), an exhaustive work-place environmental study failed to uncover any relevant factor. The mine and the characteristics of the work force of the colliery were similar to those elsewhere.

It has been hypothesized that chronic occupational exposure to environmental agents results in persistent antigenic stimulation, leading to a break-down in immune surveillance and eventual malignancy, but no such agent has been identified (Tuyp *et al.*, 1987; Reif *et al.*, 1989).

A number of drugs such as dapsone and combination therapy in HD are associated with various benign lymphadenopathies. These can only be responsible for a very small number of cases.

Infectious agents – viruses

Although a viral origin has long been suspected based on analogies with animal lymphomas, the situation in humans is uncertain. So far most studies have not been informative. EBV–DNA has been identified in AIDS-related lymphoma. In Japan, adult T-cell leukemia/

lymphoma has been reported associated with HTLV Type 1 carriers (Tokudome *et al.*, 1989). It is recognized that an interaction may occur between immunodeficiency and viral infection (Chapter 58).

Miscellaneous

A postulated link between tonsillectomy, appendectomy and malignant lymphomas has not been substantiated.

Case control studies of a wide range of factors fail to uncover any strong prenatal exposure (Greene, 1982), although a variety of occupational exposures have been suspected.

55.6 Relevant laboratory studies

Although such tumors can be induced by several chemicals, such studies have not been informative in relation to the human disease. Much laboratory work has been directed to identification of viruses. Cytological studies have been largely directed to improved identification of cell of origin with resultant better classification and prognosis assessment (Sheibani *et al.*, 1988).

55.7 Attributable risks

No relevant data are available.

55.8 Conclusions

The causes of these neoplasms for the most part remain unknown and there is no definitive explanation for the increased frequency in recent years.

55.9 References

Bernstein, L., Levin, D., Menck, H. & Ross, R.K. (1988). AIDS-related secular trends in cancer in Los Angeles County men: a comparison by marital status. *Cancer Res.*, **49**, 466–70.

Greene, M.H. (1982). Non-Hodgkin's lymphoma and mycosis fungoides. *In Cancer Epidemiology and Prevention*, ed. D. Schottenfeld & J.F. Fraumeni, Jr., pp. 754–78.

Hamilton-Dutoit, S.J., Pallesen, G., Karkov, J., Skinhj, P., Franzmann, M.B. & Perdersen, C. (1989). Identification of EBV-DNA in tumour cells of AIDS-related lymphomas by *in-situ* hybridisation. *Lancet*, **i**, 554–5.

Hardell, L. & Axelson, O. (1986). Phenoxyherbicides and other pesticides in the etiology of cancer: Some comments on the Swedish experiences. In *Cancer Prevention. Strategies in the Workplace*, ed. C.E. Becker & M.J. Coye, pp. 107–19. Washington: Hemisphere.

Harnly, M.E., Swan, S.H., Holly, E.A., Kelter, A. & Padian, N. (1988). Temporal trends in the incidence of non-Hodgkin's lymphoma and selected malignancies in a population with a high incidence of acquired immunodeficiency syndrome (AIDS). *Am. J. Epidemiol.*, **128**, 261–7.

Hoar, S.K., Blair, A., Holmes, F.F., Boysen, C.D., Robel, R.J., Hoover, R. & Fraumeni, J.F., Jr. (1986). Agricultural herbicide use and risk of lymphoma and soft-tissue sarcoma. *JAMA*, **256**, 1141–7.

IARC (1983). *IARC Monographs on the Evaluation of the Carcinogenic Risk of Chemicals to Humans*, Miscellaneous pesticides, volume 30. Lyon: International Agency for Research on Cancer.

Kristal, A.R., Nasca, P.C., Burnett, W.S. & Miki, J. (1988). Changes in the epidemiology of non-Hodgkin's lymphoma associated with epidemic human immunodeficiency virus (HIV) infection. *Am. J. Epidemiol.*, **128**, 711–18.

Locker, J. & Nalesnik, M. (1989). Molecular genetic analysis of lymphoid tumors arising after organ transplantation. *Am. J. Pathol.*, **135**, 977–87.

Muir, C., Waterhouse, J., Mack, T., Powell, J. & Whelan, S. (eds.) (1987). *Cancer Incidence in Five Continents*, volume V, IARC Scientific Publication No. 88. Lyon: International Agency for Research on Cancer.

Reif, J., Pearce, N., Kawachi, I. & Fraser J. (1989). Soft tissue sarcoma, Non-Hodgkin's lymphoma and other cancer in New Zealand forestry workers. *Int. J. Cancer*, **43**, 49–54.

Sheibani, K., Burke, J.S., Swartz, W.G., Nademanee, A. & Winberg, C.D. (1988). Monocytoid B-cell lymphoma. Clinicopathologic study of 21 cases of a unique type of low-grade lymphoma. *Cancer*, **62**, 1531–8.

Tokudome, S., Tokunaga, O., Shimamoto, Y., Miyamoto, Y., Sumida, I., Kikuchi, M., Takeshita, M., Ikeda, T., Fujiwara, K., Yoshihara, M., Yanagawa, T. & Nishizumi, M. (1989). Incidence of adult T-cell leukemia/lymphoma among human T-lymphotropic virus type I carriers in Saga, Japan. *Cancer Res.*, **49**, 226–8.

Tuyp, E., Burgoyne, A., Aitchison, T. & MacKie, R. (1987). A case-control study of possible causative factors in mycosis fungoides. *Arch. Dermatol.*, **123**, 196–200.

Weinstock, M.A. & Horm, J.W. (1988). Population-based estimate of survival and determinants of prognosis in patients with mycosis fungoides. *Cancer*, **62**, 1658–61.

Woods, J.S., Polissar, L., Severson, R.K., Heuser, L.S. & Kulander, B.G. (1987). Soft tissue sarcoma and non-Hodgkin's lymphoma in relation to phenoxy herbicide and chlorinated phenol exposure in western Washington. *J. Natl. Cancer Inst.*, **78**, 899–90

56

Multiple Myeloma and macroglobulinemia

ICD-9 203

56.1 Introduction

Multiple myeloma (MM) was the first of several conditions known as monoclonal gammopathies to be recognized. With newer and more precise methods of diagnosis, there has been increased interest in these tumors which seem to be increasing in incidence.

56.2 Histology, classification and diagnosis

Multiple myeloma is basically a malignant proliferative disorder of B-cells that secrete abnormal immunoglobulins, usually IgG or IgA. The diagnosis was formerly clinical, based on X-rays and a specific test for Bence Jones proteinuria. Today, confirmation of diagnosis is made by immuno-electrophoresis to detect free light chain globulins in the blood and urine, and by the demonstration of abnormal plasma cells in the bone marrow. On occasion, the disorders present as localized solitary masses in soft tissue. Waldenström's macroglobulinemia is a related condition.

56.3 Descriptive epidemiology
Incidence

Originally considered rare, in recent years the diagnosis of myeloma has become increasingly common. In the US SEER program, MM accounts for 1.1% of all cancers in whites and 2.1% in blacks. The incidence rates are 3–5 in white males and twice that in black males, in whom it is the most common hemopoietic neoplasm. Rates in Maoris and Hawaiians of both sexes are higher than in non-Maoris and white Hawaiians.

Geographical variations, however, must be evaluated with care in view of uncertainties of diagnosis. Though originally said to be rare in Africa, some reports suggest the rates are comparable to those in the USA. Rates

Fig. 56.1 Incidence rates around 1980: Multiple myeloma (ICD-9 203).

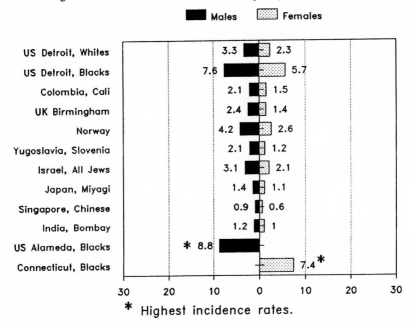

(after Muir *et al.*, 1987)

from Asia, including China, India and Japan are low. The higher rates in the upper social strata may reflect underdiagnosis in lower income groups (Johnston *et al.*, 1985).

Age and sex distribution

The tumor occurs in late life, the median age of diagnosis in the USA being 68 years in males and 69 in females. Rates increase with advancing age, those in US blacks being higher than in whites at all ages except over the age of 85. Patterns for other gammopathies are similar, but, generally, these are too rare to measure incidence rates.

Time trends

In general, the incidence of the disease appears to be increasing in all countries, especially in the older age-groups. In Denmark a two to three fold increase in incidence from 1943 to 1962 was reported for both sexes but after 1963 the rates have been rather stable with a recent tendency to decrease (Hansen et al., 1989). However, the mortality rates have been steadily increasing over recent decades in the U.S. (Devesa *et al.*, 1987). It is uncertain how much of these changes in incidence are due to diagnostic artefact.

56.4 Etiological inferences

Geographic variations have been relatively uninformative and suggest no environmental explanation for the unusually high frequencies reported in certain black populations.

56.5 Known and suspected causes

Possible causes have recently been reviewed by Pottern and Blattner (1985).

Familial and hereditary factors

Genetic factors are believed to contribute to racial and ethnic variations and some familial cases have been reported.

Radiation exposure

This is the only cause so far identified. An increase has been reported among atomic bomb survivors in whom raised levels of serum immunoglobulin and chromosome aberrations possibly represent a sub-clinical state. Increases have also been reported among radiologists (Cuzick, 1981).

Chemical agents

A range of chemicals has been suspected to be associated with MM, such as benzene. A significant trend was observed between the risk of MM and duration of exposure to this and other solvents (La Vecchia *et al.*, 1989). An association with other occupational exposures such as those in wood, rubber and petroleum industries and asbestos, has been suggested (Linet *et al.*, 1987), but not confirmed. A history of a medical implant and heavy alkali and carbon monoxide exposures were found to be significantly associated with light chain myeloma (about 15% of MM patients) but not with all types of MM combined. It is possible that these differences may have occurred by chance or they might indicate that the light chain type of the disease may be in part etiologically different (Williams *et al.*, 1989). At present, it would be premature to ascribe with certainty this cancer to any particular chemical agent.

Farming

Reports have suggested increased rates in farming areas but the data are not entirely consistent, rates in urban Vaud being twice those of rural regions of this Swiss canton. For females the converse is observed. Case-control studies, however, in various populations have consistently reported an increased risk associated with farming or agricultural work

(Pearce *et al.*, 1986), but the reason remains unknown. Thus, while a recent case-control study showed a significant increased risk of MM among farmers (RR 4.3; 95% CI 1.7 to 10.9) exposed to pesticides and herbicides (Boffetta *et al.*, 1989), this association has not been confirmed by others (Cuzick & De Stavola, 1988; La Vecchia *et al.*, 1989).

Miscellaneous

A history of 'immune-stimulating conditions' such as rheumatoid arthritis, chronic bacterial infections, asthma and allergies, has been reported slightly more often in cases than controls in some studies (Koepsell *et al.*, 1987) but not in others (Linet *et al.*, 1987; Cohen *et al.*, 1987). A previous history of diabetes was found to be significantly associated with MM in a recent study (Bofetta *et al.*, 1989).

56.6   Relevant laboratory studies

It is possible that better information regarding these lesions will develop through better sub-classification through modern immunogenetic approaches. No virus similar to those causing myeloma-related diseases in animals has been demonstrated in humans.

56.7   Attributable risks

No relevant data are available.

56.8   Conclusions

In summary, the causes of these syndromes are not known with certainty but it is possible that the increases observed in blacks in the older age-groups represent an environmental factor. Radiation and a farming occupation are the main risk factors so far identified.

56.9   References

Boffetta, P., Stellman, S.D. & Garfinkel, L. (1989). A case-control study of multiple myeloma nested in the American Cancer Society prospective study. *Int. J. Cancer*, **43**, 554–9.

Cohen, H.J., Bernstein, R.J. & Grufferman, S. (1987). Role of immune stimulation in the etiology of multiple myeloma: a case-control study. *Am. J. Hematol.*, **24**, 119–26.

Cuzick, J. (1981). Radiation induced myelomatosis. *N. Engl. J. Med.*, **304**, 204–10.

Cuzick, J. & De Stavola, B. (1988). Multiple myeloma – A case-control study. *Br. J. Cancer*, **57**, 516–20.

Devesa, S.S., Silverman, D.T., Young, J.L., Pollack, E.S., Brown, C.C., Horm, J.W., Percy, C.L., Myers, M.H., McKay, F.W. & Fraumeni, J.F. (1987). Cancer incidence and mortality trends among whites in the United States, 1947–84. *J. Natl. Cancer Inst.*, **79**, 701–70.

Hansen, N.E., Karle, H. & Olsen, J.H. (1989). Trends in the incidence of multiple myeloma in Denmark 1943–1982: a study of 5500 patients. *Eur. J. Haematol.*, **42**, 72–6.

Johnston, J.M., Grufferman, S., Bourquet, C.C., Delzell, E., Delong, E.R. & Cohen, H.J. (1985). Socioeconomic status and risk of multiple myeloma. *J. Epidemiol. Community Health*, **39**, 175–8.

Koepsell, T.D., Daling, J.R., Weiss, N.S., Taylor, J.W., Olshan, A.F., Lyon, J.L., Swanson, G.M. & Child, M. (1987). Antigenic stimulation and the occurrence of multiple myeloma. *Am. J. Epidemiol.*, **126**, 1051–62.

La Vecchia, C., Negri, E., D'Avanzo, B. & Franceschi, S. (1989). Occupation and lymphoid neoplasms. *Br. J. Cancer*, **60**, 385–8.

Linet, M.S., Harlow, S.D. & McLaughlin, J.K. (1987). A case-control study of multiple myeloma in whites: chronic antigenic stimulation, occupation, and drug use. *Cancer Res.*, **47**, 2978–81.

Muir, C., Waterhouse, J., Mack, T., Powell, J. & Whelan, S. (eds) (1987). *Cancer Incidence in Five Continents*, Volume V, IARC Scientific Publication No. 88. Lyon: International Agency for Research on Cancer.

Pearce, N.E., Smith, A.H., Howard, J.K., Sheppard, R.A., Giles, H.J. & Teague, C.A. (1986). Case-control study of multiple myeloma and farming. *Br. J. Cancer*, **54**, 493–500.

Pottern, L.M. & Blattner, W.A. (1985). Etiology and epidemiology of multiple myeloma and related disorders. In *Neoplastic Diseases of the Blood*, ed. P.H. Wiernik, G.P. Canellos, R.A. Kyle & C.A. Schiffer. New York: Churchill Livingstone.

Williams, A.R., Weiss, N.S., Koepsell, T.D., Lyon, J.L. & Swanson, G.M. (1989). Infectious and noninfectious exposures in the etiology of light chain myeloma: A case-control study. *Cancer Res.*, **49**, 4038–41.

57

The leukemias

ICD-9 204–208

57.1 Introduction

The term leukemia covers a group of malignant diseases of the blood. As a whole, these constitute less than 5% of all cancers. Despite extensive studies over the last several decades, relatively little is known regarding causation. Childhood leukemias are discussed in Chapter 58.

57.2 Histology, classification and diagnosis

Leukemias have been classified traditionally according to the cytology and origin of the leukemic cells. The common types are *lymphocytic* and *myelocytic* in origin. The rarer varieties are *monocytic, basophilic, eosinophilic, plasma cell, erythro-* and *hairy-cell* leukemias. Each cell type can be further divided into two major groups: acute and chronic depending on the degree of cellular differentiation.

Modern classification is dependent on a growing number of histological, cytochemical and immunological techniques to identify specific cellular biomarkers. None the less, the classification of acute leukemia by cell type can be difficult and a number are described as stem cell. From an epidemiological point of view, it is sufficient to discuss leukemias as acute lymphocytic (ALL), chronic lymphocytic (CLL), and chronic myelocytic (CML).

In certain cases of CLL, there is a close association with lymphomas and a number of lymphomas terminate in a leukemic phase whether or not the bone marrow is initially involved.

57.3 Descriptive epidemiology
Incidence

Incidence rates for all leukemias combined vary from 2.2 to 11.6 in males and from 1.1 to 10.3 in females, and tend to be higher in North

America, Western Europe and Israel, and low in Asia and Africa (Appendix I, Table 1). In general, similar patterns are observed for both lymphoid and myeloid leukemias, the highest rates being found in western countries whereas rates are lower in Asia. Chronic lymphocytic leukemia is, however, rare in Chinese and Japanese populations but a specific type of T cell leukemia is reported to be unduly common in South Japan and the Caribbean. Monocytic leukemia is uniformly rare with rates well below unity in practically all countries for both sexes.

The majority of leukemias in children are either acute lymphocytic leukemias or stem cell leukemias. Parkin *et al.* (1988) have reviewed lymphoma/leukaemia ratios in childhood. These are around 0.5 in most populations, rising to unity in several developing countries. The very high ratios observed in East Africa may be due to under-diagnosis (Chapter 58).

Time trends

The overall incidence and mortality from leukemia has been virtually stable in the USA over the past ten years, but in children there have been substantial declines in mortality following advances in therapy (NCI, 1988).

Age distribution

The incidence rises with age from a low of 1 to 2 per 100,000 to 30 or more over 50 years of age. However, there is a distinct childhood peak between 2 and 4 years. This is especially seen in white populations.

Sex distribution

In general, males are more affected by leukemia than females.

57.4   Etiological inferences

The relatively modest variation in incidence of leukemia suggests that environmental factors are relatively weak or ubiquitous. Modest variations between ethnic groups suggest that ethnic factors may be involved as does the rarity of CLL in Asia. Clusters have been reported which have been ascribed to viruses, toxic wastes, radiation, etc. In no case has the evidence of a cause been convincing and it is probable that most such clusters are random.

57.5   Familial or hereditary factors

Although possible familial leukemia cases have occurred (Heath, 1985), the evidence, including suggestive but inconclusive results in concordant twins, is inconsistant. Certain immunological conditions, some of which are hereditary, predispose to leukemia (Chapter 58).

57.6   Known and suspected causes

There are several recent reviews (Heath, 1985; Bloomfield, 1985; Li, 1985; Wiernik *et al.*, 1985) but, in general, little is known about the etiology of most leukemias.

Radiation

The most important etiological factor is ionizing radiation (Chapter 16). Evidence comes from a number of sources, including increases in early radiologists, also in men receiving X-ray therapy for ankylosing spondylitis. Cases have been reported following occupational exposure and modest increases in children following prenatal diagnostic X-rays.

Increases were also observed in Japanese populations surviving the atomic bomb explosions in Hiroshima and Nagasaki and in those exposed to atom bomb testing (Caldwell *et al.*, 1980). The significance of an increase in leukemia among children in Utah, however, following experimental testing of atomic bombs is uncertain and controversial, since it occurred in areas where rates previously below the national average returned to normal.

The possibility that ambient radiation around nuclear power plants may cause leukemia and other cancer is a matter of great concern. Gardner *et al.* (1990*a, b*) reported that the relative risks for leukemia and non-Hodgkin's lymphoma were higher in children born near the Sellafield nuclear plant and in children whose fathers were employed at the plant, particularly those with high radiation dose recordings before conception of the child (Chapter 12). It will be interesting to see whether comparable findings emerge from studies at other nuclear installations. In the UK an earlier report of increases around nuclear power plants became difficult to interpret when later studies showed the same phenomenon around proposed plants which were never built. No definite evidence for an etiological role of electromagnetic radiation is available.

Therapeutic drugs

There is some evidence that certain drugs such as chloramphenicol and phenylbutazone may be associated with leukemia. There are similar reports for melphalan and other agents used to treat malignant neoplasms (IARC, 1987; Kaldor *et al.*, 1990*a,b*).

Other chemicals

In view of its ubiquity in industry and ambient environment, the reported association of exposure to benzene and leukemia is of interest (IARC, 1987). Risk appears to be considerable in artisanal use, as in shoe repairers in Turkey. Such leukemias tend to be acute myelocytic in type, but some cases of CML and CLL have reported. However, the number of cases reported is very small. Although the association is accepted, it is not possible to determine the level of exposure that is hazardous. Leukemia has been related to a number of occupations, including the offspring of workers in hydrocarbon-related industries (Hakulinen *et al.*, 1976). These reports have not been confirmed.

Infectious agents

Following demonstration of viral leukemia in rodents and other animals, there has been considerable interest in the role of viruses in humans (Gelmann et al., 1985). To date, studies of clusters have yielded equivocal results and there is little evidence to indicate that such viruses as the Epstein–Barr (EBV) are in fact involved (Heath, 1985). Kinlen (1988) has suggested a possible infectious cause due to internal population movements to explain the inconsistent findings near nuclear power plants. No correlation has been observed between the incidence of bovine leukemia of viral origin and human leukemia.

Recently, a human retro-virus, HTLV has been shown to cause adult T-cell leukemia and lymphoma in Japan, and this association is now accepted. In a review of retro-viruses, Westin *et al.* (1985) postulated that expression of viral genes, the genes for TGGF, and the many homologues of known viral oncogenes does not appear necessary for maintenance of the leukemic state, although any of the latter may be necessary early in the disease.

57.6   Relevant laboratory studies

Recent studies have concentrated on the role of retro-viruses (Robert-Guroff & Gallo, 1986). A number of leukemias are associated with cytogenetic markers of which the best known is the Ph chromosome in chronic myelocytic leukemia. While further sub-classification of leukemias will be possible by newer methods, including use of monoclonal antibody techniques, this may be eventually of greatest value in determining treatment rather than in identifying etiological factors (Kyle

& Greipp, 1985; Stanley *et al.*, 1985). The study of chromosomal abnormalities as possible guides to precursor lesions following exposure to carcinogenic agents, such as chemicals, has been discussed (Sandler & Collman, 1987) (Chapter 5).

57.7   Attributable risks
While a few cases may be related to inherited chromosomal abnormalities, the most important known cause is exogenous radiation which could account for up to 10% of cases in some communities. Chemical-related cases are probably less than 1% of the total. The role of background radiation is unknown.

57.8   Conclusions
Although forming a small portion of total cancer incidence, leukemias have been extensively investigated, possibly because of their frequency in children. To date, no practical preventative measures can be suggested, apart from control of ionizing radiation exposures, e.g. diagnostic X-rays.

57.9   References

Bloomfield, C.D. (ed.) (1985). *Chronic and Acute Leukemias in Adults*. Boston: Martinus Nijhoff.

Caldwell, G.G., Kelley, D.B. & Heath, C.W., Jr. (1980). Leukemia among participants in military maneuvers at a nuclear bomb test (Smoky). *JAMA*, **244**, 1575–8.

Gardner, M.J., Snee, M.P., Hall, A.J., Powell, C.A., Downes, S., Terrell, J.D. (1990*a*). Results of case-control study of leukemia and lymphoma among young people near Sellafield nuclear plant in West Cumbria. *Br. Med. J.*, **300**, 423–9.

Gardner, M.J., Hall, A.J., Snee, M.P., Downes, S., Powell, C.A., Terrell, J.D. (1990*b*). Methods and basic data of case-control study of leukaemia and lymphoma among young people near Sellafield nuclear plant in West Cumbria. *Br. Med. J.*, **300**, 429–34.

Gelmann, E.P., Wong-Staal, F. & Gallo, R.C. (1985). The etiology of acute leukemia: molecular genetics and viral oncology. In *Neoplastic Diseases of the Blood*, ed. P.H. Wiernik, G.P. Canellos, R.A. Kyle & C.A. Schiffer, pp. 161–82. New York: Churchill Livingstone.

Hakulinen, T., Salonen, T. & Teppo, L. (1976). Cancer in the offspring of fathers in hydrocarbon-related occupations. *Br. J. Prev. Soc. Med.*, **30**, 138–40.

Heath, C.W., Jr. (1985). Epidemiology and hereditary aspects of acute leukemia. In *Neoplastic Diseases of the Blood*, ed. P.H. Wiernik, G.P. Canellos, R.A. Kyle & C.A. Schiffer, pp. 183–200. New York: Churchill Livingstone.

IARC, (1987). *IARC Monographs on the Evaluation of Carcinogenic Risks to Humans*, Overall Evaluations of Carcinogenicity: An Updating of IARC Monographs Volumes 1 to 42, Supplement 7. Lyon: International Agency for Research on Cancer.

Kaldor, J.M., Day, N.E., Pettersson, F., Clarke E., Pedersen, D., Mehnert, W., Bell, J., Host, H., Prior, P., Karjalainen, S., Neal, F., Koch, M., Band, P., Choi, W., Pompe Kirn, V., Arslan, A., Zarén, B., Belch, A.R., Storm, H., Kittlemann, B.,Fraser P., Stovall, M. (1990*a*). Leukemia following chemotherapy for ovarian cancer. *N. Engl. J. Med.*, **322**, 1–6.

Kaldor, J.M., Day, N.E., Clarke, E., Van Leeywen, F.E., Henry-Amar, M., Fiorentino, M.V., Bell, J., Pedersen, D., Band, P., Assouline, D., Koch, M., Choi, W., Prior, P., Blair,

V., Langmark, F., Pompe Kirn, V., Neal, F., Peters, D., Pfeiffer, R., Karjalainen, S., Cuzick, J., Sutcliffe, S.B., Somers, R., Pellae-Cossett, B., Pappagallo, G.L., Fraser, P., Storm, H., Stovall, M. (1990*b*). Leukemia following Hodgkin's Disease. *N. Engl. J. Med.*, **322**, 7–13.

Kinlen, L. (1988). Evidence for an infective cause of childhood leukaemia: comparison of a Scottish new town with nuclear reprocessing sites in Britain. *Lancet*, **ii**, 1323–6.

Kyle, R.A. & Greipp, P.R. (1985). Immunoglobulins and laboratory recognition of monoclonal proteins. In *Neoplastic Diseases of the Blood*, ed. P.H. Wiernik, G.P. Canellos, R.A. Kyle & C.A. Schiffer, pp. 431–59. New York: Churchill Livingstone.

Li, F.P. (1985). The chronic leukemias: Etiology and epidemiology. *In Neoplastic Diseases of the Blood*, ed. P.H. Wiernik, G.P. Canellos, R.A. Kyle & C.A. Schiffer, pp. 7–17. New York: Churchill Livingstone.

NCI (National Cancer Institute) (1988). *Annual Cancer Statistics Review Including Cancer Trends*: 1950–1985, NIH Publication No. 88–2789, U.S. Department of Health and Human Services, Public Health Service, National Institutes of Health. Washington: U.S. Government Printing Office.

Parkin, D.M., Stiller, G.J., Draper, C.A., Bieber, B., Terracini & Young, J.L. (eds.) (1988). *International Incidence of Childhood Cancer*, IARC Scientific Publications No. 97. Lyon: International Agency for Research on Cancer.

Robert-Guroff, M. & Gallo, R.C. (1986). HTLV: The family of human T lymphotropic retroviruses and their role in leukemia and AIDS. In *Biochemical and Molecular Epidemiology of Cancer*, pp. 293–301. New York: Alan R. Liss.

Sandler, D.P. & Collman, G.W. (1987). Cytogenetic and environmental factors in the etiology of the acute leukemias in adults. *Am. J. Epidemiol.*, **126**, 1017–32.

Stanley, M., McKenna, R.W., Ellinger, G. & Brunning, R.D. (1985). Classification of 358 cases of acute myeloid leukemia by FAB criteria: Analysis of clinical and morphologic features. In *Chronic and Acute Leukemias in Adults*, ed. C.D. Bloomfield, pp. 147–74. Boston: Martinus Nijhoff.

Westin, E.H., Wong-Staal, F. & Gallo, R.C. (1985). Retroviruses and *onc* genes in human leukemias and lymphomas. In *Chronic and Acute Leukemias in Adults*, ed. C.D. Bloomfield, pp. 1–25. Boston: Martinus Nijhoff.

Wiernik, P.H., Canellos, G.P., Kyle, R.A. & Schiffer, C.A. (1985). *Neoplastic Diseases of the Blood*. New York: Churchill Livingstone.

Part XIII

Cancers in children and multiple primary cancers

58

Cancers in children

58.1 Introduction

It is well known that cancer patterns are different between children and adults, and considerable information has accrued in recent years. This chapter reviews the epidemiological and etiological features of the main tumor types.

58.2 Descriptive epidemiology

Incidence rates in this chapter are given in *cases per million population*.

Incidence

Population-based data on the incidence of childhood cancer has recently been reported (Parkin *et al.*, 1988). Table 58.1 shows the age-standardized incidence rates for all childhood cancers combined from selected registries around the world. As in adults, there is only a modest three-fold difference between the highest and the lowest rates. The highest rates in boys (over 160 per million) are reported from Nigeria (Ibadan), New Zealand (Maoris), Spain (Zaragoza) and Brazil (Sao Paulo). The lowest rates (below 80 per million) are seen in Kuwait (Kuwaitis) and in Fiji. There may be some under-reporting, especially in developing countries. In general, boys are affected more often than girls.

Mortality

In developed countries, in children under 15 years of age, cancer is the second cause of death, after accidents. Mortality rates have been declined steadily in most countries, largely due to advances in the treatment of acute lymphocytic leukemia and certain lymphomas.

Table 58.1. *Age-standardized cancer incidence rates for all sites (per million) for children under 15 years of age.*

	Males	Females		Males	Females
Africa			**Europe**		
Nigeria – Ibadan	198.5	111.7	Czechoslovakia –	138.2	111.4
Uganda – Kampala	101.3	79.9	Slovakia		
Zimbabwe – Bulawayo	87.2	82.1	Denmark	143.5	110.6
America			FRG – Saarland	122.0	102.6
Canada –			Finland	150.4	118.1
Atlantic Prov.	102.6	90.4	France – Bas Rhin	136.4	123.5
Western Prov.	148.7	119.4	German Demo. Rep.	132.9	113.8
USA, SEER – white	143.9	126.9	UK, England & Wales	119.6	96.8
SEER – black	107.2	107.9	Hungary	113.5	82.2
Brazil – S. Paulo	164.1	126.4	Italy – Torino	157.0	124.9
Colombia – Cali	130.1	107.9	Norway	138.1	105.9
Costa Rica	154.7	119.3	Poland – Warsaw City	107.5	86.9
Cuba	103.1	78.7	Spain – Zaragoza	169.9	101.9
Puerto Rico	116.8	99.0	Sweden	149.9	129.9
Asia			Switzerland	136.0	114.4
China – Shanghai	115.2	98.9	Yugoslavia – Slovenia	126.0	86.6
India – Bombay	86.3	54.5	**Oceania**		
Israel – Jews	148.8	118.9	Australia – N.S. Wales	153.0	122.2
Japan – Osaka	127.0	100.5	Fiji – Fijian	60.0	61.0
Kuwait – Kuwaits	75.4	63.2	– Indian	50.6	28.6
Philippines – Manila	95.6	80.9	N. Zealand – Maori	173.9	111.5
Singapore – Chinese	105.2	88.8	– non-Maori	140.7	121.6
– Malays	89.0	74.7			

(After Parkin *et al.*, 1988.)

58.3   Epidemiologic features of specific tumors

Leukemia (Chapter 57)

Leukemia is relatively more common in children than in adults and accounts for about one-third of all childhood cancers in most populations except in Africa and in some Asian countries (e.g. Bangladesh and Kuwait) where it represents only 10–15% (Parkin *et al.*, 1988). Over 50% of childhood leukemias in most populations are acute lymphocytic leukemias (ALL). The age-adjusted incidence rates for ALL and acute non-lymphocytic leukemia (ANLL) in selected populations are given in Tables 58.2 and 58.3. The highest rates of ALL (over 30) are reported from Costa Rica, Colombia, whites in certain registries from the USA and Canada, Switzerland, The Netherlands, Germany and Australia. The lowest rates (below 15) are seen in most African and Asian countries and in blacks in the USA. Rates are slightly higher in boys than in girls. A peak

Table 58.2. *Acute lymphocytic leukemia: age-standardized incidence rates per million (0–14 years).*

	Males	Females
Costa Rica	47.5[a]	41.9[a]
Colombia – Cali	40.0	23.2
USA – SEER – whites	35.9	29.7
UK – England and Wales	33.7	25.5
Singapore – Chinese	25.5	20.5
France – Bas Rhin	24.7	27.5
Norway	24.4	20.3
Israel – Jews	21.2	20.0
Yugoslavia – Slovenia	17.4	18.1
Japan – Miyagi	17.3	15.5
USA – SEER – blacks	14.4	15.3
India – Bombay	13.2	8.6
Kuwait – Kuwaitis	10.9	12.9
Nigeria – Ibadan	6.5	4.6

[a] highest incidence rates.
(After Parkin *et al.*, 1988.)

Table 58.3. *Acute non-lymphocytic leukemia: age-standardized incidence rates per million (0–14 years).*

	Males	Females
China – Shanghai	13.5[a]	10.5[a]
Japan – Miyagi	11.7	10.1
Yugoslavia – Slovenia	10.1	4.3
Israel – Jews	9.8	3.3
Norway	7.7	8.4
Nigeria – Ibadan	7.5	2.1
Singapore – Chinese	6.7	6.5
UK – England and Wales	6.1	5.7
USA – SEER – whites	5.6	6.5
France – Bas Rhin	4.6	3.9
USA – SEER – blacks	4.3	6.2
India – Bombay	3.6	3.1
Colombia – Cali	2.5	7.2
Kuwait – Kuwaitis	1.0	1.1

[a] highest incidence rates.
(After Parkin *et al.*, 1988.)

in the incidence of ALL at four years of age emerged first in Great Britain in the 1920s, in the USA in the 1940s, in Japan in the 1960s, but not in black children in the USA or in Africa.

The highest rates of ANLL (over 10.0 per million) are seen in certain

Asian countries (e.g. China, Japan), and Maoris in New Zealand; low rates (under 3.0 per million) in other Asian countries (India), the Middle East (Kuwait), in Africa, in some Latin American countries (Brazil, Cuba), and Poland. Maoris in New Zealand have similar rates of ALL and ANLL.

Chronic myelocytic leukemia (CML) is uncommon and only represents 1–2% of all childhood leukemias in America, Africa and Europe but it accounts for a relatively high proportion of all leukemias in Sudan (30%), in Bangladesh (20%) and in Chinese in Singapore (10%). In Ankara, Turkey, acute monomyelocytic leukemia (AML) accounts for about 40% of all leukemias as compared to only 4% among US white children. These high frequencies are not believed to be due to an artefact of registration.

Risk factors

Radiation   Ionizing radiation (Chapter 16) from the atomic bomb in Japan caused an increased frequency of the usual acute leukemias of childhood and of CML peaking five years after exposure.

Children under 10 years were more susceptible than adults to radiation-induced leukemia, the relative risk being two to three times greater. By the fifteenth year after exposure, the excess of CML was no longer detectable nor that of AML a few years later.

Stewart and co-workers (1956) reported on the increased frequency of leukemia and of other childhood cancers after maternal exposure to diagnostic irradiation during pregnancy. Much of the evidence supports a causal relationship (Miller & Boice, 1986). The biological plausibility of a radiation-induced increase of the same magnitude (RR 1.5) for both leukemia and various solid tumors of childhood has been questioned (since the dissimilar epidemiological characteristics of each type suggest different etiologies). Studies of atomic bomb survivors have not confirmed an increased risk of leukemia after low-dose intrauterine or preconception irradiation (Yoshimoto *et al.*, 1988). Increase may reflect subtle abnormalities of maternal physiology or lifestyle associated with diagnostic radiation during pregnancy and thus be independently related to cancer in the offspring. MacMahon (1985) concluded that the association will probably never be completely resolved. It is not yet possible to evaluate a recent report of increased leukemia in the offspring of irradiated fathers (Evans, 1990) (Chapter 57).

Viruses (Chapter 17)   The association with viruses has recently been reviewed by Miller (1989). In the 1960s several clusters of leukemia attracted great publicity, and suggested the possibility of some horizontal virus infection. The development of statistical procedures to test objectively the significance of such clusters showed that they occurred no more often than expected by chance.

The leukemias related to HTLV-I and HTLV-II seen in Japan rarely, if ever, occur in children, although they may harbor the virus due to vertical transmission or infected blood products.

Chromosomal abnormalities (Chapter 18) Children at high risk of leukemia often have common inborn or acquired chromosomal anomalies. Down's syndrome typically has an extra chromosome 21. Two heritable disorders, Bloom's syndrome (sun-sensitive rash of the face and dwarfism) and Fanconi's aplastic anemia are characterized by chromosomes with marked instability in culture. Exposures to ionizing radiation or benzene produce long-lasting chromosomal abnormalities. Certain subtypes of leukemia have a consistent chromosomal abnormality, such as the Philadelphia chromosome (partial deletion of chromosome 22) observed in about 90% of patients with chronic myelocytic leukemia (Miller, 1986).

Lymphomas (Chapters 53, 54, 55)

This group comprises a heterogeneous group of diseases that accounts for 10–15% of all childhood cancer in most populations. In some countries in Africa, in the Middle East (Kuwait, Iraq) and in Papua New Guinea they represent 30–80% of all childhood malignancies (Parkin *et al.*, 1988). Table 58.4 shows the distribution of the major lymphoma types in selected populations. Hodgkin's lymphoma represents over 50% of all lymphomas among blacks in the USA and in Pakistan, while Burkitt's lymphoma accounts for 60–90% of all lymphomas in Sub-Saharan African countries and in Papua New Guinea (Chapter 53).

Tables 58.5 and 58.6 give the age-adjusted incidence rates for Hodgkin's and non-Hodgkin's lymphomas (NHL) in selected populations. High rates of Hodgkin's disease (over 10 per million) are reported from Costa Rica and Kuwait. The lowest rates (below 3 per million) are seen in China, Philippines, Singapore, Japan, Finland and France. High rates of NHL (over 10 per million) are reported from Brazil, Cuba, Israel, Kuwait and Spain and the lowest rates (below 3 per million) from Japan, the Philippines, blacks in the USA, Denmark and Hungary. Boys are affected slightly more frequently than girls by both types of lymphoma.

Risk factors

Epstein–Barr virus (*EBV*) In Africa, Burkitt's lymphoma is related to infection with EBV, and exhibits temporal and geographical

Table 58.4. *Distribution of lymphomas in male children from selected populations.*

	Hodgkin's (%)	Burkitt's (%)	Others (%)
Africa			
Malawi	5.3	63.2	31.6
Morocco – Rabat	36.6	15.2	48.2
Nigeria – Ibadan	8.0	78.8	13.2
Tunisia	45.0	22.5	32.4
Uganda – West Nile	1.1	90.3	8.6
America			
Canada – Western Prov.	24.2	2.7	73.1
USA, SEER – whites	34.6	16.6	48.7
USA, SEER – blacks	54.5	4.5	40.9
Brazil – S. Paulo	32.5	2.1	65.4
Colombia – Cali	31.0	41.4	27.6
Asia			
China – Shanghai	19.7	—	80.3
India – Bombay	40.7	1.0	58.3
Israel – Jews	24.2	15.5	60.2
Japan – Miyagi	9.1	9.1	81.8
Pakistan	67.8	1.7	30.5
Europe			
Denmark	27.5	25.5	47.1
UK – England and Wales	39.4	1.9	58.8
Norway	27.1	8.5	64.4
Yugoslavia – Slovenia	42.9	—	57.1
Oceania			
Australia – N.W. Wales	28.2	1.9	69.9
New Zealand – Maori	37.5	—	62.5
Papua New Guinea	3.6	55.4	41.1

% of all lymphoma.
[a] Others include non-Hodgkin lymphoma, unspecified lymphoma, histiocytosis X and other reticuloendothelial tumors.
(After Parkin *et al.*, 1988.)

changes in occurrence that reflect environmental influences (O'Conor, 1988). It is thought that holo-endemic malaria causes a continuous intense antigenic stimulus that alters susceptibility to EBV so that it gives rise to the lymphoma in Africa (Chapter 17).

In 1975, families were first recognized in which more than one boy developed B-cell lymphoproliferative disorders including: lymphoma, chronic or fatal infectious mononucleosis, or acquired agammaglobulinemia. These lymphomas probably occur due to overwhelming infection with EBV due to an X-linked genetic susceptibility in this syndrome (Purtilo *et al.*, 1988).

Table 58.5. *Hodgkin's disease: age-standardized incidence rates per million (0–14 years).*

	Males	Females
Costa Rica	14.0[a]	7.3[a]
Kuwait – Kuwaitis	13.7	7.0
Nigeria – Ibadan	10.8	2.3
Yugoslavia – Slovenia	9.2	4.6
Israel – Jews	8.7	6.0
Colombia – Cali	7.8	4.3
USA – SEER – blacks	7.5	1.9
India – Bombay	7.0	1.2
USA – SEER – whites	6.5	5.9
UK England and Wales	5.6	2.4
France – Bas Rhin	4.0	1.6
Norway	3.0	1.8
Singapore – Chinese	2.5	0.7
Japan – Miyagi	0.4	—

[a] highest incidence rates.
(After Parkin *et al.*, 1988.)

Table 58.6. *Non-Hodgkin's lymphoma: age-standardized incidence rates per million (0–14 years).*

	Males	Females
Brazil – Fortaleza	23.9[a]	11.9[a]
Israel – Jews	16.8	6.0
Kuwait – Kuwaits	15.2	4.9
Nigeria – Ibadan	10.8	4.5
France – Bas Rhin	9.2	8.2
UK England and Wales	7.9	3.4
India – Bombay	7.2	1.8
Singapore – Chinese	7.1	5.4
USA – SEER – whites	6.9	2.8
Norway	5.0	2.1
USA – SEER – blacks	3.9	1.5
Colombia – Cali	3.4	5.5
Japan – Miyagi	1.8	—
Hungary	0.6	0.3

[a] highest incidence rates.
(After Parkin *et al.*, 1988.)

Immunodeficiency While groups at high risk of leukemia have chromosomal anomalies in common, in contrast groups at high risk of lymphoma tend to show evidence of inborn or acquired immuno-deficiency. Included in this category are children with heritable immuno-

Table 58.7. *Brain and spinal tumors: age-standardized incidence rates per million (0–14 years).*

	Males	Females
Sweden	37.0[a]	30.3[a]
Norway	30.2	22.6
Yugoslavia – Slovenia	27.2	14.5
UK – England and Wales	26.4	22.4
USA – SEER – whites	26.4	23.3
Israel – Jews	25.1	22.6
France – Bas Rhin	25.0	28.9
USA – SEER – blacks	21.0	23.3
Colombia – Cali	16.8	16.9
Singapore – Chinese	11.0	12.4
Japan – Miyagi	8.6	10.4
India – Bombay	8.5	6.9
Nigeria – Ibadan	5.5	4.6
Kuwait – Kuwaitis	4.7	5.1

[a] highest incidence rates.
(After Parkin *et al.*, 1988.)

deficiency disorders (Wiskott–Aldrich syndrome, ataxia telangiectasia, and the X-linked immunodeficiency syndrome), as well as those with severe immunosuppression due to drugs for organ transplantation. Chromosomal translocations are also involved in the development of lymphoma in patients with heritable immunodeficiency, as well as in Burkitt's lymphoma, which is not heritable (Miller, 1986).

A deficiency of certain forms of lymphoma occurs in Japan and perhaps other Asian countries. A lower rate of B-cell lymphoma there, and a seemingly reciprocal higher rate of certain autoimmune diseases (such as lupus erythematosus), suggest that Japanese have a subset of lymphocytes that protects against the lymphomas but predisposes to B-cell mediated autoimmune disease.

Central nervous system tumors (Chapter 51)

Tumors of the central nervous system (CNS) account for 15–20% of all childhood cancers in most populations except in Africa where they represent 1–5%. The most common types are medulloblastoma, astrocytoma, glioblastoma, and ependymoma. The age curve of these tumors shows a peak during the first decade followed by peaks in adults except for medulloblastoma, which is rare after the age of eight. Table 58.7 shows the age-adjusted incidence rates for selected populations. High rates (over

Table 58.8. *Neuroblastoma: age-standardized incidence rates per million* (*0–14 years*).

	Males	Females
France – Bas Rhin	16.7[a]	6.5
Israel – Jews	14.6	10.4
USA – SEER – whites	12.6	12.3[a]
Nigeria – Ibadan	9.8	2.2
USA – SEER – blacks	9.6	10.8
Norway	7.4	6.6
Japan – Miyagi	7.3	6.9
Singapore – Chinese	7.0	3.9
Yugoslavia – Slovenia	6.0	5.0
Kuwait – Kuwaitis	5.8	4.9
Colombia – Cali	5.7	5.2
India – Bombay	3.8	2.4
Philippines – Manila	0.5	1.5

[a] highest incidence rates
(After Parkin *et al.*, 1988.)

25.0) are seen in the Scandinavian countries, France, Spain (Zaragoza) and Italy (Torino): the lowest rates (below 10) in African countries, India, Japan (Miyagi), the Philippines and Fiji. Astrocytomas are the most common CNS tumors in childhood representing about 30–50%, followed by medulloblastoma (about 20%) and ependymomas (5–15%). Both sexes are equally affected by astrocytomas but medulloblastomas are more frequent in boys.

Risk factors

Genetic predisposition Certain autosomal dominant single-gene disorders predispose to CNS tumors in children, e.g. patients with neurofibromatosis and tuberous sclerosis are at high risk for gliomas.

Ionizing radiation An increase of brain tumors following radiotherapy for ringworm of the scalp is described (Chapter 16).

Neuroblastomas (Table 58.8)

These are embryonal tumors derived from the sympathetic nervous system arising mainly in the adrenal medulla and which account for 5–10% of all childhood tumors. Relatively high rates (over 10) are reported from France, Italy, Switzerland, Germany, whites in the USA, Israel and Australia. The lowest rates (below 3) are seen in India and the

Philippines. It has been suggested that neuroblastoma is unusually rare in Africa and blacks in the USA. However, population-based data show that, although low, rates in Africa are higher than in India and the Philippines; rates in blacks (SEER 10.2) are only sightly lower than in whites (SEER 12.5) in the USA (Parkin *et al.*, 1988). In Latin America, the rest of Europe and Asia, the rates range from 4–9 per million. In most populations the rates are slightly higher in boys than in girls, about half of the cases are diagnosed before two years of age and 80% before five years.

Risk factors
This tumor can develop in multiple generations within families. Several inborn defects have been reported associated with neuroblastoma (neurofibromatosis, aganglionosis of the colon), suggesting a genetic factor. The latter, however, would probably account for only a minority of these tumors.

Retinoblastoma (Chapters 18 and 50)
This tumor accounts for 2–4% of childhood malignancies in most populations except in Africa where it represents 10–15%. The age-adjusted rates vary from 5–8 per million in Africa, Brazil, Colombia (Cali), American blacks, Japan (Osaka), the Philippines (Manila), Czechoslovakia, Australia (Queensland) and New Zealand, to 1–2 per million in Singapore (Malay), Germany and Hungary (Parkin *et al.*, 1988). The sex ratios are close to unity.

Risk factors (Chapter 18)
Two types of retinoblastoma are recognized: heritable and non-heritable forms. It has been estimated that 40–45% of the cases are hereditary (Bunin *et al.*, 1989; Draper *et al.*, 1986; Briard Guillemot *et al.*, 1974). Most genetic tumors are bilateral and are associated with a deletion of chromosome 13q, sometimes with mental retardation and other birth defects.

Nephroblastoma (Wilms' tumor)
It accounts for about 10% of childhood cancers in Africa and blacks in the USA but only for 2–5% in most Caucasian populations in America, Europe and Asia. Originally considered as an index tumor with little geographical variation, this is not true. Table 58.9 shows the age-adjusted incidence rates for selected populations. The highest incidence rates (over 10) are observed in France (Bas Rhin), some African countries,

Table 58.9. *Wilms' tumor: age-standardized incidence rates per million (0–14 years).*

	Males	Females
France – Bas Rhin	15.4[a]	7.8
Nigeria – Ibadan	15.1	6.5
USA – SEER – blacks	9.9	12.3
Norway	8.5	6.1
Yugoslavia – Slovenia	8.4	6.4
USA – SEER – whites	7.9	10.0
UK – England and Wales	6.9	7.5
Israel – Jews	6.2	7.4
Brazil – Fortaleza	4.0	16.6[a]
Colombia – Cali	4.0	8.0
India – Bombay	3.7	3.9
Japan – Miyagi	3.7	2.2
Singapore – Chinese	3.7	3.8
Kuwait – Kuwaitis	2.8	4.9
China – Shanghai	0.9	—

[a] highest incidence rates.
(After Parkin *et al.*, 1988.)

blacks in the USA and Brazil (Fortaleza). The lowest rates (below 3) are seen in China, Japan, the Philippines and Malays in Singapore. The sex ratios are close to 1.0. Two-thirds of the cases occur before the age of five.

Risk factors

These tumors can be classified as heritable or genetic and non-heritable (Chapter 18). The former is frequently bilateral, but it can be unilateral, occurring in families or in association with congenital anomalies (aniridia, mental retardation, hemihypertrophy, skin hamartomas). It accounts for 4–13% of all tumors (Li *et al.*, 1988; Breslow *et al.*, 1988; Bonatai-Pellié *et al.*, 1988).

Sarcomas of the bone and soft tissues (Chapters 36 and 37)

The majority of bone tumors in children are osteosarcomas and Ewing's sarcomas. For osteosarcomas, the age-adjusted rates range from 5.4 per million in Spain (Zaragoza) to less than 0.8 in Australia (Queensland) and for Ewing's sarcoma from 3.0 in Germany and Denmark to 0.3 in US blacks and in Chinese populations.

Rates of osteosarcoma in blacks in the USA (SEER) are somewhat higher (3.4) than in whites (2.5) but the incidence of Ewing's sarcoma is much less than in whites (0.4 vs 2.4). In India and Israel the rates are similar to those of most European countries (about 2). In Sub-Saharan Africa, in Chinese populations, in Japan and the Philippines, Ewing's sarcoma is very rare with rates below 1.0. The incidence of osteosarcoma is higher in girls in early adolescence but greater in boys thereafter. The rates for Ewing sarcoma are equal in both sexes.

Most soft tissue sarcomas in children are rhabdomyosarcomas or fibrosarcomas.

Rhabdomyosarcomas which include embryonal sarcomas and soft tissue Ewing's sarcomas have age-adjusted rates varying from 6–7 in Spain (Zaragoza), France and Australia (New South Wales) to less than 1.0 in Singapore (Malays) and Brazil (Recife). In most European populations and among whites in the USA the rates are around 3 to 5. In the USA rates are slightly higher in whites (4.7) than in blacks (3.5). There is a slight male excess and two age peaks, under five years of age and in adolescence.

In contrast to the cutaneous form of Kaposi seen mainly in African men, the classical disease in African children before the AIDS epidemic was usually generalized with only slight male predominance.

Risk factors

Genetic factors   Familial and genetic factors play a role in a small proportion of osteosarcomas and soft tissue sarcomas as they can occur as components of several family cancer syndromes such as the Li–Fraumeni syndrome and in certain congenital disorders, e.g. neurofibromatosis and tuberous sclerosis.

Viruses   The role of HIV viruses in African Kaposi is not yet established and the possibility of a second virus has been considered.

Other childhood neoplasms

Epithelial neoplasms are relatively rare in children, but there are a few exceptions. Thus a high frequency of skin and nasopharyngeal carcinomas (NPC) has been reported in North Africa. In Tunisia, each of these two carcinomas accounts for 10% of the childhood cancers and in Sudan NPC represents 20% of all tumors in children (Parkin *et al.*, 1988). In Africa many skin cancers in children are associated with Xeroderma pigmentosum (Chapter 18).

Thyroid and adrenocortical carcinomas and hepatoblastomas are rare in most populations with age-adjusted rates ranging from 0.5 to 1.5 per million. Relatively high frequencies of hepatocellular carcinoma have been recorded in populations where adult hepatocellular carcinoma is common, such as in China and sub-Saharan Africa. A rare cancer, clear cell adenocarcinoma of the vagina and cervix has been described in adolescent girls and young women associated to prenatal exposure to diethylstilbestrol. Germ cell and gonadal tumors are relatively rare accounting for less than 2% of all cases in boys and less than 4% in females.

58.4   Childhood susceptibility

It is commonly assumed that children possess a general susceptibility of their tissues to cancer. However, this has only been demonstrated in radiation-induced cancers and there is no epidemiological evidence for a general increased susceptibility to cancer in childhood which cannot be explained by degree or duration of carcinogenic exposure, or by a specific genetic or familial defect. The latter do not necessarily reflect increased non-specific childhood susceptibility *per se*. The data from the study of second cancers following chemotherapy in children are uninformative due to the confounding effect of radiotherapy.

58.5   Perinatal and multigeneration carcinogenesis

A recent overview of perinatal and multi-generation carcino-genesis has recently been published by Napalkov *et al.* (1989). Prenatal events can contribute to cancer induction due to: (i) direct exposure of embryonal or fetal cells to carcinogenic factors; (ii) prezygotic exposure of the germ cells of one or both parents to a carcinogen/mutagen; (iii) genetic instability and/or a genetic rearrangement resulting from in-breeding.

Transplacental carcinogenesis has been demonstrated in rodents for certain carcinogens administered at specific periods during gestation in fetal life, e.g. *N*-nitroso compounds. DNA adducts of recognized carcinogens (PAH), have been demonstrated in human chorionic villi. None the less, convincing evidence of prenatal carcinogenesis apart possibly from radiation has proved extraordinarily difficult to document in humans (Preston-Martin, 1989), and the data remain inconsistent. Convincing evidence, for example, of increased tumors in the offspring of smokers has not been demonstrated. On the other hand, the effects of DES (a hormone), which causes developmental abnormalities, were relatively easily identified once the rare vaginal cancer and associated malformations had been recognized in children and young adults (Chapter 41). It has been postulated that some germ cell tumors may also be related to intrauterine exposure to hormones.

Prenatal exposure to a number of other agents has been hypothesized as causing cancer but the data are uncertain being largely based on sporadic case reports. Draper (1986) has concluded that available studies in humans, so far, gave no evidence for transgenerational carcinogenesis.

58.6   References

Bonatai-Pellié, C., Chompret, A., Tournade, M.F., Zucker, J.M. & Lemerle, J. (1988). Etude génétique et épidémiologique française sur le nephroblastome: resultats préliminaires. *Bull. Cancer*, **75**, 131–3.

Breslow, N.E., Beckwith, J.B., Ciol, M. & Sharples, K. (1988). Age distribution of Wilm's tumor: report from the National Wilm's Tumor Study. *Cancer Res.*, **48**, 1653–7.

Briard Guillemot, M.L., Bonatai-Pellié, C., Feingold, J. & Frézal, J. (1974). Etude génétique du rétinoblastome. *Humangenetik*, **24**, 271–84.

Bunin, G.R., Emanuel, B.S., Meadows, A.T., Buckley, J.D., Woods, W.G. & Hammond, G.D. (1989). Frequency of 13q abnormalities among 203 patients with retinoblastoma. *J. Natl. Cancer Inst.*, **81**, 370–4.

Draper, G.J., Sanders, B.M. & Kingston, J.E. (1986). Second primary neoplasms in patients with retinoblastoma. *Br. J. Cancer*, **53**, 661–71.

Evans, H.J. (1990). Leukaemia and radiation. *Nature*, **345**, 16–17.

Li, F.P., Williams, W.R., Gimbrere, K., Flamant, F., Green, D.M. & Meadows, A.T. (1988). Heritable fraction of unilateral Wilm's tumour. *Pediatrics*, **81**, 147–9.

MacMahon, B. (1985). Prenatal x-ray exposure and twins [editorial]. *N. Engl. J. Med.*, **312**, 576–7.

Miller, R.W. (1986). Genes, syndromes and cancer. *Pediatr. Rev.*, **8**, 153–8.

Miller, R.W. (1989). Frequency and environmental epidemiology of childhood cancer. In *Principles and Practice of Pediatric Oncology*, ed. P.A. Pizzo & D.G. Poplack, pp. 3–18. Philadelphia: J.B. Lippincott.

Miller, R.W. & Boice, J.D., Jr. (1986). Radiogenic cancer after prenatal or childhood exposure. In *Radiation Carcinogenesis*, ed. A.C. Upton, R.E. Albert, F.J. Burns *et al.*, pp. 379–86. New York: Elsevier.

Napalkov, N.P., Rice, J.M., Tomatis, L. & Yamasaki, H. (eds.) (1989). *Perinatal and Multigeneration Carcinogenesis*, IARC Scientific Publications No. 96. Lyon: International Agency for Research on Cancer.

O'Conor, G.T. (1988). Malignant lymphoma in African children: Three decades of discovery. In *Unusual Occurrences as Clues to Cancer Etiology*, ed. R.W. Miller, S. Watanabe, J.F. Fraumeni, Jr., T. Sugimura, S. Takayama & H. Sugano, pp. 137–47. New York: Taylor & Francis.

Parkin, D.M., Stiller, C.A., Draper, G.J., Bieber, C.A., Terracini, B., & Young, J.L. (eds.) (1988). *International Incidence of Childhood Cancer*, IARC Scientific Publications No. 87. Lyon: International Agency for Research on Cancer.

Preston-Martin, S. (1989). Epidemiological studies of perinatal carcinogenesis. In *Perinatal and Multigeneration Carcinogenesis*, IARC Scientific Publications No. 96, ed. N.P. Napalkov, J.M. Rice, L. Tomatis & H. Yamasaki, pp. 289–314. Lyon: International Agency for Research on Cancer.

Purtilo, D.T., Yasuda, N., Grierson, H.L., Okano, M., Brichacek, B. & Davis, J. (1988). X-linked lymphoproliferative syndrome provides clues to the pathogenesis of Epstein-Barr virus-induced lymphomagenesis. In *Unusual Occurrences as Clues to Cancer Etiology*, ed. R.W. Miller, S. Watanabe, J.F. Fraumeni, Jr., T. Sugimura, S. Takayama & H. Sugano, pp. 149–58. Tokyo: Japan Scientific Societies Press.

Stewart, A., Webb, J., Giles, D. & Hewitt, D. (1956). Malignant disease in childhood and diagnostic irradiation *in utero*. *Lancet*, **ii**, 447.

Yoshimoto, Y., Kato, H. & Schull, W.J. (1988). Risk of cancer among children exposed *in utero* to A-bomb radiations, 1950–84. *Lancet*, **ii**, 665–9.

Multiple primary cancers: second cancers

59.1 Introduction

It has been known for many years that two or more independent primary tumors can arise in the same patient. Schoenberg (1977), who surveyed multiple cancers in Connecticut between 1935–1964, appears to have been the first to make a comprehensive quantitative analysis of the risk of developing a second tumor through the investigation of 120,195 cancer patients from a well-defined population.

Second cancers may arise in the same individual for a number of reasons (Table 59.1). The major issue is usually whether an excess risk represents a common causal factor or some degree of genetic susceptibility. Among relevant issues are the following: (i) the recognition of syndromes of associated sites which may suggest a common etiology; (ii) identification of the regions of the body to which special attention should be paid when following up individuals with the first cancer; (iii) assessment of the carcinogenicity of treatments used for a first cancer.

59.2 Common etiological factors

The combined effects of tobacco and alcohol largely account for the constellation of cancers arising in the oral cavity, larynx and oesophagus. In contrast the association between retinoblastoma and osteosarcoma is most likely to reflect the influence of common hereditary factors. The interplay of both exogenous and endogenous factors in multiple cancers of the breast, uterine corpus, ovary and colon has long intrigued investigators. Both reproductive factors and dietary habits are believed to be involved. Bülow *et al.* (1990) report metachronous colorectal cancers can be as high as 30% after 40 years.

Table 59.1. *Etiological factors involved in multiple primary cancers.*

Etiological factors	Associated cancer sites
Tobacco or alcohol consumption, or both	Cancers of the oral cavity, respiratory and upper digestive tracts and cancer of the bladder
Endocrine or dietary factors, or both	Multicentric cancers of the colon; bilateral breast cancer; and clusters of cancers of the breast, uterine corpus, ovary, and colon
Genetic predisposition	Retinoblastoma and osteosarcoma, among others
Treatment effects	
Radiation	Cancer of the rectum and bladder, following cervical cancer, among others
Chemotherapy	ANLL and lymphomas, following Hodgkin's disease, NHL, multiple myeloma, and cancers of the ovary, breast, gastrointestinal tract, and lung, and childhood cancers
Immunological defects	Non-melanoma skin cancer, chronic lymphocytic leukemia, following immunosuppression

59.3   Effects of treatment

The carcinogenic effect of a number of therapeutic agents used in treating cancer has been known for many years, e.g. radiation.

Today an increasing number of cancer patients treated by radiation or by chemotherapeutic agents survive to develop an excess of malignancies at other sites. The increased risk of cancers of the rectum and bladder in patients treated by radiation for cancer of the cervix uteri is well established. The relatively low-dose total body radiation given for non-Hodgkin's lymphoma increases the risk of leukemia. Akylkating agents used to treat cancers of the ovary, intestine, breast, multiple myeloma, lung, Hodgkin's disease and childhood cancers result in an excess of leukaemia and malignant lymphoma (Kaldor *et al.*, 1987).

59.4   Immunodeficiencies

Treatment by immunosuppressive agents results in an excess of non-melanoma skin cancers in renal transplant patients. Other cancers resulting from immunodeficiencies include leukemia in Bloom's syndrome.

59.5   Criteria for identifying a second cancer

As the frequency of recognition of multiple tumors in the same individual is clearly a function of the time elapsed since diagnosis of the first cancer, such cases are more likely to occur in cancer registries which have been operative for several decades, rather than those recently established. For patients with a particular first cancer, the number of observed second cancers is tabulated over time and compared with those to be expected if the cancer patient had experienced the same rates as prevailed in the corresponding general population. Unfortunately, there is no international agreement on the criteria for the recognition for multiple primary cancers in the same individual. The International Agency for Research on Cancer has suggested the following:

(a) A primary cancer is one which originates in a primary site or tissue and is neither an extension, nor a recurrence, nor a metastasis of another primary cancer.

(b) An organ or tissue is as defined by the three digit categories of ICD-9 or the topography of ICD-O.

(c) Recognition of the existence of two or more primary cancers in the same individual does not depend on time of appearance. This avoids the need to apply rather arbitrary rules for distinguishing between synchronous and metachronous tumors.

(d) Only one primary cancer shall be recognized as arising in an organ, or paired organ, or tissue, unless the tumors are of 'different' morphological type. This rule raises the question as to how 'different' does one morphological type of neoplasm need to be from another before they are considered as independent primaries. Berg (1982) has outlined certain criteria.

(e) Multifocal tumors occurring within an organ or other tissue, such as polyps of the bladder and bowel, are counted once only, as is Hodgkin's disease of several lymph nodes. The US SEER program however, has less rigid rules: thus, independent non-contiguous tumors arising in differing sub-sites of the colon, for example, transverse and sigmoid colon, would each be counted separately.

The forthcoming tenth Revision of the ICD, which has elevated several sub-sites to full site status, will probably mean modification of the IARC position.

The problems of methodology and interpretation are discussed extensively in a recent report on multiple primary cancers in Connecticut and Denmark (Boice *et al.*, 1985). This contains numerous tables describing nearly 40,000 second cancers seen in about 600,000 cancer patients.

59.6   References

Berg, J.W. (1982). Morphologic Classification of Human Cancer. In *Cancer Epidemiology and Prevention*, ed. D. Schottenfeld & J.F. Fraumeni, Jr., pp. 74–89. Phildelphia: W.B.Saunders Company.

Boice, J.D., Curtis, R.G., Kleinerman, R.A., Storm, H.N., Jensen, V.M., Jensen, H.S., Flannery, J.T. & Fraumeni, J.F., Jr. (1985). *Multiple Primary Cancers in Connecticut and Denmark*. National Cancer Institute Monograph 68. Bethesda: National Cancer Institute, US Department of Health and Human Services.

Bülow, S., Svendsen, L.B. & Mellemgaard, A. (1990). Metachronous colorectal carcinoma. *Br. J. Surg.*, **77**, 502–5.

Kaldor, J.M., Day, N.,E., Rand, P., Choi, N.W., Clarke, E.A., Coleman, M.P., Haklama, M., Coch, M., Langmark, F., Neal, F.E., Pettersson, F., Pompe'Kirn, V., Prior, P. & Storm, H.H. (1987). Second malignancies following testicular cancer, ovarian cancer and Hodgkin's Disease: An international collaborative study among cancer registries. *Int. J. Cancer*, **39**, 571–85.

Schoenberg, B.S. (1977). *Multiple Primary Malignant Neoplasms: The Connecticut Experience*, 1935–1964. New York: Springer-Verlag.

Conclusions: future priorities for research

Overview

The geographical and temporal variations in cancer incidence and migrant studies, complemented by analytical epidemiological investigations on cultural and occupational cancers, led to the view that most human cancers have a significant environmental component (pp. xxi–xxiv). Such studies indicated the considerable possibilities of cancer prevention, either by removal or reduction of exogenous carcinogens, through modification of 'lifestyle' factors, especially tobacco and diet, or by active intervention using vaccines, drugs or other agents during the pre-neoplastic phase. Today, it is recognized that interaction between environmental and genetic factors may also be of great importance for specific subsets of the population (Chapter 18). None the less, while there is a general consensus on the probable causes of many human cancers, specific preventive measures cannot yet be recommended with any certainty for about 50% of cancers in males and 70% in females in industrial states (Higginson, 1988; Muir, 1990; Schmähl et al., 1989).

Contribution of known or suspected causes

Estimates based on the available literature have been made in a number of countries of the contribution to the total cancer burden of a variety of defined or suspected causes. Such estimates include those of Wynder and Gori (1977), Higginson and Muir (1979) for morbidity and Doll and Peto (1981) for mortality (Tables 1 and 2).

These estimates had a common base in recognizing that while it might not be possible to specify all causes of a particular cancer with precision, it may be possible to make a reasonable estimate of the contribution of a predominant factor, such as smoking or an occupation (see Chapter 6). These calculations contained a number of assumptions. Thus, for some

Table 1. *Estimates of the proportion (%) of cancer cases attributable to various major factors[a] (Chapter 6).*

Factors	United[b] States		Birmingham[c] UK		Bombay[c] India		Bulawayo[c] Zimbabwe	
	M	F	M	F	M	F	M	F
	%	%	%	%	%	%	%	%
Tobacco	28	8	30	7	9	2	14	2
Tobacco/Alcohol	4	1	5	3	—	—	2	< 1
Tobacco/betel	—	—	—	—	41	19	—	—
Diet/lifestyle[d]	40	57	30	63	18	58	13	51
Discrete dietary[e]	—	—	—	—	—	—	44	13
Occupation	4	2	6	2	6	1	2	< 1
Sunlight	{ 8	8 }	10	10	1	< 1	< 1	< 1
Ionizing Radiation			1	1	1	1	< 1	< 1
Iatrogenic Exogenous hormones	—	4	1	1	—	—	—	—
Congenital	2	2	2	2	2	2	2	2
Parasites	—	—	—	—	—	—	6	4

[a] These estimates do not add up to 100 (see Chapter 6).
[b] (After Wynder & Gori, 1977.)
[c] (After Higginson & Muir, 1979.)
[d] Non-tobacco related, includes reproductive factors.
[e] Includes the hepatitis virus.

sites or types, where there was evidence that an occupational exposure was predominately responsible, such cancers were classified as due to occupation only (Higginson & Muir, 1979), and other attributable risks ignored. Thus, all mesotheliomas occurring in the population, whether in asbestos workers or not, were ascribed to occupation. Eighty-five per cent of lung cancers were ascribed to cigarette smoking and other attributable risks considered separately. The proportions attributed by Doll and Peto (1981) to pollution, food additives, industrial products or geophysical factors, etc, were estimated ranges based on interpretation of data from several sources.

No allowance was made in these studies for temporal changes in exposures to suspected risk factors, although this point was discussed (Doll & Peto, 1981). Thus, comparable estimates made today, a decade later, would probably show increases in the proportion of tobacco-related cancers, notably in third world countries and in women. A continuing increase in melanoma in both sexes and breast cancer in females in many countries, presumably due to lifestyle changes, would also be found. Thus, increases in young women of cervix uteri cancer have been ascribed to

Table 2. *Proportions of cancer deaths attributed to various factors*[ab].

Factors	% of all cancer deaths	
	Best estimate	Range of acceptable estimates
Tobacco	30	25–40
Alcohol	3	2–4
Diet	35	10–70
Food additives	< 1	− 5–2[c]
Reproductive/sexual behavior	7	1–13
Occupation	4	2–8
Pollution	2	< 1–5
Industrial products	< 1	< 1–2
Medicine/medical procedures	1	0.5–3
Geophysical factors	3	2–4
Infection	10?	1–?
Unknown	?	?

[a] Applies to western industrial states only.
[b] These estimates exclude the very common non-fatal skin cancers.
[c] Allows for protective effect of preservatives.
(After Doll & Peto, 1981.)

change in sexual customs. In contrast, Muir *et al.*, (1981) and Doll (1988) have pointed out there is little evidence that new carcinogenic stimuli have affected individuals below 45 years, in industrial states, in whom, on the whole, significant decreases in incidence are observed, especially in males.

None the less, despite variations in methodology, the conclusions of the above authors were remarkably consistent, and these estimates provide reasonable overall approximations on which to base cancer control policies and priorities. It is anticipated that, with further knowledge of etiological factors and attributable risks, estimates will continually be refined covering various countries and communities.

Future developments in prevention

The widely differing global and national cancer patterns described in this monograph indicate that major possibilities for primary prevention still exist (Lerman *et al.*, 1989). The black male in Los Angeles has nearly double the risk of developing cancer compared to his countryman of Japanese ethnic origin. Further, certain religious groups and occupations have rates lower than the general US population (Chapter 19). The low rates for African blacks contrast with the very high rates in American blacks. Japan with the present culture remains one of the lowest cancer rate countries in the world (Wynder & Hiyama, 1987), but patterns are changing. Norway, where the overall cancer incidence is increasing rapidly, can no longer be regarded as a low-risk country. Lynge & Thygeson (1990), using the Danish cancer registry showed that comparing 20 social groups, based on type of work, that the difference between the group with lowest and the highest rates was almost two-fold for men and 1.5 fold for females (Table 19.3). Thus, the study of such populations continues to offer major opportunities to the investigator.

Primary cancer prevention has been most successful where discrete critical causes, such as tobacco or specific chemicals, have been identified (Hakama *et al.*, 1990). Control strategies are more controversial for cancers allegedly due to exposures to low-level ambient carcinogenic hazards (Chapter 7) and those due to complex 'lifestyle' and dietary factors (Chapter 6 and 12). For these reasons, some believe that there are limitations to cancer prevention based solely on traditional eliminatory approaches, whether related to low-level chemical exposures or isolated changes in diet (Higginson, 1988).

The authors believe that the classical epidemiological approaches including descriptive studies, case-control and cohort investigations, will continue to contribute significantly to cancer control and to the evaluation of potential carcinogenic factors. However, these will be supplemented by more effective use of modern laboratory technology (molecular or biochemical epidemiology) to identify and measure potential etiological variables (Harris, 1986; Muir, 1990), and to increase understanding of genetic influences (Chapter 18).

Contribution of observational epidemiology studies to cancer control

It is clear that many of the more obvious discrete etiological factors for human cancer have been identified. Improved public health measures in most modern states make it unlikely that many strong new carcinogens will enter the environment, but such possibilities cannot be completely excluded. Well-recognized 'old' carcinogenic hazards may surface unexpectedly in new 'high-tech' industries, especially in unregulated small manufacturing plants. This is most true in third world countries, where effective controls may be limited or absent. In investigating such risks, traditional epidemiological approaches are effective. They are also valuable in the investigation of widespread risks such as domestic air pollution despite the logistical problems involved. None the less, in certain situations, epidemiological studies require more sophisticated biostatistical and laboratory approaches, such as where a virus affecting the majority of a population is suspected. Thus in evaluating the role of the EB virus in Burkitt's lymphoma, knowledge of prior antigen titer patterns was necessary. This required the follow-up of a large number of children for over seven years as well as the development of adequate auxiliary clinical and laboratory support. Other studies may require simultaneous efforts in several locations as in the IARC SEARCH program, both to provide a population of adequate size and to reduce the impact of confounding variables. Large-scale studies depending on use of biomarkers, possibly requiring interventional techniques also pose large logistic and technical problems (see below).

With growth in cancer monitoring, an increased need for accurate exposure data, on suspected chemical carcinogens both man-made and natural is foreseen, in both the work-place and general environment. It is essential that such data be collected systematically and in a form suitable for epidemiological investigations, if meaningful evaluations are to be made. Scattered random measurements of exposures are likely to be uninformative and even misleading, irrespective of the elegance and sensitivity of the analytical techniques used.

It is to be expected that many such monitoring studies will be 'negative' or uninformative, whether cancer or some biomarker is used as an end-point (Chapter 4). This will be especially true where exposures are several orders of magnitude lower than in an occupational setting, as around a waste disposal site (Grisham, 1986). None the less, public concern may justify routine monitoring and surveillance studies in some situations, especially where exposures to a potential carcinogen are suspected. Such efforts essentially represent the equivalent in cancer control of the classical public health surveillance procedures routinely used to combat communicable diseases. They may, moreover, provide data on the upper levels of risk and the effectiveness of industrial exposure standards. Such surveillance studies, however, must not be undertaken without a good reason, whether oriented to social concern or to public health, and must be interpreted with care. Over-emphasis of spurious causal associations or random cancer clusters may lead to unnecessary public anxiety which will not always be allayed later, even by well-conducted epidemiological studies, and may divert resources from more important objectives.

Biochemical and molecular epidemiology

The potential of biochemical (metabolic) epidemiology in permitting the more objective analysis of such variables as hormonal or immunological status, etc., has been increasingly recognized since the late

1950s (Higginson, 1968). In early days, however, techniques suitable for application in field studies on cancer were limited, although biochemical methods have been effectively used in the study of cardiovascular disease. Today, the term molecular epidemiology is applied to the utilization of elegant laboratory techniques based on knowledge of carcinogenic mechanisms at a fundamental level. As pointed out in Chapters 5 and 18, such techniques permit not only the direct or indirect identification and measurement of exposures to chemicals and biological agents but also metabolic variations in host susceptibility, whether of genetic or environmental origin, of relevance to cancer induction.

Biomarkers

Much research effort is presently focused on biomarkers (Montesano, 1990). However, it is important to recognize that the epidemiological evaluation of such markers is subject to the same biostatistical and biological limitations as occur in the study of any other causal parameter. It is anticipated that biomarkers will be of greatest value relative to: (a) objective identification of high-risk groups in an occupational or equivalent situation; (b) comparative geographical pathology studies of biochemical and biological variations in different populations; (c) the provision of objective support for a 'negative' epidemiological study when the 'exposed' and 'unexposed' population may show no obvious differences, as for example in routine monitoring and surveillance of a large plant; (d) the identification and definition of individual susceptibility whether genetic or acquired; (e) early predictors of cancer induction, although the predictive value of most biomarkers remains to be established; and (g) comparative evaluation of certain metabolic differences possibly related carcinogenic mechanisms, e.g. enzyme induction.

Oncogenes

To date, about 50 oncogenes have been identified from a variety of animal and human tumors, consistently appearing, sometimes with high frequency, in many cancers, e.g. Ki-*ras* in pancreas cancer. Taylor (1989) has suggested that oncogenes may serve as indicators of etiology. Unlike DNA adducts, which are transient and reflect only recent exposure, oncogene mutations persist and may be detectable in the tumor tissue. The biochemical consequences of oncogene activation are being intensely studied. Experimental studies strongly suggest that chemical carcinogens can directly activate oncogenes with considerable specificity. Thus, one chemical will produce a characteristic mutation in the activated oncogene, while another will produce a different activating mutation. These findings are held to be in line with the multistage model of carcinogenesis.

Individual susceptibility

A major objective of the program on the mapping of human genome is the identification of populations at unusual risk to a disease in the hope of developing effective preventive or secondary control strategies. It should be recognized that prevention or control usually depends on the existence and identification of a sub-group with a sufficiently high risk of a cancer to permit a specific targeted approach. On the other hand, polygenic susceptibility affecting a large segment of the population will offer little better odds than a prevention program developed for the total population.

In the immediate future, most effort is being directed to identifying individuals born with a specific defective gene who are highly susceptible to cancer. Considerable interest relates to gene p 53, since defective versions of this gene are passed from parent to child. For example, many relatives of such individuals develop several types of cancer by early adulthood, as in the Li–Fraumeni syndrome in which sisters develop breast cancer before 30 and their children develop a number of cancers before puberty. While such findings are expected to lead to major advances in diagnosis, prevention and treatment, the identification of such genes will give rise to ethical problems in dealing with the apparently healthy, since little practical help can be offered for the moment.

Other Studies

The last two decades have seen enormous growth in knowledge on carcinogenic mechanisms and the potential of eventually controlling cell growth (Huber, 1989). There is an expanding literature on the role of receptors, growth hormones, etc., whose role in modulating carcinogenesis is gradually being analyzed in molecular terms. At present, from an epidemiological viewpoint, much of the new data generated appear more relevant to intervention studies than to the identification of etiological agents.

Intervention strategies and prevention

The future role and value of chemoprevention has been reviewed in a recent symposium (Proceedings of the Third International Conference on the Prevention of Human Cancer: Chemoprevention, 1989).

Major changes in diet, cultural or sexual habits, may prove difficult to implement and may not be readily acceptable by the public unless convinced of unequivocal benefits for the individual. Enthusiastic advocacy of measures supported by a poorly defined scientific base, even with the best intentions, raise a number of important medical and ethical issues. Thus, the effectiveness in cancer control of changes in the dietary environment, such as the administration of retinoids and anti-oxidants or modification of fat and fiber intake, all subjects of considerable current interest (Wattenberg, 1985), remains to be definitively established in humans. Studies on endocrine-dependent tumors such as the impact of oral contraceptives on ovarian and endometrial cancers, have raised the possibilities of control through hormonal therapy. The concept of a drug mimicking the critical determinants of a first pregnancy or the menarche that could reduce breast cancer appears theoretically feasible. However, the widespread use of such a drug in healthy or even in patient sub-groups requires extensive testing, as illustrated by the discussion surrounding the use of tamoxifen to control breast cancer metastases (Powles *et al.*, 1990). Any side-effects must be ethically and socially acceptable. For some cancers such as primary liver carcinoma or cervical cancer, viruses may be necessary determinants and antiviral vaccines or therapy for non-A non-B hepatitis, represent obvious approaches. There are, however, many biostatistical and logistic problems in evaluating a protective vaccine or other antiviral agent of uncertain efficacy especially for rarer cancers (Higginson *et al.*, 1971).

Epidemiology can contribute to such efforts through well-executed, integrated laboratory and field studies and rigorously controlled clinical trials such as those carried out by the IARC in China (Chapter 25) and in Gambia (Chapter 29).

Evaluation of cancer risks: scientific judgement
The difficulty of measuring very small cancer risks in humans is discussed in Chapters 4 and 7. Uncertainty as to cause is greatest in situations where, for example, widespread exposure to a suspected chemical occurs at levels below which a definite effect is unlikely to be demonstrable or expected. This is illustrated by experience with dioxin. The latter, although a powerful toxic agent and promoter in some species, has never been convincingly demonstrated to carry a cancer risk to humans. However, its ubiquity and the fact that today techniques exist for measuring its presence in parts per quadrillion continues to generate public concern. Similar problems and issues also relate to pesticides and herbicides, ambient pollutants, radiation, etc., also certain oncogenic viruses infecting most of the population.

Competent scientists, however, using data on types of carcinogen, exposure levels, pharmacokinetics, comparative metabolism, etc., can often provide a sound opinion as to the probable significance to humans of a potential carcinogenic hazard, which may permit the distinction of the trivial from the significant. Such scientific judgments may be more meaningful than theoretical estimates based on biomathematical models. However, the latter may contribute input to the analysis of complex carcinogenic mechanisms and improve modelling based on pharmacokinetics and pharmacodynamic mechanisms. An essential ingredient, however, of such risk characterizations whether based on scientific judgement or biomathematical modelling, is the availability of accurate data on exposures, an area where at present there are many deficiencies (Chapter 5, 7 and 8). In such decisions, the epidemiologist will continue to have a major role in describing and evaluating the available epidemiological data.

Conclusion

While most epidemiological studies are directed to the identification of carcinogenic risk factors, it is necessary to give attention to inverse relationships and the characteristics of populations at a low risk for cancer, with a view to seeking leads to cancer control.

Despite the current enthusiasm for molecular epidemiology, which covers a range of laboratory methods, nevertheless, the input of traditional epidemiological approaches including both case history and cohort studies will be an essential ingredient in generating human data of relevance to cancer causation and determining public health priorities (Muir, 1990). None the less, there will be increased reliance on laboratory methods of varying sophistication to define suspected causal factors more accurately whether related to chemical exposures, dietary manipulation, viruses or the role of host factors.

References

Doll, R. & Peto, R. (1981). *The Causes of Cancer: Quantitative Estimates of Avoidable Risks of Cancer in the United States Today.* New York: Oxford University Press.

Doll, R. (1988). Epidemiology and the prevention of cancers: Some recent developments. *J. Cancer Res. Clin. Oncol.*, **114**, 447–58.

Grisham, J.W. (1986). *Health Aspects of the Disposal of Waste Chemicals.* Elmsford, NY: Pergamon Press.

Hakama, M., Beral, V., Cullen, J.W. & Parkin, D.M. (eds.) (1990). *Evaluating Effectiveness of Primary Prevention of Cancer*, IARC Scientific Publications No. 103. Lyon: International Agency for Research on Cancer.

Harris, C.C. (ed.) (1986). *Biochemical and Molecular Epidemiology of Cancer.* New York: Alan R. Liss.

Higginson, J. (1968). Present trends in cancer epidemiology. In *Canadian Cancer Conference*, Proceedings of the Eighth Canadian Cancer Conference, Honey Harbour, Ontario, pp. 40–75.

Higginson, J. (1980). Proportion of cancers due to occupation. *Prev. Med.*, **9**, 180–8.

Higginson, J. (1988). Changing concepts in cancer prevention: Limitations and implications for future research in environmental carcinogenesis. *Cancer Res.*, **48**, 1381–9.

Higginson, J. & Muir, C.S. (1979). Environmental carcinogenesis: Misconceptions and limitations to cancer control. *J. Natl. Cancer Inst.*, **63**, 1291–8.

Higginson, J., de-Thé, G., Geser, A. & Day, N.E. (1971). An epidemiological analysis of cancer vaccines. *Int. J. Cancer*, **7**, 545–74.

Huber, B., (1989). Therapeutic opportunities involving cellular oncogenes: novel approaches fostered by biotechnology. *FASEB J.*, **3**, 5–13.

Knudson, A.G., Jr. (1985). Hereditary cancer, oncogenes, and antioncogenes. *Cancer Res.*, **45**, 1437–43.

Lerman, C., Rimer, B. & Engstrom, P.R. (1989). Perspectives in cancer research: Reducing avoidable cancer mortality through prevention and early detection regimens. *Cancer Res.*, **49**, 4955–62.

Lynge, E. & Thygesen, L. (1990). Occupational cancer in Denmark. Cancer incidence in the 1970 census population. *Scand. J. Work. Environ. Health*, **16** Suppl. 2, 1–35.

Montesano, R. (1990). Approaches to detecting individual exposure to carcinogens. In *Complex Mixtures and Cancer Risk*, IARC Scientific Publications No.104, ed. H. Vainio, M. Sorsa & A.J. McMichael, pp. 11–19. Lyon: International Agency for Research on Cancer.

Muir, C.S., Choi, N.W. & Schifflers, E. (1981). Time trends. Cancer mortality in some countries – their possible causes and significance. In *Medical Aspects of Mortality Statistics* (Proceedings of the Skandia International Symposium), pp. 269–309. Stockholm: Almqvist & Wiksell.

Muir, C.S. (1990). Epidemiology, basic science and the prevention of cancer: Implications for the future. *Cancer Res.*, **50**, 6441–8.

Powles, T.J., Tillyer, C.R., Jones, A.L., Ashley, S.E., Treleaven, J., Davey, J.B. & McKinna, J.A. (1990). Prevention of breast cancer with Tamoxifen – an update on the Royal Marsden Hospital Pilot Programme. *Eur. J. Cancer*, **26**, 680–4.

Proceedings of the Third International Conference on the Prevention of Human Cancer: Chemoprevention. (1989). Guest editor: F. KL. Meyskens, Jr. *Prev. Med.*, **18**, 5.

Schmähl, R., Preussmann, R. & Berger, M.R. (1989). Causes of cancer – An alternative view to Doll and Peto (1981). *Klin Wochenschr.*, **67**, 1169–73.

Taylor, J.A. (1989). Oncogenes and their applications in epidemiologic studies. *Am. J. Epidemiol.*, **130**, 6–30.

Wattenberg, L.W., (1985). Chemoprevention of cancer. *Cancer Res.*, **45**, 1–8.

Wynder, E.L. & Gori, G.B. (1977). Contribution of the environment to cancer incidence: an epidemiologic exercise. *J. Natl. Cancer Inst.*, **58**, 825–32.

Wynder, E.L. & Hiyama, T. (1987). *Comparative Epidemiology of Cancer in the United States And Japan: Preventive Implications*, Gann Monograph on Cancer Research No. 33, ed. M. Kurihara, K. Aoki, R.W. Miller & C.S. Muir. Tokyo: Japan Scientific Societies Press.

Appendix 1

Cancer statistics

Table 1.1. *Age-standardized incidence rates by site for selected registries.*
(*a*)

	Lip (ICD-9 140)		Tongue (ICD-9 141)		Mouth (ICD-9 143–5)		Oropharynx (ICD-9 146)		Nasopharynx (ICD-9 147)		Hypopharynx (ICD-9 148)		Esophagus (ICD-9 150)	
	Male	Female	Male	Female	Male	Female	Male	Female	Male	Female	Male	Female	Male	Female
Senegal, Dakar	0.2	0.4	0.9	0.3	1.0	1.3	0.4	0.0	0.1	0.0	0.1	0.0	0.2	0.2
Columbia, Cali	1.0	0.3	1.8	0.5	1.9	1.6	1.2	0.7	0.4	0.4	0.3	0.2	3.1	1.9
Canada	5.5	0.5	1.9	0.8	2.9	1.2	1.5	0.5	0.7	0.3	1.1	0.2	3.7	1.3
US, Bay Area:														
White	2.3	0.3	2.8	1.7	3.7	2.4	2.4	1.3	0.6	0.3	1.7	0.7	3.4	1.8
Black	—	—	3.6	1.3	6.2	2.6	4.6	2.2	1.1	0.5	3.1	1.6	13.3	4.4
Chinese	0.2	—	2.1	0.8	1.8	0.3	0.8	—	14.8	8.0	1.1	—	6.3	0.6
Japanese	—	—	—	—	0.7	—	—	—	1.1	—	1.4	—	3.9	1.3
US, Detroit:														
White	1.3	0.2	3.0	1.3	4.2	1.7	1.7	0.8	0.5	0.2	1.8	0.4	4.4	1.1
Black	0.1	0.1	4.6	1.2	7.0	2.0	2.9	1.0	0.9	0.2	3.2	0.5	16.9	5.0
US, Utah	8.1	0.9	1.7	0.7	2.0	1.3	0.9	0.3	0.5	0.4	0.5	0.2	2.1	0.5
China, Shanghai	0.2	0.1	0.5	0.5	1.2	0.8	0.4	0.2	4.4	2.0	0.2	0.1	20.8	8.9
Hong Kong	0.2	0.1	2.6	1.0	2.6	0.9	1.0	0.3	30.0	12.9	1.4	0.2	18.7	4.3
India, Bombay	0.3	0.2	9.4	3.4	6.5	5.0	3.5	0.8	0.8	0.3	9.9	2.2	14.7	10.3
Israel:														
All Jews	3.6	0.8	0.7	0.4	0.9	0.6	0.2	0.1	1.2	0.4	0.3	0.1	1.9	1.4
Eur. Amer.	4.3	0.9	0.6	0.4	0.6	0.4	0.1	0.1	0.3	0.2	0.2	0.1	1.9	1.2
Non-Jews	2.7	0.2	0.5	0.3	1.9	0.4	—	—	1.0	0.2	0.2	0.6	1.0	0.9
Japan, Miyagi	0.1	0.0	1.1	0.4	0.5	0.2	0.1	0.0	0.5	0.2	0.4	0.1	13.3	3.1
Kuwait: Kuwaitis	—	0.1	0.5	0.3	0.9	0.8	1.6	0.1	2.1	1.3	0.2	2.0	2.0	2.0
Singapore:														
Chinese	0.1	0.0	1.5	0.6	2.4	0.6	1.1	0.4	18.1	7.9	1.3	0.2	13.5	3.7
Malay	0.3	—	1.1	0.6	0.8	1.2	0.8	0.2	4.0	1.5	0.5	—	1.2	1.0
Indian	0.3	—	4.6	3.3	4.4	9.6	3.7	2.1	0.3	1.3	3.6	1.6	8.6	3.9

Czech., Slovakia	6.6	0.8	2.8	0.2	3.4	0.4	2.1	0.2	0.5	0.2	1.4	0.1	4.1	0.3
Denmark	3.8	0.4	0.7	0.4	1.6	1.1	1.1	0.4	0.5	0.2	0.5	0.1	2.9	1.2
France, Bas-Rhin	0.7	—	7.4	0.8	13.5	0.8	10.7	0.5	1.1	0.1	11.9	0.3	16.7	1.0
FRG, Saarland	0.9	0.1	3.4	0.8	2.7	0.4	2.0	0.6	0.5	0.1	1.4	0.1	4.9	0.7
Finland	4.8	0.5	0.9	0.5	0.9	0.5	0.4	0.1	0.4	0.2	0.5	0.2	3.7	2.4
German Dem. Rep.	1.7	0.2	1.0	0.3	1.1	0.3	0.9	0.2	0.3	0.1	0.4	0.0	3.0	0.5
Hungary, Szabolcs	8.4	1.1	2.5	0.1	0.8	0.1	1.2	—	1.3	0.3	0.5	—	2.5	0.1
Iceland	4.2	0.4	0.4	0.8	0.4	0.8	0.4	0.2	1.2	0.3	0.1	0.1	4.2	2.4
Ireland, Southern	11.6	1.2	1.4	0.1	1.2	0.4	0.8	0.1	0.6	0.1	0.4	0.2	6.5	4.6
Italy, Ragusa	10.9	—	0.9	0.2	0.7	0.2	0.5	—	1.0	0.2	—	—	3.3	0.4
Italy, Varese	2.4	0.4	3.1	0.4	3.6	0.5	4.5	0.2	1.3	0.4	2.9	0.1	8.0	0.7
Norway	3.2	0.3	1.0	0.4	1.5	0.8	0.5	0.1	0.3	0.1	0.7	0.1	2.7	0.7
Poland, Cracow city	2.7	0.3	1.2	0.4	1.6	0.4	0.9	0.8	0.4	0.4	0.2	0.1	3.7	0.9
Spain, Navarra	7.7	0.7	2.9	0.2	2.8	0.4	1.3	0.1	1.1	0.2	0.7	0.0	6.9	0.7
Sweden	2.5	0.3	0.9	0.5	1.5	0.6	0.6	0.2	0.5	0.2	0.7	0.2	3.0	0.8
Switzerland, Geneva	1.5	0.2	4.0	0.4	7.2	2.0	5.4	1.0	0.5	0.3	4.5	0.1	9.0	1.0
UK, Birmingham	0.2	0.0	0.9	0.4	1.2	0.4	0.9	0.2	0.4	0.2	0.7	0.5	5.2	3.3
UK, West Scotland	1.7	0.1	1.1	0.7	2.1	0.9	0.6	0.2	0.3	0.2	0.7	0.5	8.7	4.4
Yugoslavia, Slovenia	3.1	0.6	3.5	0.2	4.3	0.3	4.6	0.2	0.5	0.2	3.7	0.1	7.1	0.8
Australia, Victoria	7.4	1.6	2.8	1.1	2.9	1.0	2.1	0.4	1.1	0.3	1.1	0.2	4.5	2.2
New Zealand, Maori	—	—	0.3	0.5	0.9	1.3	1.3	0.5	1.9	0.6	0.5	0.2	7.4	1.4
Non-Maori	3.7	0.6	1.5	0.6	1.7	0.9	1.0	0.2	0.7	0.2	1.5	0.2	4.7	2.2
Hawaii, White	3.0	0.6	4.7	2.2	6.0	4.2	2.2	1.4	1.2	0.1	1.5	1.0	3.5	1.5
Japanese	0.3	0.1	2.2	0.5	1.5	1.0	0.2	0.2	1.0	0.2	1.2	0.1	3.7	0.4
Hawaiian	—	—	1.8	1.1	2.0	1.9	0.8	0.7	0.6	1.1	0.8	0.5	11.0	1.7

Table 1.1. (*cont.*)
(*b*)

	Stomach (ICD-9 151)		Colon (ICD-9 153)		Rectum (ICD-9 154)		Liver (ICD-9 155)		Gallbladder (ICD-9 156)		Pancreas (ICD-9 157)		Nose, Sinuses (ICD-9 160)	
	Male	Female	Male	Female	Male	Female	Male	Female	Male	Female	Male	Female	Male	Female
Senegal, Dakar	3.7	2.0	0.6	0.7	1.5	1.0	25.6	9.0	0.0	0.2	1.0	1.0	0.3	0.3
Columbia, Cali	49.6	26.3	5.2	6.3	3.4	3.7	2.8	1.4	3.0	9.4	5.2	3.6	1.2	1.0
Canada	13.2	5.9	24.1	22.5	15.3	9.8	2.1	1.0	1.9	2.3	8.6	5.5	0.7	0.4
US, Bay Area:														
White	10.4	4.8	30.6	23.7	15.4	11.0	2.9	1.3	1.7	2.2	9.2	6.9	0.7	0.3
Black	19.1	6.0	28.9	27.6	12.5	8.0	6.6	2.1	1.7	1.2	15.5	8.3	0.6	0.2
Chinese	9.1	5.4	24.7	18.0	12.3	10.1	18.8	3.7	2.4	2.0	7.0	6.2	0.5	0.5
Japanese	24.3	10.8	29.8	20.8	13.6	12.4	8.9	2.7	3.1	0.5	5.0	4.8	—	—
US, Detroit:														
White	10.2	4.2	30.9	23.6	17.6	10.3	2.1	1.0	2.0	2.2	9.2	6.2	0.8	0.4
Black	16.9	6.8	32.0	29.0	13.4	8.5	4.4	1.7	1.5	1.6	12.8	8.6	1.1	0.2
US, Utah	6.3	3.1	19.4	17.3	9.7	7.8	1.5	1.0	1.3	1.6	5.5	4.4	0.3	0.2
China, Shanghai	58.3	24.6	8.5	7.6	9.4	7.1	34.4	11.6	1.6	2.3	5.5	3.8	1.2	0.7
Hong Kong	19.2	9.6	15.8	12.5	12.4	9.2	32.3	7.4	3.6	2.5	3.5	2.4	1.9	0.8
India, Bombay	8.9	6.0	3.4	2.9	4.5	2.5	4.9	2.5	0.9	1.0	2.1	1.3	1.2	1.1
Israel:														
All Jews	16.2	9.3	16.2	15.0	16.6	13.4	3.4	1.8	2.1	4.4	8.9	5.9	0.6	0.3
Eur. Amer.	18.3	10.3	21.1	17.7	22.6	15.9	3.4	4.7	2.6	4.6	9.9	6.4	0.6	0.3
Non-Jews	7.9	4.9	4.7	4.5	3.0	2.4	2.9	1.7	1.8	3.4	3.1	2.1	0.5	0.1
Japan, Miyagi	79.6	36.0	9.8	9.4	9.9	7.4	11.2	4.0	5.9	5.3	9.0	5.1	1.7	0.7
Kuwait: Kuwaitis	3.7	1.6	0.2	0.8	3.0	1.3	4.4	0.7	1.1	0.5	1.2	1.3	—	0.2
Singapore:														
Chinese	37.3	15.4	16.4	15.9	14.6	10.6	31.6	7.2	2.1	1.6	4.5	2.8	1.0	0.6
Malay	9.4	6.8	5.2	7.7	4.9	4.9	15.6	5.3	1.0	1.2	1.9	2.2	1.1	1.5
Indian	15.5	16.6	7.9	20.1	6.3	9.3	14.1	2.8	2.4	2.0	2.6	2.4	0.9	—

Czech., Slovakia	31.7	14.5	11.8	9.3	15.2	8.8	5.1	2.8	3.0	6.3	8.3	4.5	0.8	0.3
Denmark	14.3	6.7	18.9	18.9	17.4	11.2	3.6	2.3	1.9	3.1	9.0	7.0	0.8	0.5
France, Bas-Rhin	15.5	7.4	23.1	14.6	18.0	8.5	6.9	1.2	2.1	3.0	5.5	2.2	0.8	0.2
FRG, Saarland	23.6	12.1	21.1	17.2	21.5	13.2	2.9	1.6	2.4	5.4	6.7	3.8	0.6	0.1
Finland	24.6	12.9	10.0	10.3	10.1	6.7	4.0	2.3	2.3	4.1	10.0	6.3	0.6	0.4
German Dem. Rep.	25.2	12.3	11.6	11.4	13.9	9.9	3.6	1.4	3.5	7.2	7.1	4.0	0.6	0.3
Hungary, Szabolcs	32.4	12.8	7.8	7.1	10.9	6.3	3.5	1.2	2.1	6.3	5.4	3.4	0.5	0.2
Iceland	31.4	14.0	14.5	14.6	7.7	6.0	2.7	1.5	1.7	1.6	9.4	6.4	0.9	0.2
Ireland, Southern	12.4	4.2	17.8	17.1	13.0	8.6	0.1	0.3	1.3	1.5	6.6	4.6	0.2	—
Italy, Ragusa	19.8	8.4	12.1	10.4	9.1	5.1	5.9	4.1	4.0	2.7	5.3	3.3	—	—
Italy, Varese	39.0	17.1	20.8	16.6	17.3	9.0	7.1	2.7	2.9	3.7	8.3	4.3	0.9	0.4
Norway	18.1	9.2	17.4	17.7	14.8	10.2	1.8	1.1	1.1	1.5	8.5	5.3	0.8	0.4
Poland, Cracow city	32.9	13.4	8.1	6.2	10.2	6.2	5.9	4.7	3.9	8.0	9.3	5.9	0.6	0.4
Spain, Navarra	31.6	13.5	11.2	8.1	11.2	7.5	7.9	4.7	2.0	4.4	5.2	2.9	0.5	0.3
Sweden	15.0	7.5	16.8	15.8	11.6	7.8	4.7	2.7	2.8	4.9	8.7	6.3	0.5	0.3
Switzerland, Geneva	13.5	6.3	24.3	16.2	12.8	9.8	10.2	1.5	2.8	3.2	8.4	5.2	0.4	0.4
UK, Birmingham	20.3	8.4	16.9	14.6	15.3	8.7	1.3	0.6	1.3	1.4	7.7	4.4	0.6	0.3
UK, West Scotland	21.7	10.0	20.4	17.9	13.3	8.1	2.7	1.1	1.6	1.8	8.0	6.0	0.4	0.3
Yugoslavia, Slovenia	34.9	15.1	8.7	7.8	14.4	8.7	2.0	1.2	2.3	4.5	6.8	3.9	0.6	0.4
Australia, Victoria	14.8	6.2	27.6	24.6	19.2	12.5	3.1	0.9	2.5	2.3	7.9	4.8	1.4	0.2
New Zealand, Maori	29.8	19.7	10.5	11.5	11.6	4.8	11.2	4.2	2.1	2.4	12.1	5.0	0.8	0.6
Non-Maori	13.7	6.0	26.5	28.4	17.1	11.7	2.4	1.1	1.4	1.8	7.5	4.7	0.7	0.3
Hawaii, White	11.8	6.0	28.1	21.2	13.7	7.6	4.2	1.3	1.2	1.7	8.5	8.0	0.9	0.5
Japanese	28.4	14.1	34.1	22.0	17.9	9.1	6.2	1.5	3.5	2.6	7.3	5.1	0.7	0.3
Hawaiian	31.2	14.9	19.9	12.0	16.1	6.9	7.3	2.7	2.5	2.8	9.0	7.8	0.4	—

Table 1.1. (cont.)

(c)

	Larynx (CD-9 161)		Bronchus, Lung (ICD-9 162)		Bone (ICD-9 170)		C. tissue (ICD-9 171)		Melanoma (ICD-9 172)		Other Skin (ICD-9 173)		Breast (ICD-9 174)	
	Male	Female	Male	Female	Male	Female	Male	Female	Male	Female	Male	Female	Male	Female
Senegal, Dakar	1.3	0.1	1.1	0.1	0.2	0.3	2.7	1.5	1.2	1.3	10.3	7.9	0.7	11.8
Colombia, Cali	5.5	1.2	25.4	9.7	1.3	0.7	3.1	2.8	3.3	3.0	56.2	58.9	0.0	34.8
Canada	6.9	1.0	61.3	16.9	1.4	1.0	2.3	1.8	5.3	6.0	80.1*	58.7*	0.6	66.4
US, Bay Area:														
White	6.5	1.4	65.8	33.3	1.2	1.0	2.0	2.0	10.3	9.0	—	—	0.8	87.0
Black	9.9	1.5	101.2	29.9	0.5	0.5	2.7	2.0	0.7	0.7	—	—	1.3	66.4
Chinese	2.2	0.8	54.0	24.0	0.7	0.5	1.9	1.8	0.3	0.2	—	—	0.4	43.7
Japanese	2.3	—	33.0	12.1	0.6	—	—	—	0.6	—	—	—	0.7	48.9
US, Detroit:														
White	8.4	1.5	75.5	27.9	0.9	0.7	2.0	1.7	7.4	6.4	—	—	0.6	74.9
Black	10.6	2.2	102.3	29.7	0.5	0.6	2.1	2.1	0.7	0.6	—	—	0.7	63.4
US, Utah	3.8	0.6	32.6	10.0	0.5	0.7	1.9	1.4	9.8	8.8	—	—	0.4	63.8
China, Shanghai	3.1	0.7	54.7	18.5	2.1	1.5	1.5	1.4	0.3	0.2	1.8	1.2	0.3	19.1
Hong Kong	9.5	1.3	58.5	24.2	1.4	1.1	2.0	1.5	0.9	0.7	4.7	4.0	0.3	28.7
India, Bombay	10.0	2.0	15.7	3.5	0.9	0.7	1.5	1.0	0.2	0.2	1.5	1.4	0.4	24.1
Israel:														
All Jews	5.5	0.6	27.9	9.0	1.6	1.1	2.2	1.9	5.8	7.4	—	—	0.8	61.3
Eur. Amer.	5.1	0.8	29.9	10.6	1.3	1.0	2.5	1.7	7.3	9.3	—	—	1.0	69.8
Non-Jews	4.9	0.5	23.4	3.6	0.6	1.1	1.6	1.5	0.3	0.4	—	—	0.3	14.0
Japan, Miyagi	2.2	0.2	29.6	8.7	0.9	0.7	1.1	0.9	0.6	0.3	1.6	1.3	1.0	22.0
Kuwait: Kuwaitis	3.4	0.5	13.8	6.4	0.5	0.6	1.5	0.7	—	—	4.4	2.6	0.5	15.9
Singapore:														
Chinese	8.2	0.8	73.4	22.8	0.8	0.7	1.2	1.1	0.8	0.4	9.1	7.8	0.5	27.1
Malay	1.1	0.2	26.7	6.9	1.0	1.0	2.4	1.4	1.5	0.2	3.2	3.2	0.1	21.1
Indian	8.2	1.6	21.2	6.6	1.3	1.8	1.0	1.0	1.3	0.4	2.2	4.6	—	27.6

Czech, Slovakia	10.5	0.4	70.0	6.8	1.1	0.8	1.8	1.4	3.0	3.4	31.9	24.6	0.4	31.2
Denmark	5.3	0.8	56.5	16.7	0.9	0.6	1.6	1.0	5.9	8.4	38.1	27.1	0.5	63.1
France, Bas-Rhin	12.4	0.5	60.2	3.9	1.6	1.2	1.3	1.7	3.1	4.6	11.4	6.2	0.6	62.4
FRG, Saarland	7.3	0.5	72.7	7.1	1.1	0.9	3.0	2.4	3.7	4.2	20.7	13.4	0.8	56.8
Finland	4.5	0.3	74.2	7.0	1.3	0.7	1.6	1.4	4.7	4.9	5.1	3.3	0.2	44.7
German Dem. Rep.	5.2	0.3	58.9	5.8	1.0	0.7	1.3	1.2	2.9	3.6	22.2	13.4	0.4	41.4
Hungary, Szabolcs	9.4	0.7	53.2	7.1	1.3	0.7	1.3	1.2	1.5	2.2	24.0	21.1	0.2	22.9
Iceland	3.7	1.2	24.7	18.4	1.4	0.8	2.5	1.5	2.7	5.0	5.4	3.2	0.6	60.1
Ireland, Southern	3.2	0.7	36.3	11.8	1.7	1.1	2.0	1.4	2.7	6.3	62.8	48.1	0.8	59.7
Italy, Ragusa	10.7	0.5	32.9	2.8	0.5	—	3.5	2.0	3.4	1.8	37.6	15.3	0.5	46.7
Italy, Varese	16.2	0.5	80.5	6.2	0.8	1.0	2.2	1.3	3.5	3.7	28.7	15.3	0.6	59.6
Norway	3.1	0.3	30.9	7.3	1.0	0.6	2.7	1.7	8.9	10.5	7.5	4.3	0.4	51.8
Poland, Cracow city	9.3	0.8	73.1	12.3	1.1	1.1	1.7	1.2	2.2	3.8	20.5	14.8	0.8	39.6
Spain, Navarra	17.2	0.2	34.9	4.0	1.1	1.0	2.8	2.0	2.2	2.4	30.7	14.9	0.5	38.7
Sweden	2.8	0.3	25.3	7.6	1.0	1.5	2.0	1.8	7.2	8.2	8.0	3.5	0.4	60.7
Switzerland, Geneva	8.8	1.3	72.9	10.8	0.6	0.7	2.8	1.1	8.9	9.6	52.5	35.6	0.6	72.2
UK, Birmingham	3.7	0.6	70.9	15.3	0.8	0.5	1.2	1.1	1.6	3.3	31.2	19.7	0.4	55.0
UK, West Scotland	4.9	1.2	100.4	28.6	0.9	0.7	1.5	1.1	2.7	4.3	28.1	18.4	0.5	58.7
Yugoslavia, Slovenia	8.7	0.6	57.6	6.7	0.7	0.8	1.2	1.2	2.4	2.7	21.0	17.8	0.5	37.7
Australia, Victoria	5.9	0.8	55.9	12.9	1.2	0.8	2.4	2.0	13.9	16.0	—	—	0.7	62.9
New Zealand, Maori	4.2	0.4	101.3	68.1	1.4	1.4	1.6	1.7	3.7	1.3	—	—	0.4	59.5
Non-Maori	4.1	0.5	52.2	13.5	1.0	0.8	2.0	1.4	15.6	21.4	—	—	0.5	57.7
Hawaii, White	10.0	1.7	66.2	32.7	1.0	0.1	1.9	0.9	22.7	18.8	—	—	0.6	84.4
Japanese	4.2	0.4	36.0	10.3	0.4	0.5	1.3	1.2	1.7	1.2	—	—	0.2	50.1
Hawaiian	6.0	1.5	82.8	39.7	0.5	1.5	4.3	1.6	1.2	1.2	—	—	0.6	93.9

Table 1.1. (cont.)
(d)

	Cervix uteri (ICD-9 180) Male	Cervix uteri (ICD-9 180) Female	Corpus uteri (ICD-9 182) Male	Corpus uteri (ICD-9 182) Female	Ovary (ICD-9 183) Male	Ovary (ICD-9 183) Female	Prostate (ICD-9 185) Male	Prostate (ICD-9 185) Female	Testis (ICD-9 186) Male	Testis (ICD-9 186) Female	Penis (ICD-9 187) Male	Penis (ICD-9 187) Female	Bladder (ICD-9 188) Male	Bladder (ICD-9 188) Female
Senegal, Dakar		17.2		1.5		4.3	4.3		0.2		0.4		3.0	1.7
Colombia, Cali		48.2		6.0		7.8	30.6		1.5		2.4		9.6	2.7
Canada		10.5		16.7		11.5	43.7		3.0		0.9		20.1	5.5
US, Bay Area:														
White		8.9		25.7		12.9	50.0		4.9		0.6		21.8	6.8
Black		14.2		11.1		9.0	82.5		1.1		1.3		12.2	3.8
Chinese		12.0		14.8		8.5	14.9		1.3		0.7		10.0	2.0
Japanese		5.9		19.6		8.8	16.5		0.6		—		8.9	3.4
US, Detroit:														
White		8.9		22.0		12.3	51.2		4.1		0.5		25.9	6.2
Black		19.0		10.0		8.8	91.1		1.1		1.2		11.4	4.4
US, Utah		6.7		21.4		10.9	70.2		4.0		0.7		16.8	4.3
China, Shanghai		8.5		3.0		5.0	1.8		0.7		0.6		7.1	1.7
Hong Kong		23.7		6.3		5.8	6.2		1.2		1.2		16.0	4.8
India, Bombay		20.6		2.0		7.2	8.2		1.0		2.3		4.3	1.0
Israel:														
All Jews		4.0		9.8		11.9	18.8		2.2		0.2		20.3	4.3
Eur. Amer.		4.0		12.5		15.2	22.5		3.8		0.2		20.8	4.6
Non-Jews		3.0		3.1		3.8	6.5		0.7		0.1		12.5	1.5
Japan, Miyagi		10.0		2.8		4.2	6.3		1.0		0.6		6.4	1.9
Kuwait: Kuwaitis		3.9		1.8		3.3	6.0		1.1		0.1		4.4	1.7
Singapore:														
Chinese		17.0		5.1		8.6	6.6		0.9		0.9		7.8	2.2
Malay		9.9		3.9		9.9	7.6		0.4		0.4		3.8	1.7
Indian		28.0		2.7		4.2	8.9		0.6		1.0		5.8	1.7

Czech, Slovakia	15.0	13.7	9.2	15.8	2.7	1.0	11.9	2.0
Denmark	18.5	15.3	14.5	27.7	7.8	1.2	24.7	6.2
France, Bas-Rhin	15.7	12.7	11.2	27.4	4.3	0.6	22.0	3.7
FRG, Saarland	13.9	14.3	9.1	28.7	5.4	0.9	20.9	3.8
Finland	5.5	12.2	9.8	34.2	1.5	0.5	12.7	2.5
German Dem. Rep.	24.6	13.9	12.1	19.9	5.5	0.9	11.6	2.1
Hungary, Szabolcs	9.5	7.8	5.8	12.6	1.2	0.5	7.6	1.3
Iceland	11.7	13.4	13.9	36.2	3.2	0.3	15.2	5.1
Ireland, Southern	6.3	5.4	9.0	20.3	3.0	0.8	8.6	3.0
Italy, Ragusa	9.6	12.3	7.9	18.8	0.6	0.9	11.7	0.5
Italy, Varese	10.1	12.5	10.2	20.3	3.3	0.8	27.3	4.0
Norway	15.6	12.1	15.3	42.0	5.9	0.9	17.0	4.8
Poland, Cracow city	20.2	9.2	12.0	13.8	2.4	1.2	10.4	2.1
Spain, Navarra	5.7	12.5	6.4	20.5	1.2	0.8	21.5	2.7
Sweden	9.9	13.2	15.2	45.9	3.3	0.9	15.5	4.2
Switzerland, Geneva	8.1	15.2	12.0	39.6	6.3	0.5	19.8	3.8
UK, Birmingham	12.3	9.1	11.1	18.9	3.1	1.2	16.9	4.4
UK, West Scotland	12.2	5.7	11.0	21.5	3.9	1.1	20.1	6.5
Yugoslavia, Slovenia	13.5	11.6	9.5	18.7	2.8	0.7	9.3	1.6
Australia, Victoria	10.4	9.6	9.9	41.4	4.2	0.7	23.4	6.5
New Zealand,								
Maori	28.9	15.4	10.9	35.4	7.9	1.0	4.6	3.2
Non-Maori	11.8	10.0	10.5	33.3	5.3	0.6	13.6	3.3
Hawaii,								
White	8.1	23.4	11.0	58.3	4.2	0.9	24.9	6.0
Japanese	6.4	15.5	8.0	31.2	1.4	0.3	9.6	3.8
Hawaiian	12.3	25.2	14.1	40.9	3.3	0.4	10.0	4.5

Table 1.1. (cont.)
(e)

	Eye (ICD-9 190)		Brain/CNS (ICD-9 191–2)		Thyroid (ICD-9 193)		Lymphosarcoma (ICD-9 200)		Hodgkins dis. (ICD-9 201)		Other Reticuloses (ICD-9 202)		Mult. Myeloma (ICD-9 203)	
	Male	Female	Male	Female	Male	Female	Male	Female	Male	Female	Male	Female	Male	Female
Senegal, Dakar	1.5	0.9	2.0	1.3	0.6	1.1	3.5	1.2	1.4	0.7	0.0	0.0	0.2	0.2
Colombia, Cali	0.5	0.5	4.6	2.6	1.4	5.3	1.1	0.0	2.9	1.1	4.3	3.5	2.1	1.5
Canada	0.9	0.7	6.6	5.0	1.5	3.6	5.8	4.2	3.5	2.2	3.9	3.0	3.3	2.4
US, Bay Area:														
White	0.9	0.8	7.1	5.4	2.6	5.9	6.3	5.2	3.3	2.4	5.0	3.5	3.1	2.5
Black	0.9	0.3	4.9	4.0	1.0	3.1	4.1	3.6	3.3	1.4	3.6	1.4	7.9	4.5
Chinese	1.3	—	1.8	3.7	2.2	3.9	4.5	3.8	0.6	1.7	3.4	3.6	1.5	1.3
Japanese	—	—	4.4	4.6	1.6	3.1	9.5	1.9	—	—	1.1	0.7	—	0.5
US, Detroit:														
White	0.7	0.6	6.2	4.6	2.1	5.8	6.5	4.6	3.5	2.6	4.7	3.7	3.3	2.3
Black	0.3	0.2	4.1	2.4	1.3	3.4	4.8	3.2	2.1	1.3	3.1	2.2	7.6	5.7
US, Utah	1.4	1.1	6.1	4.4	1.9	6.3	5.0	3.7	3.1	2.1	4.7	3.2	2.8	2.2
China, Shanghai	0.1	0.3	3.6	2.9	1.2	3.3	2.0	1.2	0.5	0.3	1.5	0.9	0.7	0.4
Hong Kong	0.3	0.3	2.0	1.6	1.4	4.8	6.5	5.0	0.7	0.3	0.0	0.0	1.3	0.8
India, Bombay	0.3	0.1	2.1	1.5	0.6	1.7	2.0	1.0	1.1	0.5	1.6	1.0	1.2	1.0
Israel:														
All Jews	0.6	0.5	9.0	8.5	2.5	6.0	6.8	4.7	2.5	2.0	3.1	2.4	3.1	2.1
Eur. Amer.	0.6	0.6	10.9	8.8	2.8	5.3	7.1	5.3	2.7	2.1	3.4	2.5	3.1	2.1
Non-Jews	0.8	0.8	5.5	3.3	1.3	2.5	4.4	2.6	1.9	0.6	2.2	1.6	1.6	1.4
Japan, Miyagi	0.2	0.4	2.0	1.7	1.1	3.9	1.0	0.4	0.5	0.3	3.1	1.7	1.4	1.1
Kuwait: Kuwaitis	0.4	—	1.1	1.0	2.0	6.3	2.3	1.3	1.5	1.4	0.6	0.5	1.6	1.6
Singapore:														
Chinese	0.2	0.3	1.7	1.1	1.5	4.3	3.0	1.6	0.8	0.4	2.1	1.3	0.9	0.6
Malay	0.2	—	1.7	0.7	2.7	5.0	3.7	2.0	0.7	0.8	1.7	1.2	1.1	1.0
Indian	0.5	—	1.7	1.7	0.7	1.1	3.5	1.3	0.2	—	3.8	2.1	2.6	—

Region													
Czech., Slovakia	0.9	0.6	4.9	3.4	0.9	2.3	3.3	1.5	2.6	1.7	1.2	2.1	2.0	1.5
Denmark	1.0	0.7	8.5	7.8	0.9	1.9	2.9	1.9	2.6	1.6	3.9	2.5	2.7	1.8
France, Bas-Rhin	0.4	0.4	5.9	4.0	1.0	2.8	5.8	4.4	2.1	2.2	1.7	1.1	2.4	1.5
FRG, Saarland	0.7	0.4	5.7	5.4	1.6	3.7	2.4	1.2	2.8	1.2	4.0	2.9	1.2	1.0
Finland	1.0	0.7	6.4	5.2	1.6	5.2	7.4	4.7	2.8	1.7	0.2	0.1	2.8	2.1
German Dem. Rep.	0.9	0.7	5.0	4.2	1.1	2.4	1.4	0.9	2.5	1.8	3.6	2.2	1.7	1.2
Hungary, Szabolcs	0.3	0.5	2.4	1.3	0.7	2.0	0.4	0.2	1.0	0.8	2.0	0.9	1.0	0.2
Iceland	1.2	0.9	8.5	10.0	5.6	13.3	2.9	2.4	3.4	1.9	1.1	0.8	4.0	2.0
Ireland, Southern	0.5	0.7	7.0	5.3	1.1	2.1	0.8	0.3	3.1	0.8	3.7	3.6	1.6	0.7
Italy, Ragusa	0.3	0.2	6.5	1.8	0.8	1.7	4.6	1.9	4.5	2.1	—	0.3	2.3	1.8
Italy, Varese	0.7	0.5	5.5	4.4	1.9	3.7	4.3	2.3	4.7	2.5	5.5	2.1	2.4	1.7
Norway	1.0	0.8	8.3	7.5	1.7	5.1	3.7	2.6	2.6	1.6	2.4	1.7	4.2	2.6
Poland, Cracow city	0.9	0.8	8.6	5.4	0.7	1.4	0.7	0.1	2.4	1.7	2.2	1.1	2.8	1.1
Spain, Navarra	1.0	0.3	7.9	5.7	0.3	2.7	3.7	1.6	2.4	1.2	1.8	1.8	1.8	1.3
Sweden	0.9	0.6	9.4	9.3	1.6	4.3	7.1	4.7	2.3	1.5	0.3	0.2	3.5	2.3
Switzerland, Geneva	0.6	1.1	4.5	4.4	1.6	3.2	3.8	2.1	2.9	2.4	5.0	2.6	3.8	2.1
UK, Birmingham	0.4	0.3	6.1	5.0	0.5	1.4	2.4	1.3	2.6	1.6	2.9	1.9	2.4	1.4
UK, West Scotland	1.1	0.9	5.6	3.9	0.5	1.5	1.8	1.2	2.9	2.0	4.5	3.4	2.9	2.0
Yugoslavia, Slovenia	0.4	0.5	4.1	2.6	0.8	2.5	3.8	2.0	1.8	1.6	0.7	0.5	2.1	1.2
Australia, Victoria	1.1	0.4	7.0	4.5	0.8	2.4	6.4	4.3	2.9	1.9	4.4	4.0	3.2	2.0
New Zealand, Maori	0.6	0.3	9.1	4.8	2.3	3.1	4.5	2.9	2.5	1.1	3.4	2.3	5.6	4.3
Non-Maori	1.2	0.8	7.2	4.8	1.0	2.9	4.0	2.9	2.5	1.9	3.2	2.2	3.1	2.1
Hawaii, White	1.0	—	6.9	3.6	2.2	5.9	6.8	5.0	2.4	2.5	4.0	1.7	3.9	1.8
Japanese	0.5	0.1	2.3	1.6	5.3	6.0	4.9	4.4	0.9	0.2	1.7	1.1	0.6	1.4
Hawaiian	—	0.4	3.0	4.1	5.9	10.5	8.6	4.4	1.6	0.6	1.5	2.1	5.3	5.4

Table 1.1. (cont.)

(f)

	Lymphoid leukemia (ICD-9 204)		Myeloid leukemia (ICD-9 205)		Monocytic leukemia (ICD-9 206)		All Sites		All sites but 173	
	Male	Female	Male	Female	Male	Female	Male	Female	Male	Female
Senegal, Dakar	0.5	0.0	0.1	0.2	0.0	0.0	76.3	75.9	66.1	68.0
Colombia, Cali	2.4	1.8	2.7	2.1	0.2	0.4	266.1	279.6	209.9	220.8
Canada	4.8	2.8	3.3	2.3	0.2	0.1	—	—	289.1	236.2
US, Bay Area:										
White	3.7	2.6	4.3	2.8	0.2	0.1	—	—	312.0	295.0
Black	3.4	2.1	4.7	3.3	0.1	0.2	—	—	389.4	249.2
Chinese	3.6	1.3	0.8	1.3	—	0.2	—	—	224.4	197.5
Japanese	2.0	—	2.3	2.5	—	—	—	—	189.0	176.5
US, Detroit:										
White	5.5	3.1	4.4	3.2	0.4	0.3	—	—	328.3	264.5
Black	4.4	2.4	4.3	3.6	0.2	0.2	—	—	400.1	252.2
US, Utah	4.8	3.2	4.1	2.1	0.1	0.0	—	—	256.1	213.1
China, Shanghai	1.4	1.3	2.1	1.6	0.4	0.5	246.5	155.9	244.7	154.7
Hong Kong	2.6	1.4	2.8	2.3	0.1	0.1	288.4	201.4	283.7	197.4
India, Bombay	1.4	0.9	1.9	1.2	0.1	0.0	145.0	126.0	143.5	124.6
Israel:										
All Jews	3.9	2.7	3.0	2.1	0.6	0.5	—	—	215.3	216.8
Eur. Amer.	3.7	5.7	3.1	2.5	0.5	0.6	—	—	248.5	251.9
Non-Jews	2.1	0.8	1.3	0.5	0.6	0.2	—	—	117.3	80.1
Japan, Miyagi	1.3	1.1	2.5	2.1	0.3	0.4	216.7	146.0	215.1	144.8
Kuwait: Kuwaitis	2.0	1.4	1.8	1.8	0.2	—	76.3	74.6	71.9	72.0
Singapore:										
Chinese	1.5	1.2	2.5	2.2	0.0	0.0	282.6	183.1	273.6	175.3
Malay	1.2	0.7	2.8	2.1	0.2	—	121.0	114.2	117.8	111.0
Indian	1.3	—	3.0	2.2	0.3	—	155.9	175.8	153.7	171.2

Czech, Slovakia	4.4	2.5	3.1	2.4	0.1	0.1	291.0	190.0	259.1	165.4
Denmark	4.6	2.5	3.7	2.8	0.1	0.2	298.9	267.8	260.7	240.7
France, Bas-Rhin	4.2	2.9	2.5	1.7	0.1	0.0	341.6	208.6	330.2	202.4
FRG, Saarland	3.4	1.5	1.7	1.6	0.4	0.1	317.1	226.7	296.3	213.0
Finland	4.3	2.6	3.3	2.5	0.1	0.1	261.4	178.7	256.2	175.4
German Dem. Rep.	3.0	1.8	2.5	1.9	0.1	0.1	242.8	198.1	220.7	184.7
Hungary, Szabolcs	1.6	1.3	1.3	1.3	—	—	212.4	135.3	188.4	114.2
Iceland	2.2	1.3	2.9	2.1	—	—	230.0	236.9	224.6	233.7
Ireland, Southern	1.6	1.2	2.8	1.9	0.1	0.1	255.2	229.4	192.4	181.3
Italy, Ragusa	3.2	2.7	1.9	1.9	—	—	230.8	159.9	193.2	144.6
Italy, Varese	4.4	3.7	4.4	3.7	0.1	0.2	363.2	219.7	334.5	204.3
Norway	3.2	1.9	3.5	2.5	0.1	0.1	245.8	216.4	238.3	212.2
Poland, Cracow city	4.4	1.9	1.8	1.8	0.1	0.0	263.1	197.1	242.6	182.3
Spain, Navarra	4.0	2.3	3.3	1.8	0.1	0.2	273.7	168.9	243.0	153.7
Sweden	4.3	2.8	3.2	2.4	0.2	0.1	241.1	227.6	233.2	224.1
Switzerland, Geneva	3.5	3.5	3.5	2.4	0.3	0.1	372.4	257.8	319.9	222.3
UK, Birmingham	3.2	1.6	2.6	1.9	0.1	0.0	266.3	208.5	235.1	188.8
UK, West Scotland	3.5	1.9	3.1	2.4	0.2	0.1	319.6	238.9	291.5	220.5
Yugoslavia, Slovenia	3.1	1.9	1.7	1.5	0.7	0.5	256.0	176.9	235.0	159.1
Australia, Victoria	3.8	2.8	3.4	2.2	0.2	0.0	—	—	308.2	233.2
New Zealand,										
Maori	2.8	2.7	6.1	2.7	0.0	0.4	—	—	322.9	297.6
Non-Maori	4.0	2.2	3.7	2.7	0.2	0.1	—	—	265.5	229.6
Hawaii, White	6.0	3.7	3.8	3.5	—	—	—	—	346.1	289.1
Japanese	1.4	1.7	4.0	1.7	0.2	—	—	—	231.0	180.1
Hawaiian	2.0	0.6	6.3	3.6	—	0.3	—	—	311.9	297.6

(After Waterhouse *et al.*, 1982; Muir *et al.*, 1987.)
* Alberta.

Table 1.2. *Range of age-standardized incidence for selected sites of cancer 1978–1982, by sex.*

Site	ICD 9	Greatest reported incidence[a]		Lowest reported incidence		Ratio	Greatest reported incidence		Lowest reported incidence		Ratio
		Males					**Females**				
Lip	140	Canada Newfoundland	15.1	Detroit Black	0.1	150	South Australia	1.6	UK SW Region	0.1	16
Tongue	141	India Bombay	9.4	China Jianjin	0.4	24	India Bombay	3.4	Hungary Szabolcs	0.1	34
Oral cavity	143–5	France Bas-Rhin	13.5	Iceland	0.4	34	India Bangalore	15.7	Spain Zaragoza	0.1	160
Nasopharynx	147	Hong-Kong	30.0	Brazil Fortaleza	0.2	150	Hong-Kong	12.9	Switzerland Vaud	0.1	130
Esophagus	150	France Calvados, Rural	35.8	Israel Non-Jews	1.0	360	India Poona	12.4	Hungary Szabolcs	0.1	125
Stomach	151	Japan Nagasaki	82.0	Kuwait Kuwaitis	3.7	22	Japan Nagasaki	36.1	Kuwait Kuwaitis	1.6	23
Colon	153	USA/Conn. Whites	34.1	Kuwait Kuwaitis	0.2	170	USA/Detroit Blacks	29.0	India Madras	0.7	41
Rectum	154	Israel, Jews[b] born EU/AM	22.6	Kuwait Kuwaitis	2.0	75	Israel, Jews[b] born EU/AM	15.9	Kuwait Kuwaitis	1.3	12
Liver	155	China Shanghai	34.4	Canada Nova Scotia	0.7	49	China Shanghai	11.6	Australia NSW	0.4	29
Pancreas	157	USA/Detroit Blacks	12.8	India Bangalore	0.7	18	USA/Atlanta Blacks	8.7	India Madras	0.4	22
Larynx	161	Brazil Sao Paulo	17.8	Japan Miyagi	2.2	8	India Nagpur	2.3	Switzerland Zurich	0.1	23
Lung	162	USA/Detroit Blacks	102.3	India Madras	5.8	18	USA/Atlanta Whites	33.3	India Nagpur	0.5	67

Site		High		Low		Ratio	High		Low		Ratio
Melanoma of skin	172	Australia Queensland	30.9	India Madras	0.1	310	Australia Queensland	28.5	China Tianjin	0.1	285
Breast	174	—	—	—	—	—	USA/Whites S Franc. B.A.[c]	87.0	Israel Non-Jews	14.0	6
Cervix Uteri	180	—	—	—	—	—	Columbia Cali	48.2	Israel Non-Jews	3.0	16
Corpus	182	—	—	—	—	—	USA/Whites S. Franc. B.A.[c]	25.7	India Nagpur	1.2	21
Ovary	183	—	—	—	—	—	Norway	15.3	Kuwait Kuwaitis	3.3	5
Prostate	185	USA/Atlanta Blacks	91.2	China Tianjin	1.3	70					
Bladder	188	Italy Varese	27.3	India Nagpur	1.7	16	Kuwait Non-Kuwaitis	8.5	India Nagpur	0.3	28
Kidney etc.	189	Iceland	12.2	India Poona	0.7	17	Iceland	7.6	India Madras	0.4	19
Brain etc.	191–2	Israel/Jews[b] born EU/AM	10.9	India Nagpur	1.1	10	Israel/Jews[d] born AF/AS	15.7	India Nagpur	0.1	157
Thyroid	193	Iceland	5.6	Spain Navarra	0.3	19	Iceland	13.3	UK Oxford	0.0	—
Lymphoma	200/2	Switzerland Vaud	11.5	India Nagpur	1.5	8	USA/Whites S. Franc. B.A.[c]	8.7	India Nagpur	0.7	12
Hodgkin's Disease	201	Canada Quebec	4.8	China Tianjin	0.2	24	Canada Quebec	3.1	India Nagpur	0.2	16
Multiple Myeloma	203	USA/Atlanta Blacks	7.7	India Nagpur	0.1	77	USA/Detroit Blacks	5.7	India Madras	0.1	57
Leukemia	204–8	Canada Ontario	11.6	India Nagpur	2.2	5	Italy Varese	7.9	India Madras	1.1	8

[a] Rates are age-standardized to the world population and are based on at least one million person–years of observation.
[b] Jews born in Europe or America.
[c] San Francisco Bay Area.
[d] Jews born in Africa or Asia.

Appendix 2

A glossary of epidemiological terms

MICHAEL J. SHERIDAN

Introduction
This glossary contains a sample of the terms used in epidemiology. The definitions given below are based on those provided by Last (1988). For further details, other sources should be consulted (Stedman, 1982; Friedman, 1980; Lilienfeld & Lilienfeld, 1980; Kendall & Buckland, 1982; Abramson, 1984; Murphy, 1985; Pressat, 1985; Last, 1986; Schuman, 1986; Jammal *et al.*, 1988).

Glossary of terms
Adjustment a procedure in which potentially misleading effects of differences in the composition of populations being compared have been minimized – as much as is possible – by statistical methods. The mathematical procedure commonly used to adjust incidence or mortality rates for age differences is direct or indirect standardization.

Age-specific rate a rate calculated for a specific age-group, i.e., the numerator and denominator refer to the same age group. A multiplier, usually 100,000, is chosen to produce a rate that can be expressed as a convenient number.

Analytical study a study designed to examine hypothesized causal relationships. An analytical study is usually concerned with identifying the health effects of specific risk factors. In this type of study, individuals are classified either according to the absence or presence of a specific disease and/or according to the presence or absence of risk factors presumed to influence disease occurrence.

Attributable risk the rate of an outcome, usually a disease, in exposed individuals that can be attributed to the exposure alone. In calculating this rate, it is assumed that causes other than the one under study have had equal effects on the exposed and unexposed groups. Population attributable risk percent is often used to denote that proportion of a disease that would not occur if the risk factor was absent, e.g. 85% of lung cancer in a population is attributable to tobacco use.

Bias any trend in the collection, analysis, or interpretation of data that can lead to conclusions that are systematically different from the true state of affairs. Common types of systematic error or bias include: ascertainment (due to type of patient being observed or type of diagnostic process being employed); interviewer (due to selective data gathering); measurement (due to inaccurate classification of subjects); observer (due to inter- or intra-variability); recall (due to inaccuracy or incompleteness of memory); response (due to differences between those who volunteer and those who do not); selection (due to differences between those who are chosen and those who are not) and sampling (due to the use of nonprobability samples).

Case-control study a type of analytical study that starts with the identification of persons with a disease (or another outcome) and an appropriate control (comparison) group of persons without the disease. The relationship of a risk factor to the disease is examined by comparing the diseased and non-diseased with regard to how frequently the risk factor is present. Such a study is sometimes called 'retrospective' because it starts after the onset of disease and looks backward to uncover the postulated causal factors.

Causality the relating of causes to the effects they produce. Much of epidemiology concerns causality, but epidemiological evidence by itself is insufficient to establish causality.

Classification assignment to predesignated classes on the basis of common characteristics. This is useful to achieve standardization, and hence comparability in the presentation of data – mortality, morbidity, histopathological – from different sources. Many classifications provide a systematic numerical notation or code for each entity as in the ICD (International Classification of Diseases) and ICD-O (International Classification of Diseases for Oncology).

Clinical trial a type of experimental study that involves the administration of a therapeutic regimen to evaluate its efficacy and safety.

Generally these studies are rigorously designed and executed, involving random allocation of subjects to experimental and control groups.

Cluster aggregation of relatively uncommon events or diseases in time and/or space, e.g. leukemia.

Cohort study a type of analytical study in which the population is identified according to the presence or absence of risk factors associated with the probability of disease occurrence. The term is frequently used to describe any designated group of persons followed over a period of time and is sometimes called prospective or longitudinal.

Confounding the distortion of the apparent effect of an exposure or risk due to the association of that exposure to others that can influence the outcome.

Control group a comparison group that differs in disease experience or therapeutic regimen from the primary study group. Control groups may be assembled from several sources, including: hospital, neighborhood, siblings and the general population. The source of the control group can introduce systematic error into a study and so the issue of bias due to choice of control group must always be carefully addressed.

Cross-sectional study a type of study that simultaneously examines the relationship between a disease and risk factors of interest as they exist in a defined population at a specific point in time. Such studies cannot determine the temporal sequence of cause and effect.

Death rate the proportion of a population that dies during a specified period: the numerator is the number dying, the denominator is the size of the population. Age-specific death rates and age adjusted death rates, usually expressed per 100,000, are frequently calculated.

Descriptive study a type of study concerned with general relationships between disease and the distribution of such variables as age, sex, race, occupation and social class. Such studies may suggest causal hypotheses.

Ecological study a type of descriptive study based on grouped data in which the unit of analysis is populations and not individuals. Correlations based on aggregate data may mask a true association at the individual level and so such studies cannot assess a causal relationship.

Epidemiology the study of the distribution and frequency of diseases to search for determinants, and the application of this information to the control of health problems.

Experimental study a study in which conditions are under the direct control of the investigator and the subjects are randomly allocated to treatment or control groups to test the effect of a therapeutic regimen. This type of study provides the most direct and conclusive evidence for a causal relationship.

Factor an event, characteristic, exposure or other definable entity that brings about a change in a health condition or other defined outcome.

Follow-up observation over a period of time of an individual, group or defined population exposed to some risk, possessing a characteristic, or receiving a specified preventive or therapeutic procedure to assess outcome, e.g. occurrence of disease.

Geographic pathology the comparative study of countries, or of regions within them, with regard to variations in incidence or mortality. The implied aim of such studies is to demonstrate that variations are due to environmental differences.

Healthy worker effect workers usually exhibit lower overall death rates than the general population as the severely ill and disabled are usually excluded from employment.

Historical cohort study a type of analytical study conducted by reconstructing data about persons some time in the past. This method uses existing records about the past health or disease experience of a population and determines its current or subsequent health status with respect to the condition of interest. This type of study may also be referred to as a non-concurrent or historical prospective study.

Hypothesis a conjecture, usually on causation, cast in a form that will allow it to be tested and refuted.

Incidence the number of new events occurring in a specified population during a specific time interval. An incidence rate is the rate at which new events occur in a population. The numerator is the number of new events occurring in a defined period and the denominator is the population at risk of experiencing the event during this period, sometimes expressed as person–years. Incidence is a true measure of risk and is always to be preferred to prevalence when available.

Induction period   the period required for a specific cause to produce disease. Also referred to as latent period.

International Classification of Disease (ICD)   a classification of specific conditions determined by an internationally representative group of experts who advise the World Health Organization, which publishes the complete list in a periodically revised book entitled *Manual of the International Statistical Classification of Diseases, Injuries and Death* (WHO, 1977). Neoplasms are contained in Chapter II. The current version is the ICD-9, published in 1977. A new version is expected around 1992. There is a specialized adaption for oncology revised in 1990, i.e. ICD-O, which gives code numbers for morphological terms used to describe neoplasms.

Matching   the process of making a study group and a comparison group comparable with regard to selected extraneous factors, e.g. age and sex.

Meta-analysis   a process of using statistical methods to combine results of different studies, none of which individually may be large enough to demonstrate a statistically significant difference, but which, in the aggregate, may be capable of doing so. The potential of serious biases must be addressed in using and reporting the results of this process.

Migrant study   a study which takes advantage of migration to one country by those from another with different physical and biological environments, cultural backgrounds, genetic make-up and different mortality or morbidity experience. The mortality or morbidity experience of the migrants in their new country is compared with that of their country of origin.

Misclassification   assignment of an individual, value or attribute to the wrong category.

Natural experiment   a naturally occurring circumstance – resembling a true experiment – in which population groups have different exposures to a supposed causal factor but are not randomly allocated to treatment and control groups.

Nested case-control study   a case-control study in which cases and controls are drawn from the defined population in a cohort study. As some data are already available about both cases and controls, the confounding effects of some variables can be reduced or eliminated.

Nomenclature   a list of approved terms for describing and recording observations.

Observational study   a non-experimental study in which differences in one factor are studied in relation to differences in other factors without manipulation by the investigator.

Odds ratio   the ratio of the probability of the occurrence of an event to that of non-occurrence. The odds ratio is the ratio of two odds. In a case-control study, the exposure odds ratio is the ratio of the odds in favor of exposure among cases to the odds in favor of exposure among non-cases. The odds ratio is frequently regarded as synonymous with the relative risk.

Pathogenesis   the postulated mechanism by which an etiological agent produces disease.

Randomization   assignment of individuals to groups, by chance. Within the limits of chance variables, randomization should make control and experimental groups similar at the start of an investigation and ensure that the investigator does not influence allocation.

Rates   the measure of the frequency of a phenomenon, usually in a defined population.

Registry   a repository for the systematic recording of vital documents, which can then be tabulated, summarized and published. The most common types of registries are those maintained for cancer and for twins and birth defects.

Relative risk   see odds ratio.

Retrospective study   see case-control study

Risk Factor   an aspect of personal behavior or lifestyle, an environmental exposure or an inborn or inherited characteristic which is known or suspected to be associated with adverse effects or health.

Socio-economic status description of a person's position in society which may be placed on an ordinal scale using such criteria as income, educational level, occupation, location of residence, etc.

Standardization a set of statistical techniques used to remove – as far as possible – the effects of confounding variables when comparing two or more populations.

Standardized mortality ratio (SMR) the ratio of the number of events observed in a study group or population to the number that would be expected if the group under study had the same specific rates as the standard population, multiplied by 100.

Xenobiotic a foreign compound that is metabolized in the body.

References

Abramson, J.H (1984). *Survey Methods in Community Medicine*. London: Churchill Livingstone.

Friedman, G.D. (1980). *Primer of Epidemiology*. New York: McGraw-Hill.

Jammal, A., Allard, R. & Loslier, G. (eds.) (1988). *Dictionnaire d'epidemiologie*. Paris: Edisem.

Kendall, M.G. & Buckland, A.A. (1982). A *Dictionary of Statistical Terms*. London: Longman.

Last, J.M. (ed.) (1988). *A Dictionary of Epidemiology*. New York: Oxford University Press.

Last, J.M. (ed.) (1986). *Maxcy-Rosenau Public Health and Preventive Medicine*. Norwalk, CT: Appleton-Century-Crofts.

Lilienfeld, A.M. & Lilienfeld, D. (1980). *Foundations of Epidemiology*. New York: Oxford University Press.

Murphy, E.A. (1985). *A Companion to Medical Statistics*. Baltimore: Johns Hopkins University Press.

Pressat, R. (1985). *Dictionary of Demography*, English trans., C. Wilson. Oxford: Blackwell.

Schuman, S.H. (1986). *Practice-Based Epidemiology*. New York: Gordon & Breach.

Stedman, T.L. (1982). *Stedman's Medical Dictionary*. Baltimore: Williams & Wilkins.

WHO (World Health Organization). (1977). *Manual of the International Statistical Classification of Diseases, Injuries, and Causes of Death*, volume 1. Geneva: World Health Organization.

Appendix 3

Acronyms and abbreviations

AF	Aflatoxin
AF-2	2-(2-Furyl)-3-(5-nitro-2-furyl)acrylamide
AHH	Aryl hydrocarbon hydroxylase
AIDS	Acquired immunodeficiency syndrome
AL	Acute leukemia
AT	Ataxia telangiectasia
BEIR	Biological effects of Ionizing Radiation
BHA	Butylated hydroxyanisole
BL	Burkitt's lymphoma
BPDE	Benzo[a]pyrene-7,8-diol-9,10-epoxide
BS	Bloom's syndrome
CAG	Chronic atrophic gastritis
CAT	Computerized axial tomography
CI	Confidence interval
CI5C	'Cancer Incidence in Five Continents', one of a series of volumes compiling cancer registry data.
CI5V	'Cancer Incidence in Five Continents', volume V
CIN	Cervical intra-epithelial neoplasia
CIOMS	Council for the Coordination of International Congresses of Medical Sciences.
CIRC	Centre International de Recherche sur le Cancer (IARC)
CLL	Chronic lymphocytic leukemia
CML	Chronic myelocytic leukemia
CMV	Cytomegalovirus
CNS	Central nervous system
CYPIA	Cytochrome P450 IA
DDE	Dichlorodiphenyldichloroethane
DDT	Dichlorodiphenyltrichloroethane

DFMO	Difluoromethylornithine
DNA	Deoxyribonucleic acid
EBNA	Epstein–Barr nuclear antigen
EBV	Epstein–Barr Virus
EDB	Ethylene dibromide
EEC	European Economic Community
EGFR	Epidermal growth factor receptor
ELF	Extremely low frequency
ELISA	Enzyme-linked immunosorbent assay
E_{01}	A large animal experiment based on the minimum dose necessary to produce tumors in 1%
EPA	Environmental Protection Agency
ERT	Estrogen replacement therapy
ETS	Environmental tobacco smoke
FAO	Food and Agricultural Organization (United Nations)
FAP	Familial adenomatous polyposis
FB	Foreign body
FDA	Food and drug administration
FSH	Follicular stimulating hormone
GHIS	Gambia hepatitis study group
GC	Gas chromatography
GIRLS	Generalized iterative record linkage system
HAS	Hepatic angiosarcoma
HBcAg	Hepatitis B core antigen
HBeAg	Hepatitis B e antigen
HBsAg	Hepatitis B surface antigen
HBV	Hepatitis B virus
HCC	Hepatocellular carcinoma
HCV	Hepatitis C virus
HD	Hodgkin's Disease
HER-2/*neu*	An oncogene associated with breast cancer
HIV	Human immunodeficiency virus
HLA	Human leukocyte antigen
HPLC	High performance liquid chromatography
HPV	Human papilloma virus
HSV	Herpes simplex virus
HTLV	Human T-cell leukemia virus
IA	Infra-red analysis
IARC	International Agency for Research on Cancer
ICD	International classification of diseases
ICD-O	International classification of diseases–oncology

ILO	International Labor Organization
LPO	Lipid peroxidation
MEN	Multiple neuroendocrine neoplasia
MMMF	Man-made mineral fibers
MN	Micronucleus
MOPP	A specific drug combination (mechlorethamine, oncovin (vincristine), procarbazine and prednisone) used in cancer chemotherapy
MS	Mass spectrometry
NAS	National Academy of Sciences
NCI	Negative-ion chemical ionization
NCTR/SOT	National Center for Toxicological Research, Society of Toxicology
NF	Neurofibromatosis
ng	Nanogram
NIOSH	National Institute of Occupational Safety and Health
NNNG	N-methyl-N-nitro-N-nitroso guanidine
NOC	N-nitroso-compounds
NPC	Nasopharyngeal carcinoma
NPRO	N-nitrosoproline
NSP	Non-starch polysaccharides (non-starch carbohydrate)
NTP	National Toxicological Program
OC	Oral contraceptive
OSHA	Occupational Safety and Health Administration
PAH	Polycyclic aromatic hydrocarbons
PCB	Polychlorinated biphenyl
PCR	Polymerase chain reaction
PIN	Penile intra-epithelial neoplasia
PMR	Proportional mortality ratio
QF	Quality factor (in radiation)
QRA	Quantitative risk assessment
RB	Retinoblastoma
RBE	Relative biological effectiveness (in radiation)
rem	Roentgen equivalent man
RIA	Radioimmunoassay
RFLP	Restriction fragment length polymorphism
RNA	Ribonucleic acid
RR	Relative risk
SCE	Sister chromatid exchange
SCLC	Small cell lung cancer
SEARCH	Surveillance of environmental aspects related to cancer.

	An international collaborative IARC program to carry out cancer epidemiology studies
SEER	Surveillance, epidemiology and end results program of the US National Cancer Institute
SIR	Standardized incidence ratio
SM	Standardized mortality rate
SMR	Standardized mortality ratio
SNC	Sinonasal cancer
SNOMed	Standard nomenclature of medicine
SSFS	Synchronous scanning fluorescence spectrophotometry
STS	Soft tissue sarcoma
Sv	Sievert (1 sv = 100 rem)
TCDD	Chlorinated dioxin (2,3,7,8-tetrachlorodibenzo-para-dioxin)
TEA	Thermal energy analysis
UAREP	Universities Associated for Research and Education in Pathology
ug	Microgram
UICC	International Union Against Cancer
UK	United Kingdom
UNSCEAR	United Nations Scientific Committee on the effects of atomic radiation
USA	United States of America
USPHS	United States Public Health Service
UV	Ultraviolet
WBC	White blood cells
WHV	Woodchuck hepatitis virus
WHO	World Health Organization
XP	Xeroderma pigmentosum

Supplement

Introduction

Since the manuscript was completed, additional data of interest have been published. This supplement provides certain recent references that may be of value to the reader. In some cases, these amplify or confirm the information already in the text; in others, however, they provide new information on a suspected cause or potential laboratory approaches to etiological studies.

Chapter 5: Laboratory methods

Interactions of chemical carcinogens with critical genes: implications for evaluating etiological associations and possible use in courts

The reactivity of carcinogens with DNA in humans and resultant biological consequences has been fundamental to the development of modern theories and understanding of chemical carcinogenesis and principles discussed in Chapter 18. Only recently, however, has evidence of mutations in critical genes involved in control of cell proliferation and neoplastic transformation been available from tumor tissue. Such specific mutations can be induced by chemicals experimentally in animals.

Analysis of such genes in human cancers may provide clues to etiology since both mutagens as well as endogenous pro-mutagenic processes can elicit characteristic mutation patterns in defined sequences. This has now been demonstrated in such animal systems as the mouse skin tumor and the rat mammary carcinoma, and recently from analysis of mutations in the p53 tumor suppressor gene in human cancers (Hollstein *et al.*, 1991).

An analysis of chemically induced murine skin papillomas and carcinomas for activated oncogenes revealed that nearly all tumors initiated by 7,12-dimethylbenzanthracene (DMBA) harbored a mutated H-*ras* gene with a specific A to T transversion of the second base in codon 61. Tumors initiated by MNNG or benzo[*a*]pyrene, however, did not have this type of mutation, but rather G to A/T mutations of the first base in codon 12. These 'carcinogen-specific' mutations correlate with the known metabolism and DNA binding properties of the chemicals and therefore strongly support the hypothesis that the carcinogen treatment elicited the oncogene mutations by direct interaction with DNA (Balmain & Brown, 1988).

Comparable results were obtained in a mammary tumors system

induced in female rats by a variety of carcinogens including methyl-nitrosurea (MNU) and DMBA. Virtually all tumors initiated by MNU with a transforming *ras* gene contained a mutated H-*ras* allele with a mutation in codon 12, where GAA substitutes GCA. In tumors induced by DMBA an activated H *ras* gene is rarely present in these cases, the mutation is in codon 61 (Sukumar *et al.*, 1983; Zarbel *et al.*, 1985). Again, a direct interaction of the carcinogen or its metabolites with the target gene is believed probable. The 'carcinogen-specific' H-*ras* mutation can be detected in mammary tissue as early as two weeks after treatment (Kumar *et al.*, 1990).

In humans, a possible correlation between the type of base substitution and the putative carcinogen is found in tobacco-related, non-small cell lung cancers (Bos, 1989; Hollstein *et al.*, 1991), where G to T transversions predominate both in the K-*ras* gene and the p53 gene. A similar mutation also is found in mouse lung tumors induced by benzo[*a*]pyrene, a constituent of tobacco smoke (You *et al.*, 1989).

The p53 gene is considered to be a tumor suppressor gene, since the wild-type gene product regulates cell proliferation and inhibits growth of transformed cells. This nuclear protein has a short half-life and is present at low levels in normal cells. The mutant proteins are no longer effective in growth control, and thus are believed to contribute, with other oncogene anomalies, to transformation. Mutant p53 proteins in tumor cells can be detected by immunohistochemistry, due to a greatly extended half-life of the altered proteins (Levine *et al.*, 1991). Binding of the early proteins (E6 and E7) of HPV16 and 18 to Rb and p53 gene products may be a part of the mechanism triggering cell transformation in the cervical carcinomas associated with HPV.

An even more striking putative correlation between carcinogen-induced mutation specificity and human tumor mutations is seen in p53 base substitution patterns found in hepatocellular carcinomas from high-incidence populations where aflatoxins and hepatitis B virus are major risk factors.

Hepatocellular carcinomas from Qidong, People's Republic of China (Hsu *et al.*, 1991) and from southern Africa (Bressac *et al.*, 1991) showed most base substitution mutations in the p53 gene were at a single site, the third base position of codon 249, and the majority were G to T transversions. Aflatoxin B_1 forms promutagenic DNA adducts at N7 position of guanine and induces primarily G to T transversions in experimental systems (McMahon *et al.*, 1990).

The high frequency of this lesion occurring at the same codon and base pair of the p53 gene suggests that aflatoxin exposure induced these mutations and thus provides supportive evidence for a significant etiological role in humans. The initial geographical comparisons are being followed by studies in which individual exposures are estimated by macromolecule–aflatoxin adduct measurement.

Mutations in the evolutionary conserved codons of the p53 tumor suppressor gene are common in a variety of cancers. However, in groups studied to date, the p53 mutational spectrum differs among cancers of the colon, lung, esophagus, breast, liver, brain, reticuloendothelial tissues and hemopoietic tissues (Hollstein *et al.*, 1991). Accordingly, such mutational differences may reflect exposures to different exogenous factors although interpretation may be confounded by inherent biochemical differences in different cell types and the microenvironment.

The importance of p53 gene mutations, possibly as a major event driving the evolution of initiated cells to cancer, is further underlined by the findings in some families with Li-Fraumeni syndrome. These are characterized by a high-risk for certain malignancies, including leukemias, sarcomas, breast and brain tumors and carry germinal p53 mutations (Malkin *et al.*, 1990; Srivastava *et al.*, 1990).

As p53 mutations seem to be the most common genetic change in human cancers, systematic analyses of mutational spectra in tumors collected from different geographical locations and presumably associated with different etiologies, should provide a better understanding of human cancers and their origins.

These findings should be confirmed and refined in a large series of tumors of varying etiology. Such data may prove of inestimable value in indicating the probable specific cause of an individual cancer, and may be valuable to the courts in evaluating suspected chemical exposures in the ambient or occupational environment.

References

Balmain, A. & Brown, K. (1988). Oncogene activation in chemical carcinogenesis. *Adv. Cancer Res.*, **51**, 147–82.

Bos, J.L. (1989). *ras* oncogenes in human cancer: a review. *Cancer Res.*, **49**, 4682–9.

Bressac, B., Kew, M., Wands, J. & Ozstujrk, M. (1991). Selective G to T mutations of p53 gene in hepatocellular carcinoma from southern Africa. *Nature*, **350**, 429–31.

Hollstein, M., Sidranksy, D., Vogelstein, B. & Harris, C.C. (1991). p53 mutations in human cancer. *Science*, in press.

Hsu, I.C., Metcalf, R.A., Sun, T., Welsh, J.A., Wang, N.J. and Harris, C.C. (1991). Mutational hotspot in the p53 gene in human hepatocellular carcinomas. *Nature*, **350**, 427–8.

Kumar, R., Sukumar, S. & Barbacid, M. (1990). Activation of *ras* oncogenes preceding the onset of neoplasia. *Science*, **245**, 1101–14.

Levine, A.J., Momand, J. & Finlay, C.A. (1991). The p53 tumour suppressor gene. *Nature*, 351, 453–6.

Malkin, D., Li, F.P., Strong, L.C., Fraumeni, J.F., Jr., Nelson, C.E., Kim, D.H., Kassel, J., Gryka, M.A., Bischoff, F.Z., Tainsky, M.A. *et al.* (1990). Germ line p53 mutations in a familial syndrome of breast cancer, sarcomas, and other neoplasms. *Science*, 250, 1233–8.

McMahon, G., Davis, E.F., Huber, L.J., Kim, Y. & Wogan, G.N. (1990). Characterization of c-Ki-*ras* and *N-ras* oncogenes in aflatoxin B1-induced rat liver tumors. *Proc. Natl. Acad. Sci. USA*, 87, 1104–8.

Srivastava, S., Zou, Z.Q., Pirollo, K., Blattner, W. & Chang, E.H. (1990). Germ-line transmission of a mutated p53 gene in a cancer-prone family with Li-Fraumeni syndrome. *Nature*, 348, 747–9.

Sukumar, S., Notario, V., Martin-Zanca, D. & Barbacid, M. (1983). Induction of mammary carcinomas in rats by nitrosomethylurea involves malignant activation of H-*ras*-1 locus by single point mutations. *Nature*, 306, 658–61.

You, M., Candrian, U., Maronpot, R.R., Stoner, G.D. & Anderson, M.W. (1989). Activation of the Ki-*ras* protooncogene in spontaneously occurring and chemically induced lung tumors of the strain a mouse. *Proc. Natl. Acad. Sci. USA*, 86, 3070–4.

Zarbl, H., Sukumar, S., Arthur, A.V., Martin-Zunca, D. & Barbacid, M. (1985). Direct mutagenesis of Ha-*ras*-1 oncogenes by *N*-nitroso-*N*-methylurea during initiation of mammary carcinogenesis in rats. *Nature*, 315, 382–5.

Chapter 7: Chemical factors

Pollution

Reports continue to appear on the relationship of ambient exposures to pesticides and solvents to the induction of certain human cancers. While elevated risks and associations have been demonstrated for some tumors, the evidence, even in the occupational setting, remains inconclusive and inconsistent. This is illustrated by dioxin.

The impact of dioxin on cancer, especially soft tissue tumors, found in trace quantities through the environment and a contaminant of 'Agent Orange' used during the Vietnam War continues to generate controversy. Well over 1 billion dollars has been spent on research. Some epidemiologists have suggested that its carcinogenicity potential in humans is much less than previously suspected quoting not only the negativity of the Vietnam veterans studies and the fact that its effect appears to be receptor mediated and thus have a possible threshold. It is unlikely that new human data will become available in the absence of further identification of new high risk populations.

It should be emphasized that the newer techniques outlined in the supplement to Chapter 5 (pages 534–7) may provide data on which much more confident assessments as to etiology may be made either in an occupational setting or due to a suspected ambient pollutant.

References

Bailar, J.C. III (1991). How dangerous is dioxin? (editorial). *N. Engl. J. Med.*, **324**, 260–2.

Brown, L.M., Blair, A., Gibson, R., Everett, G.D., Cantor, K.P., Schuman, L.M., Burmeister, L.F., Van Lier, S.F. & Dick, F. (1990). Pesticide exposures and other agricultural risk factors for leukaemia among men in Iowa and Minnesota. *Cancer Res.*, **50**, 6585–91.

Fingerhut, M.A., Halferin, W.E., Marlow, D.A., Piacitelli, L.A., Hinchar, P.A., Sweeney, M.H., Greife, A.L., Dill, P.A., Steenland, K. & Suruda, A.J. (1991). Cancer mortality in workers exposed to 2,3,7,8-tetrachlorodiebenzo-*p*-dioxin. *N. Engl. J. Med.*, **324**, 212–18.

Letters to the Editor. (1991). Dioxin and mortality from cancer. *N. Engl. J. Med.*, **324**, 1809–13.

Water pollution

The IARC Monograph series (1991) recently has made an extensive review on cancer and water pollution with specific reference to chlorinated water and chlorination byproducts. For the latter, the working group concluded six correlation studies and one time-trend study provided some useful data. These studies showed moderately consistent patterns of a positive correlation between use of surface water or of chlorinated water and cancers of the stomach, colon, rectum, urinary bladder and lung, with the most consistent patterns for cancers of the urinary bladder and rectum. The working group, however, added the following caveats:

The studies that were considered informative, and therefore included in this summary, were nevertheless difficult to interpret in an evaluation of the carcinogenicity of chlorinated drinking-water. The water variables studied – whether surface or groundwater and others – were generally imperfect surrogates for the subject of this monograph. There is cause for some scepticism about the estimates of exposure to chlorinated drinking-water in all of these studies. Furthermore, very few attempted to document exposure over long periods of the subjects' lives. Chlorination by-products differ according to local conditions and practices of chlorination, and the health effects found in one place may not be found elsewhere. Many variables, such as smoking habits, dietary practices and environmental conditions, influence the risks for cancer, and they may differ between populations served by chlorinated and unchlorinated water supplies. Such factors should ideally be taken into account in an epidemiological study; however, in most of the studies evaluated, there was little if any information available about them. When the data are examined on the basis of individual cancer sites, the evidence of elevated risk is strongest for cancer of the urinary bladder. The strongest study of cancer at this site supports the hypothesis of an elevated risk due to drinking chlorinated surface water compared with unchlorinated groundwater. However, the sum of the evidence from other studies, although showing some degree of consistency, is severely compromised by the weaknesses outlined above.

Reference

IARC (1991). *IARC Monographs on the Evaluation of Carcinogenic Risks to Humans. Volume 52. Chlorinated Drinking-Water; Chlorination By-Products; Some Other Halogenated Compounds; Cobalt and Cobalt Compounds.* Lyon: International Agency for Research on Cancer.

Chapter 8: Occupational factors

Researchers continue to examine the attributable risk of cancers due to occupational exposure, and the difficulties of making accurate estimates have been further identified. Thus, Vineis and Simonato (1991) in a study of lung and bladder cancer confirmed their previous conclusion that, 'the proportion of lung cancer cases attributable to occupational exposure can be very elevated (up to 40%) among selected populations resident in specific areas. These estimates are strictly time- and place-dependent and certainly do not represent the true proportion of lung cancer cases due to occupational exposure in the general population at a national level. Estimates from smaller and more homogeneous communities are likely to be higher than estimates from larger populations, given that these communities were chosen because of a presumed high risk for lung cancer'.

Gaffuri (1991) has drawn attention to the discrepancies between estimated numbers and reported cancer cases and emphasizes the deficiencies of occupational histories in many countries.

References

Gaffuri, E. (1991). Disparity between estimated numbers and reported cases of occupational cancer. (Letter to editor). *Scand. J. Work Environ. Health*, **17**, 216–17.

Vineis, P. & Simonato, L. (1991). Proportion of lung and bladder cancers in males resulting from occupation: a systematic approach. *Arch. Environ. Health*, **46**, 6–15.

Chapter 13: Fiber carcinogenesis – asbestos

Asbestos and lung cancer

Although the evidence remains inconclusive, further studies suggest that most, if not all, cases of lung cancer following asbestos exposure arise in workers with some evidence (radiography or autopsy) of asbestosis (Hughes & Weill, 1991).

Reference

Hughes, J.M. & Weill, H. (1991). Asbestosis as a precursor of asbestos related lung cancer: results of a prospective mortality study. *Br. J. Indust. Med.*, **48**, 229–33.

Chapter 16: Ionizing radiation

Hatch *et al.* (1991) reported a modest association between post-accident cancer rates and proximity to the Three Mile Island Nuclear Reactor. After adjusting for a gradient in cancer risk which had been noted to exist prior to the accident, the odds ratio contrasting those closest to the plant with those living further away was 1.2 (95 % CI = 1.0 to 1.4). The post-accident increase in rates that was observed in 1982, persisted for another year, and then declined. Radiation emissions, as modeled mathematically, did not account for the observed increase. The authors suggest the increase may be due to changes in seeking care and diagnostic practice arising from post-accident concern.

References

Hatch, M.C., Wallenstein, S., Bayea, J., Nieves, J.W. & Susser, M. (1991). Cancer rates after the Three Mile Island nuclear accident and proximity of residents to the cloud. *Amer. J. Public Health*, **81**, 719–29.

Chapter 23: Lip, oral cavity and/or pharynx

La Vecchia *et al.* (1991) in confirming the causal role of tobacco and alcohol in these cancers found that frequent fruit consumption was strongly protective. While noting that the latter association may simply reflect a generally poorer nutritional status in the cases, they also pointed out that the protective role of fruit has frequently been found for many cancer sites. Harris *et al.* (1991) consider the protective factor is carotene itself rather than another component of vegetables and fruit. This remains to be confirmed.

References

Harris, R.W.C., Key, T.J.A., Silcocks, P.B., Bull, D. & Wald, J. (1991). A case control study of dietary carotene in men with lung cancer and in men with other epithelial cancers. *Nutr. Cancer* **15**, 63–8.

la Vecchia, C., Negri, E., D'Avanzo, B., Boyle, P. & Francheschi S. (1991). Dietary indicators of oral and pharyngeal cancer. *Int. J. Epidemiol.* **20** (3), 39–44.

Chapter 25: Esophagus

The incidence of adenocarcinoma of the esophagus and gastric cardia has been shown to be rising in the past decade in males in the United States by from 4% to 10% per year so that, by the mid-1980s, adenocarcinomas accounted for about one-third of all esophageal cancers. The patterns for the two sites were considered by Blot *et al.* (1991) to be sufficiently alike to implicate shared risk factors or even a single neoplastic entity.

Reference

Blot, W.J., Devesa, S.S., Kneller, R.W. & Fraumeni, J.F. (1991). Rising incidence of adenocarcinoma of esophagus and gastric cardia. *JAMA*, **265**, 1287–9.

Chapter 26: Stomach

Association with *Helicobacter pylori*

Four recent case-control studies have reported a statistically significant association between the prevalence of antibodies to *H. pylori* and the risk of gastric cancer. In one study, (Talley *et al.*, 1991), blood samples were taken after the cancers have been diagnosed and therefore the possibility that the stomach becomes more susceptible to *H. pylori* infection as a consequence of cancer development cannot be excluded. The other three studies, however, were nested case-controls in large cohorts of subjects in whom blood was collected many years prior to diagnosis; these results therefore indicate that *H. pylori* infection precedes gastric cancer development (Forman *et al.*, 1991; Parsonnet *et al.*, 1991; Nomura *et al.*, 1991). The odds ratios in these studies ranged from 2.7 to 6.0 and an attributable risk of about 60% was estimated. The lack of association of *H. pylori* with cancer of the cardia and other cancers indicate that the association is specific for gastric adenocarcinoma.

These studies thus provide strong evidence that *H. pylori* infection is associated with an increased risk of gastric cancer. It is clear, however, that infection with *H. pylori* alone cannot explain the pathogenesis of gastric carcinoma since only a very small proportion of infected subjects will ever develop gastric cancer; other co-factors should therefore play a critical role.

References

Talley, N.J., Zinsmeister, A.R., Weaver, A., DiMagno, P., Carpenter, H.A., Perez-Perez, G.I. & Blaser, M.J. (1991). Gastric adenocarcinoma and *Helicobacter pylori* infection. *J. Natl Cancer Inst.*, **83**, 1734–9.

Forman, D., Newell, D.G., Fullerton, F., Yarnell, J.W.G., Stacey, A.R., Wald, N. & Sitas, F. (1991). Association between infection with *Helicobacter pylori* and risk of gastric cancer: evidence from a prospective investigation. *Br. Med. J.*, **302**, 1302–5.

Parsonnet, J., Friedman, G.D., Vandersteen, D.P., Chang, Y., Vogelman, J.H., Orentreich, N. & Sibley, R.K. (1991). *Helicobacter pylori* infection and the risk of gastric carcinoma. *N. Engl. J. Med.*, **325**, 1127–31.

Nomura, A., Stemmermann, G.N., Chyou, P.H., Kato, I., Perez-Perez, G.I. & Blaser, M.J. (1991). *Helicobacter pylori* infection and gastric carcinoma among Japanese Americans in Hawaii. *N. Engl. J. Med.*, **325**, 1132–6.

Chapter 28: Large intestine and rectum

Exercise

Recent studies have reported a protective effect of physical activity against colon and breast cancers. Gerhardsson *et al.* (1986) report the relative risk of colon cancer in men employed in sedentary occupations was estimated at 1.3 (90% CI 1.2 to 1.5), with the highest risk for the transverse colon including flexures (RR = 1.6) and the lowest risk for the sigmoid (RR = 1.2). In contrast, le Marchand *et al.* (1991) studying lifetime occupational physical activity and prostate cancer risk, established an odds ratio of 0.5 for those who had spent much of their lives in jobs involving only sedentary or light work. This negative association was dose-dependent, consistent across ethnic groups and unrelated to socio-economic status, dietary risk factors or job-related chemical exposures.

References

Gerhardsson, M., Norell, S.E., Kiviranta, H., Pedersen, N.L. & Ahlbom, A. (1986). Sedentary jobs and colon cancer. *J. Epidemiol.*, **123** (5) 775–80.
le Marchand, L., Kolonel, L.N. & Yoshizawa, C.N. (1991). Lifetime occupational physical activity and prostate cancer risk. *Amer. J. Epidemiol.* **133**, 1033–11.

Chapter 29: Liver

Parasites

The relationship between *Opisthorchis viverrini* infestation and endogenous nitrosamines as risk factors for cholangiocarcinoma in Thailand has recently been examined by Srivatanakul *et al.* (1991). The results suggested an interaction.

Reference

Srivatanakul, P., Ohshima, H., Khlat, M., Parkin, M., Sukaryodhin, S., Brouet, I. & Bartsch, H. (1991). Endogenous nitrosamines and liver fluke as risk factors for cholangiocarcinoma in Thailand. *Int. J. Cancer*, **48**, 821–5.

Chapter 34: Bronchus and lung

Role of non-tobacco agents in Chinese women

Lung cancer mortality rates in Xuanwei County, Yunnan Province, China are among the highest in that country, there bring very little difference in age adjusted incidence rates between males (27.7) and females (25.3) although tobacco smoking is rare in Xuanwei women. A strong association of indoor combustion of 'smoking' coal with lung cancer had been demonstrated. Lung cancer was associated with (a) frequency of cooking food (in males) and duration of cooking foods (in females) even after matching on fuel type, (b) with active smoking in males. No association with passive smoking was observed in females. The tobacco association was however much weaker than reported in many previous studies possibly a reflection of the low proportion of lifetime non-smokers in the study participants. Tobacco is also frequently smoked through a long bamboo cylinder partially filled with water. The nature of carcinogens other than tobacco smoke provoking lung cancer in Chinese women needs further elucidation.

Reference

Liu, Z., He, X. & Chapman, R.S. (1991). Smoking and other risk factors for lung cancer in Xuanwei China. *Int. J. Epidemiol.*, **20**, 26–31.

Chapter 39: Skin cancers other than malignant melanoma

In a case-control study in western Australia of 226 basal cell carcinoma (BCC) and 45 squamous cell carcinoma (SCC), the risk was higher in native born Australians than in migrants. Statistical modeling showed that inability to tan, solar elastosis of the neck and number of moles on the back were independently significant risk factors for BCC.

Reference

Kricker, A., Armstrong, B.K., English, D.R. & Heenan, P.J. (1991). Pigmentary and cutaneous risk factors for non-melanocytic skin cancer – a case-control study. *Int. J. Cancer*, **48**, 650–62.

Chapter 41: Uterine cervix

Association with human papillomavirus (HPV)

A recent investigation has shown that the well-known risk factors for cervical cancer (number of sexual partners, age at first intercourse, use of oral contraceptives) were also good predictors of HPV-DNA detection (Ley *et al.*, 1991). In China, a case-control study of invasive cervical cancer in which a reliable PCR-based method was used to detect HPV-DNA has shown a strong association with HPV 16 and 23 after adjustment for other risk factors (OR = 32.9; 95% CI = 7.7–141.1; Peng *et al.*, 1991). Similar findings were observed by Morrison *et al.* (1991) in a case-control study of cervical intraepithelial neoplasia using Southern blot (OR = 17.9; 95% CI = 6.2–51.6) or PCR (OR = 10.4; 95% CI = 3.6–30.4) and in an IARC case-control study of invasive and in situ cervical cancer conducted in Spain and Colombia (Muñoz *et al.*, unpublished data).

Taken as a whole, the best current epidemiological evidence suggests a major role of HPV infection in the aetiology of cervical cancer. However, cervical HPV infection being very common among young women, other unknown factors should be important determinants of the cervical cancer risk.

References

Ley, C., Bayer, H.M., Reingol, A., Schiffman, M.H., Chambers, J.C., Tashiro, C.J. & Manos, M.M. (1991). Determinants of genital human papillomavirus infection in young women. *J. Natl Cancer Inst.*, **83**, 997–1003.

Peng, H., Liu, S., Mann, V., Rohan, T. & Rawls, W. (1991). Human papillomavirus types 16 and 33, herpes simplex virus type 2 and other risk factors for cervical cancer in Sichuan Province, China. *Int. J. Cancer*, **47**, 711–16.

Morrison, E.A.B., Ho, G.Y.F., Vermund, S.H., Goldberg, G.L., Kadish, A.S., Kelley, K.F. & Burk, R.D. (1991). Human papillomavirus infection and other risk factors for cervical neoplasia: a case-control study. *Int. J. Cancer*, **49**, 6–13.

Index

Page numbers followed by an * refer to a table; page numbers followed by ** refer to a figure; page numbers followed by an S are contained in the supplement.

Printed in the United States
40663LVS00009B/10